KV-692-570

TEXTBOOK OF
FETAL
ULTRASOUND

007545

WITHDRAWN
Robert Lamb Library
Inverclyde Royal Hospital

ROBERT LAMB LIBRARY
INVERCLYDE ROYAL
HOSPITAL

TEXTBOOK OF
FETAL
ULTRASOUND

EDITED BY

Richard Jaffe, MD

Columbia Presbyterian Medical Center, New York, USA

and

The-Hung Bui, MD

Karolinska Hospital, Stockholm and Karolinska Institute, REF 618.3204543 JAF
Huddinge, Sweden

618.3204543

The Parthenon Publishing Group

International Publishers in Medicine, Science & Technology

NEW YORK   LONDON

Library of Congress Cataloging-in-Publication Data
Textbook of fetal ultrasound / edited by Richard Jaffe
and The-Hung Bui.
   p. cm
   Includes bibliographical references and index.
   ISBN 1-85070-017-6
   1. Fetus—Ultrasonic imaging.   2. Ultrasonics in
obstetrics. 3. Fetus—Diseases—Diagnosis. I. Jaffe,
Richard. II. Bui, The-Hung.
   [DNLM: 1. Ultrasonography, Prenatal. 2. Fetal
Diseases—ultrasonography. WQ 209 T355 1998]
RG628.3.U58T48 1998
618.3'207543—dc21
DNLM/DLC
for Library of Congress   98-15514
                                CIP

British Library Cataloguing in Publication Data
Textbook of fetal ultrasound
   1. Fetus – Ultrasonic imaging
   I. Jaffe, Richard   II. Bui, The-Hung
   618.3'207543

ISBN 1-85070-017-6

Published in the USA by
The Parthenon Publishing Group Inc.
One Blue Hill Plaza
PO Box 1564, Pearl River
New York 10965, USA

Published in the UK and Europe by
The Parthenon Publishing Group Limited
Casterton Hall, Carnforth
Lancs. LA6 2LA, UK

Copyright © 1999 Parthenon Publishing Group

*No part of this book may be reproduced in any form without
permission from the publishers, except for the quotation of
brief passages for the purposes of review.*

Typeset by Speedlith, Manchester, UK.
Printed and bound by T.G. Hostench S.A., Spain

Contents

List of contributors vii

Dedication x

Preface xi

List of color plates xii

Color plates xiii

1   Physics of real-time ultrasound imaging and Doppler 1
Zvi Friedman and Richard Jaffe

2   First trimester ultrasonography 23
Richard Jaffe and Tamara Allen

3   Sonoembryology 37
John M.G. van Vugt

4   Fetal biometry and gestational age estimation 47
Bobbi Stebbins and Richard Jaffe

5   Intrauterine growth restriction 59
John J. Anthony and Patricia A. Smith

6   Macrosomia 81
Edward J. Coetzee

7   Placenta, umbilical cord and amniotic fluid 87
Moshe D. Fejgin, Ron Tepper and Dvora Kidron

8   Fetal face and central nervous system 103
Ana Monteagudo and Ilan E. Timor-Tritsch

9   Abnormalities of fetal neck and thorax 129
Oded Inbar, Reuven Achiron and Richard Jaffe

10   Abnormalities of fetal abdomen and pelvis 143
Richard Jaffe

11   Fetal echocardiography 153
Susie C. Truesdell

12   Skeletal disorders: *in utero* diagnostic approach 175
Israel Meizner

13   The fetal spine   199
      The-Hung Bui, Richard Jaffe, Henry Lindholm and Mark I. Evans

14   Hydrops fetalis   217
      Shyla Vengalil, William J. Meyer and Joaquin Santolaya-Forgas

15   Multiple gestation   227
      Steven L. Warsof, David E. Patton and Richard Jaffe

16   Antenatal fetal assessment technologies   239
      J. Christopher Glantz

17   Current perspectives and new developments in ultrasound guided invasive
      procedures for prenatal diagnosis and therapy   259
      The-Hung Bui, Jan A. Deprest, Eric Jauniaux and R. Douglas Wilson

18   Ultrasonographic screening for fetal chromosomal abnormalities in the first and
      second trimester of pregnancy   287
      The-Hung Bui, Roderick F. Hume Jr, Kypros H. Nicolaides and Richard Jaffe

19   Ultrasonography and general screening   305
      Kevin J. Gomez, Edilberto Martinez and Joshua A. Copel

20   Three-dimensional ultrasonography of the embryo and fetus   317
      Roger A. Pierson

Index   327

List of contributors

Reuven Achiron
Department of Obstetrics and Gynecology
Sheba Medical Centre
Tel Hashomer 52621
Israel

Tamara Allen
Department of Obstetrics and Gynecology
Strong Memorial Hospital
University of Rochester
601 Elmwood Avenue
Rochester, NY 14642
USA

John J. Anthony
Department of Obstetrics and Gynecology
Maternal and Fetal Medicine Unit
Groote Schuur Hospital
H45, Old Main Building
Observatory 7925
Cape Town
South Africa

The-Hung Bui
Department of Molecular Medicine
Clinical Genetics Unit
Karolinska Hospital
S-171 76 Stockholm
Sweden
and
Division of Fetal and Maternal Medicine
Department of Obstetrics and Gynecology
Huddinge University Hospital
Karolinska Institute
S–141 86 Huddinge
Sweden

Edward J. Coetzee
Department of Obstetrics and Gynecology
Maternal and Fetal Medicine Unit
Groote Schuur Hospital
H45, Old Main Building
Observatory 7925
Cape Town
South Africa

Joshua A. Copel
Department of Obstetrics and Gynecology
Yale University School of Medicine
PO Box 208063
New Haven, CT 06520-8063
USA

Jan A. Deprest
Department of Obstetrics and Gynecology
Catholic University Leuven
University Hospital Gasthuisberg
B-3000 Leuven
Belgium

Mark I. Evans
Department of Obstetrics and Gynecology
Wayne State University/Hutzel Hospital
4707 St Antoine Boulevard
Detroit, MI 48201
USA

Moshe D. Fejgin
Department of Obstetrics and Gynecology
Meir Hospital
Kfar-Sava
Israel

Zvi Friedman
Diasonics Israel
PO Box 2002
Tirat Hacarmel 30200
Israel

J. Christopher Glantz
Department of Obstetrics and Gynecology
Maternal Fetal Medicine
Strong Memorial Hospital
University of Rochester
601 Elmwood Avenue
Rochester, NY 14642
USA

Kevin J. Gomez
Department of Obstetrics and Gynecology
Yale University School of Medicine
PO Box 208063
New Haven
CT 06520-8063
USA

Roderick F. Hume
Department of Obstetrics and Gynecology
Madigan Army Medical Center
MCHJ-OG (ADC)
Tacoma, WA 98431
USA

Oded Inbar
Department of Obstetrics and Gynecology
Sheba Medical Centre
Tel Hashomer 52621
Israel

Richard Jaffe
Department of Obstetrics and Gynecology
Maternal Fetal Medicine
Columbia Presbyterian Medical Center
622 West 168th Street
New York, NY 10032
USA

Eric Jauniaux
Department of Obstetrics and Gynaecology
University College London Medical School
86-96 Chenies Mews
London WC1E 6HX
UK

Dvora Kidron
Department of Obstetrics and Gynecology
Meir Hospital
Kfar-Sava
Israel

Henry Lindholm
Department of Diagnostic Radiology
Section of Ultrasound
Karolinska Hospital
S-171 76 Stockholm
Sweden

Edilberto Martinez
Department of Obstetrics and Gynecology
Yale University School of Medicine
PO Box 208063
New Haven, CT 06520-8063
USA

Israel Meizner
Department of Obstetrics and Gynecology
Rabin Medical Centre Beilinson Campus
Ultrasound Unit
Petach Tikva 49100
Israel

William J. Meyer
Department of Obstetrics and Gynecology
University of Illinois at Chicago
820 South Wood Street
Chicago, IL 60621
USA

Ana Monteagudo
Department of Obstetrics and Gynecology
New York University Medical Center
550 First Avenue, Rm 9N20
New York, NY 10016
USA

Kypros H. Nicolaides
Department of Obstetrics and Gynaecology
Harris Birthright Research Centre for Fetal Medicine
Kings College School of Medicine and Dentistry
Denmark Hill
London SE5 8RX
UK

David E. Patton
Tidewater Perinatal Center
1080 First Colonial Road
Suite 305
Virginia Beach, VA 23454
USA

Roger A. Pierson
Department of Obstetrics and Gynecology
College of Medicine
University of Saskatchewan
Royal University Hospital
103 Hospital Drive
Saskatoon, Saskatchewan
S7N 0W8, Canada

Joaquin Santolaya-Forgas
Department of Obstetrics and Gynecology
University of Illinois at Chicago
820 South Wood Street
Chicago, IL 60621
USA

Patricia A. Smith
Department of Obstetrics and Gynecology
Maternal and Fetal Medicine Unit
Groote Schuur Hospital
H45, Old Main Building
Observatory 7925
Cape Town
South Africa

Bobbi Stebbins
Department of Obstetrics and Gynecology
Strong Memorial Hospital
University of Rochester
601 Elmwood Avenue
Rochester, NY 14642
USA

Ron Tepper
Department of Obstetrics and Gynecology
Meir Hospital
Kfar-Sava
Israel

Ilan E. Timor-Tritsch
Department of Obstetrics and Gynecology
New York University Medical Center
550 First Avenue, Rm 9N20
New York, NY 10016
USA

Susie C. Truesdell
Division of Pediatric Cardiology
Children's Hospital at Strong
601 Elmwood Avenue
Rochester, NY 14642
USA

Shyla Vengalil
Department of Obstetrics and Gynecology
University of Illinois at Chicago
820 South Wood Street
Chicago
IL 60621
USA

John M.G. van Vugt
Department of Obstetrics and Gynecology
University Hospital Vrije Universiteit Amsterdam
PO Box 7057
1007 MB Amsterdam
The Netherlands

Steven L. Warsof
Tidewater Perinatal Center
1080 First Colonial Road
Suite 305
Virginia Beach
VA 23454
USA

R. Douglas Wilson
Department of Obstetrics and Gynecology
Room 1 U3
British Columbia Women's Hospital
4500 Oak Street
Vancouver, BC V6H 3N1
Canada

Dedication

To Louise, Jaffa, Adi, Shirlee, Jonathan,
Alexander and Stephanie.

R. Jaffe

Preface

Many advances have been made in the field of obstetrical ultrasound in the last few years. There has been a need for a textbook incorporating this new knowledge and the vast clinical know-how derived from considerable experience gained in leading perinatal centers.

We wanted to achieve a comprehensive, authoritative and up-to-date text with a prospective view on new developments for all those working in the field of fetal ultrasound. The individual chapters draw from the wide experiences of a multidisciplinary group of contributors who are internationally recognized authorities. Every issue of importance in fetal ultrasonography is presented concisely.

Chapters have been devoted to the evaluation of common obstetrical problems. The tradition of ordering fetal defects according to anatomical systems, which appeared in the philosophical and medical literature of the seventeenth century, is continued here. We have attempted to connect individual anomalies to the malformation syndromes in which they are known to occur and have considered them within the context of current knowledge of embryonic and fetal development. We hope that this book takes the reader through a logical progression from knowledge of physics as applied to ultrasound and Doppler, to various clinical aspects of fetal ultrasound, and finally to the discussions on the use of this technology as a screening tool and the new development of three-dimensional ultrasound. A systematic examination of the fetus, placenta and cord is emphasized throughout this text. Useful algorithms that promote sound decision-making have been provided, while numerous tables and illustrations, some of which are in color, have been chosen to help clarify key topics, or illustrate important features. Cross-referencing between chapters has been used to reinforce and broaden the understanding of core concepts. However, each chapter can be read separately.

We believe that this textbook will be a useful resource not only to all those involved in fetal ultrasound, but to those providing genetic counseling. It is our hope that this book will help physicians to more easily identify structural malformations in the fetus, or other common obstetrical problems, take the correct diagnostic approaches, make accurate differential diagnoses, and implement the most appropriate procedures in the management of these pregnancies.

Editing this book has been an enriching experience and a privilege. We are much indebted to the many authors for their excellent contributions and for the help and support of our Publisher, in particular Ms Dinah Alam, Scientific Editor.

R. Jaffe
T.-H. Bui

Color plate 1 (a) Color velocity images of a native kidney. (b) Power Doppler image of the same kidney

Color plate 2 Histogram of pulsatility index values generated automatically by a new modality

Color plate 3 Viable 12 week tubal ectopic pregnancy with color Doppler demonstrating active blood flow

Color plate 4 Color Doppler demonstrating characteristic low resistance flow around gestational sac (arrow). Blood flow also seen in early embryo and umbilical cord

Color plate 5 Physiological midgut herniation in a 10 week fetus. (a) Sagittal plane. (b) Transverse plane

Color plate 6 Calcifications of the basal plate, term placenta (H&E, x40)

Color plate 7 Multiple infarcts of placenta, 36 weeks gestation, recent pre-eclamptic toxemia. Several small old infarcts involve the basal aspect of the cut sections. A large recent infarct is seen on the right hand side of the lower slice

Color plate 8 Intervillous hematoma measuring 2 cm in diameter, fetus at 22 weeks gestation

Color plate 9 Histologic section of an intervillous hematoma surrounded by normal appearing chorionic villi (H&E, x 10)

Color plate 10 Massive subchorionic fibrin deposits of the placenta at 33 weeks gestation. The mother had cardiomyopathy due to doxorubicine cardiotoxicity

Color plate 11 Gross appearance of complete hydatidiform mole: the entire villous tree is converted into numerous vesicles of 5mm in average diameter

Color plate 12 Histologic section of a partial hydatidiform mole: some villi are markedly distended, show cystic degeneration in the center and focal trophoblastic proliferation to various degrees (H&E, x40)

Color plate 13 Histologic section of hydropic degeneration of 14 weeks missed abortion. The chorionic villi are markedly distended but lack the cystic formation and trophoblastic proliferation of molar change (H&E, x40)

Color plate 14 Color Doppler flow demonstrating some vascularity of a placental chorioangioma

Color plate 15 Abruptio placenta at 33 weeks gestation. A large retroplacental hematoma on the right side is firmly attached to the maternal (basal) floor, covering approximately 30% of its surface

Color plate 16 Two cut sections of umbilical cord at 40 weeks gestation demonstrating single umbilical artery

Color plate 17 Color Doppler demonstrating two umbilical arteries entering umbilical cord

Color plate 18 Power Doppler demonstrating single umbilical artery around bladder

Color plate 19 Thirty-two and a half weeks fetus with a vein of Galen aneurysm. An oblique-1 section in which color Doppler has been applied and shows the turbulent flow within the aneurysm of the vein of Galen

Color plate 20 Demonstration of nuchal cord with color Doppler imaging

Color plate 21 Ebstein's anomaly of the tricuspid valve. In the transverse plane, with the right ventricle (RV) anterior, the right atrium (RA) appears quite large. Color Doppler demonstrates a wide band of retrograde flow from RV to RA (tricuspid insufficiency, TI) which begins deep in the ventricle, suggesting that the tips of the tricuspid valve hinge at that point. In addition, there is a small amount of mitral insufficiency (MI). LA, left atrium; LV, left ventricle

Color plate 22 All three panels show umbilical blood velocity waveforms in three very similar fetuses of 23 weeks gestational age. Upper panel demonstrates severe umbilical venous pulsation in a fetus with hypoplastic right heart, mid-panel demonstrates less severe umbilical venous pulsation in a fetus with bone dysplasia and a restrictive thoracic pattern, and lower panel shows normal vein waveforms in a fetus with a placental chorioangioma

Color plate 23 Fetoscopic cord ligation. The umbilical cord of an acardiac twin has been ligated with an extracorporeal knot. The fetoscopic surgeon is continuously backed up by ultrasound images projected by a twin-camera system at the right upper corner of the screen

Color plate 24 Fiber-fetoscopic image of superficial chorionic plate vessels crossing the intertwin membrane insertion (the white line crossing the image). At 8 o'clock in the image, a 400μ m Nd:YAG laser fiber is inserted to coagulate vessels. The endoscope itself is 1.2mm in diameter.

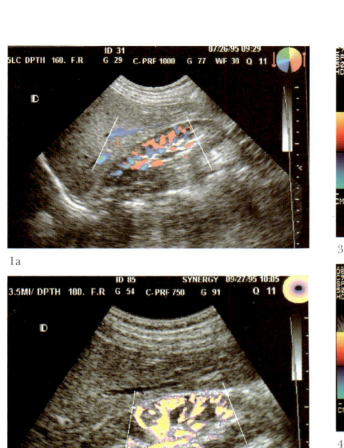

1a

1b

2

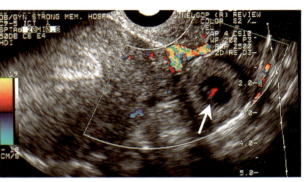

3

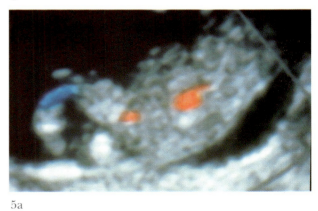

4

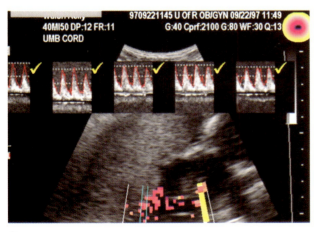

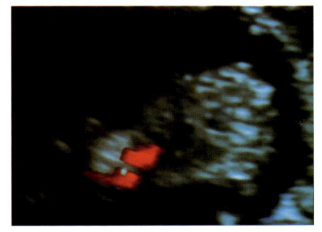

5a

5b

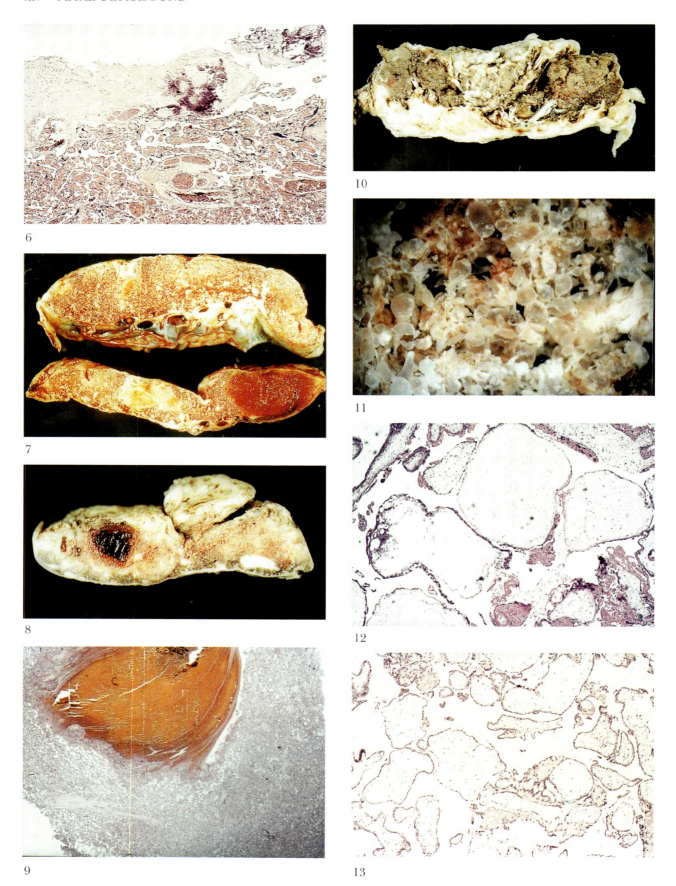

6

7

8

9

10

11

12

13

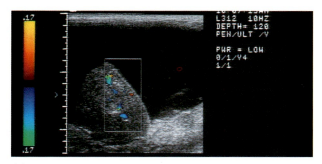

14

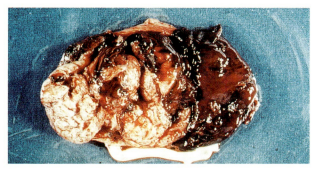

15

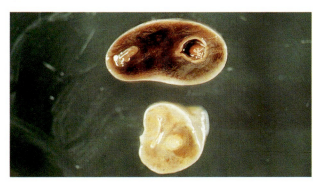

16

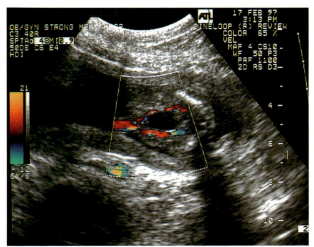

17

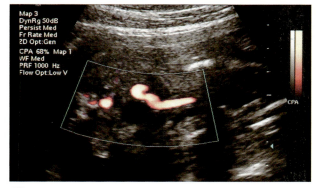

18

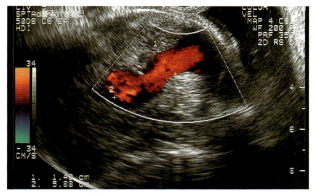

19

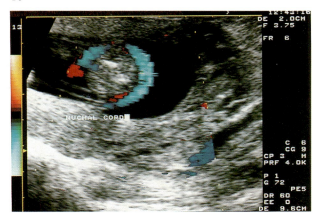

20

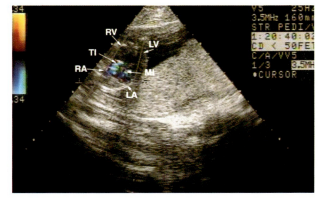

21

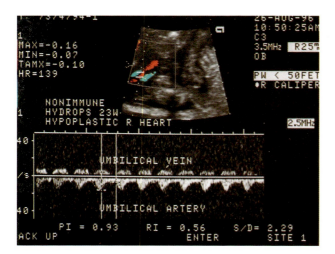

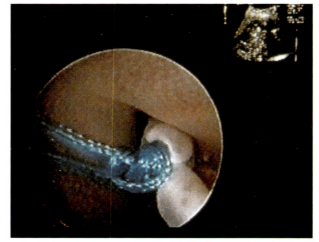

23

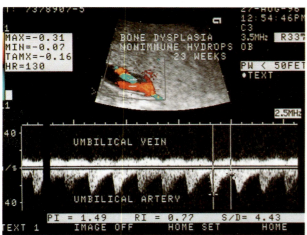

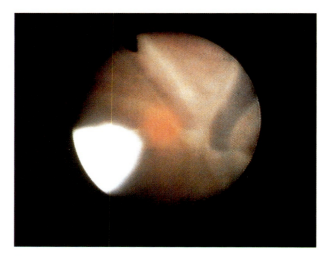

24

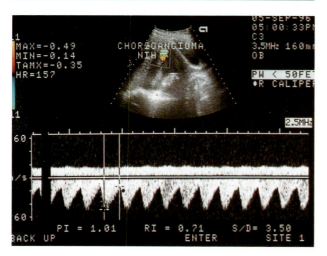

22

Physics of real-time ultrasound imaging and Doppler

1

Zvi Friedman and Richard Jaffe

This chapter reviews the physics of ultrasound imaging and the various parameters that define image quality, and subsequently shows how the image can be optimized using the system controls. Confident and reliable ultrasonographic diagnosis depends on the ability to consistently produce excellent images. Table 1 summarizes the basic concepts used in this chapter to define a 'good' image. A good image depends upon the various system parameters, and can be affected by the system controls.

GENERATION OF THE ULTRASONIC IMAGE

A short pulse of ultra-high frequency sound (between 2 and 20 MHz), lasting about 1 microsecond (one millionth of a second) is transmitted into the body. The pulse is 'focused' and portions of it are reflected back towards the transducer. By 'focused' we mean that the pulse is somehow made to travel along a very thin beam. The point in the body where the beam is thinnest will be referred to as the 'focal point' and the total length where the beam is still 'thin' is called the 'focal depth of field'. If we assume that the velocity of propagation of sound in the tissue is known, we can assign the received echo at a specific time to a definite location within the body. The quality of the image will be affected by the beam parameters detailed in Table 2[1,2].

PROPAGATION OF SOUND IN THE BODY

Interference

Sound propagates in the body in the form of pressure waves. Beams are formed utilizing the physical phenomenon of interference. These waves, a succession of high- and low-pressure regions, travel through the tissue at the speed of sound – about 1500 m/s. The *wavelength* is defined as follows: take a snap shot of the wave at any instant. The wavelength is the distance between two adjacent points along the beams having the same phase, i.e. distance between two successive minimums or two successful maximums.

Molecules crowding into a region in the tissue will generate a high-pressure zone. The molecules leaving it generate a low-pressure region. This leads to the physical concept of interference. When two or more sources send sound waves across the same volume in the tissue, the resultant sound pressure in a given region is determined by the net inflow of molecules. It is therefore determined by the algebraic sum of the individual pressures. We may also distinguish between destructive and constructive interference.

Destructive interference

If the high-pressure region from one wave coincides with the low pressure region from another wave traveling across the same region, the net resultant pressure change in that region will be lower in magnitude than any of the individual pressures.

Constructive interference

If the high-pressure regions of two waves coincide, the sound pressure at the region where the two waves cross will be higher in magnitude than that of each of the individual waves. This is called constructive interference.

Beam forming

The beam forming in modern ultrasound systems is accomplished using one- or two-dimensional transducer arrays. Beam forming allows us to better visualize minute anatomical details in the patient. The transmit beam is our 'search-light'. The receive focus is the 'microscope' with which we examine the lighted area. With one- or two-

Table 1 Parameters that define image quality

Concept	Explanation
Detail resolution	The ability to visualize minute anatomic detail
Sensitivity	The ability to adequately visualize minute anatomic detail deep in the patient
Contrast resolution	The ability to clearly and easily differentiate between tissue types (e.g. fetal lungs should be easily distinguishable from fetal liver)
Low noise	Non-echogenic objects in the image (e.g. amniotic fluid or simple cysts) should appear as totally 'black'
	Spurious echoes resulting from a variety of artifacts might cause these areas to appear as echogenic and lead to misdiagnosis
Consistency	Uniformity of all the above throughout the entire image

Table 2 Beam parameters that affect image quality

Parameter	Explanation
Beam-width – transmit	The width of the beam along which the transmitted beam travels
Beam-width – receive	The width of the beam along which the received (reflected) beam travels
Pulse length – transmit	The length (time duration) of the ultrasonic beam transmitted into the body
Pulse length – receive	The length (time duration) of the electric pulse generated by the transducer when the ultrasonic beam impinges on it
Velocity of sound in the tissue	Approximately 1540 m/s. The fact that this velocity is not the same for all tissues is one of the reasons for degradation in image quality

dimensional transducer arrays, beam forming is accomplished electronically. As can be intuitively understood, two-dimensional arrays can provide much narrower beams.

Frequency and band-width

When measuring the pressure at any given point in the body, we find a periodic temporal behavior. The number of pressure maximums (or minimums) per second at any given location within the body is defined as the *frequency* of the sound wave. An ultrasonic pulse will not persist, however, at any given point longer than 1 microsecond, (this is the typical pulse length used in diagnostic ultrasound). In order to measure the frequency, we measure the time difference between two adjacent maximums (or minimums). Thus a crude description would be: if the time difference between two adjacent maximums is T microseconds, the wave frequency (f) is f = 1/T MHz (millions of cycles per second). The main reason is that for a time signal to be described as a single frequency signal (a 'pure' sine wave), it must be long enough in time. The longer the signal lasts the 'purer' its frequency. Thus, for example, a 3.5 MHz signal lasting 1 microsecond (about three cycles) will contain signals in the frequency range 2.5 MHz to 3.5 MHz (the frequency range is inversely proportional to the time duration of the signal). The situation is illustrated in Figure 1.

To get a rough idea of the actual frequency content of the signal, we measure time differences between all adjacent peaks (maximums or minimums). Each measurement will result in a slightly different value for the frequency, thus defining the frequency range in the signal.

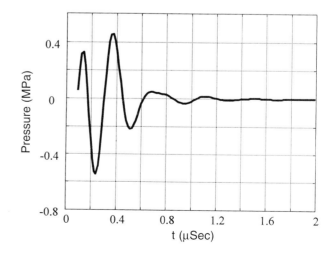

Figure 1 Pressure wave generated by a 3.5 MHz probe

Attenuation

As the signal travels across the body its intensity is continuously decreased due to absorption, scattering and specular reflection (Table 3).

Specular reflection and scattering

Only two mechanisms will eventually result in an ultrasound wave getting back to the transducer: specular reflection and scattering. Specular (mirror like) reflection occurs when the reflector is a large, extensive (relative to the wavelength – 0.44 mm at 3.5 MHz) surface. Examples of such a surface could be the boundaries of a kidney, the surface of the placenta, the diaphragm, the skin of a fetus, etc. Specular reflections are highly directional and will occur only if the reflecting surface is precisely perpendicular to the direction of the beam. The amplitude of the reflected beam depends only upon the properties of the tissues on both sides of the surface. The amplitude of the reflected wave will be large for tissues with very different properties and will be very direction dependent.

Scattering is generated by parenchymal structures. It occurs when the ultrasonic wave is reflected from particles that are of the size of one wavelength (0.44 mm at 3.5 MHz) or smaller. The intensity of the reflection will depend upon the size of the reflector relative to the wavelength. The larger the reflector, the stronger the reflection. It has been shown experimentally that the intensity of the reflection is roughly proportional to the square of the ratio between the particle size and the wavelength. This means that if the parenchymal architecture that gives rise to echoes in one organ is three times larger than that in another, the scatter will be nine times more intense. Similarly, doubling the frequency of the ultrasound (halving the wavelength) increases the relative echo strength by a factor of four.

Absorption

Absorption is a significant factor in attenuation. Unlike specular reflection and scatter, it does not result in a wave that gets back to the transducer. Rather, it represents a series of processes through which the energy in the ultrasonic wave is eventually converted into heat. In the frequency range usually used in diagnostic ultrasound, the absorption coefficient is proportional to the wave frequency. Thus for example a 7.0 MHz wave will lose 50% of its original intensity at about half the depth for which a 3.5 MHz wave loses 50% of its original intensity.

Acoustic impedance

As stated above, when an ultrasonic beam meets an interface between two types of tissues, part of the beam is reflected. The proportion of the sound that is reflected depends on the acoustic properties of the two tissues. The acoustic properties affecting reflection can be related to a single parameter in the tissue, also referred to as the acoustic impedance of the tissue. This parameter is a function of the density of the tissue and its stiffness.

Table 3 The three mechanisms causing sound attenuation in the body

Mechanism	Description	Angle dependence	Frequency dependence
Absorption	Kinetic energy of particles moving into high pressure regions and out of low pressure regions is converted into heat due to viscous friction	Angle independent	The intensity of the beam is decreased with depth, following an exponential decay law. The distance at which the beam intensity is reduced by half is inversely proportional to the frequency.
Scattering	Part of the beam is scattered (in all directions) by small microscopic particles (smaller than the wavelength)	Angle independent	Scattered intensity is proportional to the fourth power of the frequency
Specular (mirror-like) reflection	Part of the beam is reflected at the surfaces interfacing between two regions that have different acoustic properties	Strongly angle dependent	Not frequency dependent

Shadowing and enhancement

Ideally, an ultrasound image would be one for which the gray level at a given point on the screen represents unambiguously the reflection coefficient of the corresponding point in the tissue. In reality this is almost never the case due to several artifacts. Two of these sonographic artifacts will be discussed here while others will be discussed later. When an echo is so large that the sound continuing into the tissue is highly attenuated, an acoustic shadow will be cast, as in Figure 2 showing a transthoracic image of a fetus with shadows cast by the fetal ribs. A very similar situation will occur in cases where the attenuation is caused by absorption rather than by reflection as can be seen in Figure 3.

The reverse phenomenon will occur when the sound traverses through a medium with relatively small attenuation, i.e. no absorption and no scattering. Typical examples could be a cyst or a pocket of amniotic fluid. Because the beams passing through the cyst are less attenuated than the rest of the beams that pass through tissue with higher attenuation, the area behind it will be brighter. This is called posterior enhancement and is sometimes used to differentiate between fat (highly absorbing) and liquid (non-absorbing).

Resolution

Spatial (detail) resolution

The concept of resolution relates to the amount of detail that can be perceived in an image. In a high resolution image small structures can easily be seen. A simplified definition of system resolution is the separation between two target points that are just resolvable (can be seen in the image as two distinct points). The axial resolution is limited by the pulse length, and is due to the fact that two targets along the beam direction will be separable only if the echo from the first target dies off before the echo from the second target starts arriving. The lateral resolution, on the other hand, is determined by the beam width.

Both axial and lateral resolution depends on the relative intensity (reflection coefficient) of the targets. Thus, for example, for two equal targets along the beam the resolution will be relatively high since echoes arriving from the second target will be separable from those arriving from the first target after the latter are decreased by a factor of approximately two. If, on the other hand, the first

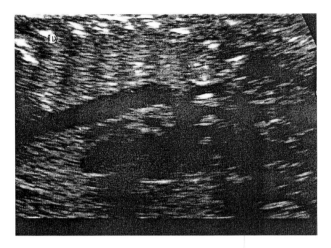

Figure 2 Fetal aortic arch. Notice the acoustic shadowing formed by the ribs

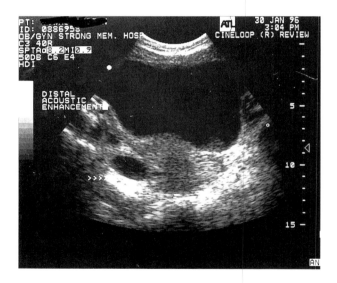

Figure 3 Acoustic shadowing formed by highly absorbing tissue

target is a thousand times stronger than the second target (a situation that very often occurs in diagnostic ultrasound), one needs to wait until the echoes from the first target are less than one thousandth of their peak value. When evaluating equipment, one should be very careful in examining and comparing resolution numbers quoted by the manufacturers. These numbers must also state the relative intensities of the targets in order to have any meaning at all.

In most state-of-the-art ultrasound systems the axial resolution is much smaller than the lateral resolution. Both axial and lateral resolution degrade with imaging depth. The degradation of the axial resolution with depth is a result of the attenuation in the tissue, and is related to the fact that higher frequencies are attenuated faster than lower frequencies. The lateral resolution for a given sound frequency and a given transducer aperture is inversely proportional to the distance. Thus, if the resolution at a distance of 50 mm is 1 mm it will be degraded to 2 mm at a distance of 100 mm. In actuality the situation will be even worse due to the dependence of the attenuation on the depth. Thus, for example, the frequency that can be used for imaging at a depth of 100 mm is half the frequency that could have been used for imaging at a depth of 50 mm. Most modern systems attempt to provide a uniform resolution throughout the entire image. In order to accomplish this, the transducer aperture is increased with the depth of imaging. This partly takes care of the dependence of the lateral resolution on the depth. However, it ignores the effects of the attenuation.

Contrast resolution

Contrast resolution is the ability to perceive tissue contrast differences in gray-scale images. Diagnostically important image contrast results from small differences in the acoustic properties of tissues, sometimes referred to as subject contrast. It is mainly determined by the spatial distribution, concentration and reflectivity of tissue structures within the scan plan. The ultrasound system translates these minute differences into low amplitude shades of gray[3].

Speckles

One of the essential tasks of diagnostic ultrasound imaging is the detection of the focal lesions of low contrast against background tissue. The capability to detect a target of any given shape (e.g. circular) depends on the 'contrast' between the target and the background, the target size and the background 'noise'. The main noise factor in diagnostic ultrasound imaging is the so-called 'speckle-noise'. This noise is superimposed on the image and appears in the form of gray 'stains' of random sizes and intensities. This noise camouflages the target, mainly by 'breaking' its contours. It has been named speckle because of its similarity to the equivalent optical phenomenon, laser speckle.

The phenomenon of speckles results directly from the use of coherent radiation for imaging. It occurs when structures in the object (tissue), which are on too small a scale to be observed by the imaging system (smaller than the imaging wavelength), cause interference to occur between different parts of the wave received from the object region that correspond to a given point in the image[4–6].

The detection of a lesion within background tissue is a psychophysical process, carried out by the eye–brain system of the observer. The observer performs an integration process by which all signals resulting from echoes from the target area are summed together. The target lesion will be discriminated from the background if (1) the number of individual speckles in the target area is large enough (i.e. the average speckle size is much smaller than a typical target dimension); and (2) if the average brightness of individual speckles in the target area is different enough from the average brightness of individual speckles in the background area. Statement (1) can also be phrased mathematically by stating that the ratio of signal to noise is proportional to $m^{1/2}$, where m is the average number of speckles in the target area.

The average speckle size depends mainly on the properties of the ultrasonic beam; i.e. the ultrasonic frequency, the transducer aperture, the distance from the transducer and the pulse length. The image sampling, i.e. the number of beams across the field of view that are used to generate the image (image line density) as well as the number of samples along the beam, can also affect the speckle pattern. Modern well-designed systems are sampled densely enough so that sampling will have minimal effects on the image. The speckle intensity will depend on the average number of scatters per unit volume in the tissue, the difference in acoustic properties between the scatters and the tissue in which they are immersed, their size, the uniformity of their distribution, as well as on the properties of the beam. However, since the amplitude and distribution of the speckles are related not only to the ultrasonic beam properties but also to the parenchymal tissue architecture, the appearance of the speckles is fairly constant for each type of tissue and shows constant difference between tissues. This allows us to use the speckle information to discriminate between tissues, despite the fact that the echo pattern is random.

Under-sampling and aliasing

As previously stated, the sampling rate (in both axial and lateral directions) must be high enough to comply with the speckle density, i.e. the distance between two samples must be much smaller the average speckle size or the average distance between two speckles in the image. One of the most severe effects of 'under-sampling' (sampling at a rate which is not high enough) on the image is called aliasing. Speckles are caused by interference of echoes from densely packed tiny parenchymal-reflecting structures that are closer than the basic system resolution. Thus, there is no one-to-one correspondence to any identifiable structures in the body, which are relatively large. Small movements of the probe will cause continuous small movements of these structures. The speckle pattern will, however, change abruptly, giving the effect of a moving background noise. Of course, the larger the change the more disturbing the effect. The amount of change will depend initially on the ratio between the sampling rate and the natural resolution of the system. Another important factor will be the gain setting of the system, where the effect will be most annoying at high gain.

Reverberations

Consider yourself in a room that has mirrors on two opposite walls. Now try to estimate your distance from one of the mirrors by just looking at it. Multiple reflections at the opposing mirrors will probably make such an attempt useless. A very similar situation occurs in acoustics. As discussed above, when the sound beam is perpendicular to an interface, part of it will be reflected. The amount of the reflected wave will depend upon the intensity of the incident wave. It will, however, also depend on the difference in the acoustic properties of the two tissues. The reflected wave will then hit the face of the transducer. Since the transducer material has acoustical properties that are very different from those of the patient tissue, only part of the wave will enter the transducer. A large portion of the wave will bounce back into the patient. It will travel to the reflecting surface and back to the transducer. Since the time for such a multiple round trip between the transducer and the patient is a multiple of the time for a single round trip, and since the system registers the axial location of an object according to the time of a single round trip, the same object will be registered in multiple positions on the image.

IMAGE FORMATION IN PREMIUM HIGH-RESOLUTION DIAGNOSTIC ULTRASOUND SYSTEMS

Introduction

Premium high-resolution ultrasound systems have become increasingly sophisticated and include many new signal-processing features. The main factors affecting diagnostic image quality have already been identified as detail resolution, sensitivity, contrast resolution, noise and consistency. In this section the entire system signal processing chain will be described in detail and the effects of the various blocks and system features on the diagnostic image quality will be elaborated.

The signal processing chain

The signal processing chain schematically described in Figure 4 begins with the scanned cross-section in the patient, the features of which are determined by the interaction of the ultrasound beam with the tissue. It ends in the eye–brain system of the examiner. The machine must, however, do a larger amount of electronic signal processing before the echo information it receives can be displayed as a clinically useful diagnostic image. The signal processing functions include: improving the lateral resolution by focusing techniques; correcting for attenuation (in order to make the image brightness uniform); adjusting the amplitude of the echoes further to emphasize particular features of interest; estimating the amplitudes of missing echoes, and inserting the results in the right places to generate a smooth pleasant image and rejecting misleading information.

Focusing

To generate a high-resolution image, the origin of each echo must accurately be determined. For this to be achieved, one needs to use high frequency, very short pulses, and make the beam as narrow as possible. Modern scanners employ multi-element electronic beam-forming and focusing. In order to

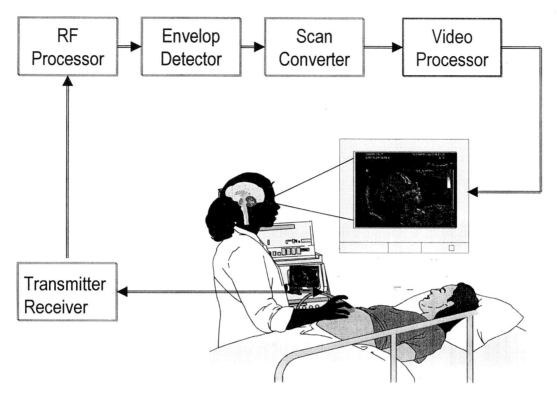

Figure 4 Signal processing chain

understand the operation and performance of these beam-forming techniques let us first review the 'fixed lens' focusing method.

Fixed lens focusing

Old technology, such as single-element mechanical sector scanners used a fixed lens to focus the beam. Focusing is accomplished by attaching a lens, usually shaped spherically (Figure 5), in which the sound wave travels slower than in the tissue. Since the wave from the edge of the transducer starts traveling in the tissue before the wave from the center of the transducer, and since the speed of sound in the lens is slower than that in the transducer, the wavefront will bend and become spherical.

Focusing with an array transducer

The same principle is used in array transducers. The effect of curving the wavefront is accomplished by dividing the transducer into a large number of very small transducers (elements). On transmit, the pulse is fired from each of the elements separately. The edge of the array is fired first and the central element is fired last. By properly adjusting the time delays between the elements a spherical wavefront, similar to that produced by the fixed lens, is obtained (Figure 6).

Confocal imaging on transmit With an electronic transducer array the focusing point is determined by the set of delays between the pulses. This results in a beam with a focal point at which lateral resolution is best. Areas close to the focal point portray good image quality. Other areas are out of focus and have much lower image resolution. In order to improve image resolution in other areas, more focal points are used. To generate an ultrasonic line several consecutive beams are fired. Each of the beams is focused at a different point. For each beam, only a segment close to the focal point is used; the rest of the beam is ignored. Combining the segments around each of the focal points then generates the entire image. The fact that many beams need to be transmitted in order to generate a single line in the image severely reduces the frame rate. Often the frame rate is further reduced, since in order to avoid mixing of reflections of the present beam from the near zone with reflections

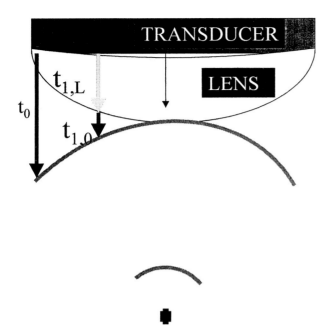

Figure 5   Focusing with a fixed focus lens

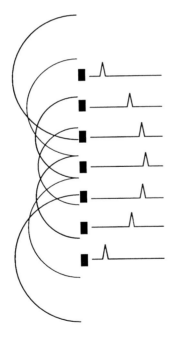

Figure 6   To focus the beam, the pulses are first applied to the outside elements and then later to the elements that are situated nearer the center of the array. Each element is a center of a circular wave. The circular wave fronts spreading from the outer elements propagated a greater distance because they were fired earlier. The varying distances of propagation result in crossing points (where constructive interference occurs) lying along a circular curve

of the previous beam by strong reflectors deep in the body, one should allow more time for all echoes from a pulse to arrive before transmitting the next pulse. This extra time can be saved if consecutive beams are transmitted along separate lines. This technique allows for some systems to achieve clinically acceptable frame rates with more than five transmitted focal zones.

Dynamic focusing on receive   Focusing a transducer array in receive mode is very similar to focusing it on transmit mode. One simply has to delay the output of each of the elements properly and then sum them together. Owing to the fact that echoes from deeper points in the patient arrive later at the surface of the transducer, one can easily optimize the image by dynamically varying the delays as functions of time so that all echo sources are focused (summed in phase to generate a constructive interference). At the summation point, echoes from all other points will not be in phase, resulting in a destructive interference.

Out-of-plane focusing and beam-width artifacts

Most array transducers available in the market today employ a single row of 128–192 very small elements. This allows for excellent focusing of the beam in the plane of scanning, which is the plane perpendicular to the transducer surface and which cuts the center points of all the elements. The beam width in the perpendicular direction is focused with a cylindrical lens along the length of the array. This allows one to focus the beam at some distance from the array. Because of practical limitations the transducer aperture in this direction is rather limited (typically 10–15 mm), and since the focus is fixed, the beam is relatively wide in this direction. The results of a wide beam in the out-of-plane may be painful[7].

Let us consider two examples. The first example comes from gynecology. It is well known that diagnosing an adnexal mass as a simple cyst may be crucial to determine its benign nature. A simple cyst appears black (non-echoic) since it does not absorb and does not scatter. If the beam is too wide, one of the portions of the beam may be interacting with the fluid (non-echoic) structure while another portion of the beam interacts with adjacent soft tissue. This could create echoes registered within the cystic structure. A second example is when one desires to detect a low contrast lesion within a tissue the contrast is even further reduced due to the width of the beam.

Side lobes and grating lobes

A serious problem in multi-element array transducers is related to image degrading artifacts referred to as side lobes and grating lobes. Generally, side lobes will appear close to the main beam, whereas grating lobes appear at a relatively large distance from the main lobe.

Side lobes

Although the majority of the sound produced by a simple transducer propagates directly away from the transducer face to generate the so-called main beam, a small portion of the energy will be concentrated outside the main central beam. These secondary, side lobes are produced because at the lateral margins of the sound source a portion of the sound energy is transmitted radially away from the beam axis. Spatial variation in side lobe intensity occurs because of interference between sound energy arising from the opposite sides of the transducer. Interference can be either constructive or destructive. As side lobes are mainly an edge effect, their intensity relative to the intensity of the main lobe will decrease with increasing size of the transducer (the size is most conveniently expressed in units of the wavelength). Also, since side lobes are caused by interference, their intensity will decrease if the pulse length is decreased.

A second source of side lobes in array transducers comes from the discontinuous nature of the aperture. The ideal shape of the aperture is a circular curve, which we now approximate with a set of linear segments. The approximation will naturally improve as we decrease the length of each of the segments and increase their number. The contribution of this source to the side lobes will therefore decrease as we increase the number of elements and decrease their size.

Side lobes mainly disturb the possibility of seeing a weak target next to a strong target since the side lobe intensity of the strong target might be larger than the echo of the second target. The effect of each of the above parameters on the side lobe intensity is summarized in Table 4.

Grating lobes

Grating lobes are caused by the constructive interference of laterally directed energy from the

Table 4 Effect of various array parameters on side lobe intensity

Parameter change	Effect on side lobe intensity
Increase total array aperture	Decreased
Increase sound frequency	Decreased
Decrease element size, but keep total aperture fixed (by increasing number of elements)	Decreased

edges of the individual array elements. Their intensity and angle from the main beam depends on the center-to-center spacing (pitch) of the elements, on the spacing between edges of adjacent elements, upon the wavelength (or sound frequency), and upon the size and curvature of the array. The effect of each of the above parameters on the grating lobe intensity and position is summarized in Table 5.

Modern, high performance systems should not produce noticeable grating lobes. As can be seen from Table 5, increasing the imaging frequency for a given transducer will produce grating lobes. Figure 7 shows an example of grating lobes in a transvaginal high-bandwidth probe that occurred when an exaggerated high frequency was used for the imaging.

Dynamic range – gray scale

The acoustic transducers used in diagnostic ultrasound are capable of recording echoes over a range of pressures in excess of 100 000 : 1 (100 dB). Presently available, state-of-the-art monitors are capable of displaying a range of no more than approximately 32 : 1 (30 dB). Generally, the information is displayed in the form of gray levels as shown in Figure 8.

In order to extract all the clinically relevant information contained in the image and display it to the diagnostician, the acoustic data must be electronically manipulated so that all the clinically relevant information is faithfully displayed on the limited range monitor. It is convenient to base the operation of the system in terms of the concept of dynamic range. As can be seen from Figure 9, all ultrasound signals start from zero level and end at the system saturation level. The lower portion of the signal lies in the range within the noise level and is therefore obscured by it. The system reject level is set just above the noise level so that only the echoes above the reject level are displayed. The

Table 5   Effect of various array parameters on grating lobe intensity

Parameter change	Effect on grating lobe intensity and position
Increase total array aperture	Increase
Increase sound frequency	Increase. Grating lobes will appear closer to the main lobe
Decrease element size, but keep total aperture fixed (by increasing number of elements)	Decrease. Grating lobes will be shifted far away from the main lobe
Increase probe radius of curvature	Decrease

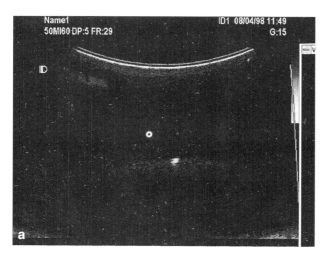

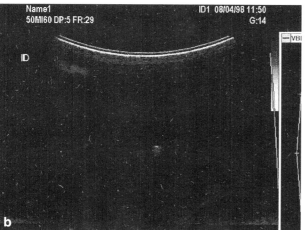

Figure 7   Effect of imaging frequency on grating lobe. Grating lobes become more apparent (**a**) when imaging frequency is increased and less apparent (**b**) when imaging frequency is decreased

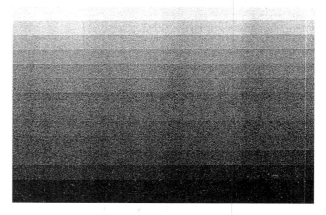

Figure 8   Shades of gray representing a dynamic range of 64:1. The brightest shade (white) represents the value 64 and the darkest shade (black) represents the value 1

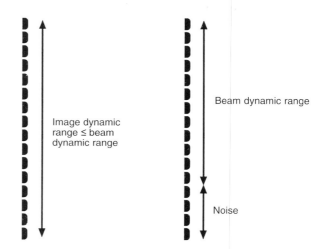

Figure 9   The dynamic range of a representative ultrasound system. All ultrasonic signals begin at a zero signal level and can increase in amplitude until they reach the system 'saturation level'. Some of the low level signals fall in the region of the background noise and will therefore be obscured. All modern systems have a built-in system-reject, which eliminates both system noise and the low-intensity echoes that lie just above the noise level. The dynamic range of the system is the ratio between the system saturation level and the system reject level

ratio between the saturation and reject level is defined as the system dynamic range. In most modern systems, the dynamic range of echoes exceeds 100 dB (a ratio of 100 000 : 1). Since the system cannot display this whole range of information, several steps are usually taken in order to reduce it with minimal diagnostic penalty. This will be most effectively accomplished by noting that the huge dynamic range of 100 000 : 1 is mainly a result of two effects. The range of each of the effects is approximately 300 : 1. The first effect is the result of the tissue attenuation, which is negligible at close range but is very high deep in the image, and the second effect is a result of the differences in the reflection coefficients. An ideal ultrasound image is a two-dimensional map of reflection coefficients, regardless of depth. Our first task would therefore be to minimize the effects of attenuation by the tissue. This task is achieved using a system function called time gain compensation (TGC).

Time gain compensation

The effect of the attenuation by tissue can be at least partly compensated for by progressively increasing the gain of the system as echoes come deeper from the body. When sound is attenuated by a large homogeneous object such as the liver, the reduction in intensity is exponential. In order to compensate for this type of attenuation, one would need to increase the gain logarithmically with time, since time is equivalent to depth. Since the attenuation coefficient may be patient dependent, one could compensate fairly well for this type of attenuation by adjusting a single parameter.

The situation in obstetrics is, however, far more complicated. The ultrasonic beam will traverse through fat, muscles (e.g. maternal abdominal wall), amniotic fluid, placenta, fetal bones and tissues etc. The attenuation is extremely heterogeneous and can by no means be represented using a single parameter. In this case, a multiple gain adjustment with some 8–12 sliding potentiometers is implemented. The image is then optimized by trial and error.

Compression

After having reduced the original 100 000 : 1 input dynamic range by the TGC to a value of about 300 : 1, the dynamic range needs to be further compressed until a displayable range of 30 : 1 is reached. Most ultrasound systems use some kind of a logarithmic function for compression of the dynamic range as described in Figure 10.

Post processing In addition to the logarithmic compression an additional post-processing function is usually applied to the resultant curve.

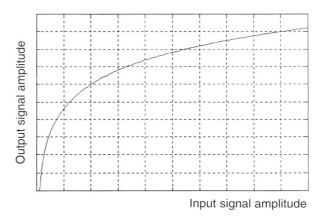

Figure 10 Logarithmic compression of the dynamic range

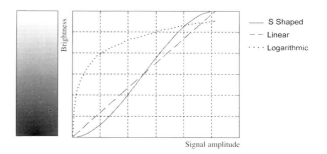

Figure 11 Examples of 3 possible post-processing functions: logarithmic (dotted line), linear (broken line) and S shaped (solid line)

This function is application specific. Examples of such functions are shown in Figure 11. The selection of the post-processing function is crucial to obtaining the desired appearance of the image. Different image appearances are optimally tuned for different diagnostic requirements and applications. Thus, for example, the type of image that is best suited to emphasize outlines of objects is different from the image that would maximize the contrast between similar tissues. The first example is characterized by large echo differences (e.g. between the fetal abdomen and the amniotic fluid, which would be relevant for measuring the fetal abdominal circumference; or between bone and soft tissue, which could be relevant for measuring fetal head circumference or femur length). In this case, the information required could be extracted even if the 30 shades of gray provided by the display are equally divided between the 300 input levels, as described in Figure 11.

For the second application the requirement will be to able to differentiate between tissue structures with only slight difference in structure. Echoes from such tissue structures are very weak to begin with, as they mainly result from scattering from tiny scatters. The requirement, therefore, is that the gain for low amplitude signals should be relatively high so that similar tissue structures with only slight differences in echo signal would still look different on the screen. On the other hand, we are less interested in the highly echogenic structures, so that the fact that they are saturated (appear as white on the screen, without any capability to resolve any structures in them) is less important. This might have an effect on the image 'cosmetics' but will not affect the diagnosis. Note, however, that we still do not wish to emphasize the extremely low signals that usually represent noise, or are obscured by noise (see Figure 9). The gain for these levels should therefore be kept very low. The overall gain curve will therefore have a shape of a logarithmic S curve as shown in Figure 11.

Persistence

As seen above, even very slight movements of the probe could change the speckle pattern in tissue texture echoes, but will cause much slighter changes in the appearance in the larger outlines. Averaging successive frames will therefore smooth the speckles but will hardly affect important outline information. During rapid search scanning or when imaging very fast moving objects, such as heart valves, this temporal averaging is undesirable. This calls for an implementation that would allow full control of the degree of averaging.

In most common implementations, the averaging is an iterative process in which the new pixel (picture element) information is averaged with the old information, with user selectable weights. In some implementations weights are allowed to change automatically to the rate of change of image data between successive frames.

GRAY SCALE SYSTEM CONTROLS AND THEIR EFFECT ON IMAGE QUALITY

As already discussed, due to inherent physical and technological limitations an 'ideal system' does not exist and the user will generally face painful compromises. Thus, for example, one would like to image at the highest possible frequency in order to improve resolution. However, high frequency ultrasound is highly attenuated. This would mean that for 'heavy patients' one needs to image at lower frequencies in order to gain penetration.

In most modern systems, the imaging parameters are preset for the various applications in most expected conditions. The situations in 'real life' will, however, always be somewhat different from those for which the presets were determined. Some adjustments by the operator will therefore almost always be required. The system controls and their effect on overall image quality are summarized in Table 6.

DOPPLER ULTRASONOGRAPHY

When a sound wave is reflected from a moving target, the reflected wave changes its frequency. The frequency change is proportional to the velocity of the moving target along the direction of the beam, and to the beam frequency. The frequency change of the reflected beam will be positive (the reflected beam will have a higher frequency than the incident beam) if the target is moving towards the transducer and will be negative (the reflected

Table 6 Gray scale system controls

Control change	Favorable effect	Adverse effect
Increase gain	See weak echoes	Strong echoes will be saturated
Set TGC	Optimize gain at all depths	
Increase imaging frequency	See more detail in the near field	Lose the image at the far field
Increase system field of view	Improve orientation. Improve the ability to measure large objects	Reduce frame rate, and smear of fast moving objects
Increase persistence	Reduce speckle and temporal noise	Smearing of fast moving objects
Add transmit focus	Increase image area that can be 'seen better'	Reduce frame rate
Move transmit focus to region of interest	Improve image resolution of object of interest	
Select required gray scale curve	Optimize image for the desired diagnosis	

TGC, time gain compensation

beam will have a lower frequency than the incident beam) if the target moves away from the transducer. The situation is described schematically in Figure 12.

When a certain 'sample volume' (see definition below) in the body is insonated, there will generally be a multitude of reflected waves at a variety of ultrasonic frequencies. Each of the red blood cell clusters, moving at a certain velocity, will scatter an ultrasonic beam with the corresponding Doppler shift. The intensities of the individual waves at given Doppler shifts will be proportional to the number of the red blood cells in each of the clusters. A Doppler signal is therefore usually composed of a range of frequencies with varied amplitudes. Note also that not only the red blood cells but also the arterial walls are moving reflectors that contribute to the Doppler signal. Since the vessel walls are usually extended in size, the reflected signals from them could be quite large. In extreme cases when the beam is perpendicular to the wall, the intensities of these signals might be more than 100 000 times stronger than the reflections from the blood cells themselves. Luckily, in most cases the velocities of the arterial walls are significantly lower than the velocities of the blood cells. This fact is used to discriminate between the two types of signal. There are cases, however, such as coronary flow, where this is not true. There is practically no way to measure blood flow in the coronaries using Doppler ultrasound methods.

There are three modes of Doppler operation: continuous wave (CW) spectral Doppler, pulsed wave (PW) spectral Doppler and Doppler color flow imaging, which are discussed below.

Continuous wave Doppler

Continuous wave (CW) Doppler is performed using a transducer composed of two separate elements. The first element functions continuously as the transmitter while the second element functions continuously as the receiver. In CW Doppler all blood flow velocities detected along the axis of the transducer will contribute to the Doppler signal. In practice this means that the operator cannot determine the origin of the Doppler signal in the body. This type of operation was used in obstetrics more than 20 years ago. It is still used in monitoring equipment and in echocardiology scanners. It is no longer found in modern imaging equipment for obstetrics and gynecology.

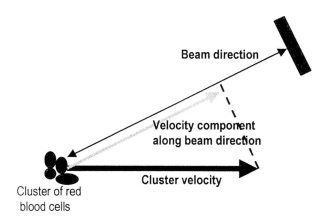

Figure 12 An ultrasonic beam, emitted by the transducer, is reflected by moving red blood cells. The change in frequency of the wave is proportional to the velocity of the red blood cells. When the reflected signal reaches the transducer, the difference between the transmitted and the returned frequency is measured. This difference in frequency is called the Doppler frequency shift. The magnitude of the Doppler frequency shift is dependent on the angle between the ultrasonic beam and the red cell velocity vector

Pulsed wave Doppler

In pulsed wave (PW) Doppler, the same transducer elements are used for both transmitting and receiving the ultrasonic beam; and in most cases also for gray scale imaging and for color flow imaging (see explanation below). The transmitted signal in this case is a relatively short pulse, although it may be several times longer than the pulse in gray scale imaging. The returned signal is 'gated', which means that only the received signal at a predefined time gate (which corresponds to a specific range gate) is processed and included in the spectral analysis.

The Doppler measurement starts by positioning a sample volume on the two-dimensional gray scale image prior to activating the PW Doppler beam. Only the signals returning from the ranges of the sample volume will be analyzed. The sample volume can be positioned anywhere on the image and may assume almost any desired size. Another difference between the two modes is that, unlike CW Doppler where insonation is continuous, insonation in PW Doppler generally lasts less than 1% of the time. This allows the use of lower signal intensities which means lower risk to the patients.

Pulse repetition frequency (PRF)

After a pulse is transmitted, the transducer will function as a receiver until the signal has returned from the specified depth. Only than can the next pulse be transmitted. This defines a minimum time between consecutive pulses or a maximum rate or repetition frequency. The depth range thus limits the pulse repetition frequency. High PRFs are required for measuring high velocities resulting in high Doppler frequency shifts. It can be shown mathematically that only when the Doppler frequency shift is less than half the sampling rate (PRF/2), can the velocity be properly assessed. When the Doppler frequency shift exceeds PRF/2 a folding artifact will occur, as illustrated in Figure 13.

Actually, for a given PRF, the measured Doppler frequency shift may be anywhere between −PRF/2 and PRF/2. This defines a total measurable range of frequencies of PRF that can be measured. Thus, for example, we could measure frequency shifts in the range −0.25PRF–0.75PRF as illustrated in Figure 13. This is accomplished by manually shifting the base line.

Doppler color flow imaging

By placing multiple gates (sample volumes) across an entire area in the gray scale image and separately processing the Doppler shift signals in each of them, a two-dimensional distribution of Doppler shift signals can be obtained. In order to achieve high enough frame rates, the 'interrogation time' at each gate is rather limited. A detailed spectral analysis at each gate would be too long if a reasonable accuracy is required and is therefore not applicable. As a result, the analysis is usually limited to the determination of the average velocity at each gate.

Slowly moving tissue will also cause a Doppler signal, which must be filtered out in order to eliminate 'flash' artifacts. A relatively sophisticated filtering to remove the tissue Doppler signal is in this case crucial since the spectral analysis used in CW Doppler or in single gate PW Doppler is not applicable.

The Doppler frequency shifts and the amplitude of the Doppler signal are then analyzed in each individual gate. The data are used to assess either the average velocity (magnitude and direction) or the total amplitude of the signal in each of the gates. There are two forms of presenting real-time blood flow information: color flow imaging, where

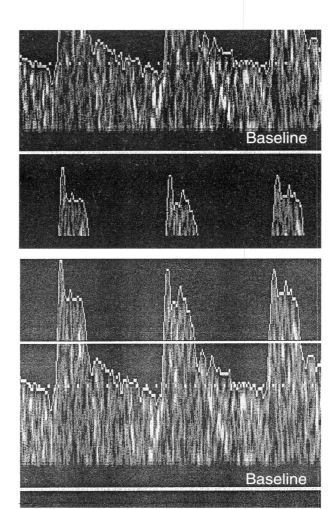

Figure 13 Spectral folding caused by aliasing. By moving the baseline upward, the measurable range of positive frequencies is increased to 0.75PRF, while that of the negative frequencies is reduced to 0.25PRF. This eliminates the 'folding'. The overall range is preserved

a color-coded velocity map is displayed on top of the gray scale image, and the second, referred to as power Doppler or 'Ultrasound Angio', where the Doppler signal amplitude, which is proportional to the density of the blood cell, is displayed as a color map on top of the gray scale image.

Color velocity imaging

In this mode a real-time image representing blood-flow velocities is displayed as an overlay on top of the gray scale two-dimensional image. Color flow imaging is based on a color scale. Similar to the gray scale presentation used in two-dimensional imaging, the velocities measured at each Doppler gate are assigned a corresponding shade of color. The scale is designed to optimize high or low velocity display. Usually a red and blue color scheme is used. According to this scheme, blood flowing towards the transducer is colored red while blood flowing away from the transducer is colored blue. An example of a color velocity image is provided in Figure 14: blood perfusion in the kidney (Color plate 1).

Power Doppler imaging

This is a relatively new way to image blood flow. What is displayed in this case is not the average velocity in the sample volume, but only the Doppler intensity. This is essentially the intensity of the reflection from moving blood particles. Most physical phenomena affecting Doppler ultrasound are not relevant in this case. There is almost no angle dependence and no aliasing effects, so that very low pulse repetition rates can be used in order to detect very low flow without risking the artifacts associated with two low PRFs. Since power Doppler is velocity independent, values do not change significantly over the heart cycle. In particular, since we are not trying to trace the fast velocity changes during the systolic phase, temporal averaging techniques can be employed to reduce noise. This generally results in a three-fold increase in sensitivity in the capability to demonstrate low flow. Figure 14 shows a side-by-side comparison of renal flow as imaged by color velocity mapping and by power Doppler (see also Color plate 1).

Doppler signal processing

The chain of the Doppler signal processing is described in Figure 15. The first function in the signal processing chain is called demodulation. The problem we are trying to solve is quite complicated. The 'frequency shifts' (the frequency difference between the incident ultrasonic wave and the waves reflected from the moving objects) involved are usually in the range of a few hundred Hertz to tens of thousands of Hertz. These are to be compared to the carrier frequency (the frequency of the incident ultrasonic beam) which is of the order of several (2–10) million Hertz. The task of determining those relatively minute frequency shifts is generally accomplished by 'mixing' (multi-

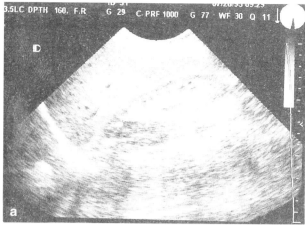
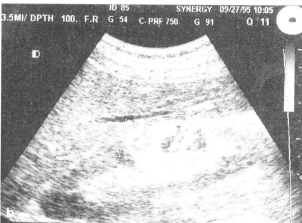

Figure 14 (**a**) Color velocity images of a native kidney. (**b**) Power Doppler image of the same kidney. (See also Color plate 1)

plying point by point) the received signal with a reference 'master clock' signal that is of the frequency of the transmitted wave. This will result in a signal, which could be written as a sum of two components having two main frequencies. The first component is a high frequency signal equal to the sum of the transmitted and reflected signals. The second component is a low frequency signal that equals the difference between the frequencies of the transmitted and reflected signals.

By passing the resultant signal through a low pass filter, the high frequency component is removed (filtered out). A high pass filter is also almost always used in order to filter out frequency components that originate from arterial wall and tissue motions. It can be shown that this process will give us only the magnitude of the frequency shift. In order to get also the sign of the shift, we also 'mix' the signal with a second 'master clock'

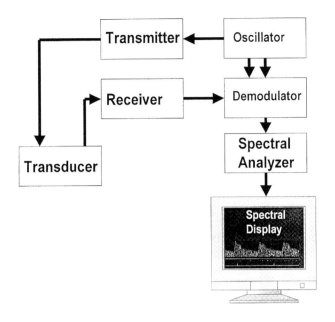

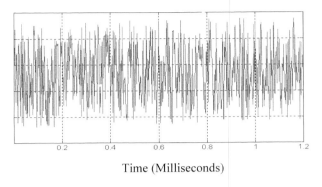

Time (Milliseconds)

Figure 16 An example of an actual recording of a demodulated acoustic Doppler signal

Figure 15 Schematic description of the Doppler processing chain

reference signal. The second signal is identical to the first master clock signal, but shifted by 90° (delayed in time by exactly one quarter of the cycle of the signal). It can be shown that using the resultant two demodulated signals, the direction of the flow can also be determined.

Our next step is to determine the frequency content of the demodulated signal. An example of such a signal is described in Figure 16. A rough idea of the frequency content of the signal can be gained simply by measuring all time differences, t_1, t_2, t_3... etc. between adjacent peaks. From these one can then calculate the corresponding frequency shifts $f_1 = 1/t_1$, $f_2 = 1/t_2$, $f_3 = 1/t_3$... etc. The number of particles in each frequency shift range is approximately proportional to the number of measurements with frequencies in that range. This process must take place over a long enough period of time (T) as demonstrated in Figure 16. The longer the measurement time T, the more 'peaks' in the signal, the more data points and the higher the accuracy. As a rule of thumb, $T \approx 1/Df$, where Df is the required resolution in frequency. However, T cannot be made too large because the frequency content of the signal changes over time. Thus for example during systole, when the velocity of the particles changes rapidly, T must be small enough so that the frequency content of the acoustic Doppler signal remains constant for the period of measurement T.

Sometimes, as will be explained later, T is severely limited by other system requirements, for example in color flow imaging. In this case, the frequency resolution becomes so coarse that a spectral analysis of the signal becomes meaningless. In situations like these, only the average frequency over a given period of time is measured. With the simplistic approach described above, we simply average out f_1, f_2, f_3... etc. The estimate is quite accurate even for a short measuring period T, as the number (N) of frequency measurements (N= T <f>, where <f> is the average frequency shift) may still be quite large. In most practical cases, N is of the order of 10. For detailed spectral analysis, much larger values of T (N = 64, 128 or 256) are used.

Spectral analysis

In practice, the methods employed for spectral analysis are much more sophisticated and accurate. Spectral analysis is mostly performed using a highly efficient computer-coded algorithm called Fast Fourier Transform (FFT). Usually there is also a certain overlap between data used for consecutive spectra (Figure 17). This overlap is required in order to update the spectra often enough, in order to follow quick changes such as during systole. Spectral Doppler analysis is usually performed at a single Doppler sample volume (gate), for consecutive periods of time of 2–10 s, in order to include several heart cycles. It is therefore 'non-real-time' in nature.

The display of spectral results

The information obtained from each spectrum is quite extensive. One actually obtains for each velocity (or Doppler frequency shift) the spectral density function. The spectral density function at each velocity is proportional to the number of blood cells that move at that velocity (and reflect a sound wave with the corresponding frequency shift). Modern systems usually repeat the calculation every 2 ms. This results in a huge amount of extensive information that must be properly displayed so that it can be easily interpreted by the sonographer. The method commonly accepted in all commercial systems is described in Figure 18.

Each 'spectrum' (the spectral density as a function of frequency shift) is displayed as a narrow vertical bar. The height along the vertical axis is proportional to the velocity (or frequency shift) and the brightness at each point is proportional to the number of particles moving with this velocity. The next spectrum is now displayed next to the previous one and so on. This is repeated until the whole area that is dedicated for the spectral display is full. When this happens the next spectrum will be displayed in the next left position, replacing the old spectrum displayed there, the next one will be displayed to its right and so on.

The spectral 'envelope'

Often, the entire overwhelming amount of information is not actually used for clinical diagnosis. In some cases, only the 'envelope' is required in order to provide the relevant hemodynamic information. The envelope actually describes the velocity of the faster cluster of cells as a function of time. In order to obtain this function one needs, for each spectrum, to mark the highest velocity (frequency shift) for which the spectral density function is not zero. It is called envelope because historically this curve was manually inscribed by the sonographer as an envelope to the spectral display (after the image was frozen). In today's modern equipment the envelope is automatically computed on-line (during scan). Figure 19 is an example of a spectral display describing the flow at a certain point of a uterine artery. The envelope, as provided automatically by the system, is marked in red.

Wave form analysis

Note that Doppler frequency shifts do not measure velocity. They are only *proportional* to velocity. In the following we shall concentrate on the hemodynamic information that can be extracted from

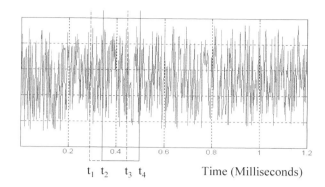

Figure 17 Two consecutive time windows, t_1–t_3 and t_2–t_4, during which the Doppler signals are processed. The two windows overlap during the time period t_2–t_3

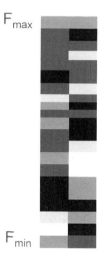

Figure 18 An illustration of a display of 2 spectra. Each spectrum is displayed as a column of bars. The bar at the bottom represents the lowest frequency (F_{min}) whereas the bar at the top represents the highest frequency (f_{max}). The vertical position of each of the bars represents its frequency. The brightness of each bar is proportional to the number of blood cells moving at a velocity resulting in the specific frequency shift

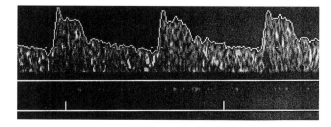

Figure 19 Spectral display and envelope

these frequency shift measurements. In doing so we are giving up the pretension to measure volume flow. The data provided by the Doppler shifts alone are, however, extensive enough to allow clinical assessment of the hemodynamic system. Obviously, the Doppler data allow a simple recognition of the existence of flow. In the following we shall show how the information embedded in the spectral envelope (maximum frequency shift curve) can be used in the evaluation of the vascular system.

Doppler waveform analysis and the Doppler indices

The maximum frequency shift curve (the spectral envelope) represents the temporal changes in the velocities of the fastest moving blood cells during the cardiac cycle. Perhaps the most important feature of the Doppler waveform is its pulsatility. Pulsatile flow, such as is often found in arteries, is characterized by a pulse-like shape with a systolic peak. This is distinctly different from the flat constant velocity waveform, usually found in veins. The amount of pulsatility carries a lot of information regarding the vascular system. The pulsatility of the waveform can be represented quantitatively in many different ways according to the vascular property under investigation. The indices defined below are mostly relevant for evaluating downstream resistance. Several different indices have been defined in the literature. They are all based on the peak systolic frequency shift (S), the end diastolic frequency shift (D) and the temporal mean frequency shift over exactly one cardiac cycle (A) (Figure 20). The most common indices are the resistance index[8], RI = (S–D)/S; the SD ratio[9], S/D; and the pulsatility index[10], PI = (S–D)/A.

It has been found that elevated values of these indices are associated with increased downsteam resistance. This has led to a multitude of clinical studies aimed at the development of clinical tools for the evaluation of the feto-placental, utero-placental and fetal cerebral circulation. Due to technical limitations, all presently available methods are based on measuring the Doppler indices in a very small number of sites, typically 1 to 3. Usually, these sites are conveniently selected in locations where the Doppler signals are relatively easy to acquire, e.g at the umbilical artery, the uterine artery or the middle cerebral artery. As a result, only major changes in the waveforms, such as reverse or no end diastolic flow in the umbilical artery or a diastolic notch in the uterine circulation, are really clinically significant. Following

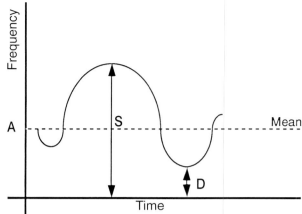

Figure 20   Typical time-velocity waveforms. S is the maximal value maximum frequency Doppler shift (peak systolic flow), D is the minimal value of maximum frequency Doppler (end diastolic flow) and A is the average of the maximum frequency Doppler shift over a heart cycle

recent advances in computer and multimedia technologies, it has become possible to perform simultaneous acquisition and analysis of a multitude of Doppler waveforms in a very short period of time. This has stimulated a wealth of new promising ideas and methods that could potentially improve the accuracy of Doppler waveform analysis as a clinical tool for evaluating various vascular systems. The limitations of the present methods and some of the new ideas are reviewed in the context of feto-placental circulation.

Umbilical-feto-placental circulation

Umbilical Doppler waveform analysis was first suggested as a non-invasive tool for the assessment of the feto-placental circulation in 1978. It has been shown that an elevated pulsatility index in the umbilical artery is indicative of increased downstream resistance within the placenta, associated with an obliterative process. Even though the clinical diagnostic value of Doppler velocimetry of the umbilical circulation has been demonstrated, there are still several factors that make interpretation of the Doppler signal difficult.

(1) It has been shown that only when two-thirds of the placental microvasculature is affected will a significant change in the PI be noticed.

(2) Pulsatility values depend also upon additional factors such as the fetal cardiac output, fetal heart rate, fetal cardiac stroke volume, etc.

(3) Although all Doppler indices defined above do not depend explicitly on direction, there still is a residual dependence, mainly due to the high pass filter, originally designed to filter out the arterial wall and tissue signals. When a vessel is approximately perpendicular to the flow direction, slow diastolic flow might be more affected by the filter than the relatively fast systolic flow. In the case of flow in the umbilical artery, the flows at the center of the arteries are always faster than the flows closer to the vessel walls, especially during diastole. One therefore expects a distribution of pulsatility values in the umbilical artery, resulting from variations in the position and orientation of the beam and Doppler sample volume relative to the vessel walls.

Recent developments

The wide distribution of pulsatility values can now be demonstrated by a new Doppler modality that allows for simultaneous measurements of Doppler waveforms by a large number of sample volumes. The system consists of an ultrasound system with pulse wave Doppler capability, to which a special scanning mode has been added. Data is continuously acquired along a group of lines. The process is repeated until the desired region of interest is scanned. For each sample volume the Doppler data are used to compute a spectra and for each spectra the maximum frequency shift curve is generated and Doppler indices computed. By generating histograms of the computed PI values it can clearly be seen that a wide distribution of these values occurs in the umbilical artery[11,12] (Figure 21 and Color plate 2).

Early detection of placental diseases

It is well known that the PI values at the umbilical artery are relatively insensitive to small variations in the placental microvasculature in the early stages of disease. At these stages, in which less than about two-thirds of the terminal arterioles are affected, umbilical PI values do not correlate well with placental disease. The question is whether Doppler methods are applicable at all to the detection of placenta diseases at their early stages. It has been shown by several researchers that in the normal placenta there is a downstream gradient in the pulsatility, from the umbilical artery down the branching, all the way to the arteriole level. It has

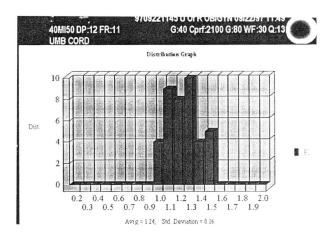

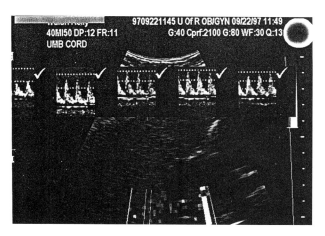

Figure 21 Histogram of pulsatility index values generated automatically by a new modality (see Color plate 2)

also been shown theoretically and observed clinically that a reversed pulsatility gradient indicates microvascular disease. Moreover, the downstream gradient is much more sensitive to small changes in microvasculature even at the early stages of the disease when only a few of the terminal arterioles are obliterated. It is hoped, therefore, that the new method could even allow 'early' screening in the low risk population.

At the later stages of the disease, after more than 70% of the placenta is already obliterated, the sensitivity of the measurement is expected to increase quite significantly. As can be seen from the figure above, a small increase of the percentage of obliteration will cause a significant change in the pulsatility. The situation however becomes complicated by the fact that in the case of a diseased placenta, one gets a rather wide distribution of the pulsatility measurements. In order to obtain reproducible meaningful results a relatively large number of measurements needs to be taken.

SYSTEM CONTROLS

An optimal Doppler signal requires optimization of quite a large number of system parameters. Thus for example, if the PRF selected is too low, high velocities will result in aliasing. If on the other hand the PRF selected is too high, the overall measurement time will be short so that the measurement resolution will be low. As discussed above, tissue and vessel wall motion need to be filtered out. This again is quite tricky. Too much filtering will also eliminate 'legitimate' low velocity blood flow signals. Color flow imaging still presents more problems. The quality of the measurement depends on the number of ultrasonic beams that are transmitted at a given direction, which defines at each gate the number of data points that are available for the calculation. Increasing the 'quality' will improve the accuracy of the calculation, but will also adversely affect the frame-rate. Table 7 lists the various controls used in the operation of the various Doppler modes. As is apparent from this table the number of controls

Table 7   System controls available to the operator for optimizing Doppler measurements

Control	PW (spectral) Doppler	Color flow imaging
Total gain	Increases signal received from moving objects of low reflectivity. Noise is also amplified	Increases signal received from moving objects of low reflectivity. Noise is also amplified
Wall motion filter	Decreases the signal from slowly moving objects such as vessel walls or surrounding tissue. Effect will increase with higher setting, but signal from slowly moving blood particles will not be observed	Decreases the signal from slowly moving objects such as vessel walls or surrounding tissue. Effect will increase with higher setting, but signal from slowly moving blood particles will not be observed
Baseline	Shifting the baseline will increase the measurement range of positive (negative) velocities and reduce the measurement range of the negative (positive) velocities	Shifting the baseline will increase the measurement range of positive (negative) velocities and reduce the measurement range of the negative (positive) velocities. Not provided by some manufacturers. Irrelevant in the power Doppler mode
Sample volume position	Defines the precise location on the anatomical gray scale image from where Doppler data are sampled	NA
ROI position	NA	Defines the part of the image where blood flow will be imaged
Sample volume size	Increasing the sample volume will increase signal intensity, as long as the sample volume size does not exceed the boundaries of the vessel	NA
Size of the ROI	NA	The size and position of the area on the image where flow will be demonstrated. Increasing the size of the ROI will reduce the frame-rate
Pulse repetition frequency (PRF)	The PRF determines the maximum velocity that can be measured without causing aliasing. The maximum PRF is depth range dependent. Aliasing could sometimes be indicated by 'copped' spectral displays	The PRF determines the maximum velocity that can be measured without causing aliasing. The maximum PRF is depth range dependent. Aliasing can sometimes be recognized when colors are mixed within the same vessel
Color 'quality'	NA	Defines the number of beams transmitted in each direction, for the computation of the velocities along the vector. Increasing the 'quality' may be required for demonstrating very low flow, but will result in reduced frame-rates

NA, not applicable; ROI, region of interest

that need to be optimized is quite large. In order to allow rapid optimization of the gray scale image, Doppler and color, most systems will use presets for all clinical applications. Proper use of the presets saves time, reduces button pushing and ensures diagnostic results. Note however that presets are usually designed for the average set of conditions in the given application. Fine adjustments are usually for the individual cases.

References

1. Maslak S. Computed sonography. In Sanders R, Hill M, eds. *Ultrasound Annual 1985*. New York: Raven Press, 1985

2. Kremkau WF. *Diagnostic Ultrasound: Principles, Instrumentation and Exercises*. Orlando: Grune & Stratton Inc., 1984

3. Wagner RF, Smith SW, Sandrick JM, *et al*. Low contrast detectibility and contrast detail analysis in medical ultrasound. *IEEE Transactions on Sonics and Ultrasonics* 1983;30:164–73

4. Wells PNT, Halliwell M. Speckle in ultrasonic imaging. *Ultrasonics* 1981;September:225–9

5. Smith SW, Wagner RF, Sandrick JM, *et al*. Statistics of speckles in ultrasound B scans. *IEEE Transactions on Sonics and Ultrasonics* 1983;30:156–63

6. Burckhart CB. Speckles in ultrasound B-mode scans. *IEEE Trans Sonics Ultrasonics* 1978;25:16–6

7. Scanlan KA. Sonographic artifacts and their origins. *Am J Radiol* 1991;156:1267–72

8. Gosling RG, King DH. Ultrasound angiology. In Macus AW, Adamson J, eds. *Arteries and Veins*. Edinburgh: Churchill Livingstone, 1975;61–98

9. Stuart B, Drumm J, Fitzgerald DE, *et al*. Fetal blood velocity waveforms in normal pregnancy. *Br J Obstet Gynaecol* 1980;87:780

10. Pourcelot L. Applications clinique de l'examen Doppler transcutanée. In Pourcelot L, ed. *Vélocimétrique Ultrasonore Doppler*. Paris: INSERM, 1974;213

11. Haberman S, Friedman Z. A new technique for improved diagnosis of local placental abnormalities: Fourier analysis of intraplacental waveforms. *Gynecol Obstet Invest* 1993;36:211–20

12. Jaffe R. Multigate spectral Doppler velocimetry in fast assessment of intraplacental fetal circulation. *J Ultrasound Med* 1996;15:309–12

Robert Lamb Library
Inverclyde Royal Hospital

First trimester ultrasonography

Richard Jaffe and Tamara Allen

Ultrasonography has had an unprecedented impact on the practice of clinical obstetrics and it is the most accurate and reliable method for evaluation of first trimester gestations and their complications. High frequency transvaginal ultrasonography (TVS) has further enhanced our ability to follow the development of early gestation and detect pathologies in its earliest stages. One of the most important tasks of the obstetrician is correct dating of pregnancies, which has changed significantly since the introduction of ultrasonography with most clinicians now relying solely on this technique for estimation of gestational age. With ultrasonography, abnormal development of early gestations can be detected before the appearance of clinical symptoms, enhancing counseling and treatment. The incidence of multiple gestations has increased significantly with the widespread use of assisted reproductive techniques (ART). Vital information regarding number of embryos, amniotic and chorionic sacs and early development may be obtained with first trimester ultrasonography. Ultrasonography has also become an invaluable tool in performance of early genetic testing and multifetal reduction.

The diagnosis and treatment of ectopic gestations have undergone significant changes over the last decade. Clinical and biochemical parameters are insufficient for timely and accurate diagnosis of ectopic gestations. With TVS the close proximity of the probe to the pelvic structures enables improved evaluation of ultrasonographic findings and improved diagnosis. Ultrasonography also has been employed in treatment of ectopic gestations by guiding the injection of KCl or methotrexate directly into the gestational sac.

Transabdominal ultrasonography (TAS) and TVS have their individual advantages and disadvantages. The general view of the pelvis and its structures obtained with TAS is superior and important in identifying the pelvic structures correctly when performing TVS. TVS has superior resolution due to the use of high frequency probes. Large uteri with pedunculated fibroids or ovaries located high in the pelvis may occasionally be beyond the field of image of TVS and imaged only with TAS due to deeper penetration of low frequency waves. It is therefore important to view these two techniques as complementary.

ULTRASONOGRAPHIC LANDMARKS OF EARLY PREGNANCY

The embryo enters the uterine cavity 4 to 6 days following fertilization in the tube when the endometrium is in its early secretory phase. Implantation subsequently occurs 1 to 1½ weeks following fertilization. Implantation is followed by increased blood flow to the uterus and thickening of the endometrium. Thickening of the endometrium is the first detectable ultrasonographic sign of the presence of a pregnancy and has been termed 'decidual reaction'.

Gestational sac

The gestational sac is the first definitive ultrasonographic sign of a developing pregnancy. On the ultrasonographic scan the gestational sac appears as a hypoechogenic area surrounded by an echogenic ring, the endometrium (Figure 1). This sac, termed the chorionic sac, contains the embryonic disc, amnion and primary yolk sac. With TVS the gestational sac may be visualized when it has obtained a diameter of 1 to 2 mm which occurs at approximately 4 to 4.5 weeks menstrual age. The gestational sac grows to 2 to 4 mm at 32 to 35 days and is 5 mm at 36 to 37 days menstrual age. A gestational sac should be viewed in normal intrauterine pregnancies when the serum β human chorionic gonadotropin (β-hCG) reaches 500 mIU/ml (2nd International Standard) but has been detected with levels as low as 150 mIU/ml[1-3].

At 13 to 14 days post-fertilization the decidua is arranged in three layers: (1) decidua basalis situated beneath the implanted embryo; (2) decidua capsularis covering the rest of the chorionic sac; and (3) decidua parietalis lining the portions of uterine cavity not involved in implantation. The double decidual ring was described by Nyberg *et al.*[4]. This important sign consists of two echogenic rings surrounding the hypoechoic gestational sac (Figure 2). The inner ring consists of the chorion, embryonic disc and decidua capsularis and the outer ring represents the decidua parietalis. Frequently a hypoechoic area may be seen between these two rings and it represents the compressed uterine cavity adjacent to the gestational sac. In the presence of an ectopic pregnancy, a single hypoechoic area may be visualized which cannot be separated from the uterine cavity. This is due to the accumulation of fluids within the uterine cavity but absence of a gestational sac. The gestational sac in normal pregnancies has been reported to grow 1.0 to 1.2 mm per day[5]. Absent or subnormal growth of the gestational sac is a poor prognostic sign even though 25–50% of abnormal intrauterine gestations will demonstrate growth within normal limits[5,6]. Therefore, observing normal intrauterine gestational sac growth does not guarantee favorable outcome.

Yolk sac

The primary yolk sac appears during the second week following fertilization. It develops as a result of growth of extra-embryonic endoderm from the ventral aspect of the embryonic disc and enclosure of a fluid-filled cavity. It cannot be seen by ultrasonography. The primary yolk sac soon degenerates and is replaced by the secondary yolk sac. It is the secondary yolk sac that is visualized by ultrasonography and appears at 5 to 6 weeks menstrual age. The yolk sac is characteristically round with a thin echogenic wall and internal hypoechoic area (Figure 3). The yolk sac is located outside the amnion within the chorionic space and is of embryonic origin. It has been shown in several studies that the yolk sac may be visualized in 70–80% of normal pregnancies[7]. The normal yolk sac measures 3 to 7 mm in diameter and is usually present until 12 weeks gestation. The appearance of a yolk sac within the gestational sac excludes blighted ova as well as ectopic gestations except for the rare cases of heterotopic pregnancies where intra- and extrauterine pregnancies coexist, a phenomenon more frequently encountered with the increased availability of ART. The normal yolk sac has a round spherical appearance. In abnormal

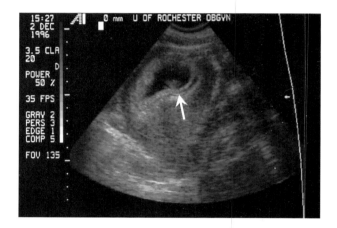

Figure 2   The 'double sac sign' showing small amount of free fluid between developing gestational sac and uterine wall (arrow)

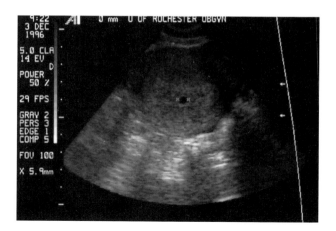

Figure 1   A gestational sac of 4 weeks and 2 days menstrual age as visualized by transvaginal ultrasonography

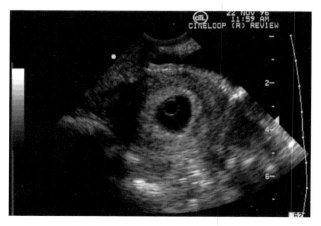

Figure 3   The yolk sac at 6 weeks and 4 days menstrual age

pregnancies the yolk sac may be an irregular shape, become calcified (Figure 4) as well as have diameters below 3 mm or above 7 mm (Figure 5). Yolk sacs measuring more than 7 mm in diameter are commonly seen in abnormal pregnancies[8,9]. Smaller than normal yolk sacs have been associated with chromosomally abnormal pregnancies as well as in the products of conception obtained from spontaneous miscarriages[10].

Embryonic pole and cardiac activity

The early embryonic disc is connected to the yolk sac at its ventral aspect. As a consequence, the identification of the yolk sac serves as a landmark for the identification of the embryonic pole and cardiac activity. At 16 days to 17 days conceptional age the embryonic pole measures approximately 1 mm. At 5 to 6 weeks menstrual age the embryonic disc measures 2 to 4 mm and can be identified by TVS. Fetal cardiac activity can be detected by TVS on day 27 to day 29 conceptional age or as soon as the embryonic pole is visualized[11,12]. The embryonic heart rate at this early stage is characteristically slower than later in pregnancy and may range from 70 to 90 beats per minute[12]. It may for this reason be confused with maternal pulse. Fetal heart activity should always be detected in a normal embryo of 4 to 5 mm at 45 days menstrual age. The detection of embryonic cardiac activity is clinically of great importance since the majority of these pregnancies have normal outcome[6,7].

Amniotic cavity

The amniotic cavity appears within the inner cell mass on the dorsal aspect of the embryonic disc. The amnion is attached to the body at the umbilical ring. During weeks 7 to 10 menstrual age the amnion can be detected as a separate sac within the chorionic space (or extra embryonic coelom) (Figure 6). By week 7 of normal pregnancies the amniotic cavity will be larger than the yolk sac. The amniotic cavity expands and will eventually fill the entire chorionic space and adhere to the chorion. In most cases this occurs approximately at week 8 to week 10 of menstrual age but may in rare cases occur as late as 16 to 17 weeks.

Early embryonic size and crown–rump length

In addition to yolk sac and gestational sac measurements the most commonly used first trimester

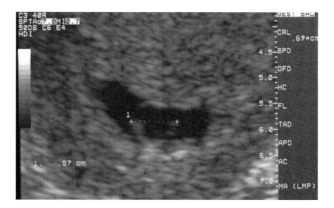

Figure 5 A large yolk sac of a missed abortion

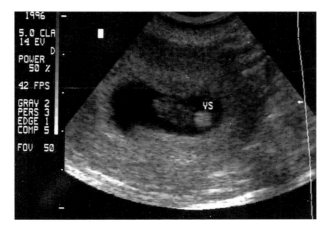

Figure 4 An 8 weeks and 2 days old pregnancy. The yolk sac is calcified (YS). This pregnancy ended in a spontaneous miscarriage

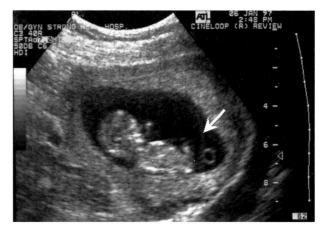

Figure 6 A 9 weeks and 2 days embryo within the amniotic cavity. Amnion (arrow)

parameter for gestational age estimation is the crown–rump length (CRL). The CRL measurement was originally established by Robinson and Fleming[13] and has been repeated in several studies[14]. Variations in measurement can be due to the natural curvature of the embryo, errors in measurement with inclusion of the yolk sac, population differences and variation in ovulation, fertilization and implantation timing[6]. Significantly smaller CRLs than expected have been associated with embryos with chromosomal abnormalities.

The CRL is the most accurate assessment of gestational age in the first trimester (Figure 7). This probably is also true for the entire pregnancy. The mean error of CRL in the first trimester was reported to be 7.73 days in one study[15] and 95% of patients delivered within ±12 days of CRL estimated delivery date in a second study[16]. Due to the presence of a natural curvature of the embryo and the inability to accurately define the crown

and rump in the early stages of the first trimester, the measurement of the greatest length of the embryo (or early embryonic size) has been suggested to replace the traditional CRL[17] during weeks 5 to 7 (Figure 8).

Embryonic and early fetal development

The first 8 weeks postovulation are referred to as the embryonic period. It is during this period that the majority of the embryonic structures appear[18]. As a consequence, many congenital abnormalities will occur at this stage. The fetal period extends from the end of the embryonic period (10 weeks menstrual age) until birth. The embryo can be identified as a distinct structure at 3 weeks postovulatory age when it has obtained the length of 1 to 2 mm[19]. Cardiac activity may be detected during the third postovulatory week. At 4 weeks the embryo is 5 to 6 mm in length with prominent cranial and caudal folds. The limb buds appear at this stage, although they are not detectable by ultrasonography before week 5 postovulation. During weeks 5 and 6, the first movements of the embryo can be detected and are mainly general and sudden movements of the whole body. During week 7, when the embryo measures 18 to 20 mm in length, the limb buds grow and fingers and toes may be visualized (Figure 9). At this stage the physiological herniation of fetal bowel into the umbilical cord is evident.

The embryonic heart activity starts during week 3 postconception[1,20]. During the third week the heart is structured as a single tube and blood flow

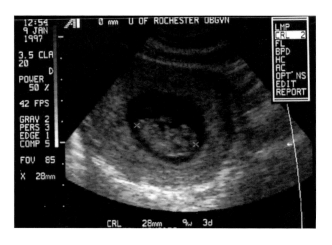

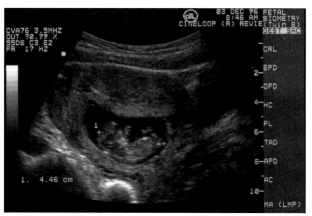

Figure 7 Two crown–rump length measurements demonstrating caliper placements

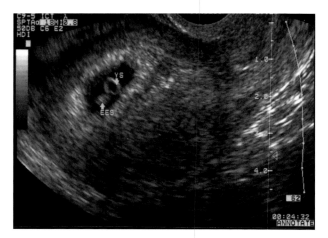

Figure 8 Early embryonic size. YS, yolk sac

is from the venous to the arterial side in a sequential manner. At this stage, Doppler signals from the embryonic heart are obtained as blood flows from the left atrium to the left ventricle into the right ventricle and from there to the aortic system. The blood flow changes to a parallel pattern with the main flow going from both atria through the atrio-ventricular valves and into their respective ventricles with the differentiation of the atria and the septation of the ventricles[20]. At this stage, the wave forms obtained show an adult pattern with flow from both sides of the heart directed the same way.

The central nervous system may also be visualized by ultrasonography during the embryonic period. During weeks 7 and 8 a single ventricle is seen on ultrasonography (Figure 10). This represents the undivided ventricular system of the early brain[19,21]. Depending on the plane of scanning, this single space represents either the lateral system, third or fourth ventricles. During week 9, partition of the ventricular system occurs and the falx cerebri and choroid plexus appear. The early spinal cord also may be visualized during weeks 7 and 8, and at 9 weeks can be traced along its whole length. Table 1 depicts the ultrasonographic landmarks and their time of appearance in menstrual weeks.

At the end of the embryonic period (8 weeks) the embryo measures approximately 30 mm and has an identifiable human appearance. By the end of the first trimester the fetus has obtained a length of 60 to 65 mm. At this stage movements of the trunk and independent movements of the limbs may be seen. At the end of the first trimester

sucking and swallowing motions as well as some breathing motions appear.

Early pregnancy failure

High-frequency TVS has enabled visualization of normal early pregnancy at approximately the time of the first missed menstrual period. The

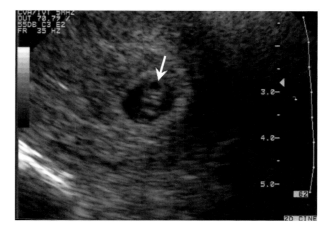

Figure 10 Single ventricle (arrow) of early brain

Table 1 Transvaginal ultrasonographic findings of early embryonic development

Menstrual age (weeks)	CRL (mm)	Ultrasonographic landmark
3–4	–	Decidual reaction
4 (+2 days)	–	Gestational sac, double sac sign
5	1–2	Yolk sac and embryonic pole, amniotic cavity
5–6	5–6	Cardiac activity
6–7	10	Single ventricle, early embryonic size
7–8	18–20	Limb buds, physiologic bowel herniation
8–9	20–25	Falx, choroid plexus, cranial and caudal poles seen, embryonic movements
9–10	30–35	Fingers, jaw and limb movements
12	40	Midgut herniation resolved, yolk sac absorbed, stomach visible

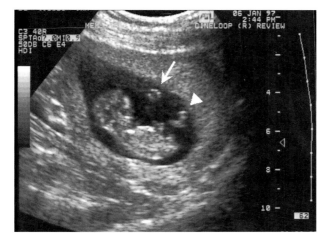

Figure 9 A 9 weeks and 5 days menstrual age gestation. Upper (arrow) and lower (arrow head) limbs are seen

development of embryonic structures may be closely followed and in many cases a diagnosis of early pregnancy failure made before the onset of clinical signs or symptoms. With TVS the assessment of the early gestation has undergone a significant change and we can now evaluate the prognosis of any pregnancy by scanning structures that are visible earlier than the embryonic pole or heart activity. First trimester vaginal bleeding is present in 10–20% of all pregnancies[6,22]; 40–50% of these will eventually end in spontaneous miscarriage[23]. In the past, with the use of TAS, the diagnosis of abnormal first trimester gestations was based on clinical symptoms and ultrasonographic findings at 6 to 7 weeks gestation. The detection of embryonic heart activity in the presence of vaginal bleeding is a good prognostic sign and most of these pregnancies will have favorable outcomes[6,7].

Evaluation of growth of the gestational sac as well as yolk sac anatomy are important in the evaluation of the status of the pregnancy. Nyberg reported a mean gestational sac growth of 1.13 mm per day between 5 weeks and 11 weeks of menstrual age[5]. Other reports have shown similar results[22]. The range of gestational sac growth in normal pregnancies was 0.71 to 1.75 mm per day[5]. In this reported series, within a group of 30 abnormal gestations six showed no sac growth and 16 demonstrated growth below that expected for gestational age. Only 8 (27%) demonstrated normal growth. Consistent with the observations of other reports, Nyberg concluded that a yolk sac should always be present in a gestational sac of > 20 mm and an embryo with heart activity present in a gestational sac of > 25 mm. The finding of a gestational sac with no identifiable yolk sac or embryo is not uncommon when patients are scanned very early in pregnancy. With the current information we can follow gestational sac growth and calculate the normal time intervals between scans to obtain optimal diagnostic information.

In addition to growth of the gestational sac, the anatomical relation of the gestational sac to the uterine cavity is important in the exclusion of ectopic gestations. When the blastocyst implants into the endometrium it very soon becomes separated from the uterine cavity by the decidua capsularis. At this stage the chorionic sac is not in direct contact with the partly collapsed uterine cavity. This sequence of events brings the decidua capsularis and parietalis very close to each other, and the area between them will appear as a small hypoechoic region in close proximity to the gestational (chorionic) sac. This sign was named the double decidual sac (DDS) and its presence correlated with an intrauterine pregnancy in approximately 98% of cases[4] (Figure 2). In the presence of an ectopic pregnancy, the uterus demonstrates the decidual reaction with fluid formation in the uterine cavity, but no gestational sac present. In these cases, the walls of the uterine cavity will appear widely separated and no other echo-free region may be visualized. In some cases, widening of the uterine cavity may be seen in the presence of a normal intrauterine pregnancy. This is often caused by subchorionic bleeding into the uterine cavity and separation of the decidual layers.

The yolk sac is essential for normal embryonic development and is normally detected by ultrasonography before the detection of heart activity. Nyberg reported that the identification of a normal yolk sac had a 100% positive predictive value for a normal gestational sac[7]. The presence of a yolk sac was also of great value in confirming an intrauterine pregnancy. When a yolk sac was detected but an embryo was not, normal outcome occurred in 84% of gestations. The normal yolk sac measures 3 to 7 mm at 7 weeks gestation and abnormally large or small yolk sacs have been associated with structural and chromosomal anomalies[6,10].

Threatened abortion

Threatened abortion is a clinical term associated with early pregnancy and vaginal bleeding. As already stated this is not an uncommon finding and probably the main reason most patients are referred for early ultrasonography, and the diagnosis depends on the ultrasonographic findings. The most common causes of first trimester bleeding with an intact intrauterine pregnancy are subchorionic hematomas, placenta covering the internal cervical os and vanishing twin phenomenon. Other rare causes are myomas in close proximity to the placenta, bleeding following removal of an intrauterine device and partial molar gestations. In many cases no specific cause for the bleeding is provided by ultrasonography and the majority of these patients will have normal pregnancy outcome if embryonic cardiac activity was detected.

The most common positive ultrasonographic finding is a subchorionic hematoma. They usually are identifiable as hypoechogenic areas adjacent to the developing placenta but outside the gestational sac (Figure 11). The bleeding typically occurs between the decidua basalis and chorion frondosum or chorion leave. The worst outcome is associated with subchorionic hematomae situated directly under the chorion frondosum. There is no good correlation between the size of the hematoma and outcome of pregnancy. It has been reported that if a subchorionic hematoma consists of more than 50 ml of blood the rate of spontaneous miscarriage is in the range of 20–40%[6].

Blighted ova

Blighted ova (anembryonic pregnancy) is characteristically defined as a gestational sac over 20 mm in diameter with no embryonic structures[6]. Since the advent of TVS we now know that some of the empty sacs probably result from early embryonic death and subsequent resorbtion of the tissue. The diagnosis depends on the time lapsed between the embryonic death and the ultrasonographic examination. It has been reported that blighted ova demonstrate gestational sacs with sub-optimal growth[24]. Chromosomal abnormalities are common in blighted ova and in many cases the placenta and gestational sac grow despite the fact that an embryo has not developed.

Missed abortion

If the ultrasonographic scan reveals an intrauterine sac with an embryo with no cardiac activity, the diagnosis of missed abortion is established. The causes of missed abortions are several. Some are associated with faulty development of uterine vascularization to the gestational sac, others due to immunological abnormalities. By incorporating color Doppler imaging into the examination we can assess the uterine circulation. Specific attention should be paid to the spiral arteries and intervillous space. In some cases increased resistance to flow in spiral arteries may be observed as a result of abnormal placentation.

Incomplete abortion

The diagnosis of an incomplete abortion is made when bleeding and passage of tissue occurs in the presence of an open cervical canal and products of conception still remain in the uterine cavity. If all

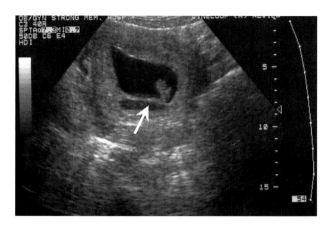

Figure 11 Seven week pregnancy with subchorionic hematoma (arrow) adjacent to placenta

products of conception were expelled and the cervix found to be closed the diagnosis would be a complete abortion.

Inevitable abortion

When bleeding occurs in association with lower abdominal pain and ultrasonography reveals an intact intrauterine pregnancy situated low in the uterus the diagnosis of an inevitable abortion is made. With an inevitable abortion uterine contractions originating in the uterine fundus may often be observed during the ultrasonographic examination.

Molar pregnancies

Molar pregnancies are associated with degeneration of placental tissue, hypervascularity of the uterus and an empty gestational sac. Vaginal bleeding is a common finding. In a complete molar pregnancy there is no embryonic or fetal tissue and therefore an empty or absent gestational sac. In a partial (or incomplete) molar gestation a gestational sac, embryo and hydropic placenta coexist and chromosomal abnormalities, specifically triploidy, are common in these patients (Figure 12). All patients with molar gestations are at high risk for developing pre-eclampsia/eclampsia and placental abruption later on in pregnancy due to the effect of the high levels of β-hCG[25]. When a cystic-hydropic placenta is detected on ultrasonography the gestational sac, if present, should be carefully scrutinized for any embryonic structures to rule out an incomplete mole. A second characteristic ultrasonographic finding in these patients is the presence of ovarian theca-lutein cysts that can obtain diameters of up to 10 cm.

ECTOPIC PREGNANCY

Ectopic pregnancy (EP) is a very significant disease in women of reproductive age and accounts for 10–15% of maternal deaths[26]. 'Think ectopic' is an important routine in any first trimester abnormality. These abnormalities include: vaginal bleeding, irregular cycles with unknown date of conception, missed menstrual period with regular cycles, abdominal or pelvic pain, dizziness, history of change in consciousness and/or a pelvic mass on bi-manual examination. Advances in TVS and increased sensitivity of quantitative β-hCG tests have greatly improved the assessment of early gestations and diagnosis of ectopic gestation.

An EP occurs when the conceptus implants anywhere outside the uterine cavity, and accounts for about 1% of all pregnancies. Recent advances in TVS combined with radioimmunoassay of the beta subunit of human chorionic gonadotropin have made the diagnosing of the presence of an EP over 90% accurate. Ninety-five per cent of EPs occur in the fallopian tube, 2–4% in the interstitium and the remaining in the ovary, abdomen and cervix. The Centers for Disease Control (CDC) have determined that EPs occur in approximately 17/1000 pregnancies. A woman with a history of a previous ectopic has a 25% chance of a recurrence[27]. Patients undergoing infertility treatments such as *in vitro* fertilization

(IVF) have a 2–8% risk of an EP[26] and a 1:100 probability of having a heterotopic (concomitant intra- and extrauterine) pregnancy. The general population has a 1:4000 risk for a heterotopic pregnancy.

Risk factors

Risk factors associated with an increased incidence of ectopic implantation are:

History of pelvic inflammatory disease (PID)
Prior tubal surgery
Previous ectopic pregnancy
Use of intrauterine contraceptive device
Infertility treatments, ovulation induction, IVF and GIFT
Heavy smoking
DES exposed women with or without uterine abnormality
Progestin-only contraceptives

Numerous factors will result in an increased probability of a fertilized ovum not reaching the uterus for normal implantation. PID, tubal surgery for patients with infertility problems or congenital developmental defects can result in scarred and abnormal fallopian tubes. Ironically, the administration of antibiotics for PID allows the tubes to remain patent but scarred, increasing the time the conceptus takes to reach the uterus and thereby resulting in a tubal implantation[28].

Beta-hCG assay

Pregnancy tests are performed on both urine and blood and measure the beta-subunit of the human chorionic gonadotropin (β-hCG). hCG is a glyco-protein produced by the syncytiotrophoblast which peaks at 6 weeks at 100 IU/l. The doubling time of the hCG in viable intrauterine pregnancies has been shown to be 1.4 to 2.1 days, or an increase of 66% over 48 hours. This doubling time is generally slower with both an abnormal intrauterine or an ectopic pregnancy possibly due to abnormal development of the trophoblast or the difference in implantation in the tube as opposed to the endometrium. A single quantitative level that falls above the discriminatory level is helpful to determine a normal intrauterine pregnancy. The initial discriminatory hCG zone was the hCG level at which a viable intrauterine pregnancy

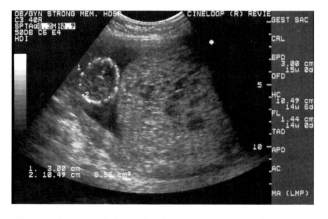

Figure 12 Partial mole demonstrating a fetus and hydropic placenta

(IUP) could be distinguished on TAS and was established by Kadar *et al.* in 1981[29]. With TVS a normal intrauterine gestational sac should be detected at serum levels of 1000 mIU/ml (IRP)[30] and all normal intrauterine pregnancies should demonstrate a gestational sac at this level. However, serial quantitative β-hCG measurements are of more value if the pregnancy location is in question. Abnormal increase in serum levels of hCG has been associated with ectopic gestations although is also seen occasionally with normal gestations. Due to the overlapping of hCG levels between intra- and extrauterine gestations serial hCG levels have to be correlated with ultrasonographic findings to make the correct diagnosis. The recently developed enzyme-linked immunoassay (ELISA) tests the β-hCG level in urine within minutes, is qualitative and is positive in 99% of patients with a symptomatic EP. The serum β-hCG radioimmunoassay (RIA) is extremely sensitive and quantitates the hCG. Both the ELISA urine and serum tests can diagnose a pregnancy as early as 10 days after conception. It is important to know which measurement standard your laboratory uses, either the International Reference Preparation (IRP) or the Second International Standard (2nd IS). The IRP value is approximately twice the value yielded by the 2nd IS.

Clinical assessment

Clinical signs and symptoms of an EP are not always typical. The classic triad of irregular menstrual bleeding, abdominal or pelvic pain, and a tender palpable adnexal mass may or may not be present. Only 60% of women complain of a missed menstrual period. Women who complain of left shoulder pain are more likely to have a significant amount of fluid in the pelvis and abdomen. This fluid causes irritation of the diaphragm which refers pain to the shoulder region. Any woman who complains of pelvic pain, has a positive pregnancy test and an empty uterus on ultrasound should have further follow-up to rule out an EP.

Differential diagnosis

There are various pelvic pathologies that could lead to suspicion of an ectopic on pelvic ultrasonography (Table 2). A uterus with congenital anomalies, pelvic inflammatory disease, the presence of myomas that cause distortion of the

uterus or a degenerating myoma may confuse the picture. Other ovarian masses or bowel pathology can also confuse the ultrasonographic image and may lead to an inaccurate diagnosis. One third of EP, however, have normal adnexa. Careful scanning and a familiarity with various pathological appearances are necessary to accurately diagnose or be highly suspicious of an ectopic, thus obtaining the proper treatment that is needed. Care must also be taken not to call fluid in the endometrium a gestational sac when there is actually an EP present elsewhere. This fluid mimicking a gestational sac is termed a pseudo-gestational sac and occurs in 5% of EPs (Figure 13). The shape of this fluid collection is usually elongated or irregular in shape without the thickened endometrial rim seen with normal IUPs. It is believed to occur due to the hormonal effects of the pregnancy on the endometrium.

Ultrasonographic evaluation

Transabdominal (TA) ultrasonography should initially be performed to obtain an overview of the pelvic organs and any adnexal masses or myomas that may lie outside the transvaginal (TV) scanning plane. The TA scan should be performed with a full but not over distended bladder which may collapse a tiny sac in the uterine cavity. If an IUP is seen, an ectopic would not be likely unless the patient had IVF or GIFT which increases the

Table 2 Differential diagnoses suggestive of an ectopic pregnancy

Ectopic location	Differential diagnosis
Abdominal	Severely retroflexed uterus
	Bicornuate uterus
Cervical	Impending abortion
	Degenerating cervical myoma
	Cervical cyst
Interstitial	Fibroid
	Bicornuate uterus
Ovarian	Endometrioma
	Bowel
	Hemorrhagic corpus luteum
	Tubal pregnancy
Tubal	Corpus luteum cyst/simple cyst
	Dermoid/other ovarian tumors
	Salpingitis/tubo-ovarian abscess
	Acute appendicitis/appendicial abscess
	Adhesive bowel
	Paraovarian cyst

chances of a heterotopic pregnancy to 1:400. The uterus and ovaries should be imaged and measured in all planes. The right upper quadrant should also be checked for the presence of free fluid. Some disadvantages of TA scanning are suboptimal visualization if obese, early IUP poorly seen, and decreased resolution due to typically using a lower frequency transducer. If an IUP is not visualized, the patient should void and a TV ultrasound should be performed. The advantages of TV scanning are: increased resolution due to higher frequency, avoidance of scanning through the maternal bladder and adipose tissue, the ability to visualize ovaries that cannot be seen on TA, and seeing an IUP one to two weeks earlier than by TA scanning. The disadvantages of TV ultrasound is that structures more than 8 cm from the transducer cannot be imaged and large myomas may

obscure the view of ovaries and even the endometrial cavity. A gestational sac in the fallopian tube with a living embryo or containing a yolk sac and nonviable embryo are 100% diagnostic of an ectopic pregnancy (Figure 14) although rarely seen. A tubal or adnexal ring is 95% diagnostic of an ectopic and a complex or solid adnexal mass is 92% diagnostic[30] (Figure 15). The adnexal ring is separate from the ovary and appears sonographically as an echogenic rim around a sonolucent area. These findings are produced by the trophoblast surrounding the gestational sac and vary in size from 1–3 cm. Recent studies have surmised that one-third of ectopic gestations have an abnormal karyotype which is evidenced by the high number of blighted EPs[31].

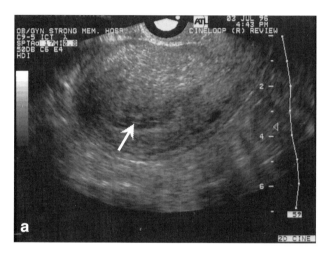

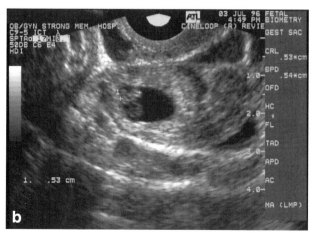

Figure 13 Ectopic pregnancy. (**a**) Uterus with fluid collection within cavity (arrow). (**b**) Gestational sac and embryo in tube

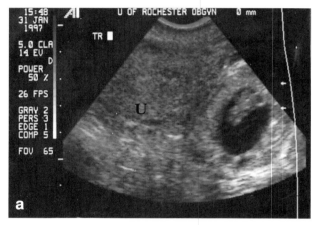

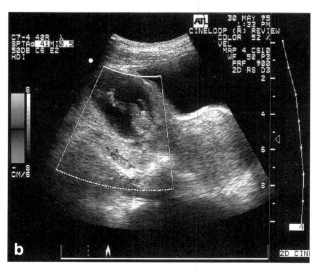

Figure 14 (**a**) Viable tubal ectopic pregnancy seen adjacent to uterus (U) on transvaginal ultrasonography. (**b**) Viable 12 week tubal ectopic with color Doppler demonstrating active blood flow (see also Color plate 3)

Chronic ruptured EPs can occur and present as a palpable solid mass. Ultrasonography will show an ill defined mass. Abdominal pregnancies may occur as a result of a tubal pregnancy aborting into the peritoneal cavity and reimplanting there. Abdominal pregnancies can go to term and are characterized by oligohydramnios, malpresentation, and pain during the pregnancy. Careful scanning will reveal a uterus with a normal endometrium but a TV ultrasound may be required to determine this. A cornual, or interstitial, EP can be diagnosed with careful assessment of the uterus and location of an ectopic sac (Figure 16). Free fluid is a nonspecific finding that if minimal is probably physiologically normal. A significant amount of free fluid, fluid in the hepatorenal space or fluid seen with echogenic debris is more suggestive of an ectopic, one that is either leaking or ruptured.

Color Doppler imaging

Circulation surrounding trophoblastic tissue, either intrauterine or extrauterine, is usually characterized by a low-resistance (high-diastolic) arterial waveform (Figure 17 and Color plate 4). Doppler can help confirm the presence of an EP when an irregular adnexal mass is identified.

Management

In recent years, the β-hCG pregnancy assay test in conjunction with the use of TVS has changed the management of patients with EP. A woman with an unruptured EP with declining β-hCG levels can now be considered for a more conservative approach. It is not unusual for EPs to spontaneously resolve, which excludes the need for invasive surgery. Current research has indicated that 64–92% will spontaneously resolve[32]. Criteria for using this method of 'wait and see' are: decreasing serum β-hCG, no signs of an IUP by TVS, adnexal mass less than 4 cm, no fetal heartbeat and no signs of bleeding or rupture. This management should be done with great care with the patient informed to call the emergency unit if symptoms become worse. The benefit of expectant management is to preserve tube function for future fertility[33].

Half of interstitial pregnancies require cornual resection and repair while the remainder require a hysterectomy due to massive bleeding caused by

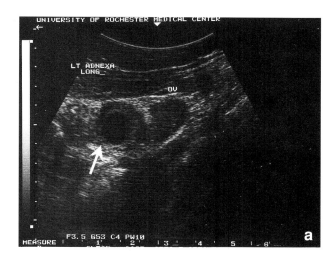

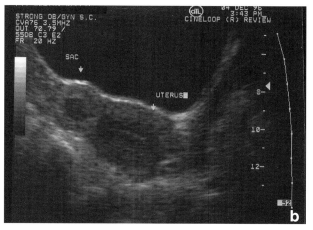

Figure 15 (a) Adnexal ring of an ectopic pregnancy (arrow) next to normal appearing ovary. (b) Adnexal ring of an ectopic pregnancy demonstrated by abdominal ultrasonography next to a normal appearing uterus

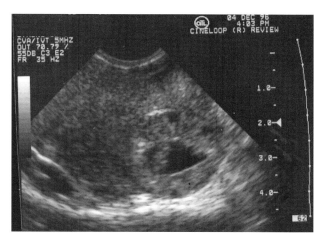

Figure 16 Interstitial ectopic pregnancy. Gestational sac is clearly part of upper uterine body

rupture of the uterine vessels. Abdominal pregnancies require a laparotomy. The placenta is usually left in the abdominal cavity and methotrexate administered. Removal of the placenta may lead to hemorrhage due to the trophoblastic invasion into bowel and omentum. Tubal ectopics can either spontaneously resolve or require a salpingostomy to remove the ectopic and the tube is then repaired.

MULTIPLE GESTATION

With the increase in pregnancies achieved by ART there has been a significant increase in the incidence of multiple gestations. This is true especially in cycles induced by clomiphene citrate and/or human menopausal gonadotropin and in pregnancies achieved by GIFT. Early ultrasonographic evaluation of multiple gestations will provide important information for assessment of the pregnancy. These include: accurate estimation of gestational age, number of gestational sacs, number of amniotic sacs in each gestational sac, anatomic location of the sacs within the uterus and viability of the embryos (see Chapter 15). It is not uncommon to find a hypoechoic area with no internal echoes adjacent to gestational sacs with viable embryos. These hypoechoic areas represent additional sacs that lag behind the other(s) in development, subchorionic hematomas or vanishing twins. The incidence of multiple gestations

detected by ultrasonography during the first trimester has been found to be significantly higher than that found in the second trimester[34]. The explanation for this finding is that many gestational sacs do not develop into a viable pregnancy and are absorbed early in pregnancy. Before the use of ultrasonography this phenomenon was not known and as these sacs disappear early in pregnancy they are termed the vanishing twin. Only follow-up ultrasonographic examinations will enable determination of the actual number of viable gestational sacs.

ANOMALY DETECTION

High-resolution TVS has moved some prenatal diagnosis into the first trimester and early stages of embryonic–fetal development. Patients with a history of pregnancies complicated by anomalies are at increased risk for recurrence. Early diagnosis of some severe anomalies is possible and can be offered to these patients. Most anomalies detectable in the first trimester are of the central nervous system, such as exencephaly and anencephaly (Figure 18), meningencephalocele and early hydrocephaly. Other detectable anomalies are cystic hygroma (Figure 19), osteogenesis imperfecta and some cardiac defects. Anomaly screening in the first trimester is feasible but not yet standard treatment in most centers.

CONCLUSIONS

Transvaginal ultrasonography has become an integral part of the evaluation of early pregnancy

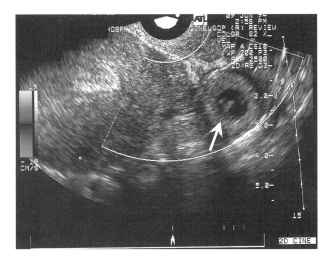

Figure 17   Color Doppler demonstrating characteristic low resistance flow around gestational sac (arrow). Blood flow also seen in early embryo and umbilical cord (see also Color plate 4)

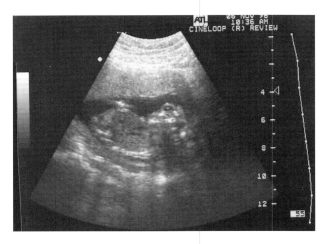

Figure 18   Anencephalic fetus of 12 weeks gestation

and its complications. With the high-frequency probes and the proximity to the pelvic organs the status of the pregnancy can be assessed before the appearance of clinical signs. With the observed increase in pregnancies achieved by ART there is also an increase in the incidence of ectopic gestations. With TVS the early gestational sac can be located approximately at the time of the first missed menstrual cycle. Less than one week later the yolk sac and with it the fetal pole and cardiac activity may be visualized. We can now follow developmental processes such as the physiological herniation of bowel and partition of embryonic cerebral ventricles and better understand the mechanism behind some congenital anomalies and the timing of their appearance. This learning process may eventually give us the ability to correctly diagnose structural anomalies during the first trimester and convey that information to the patient and her physician for further action.

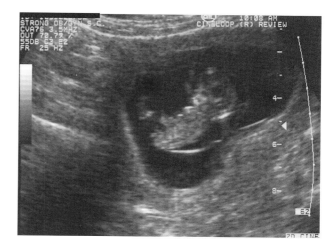

Figure 19   Cystic hygroma of 11-week-old fetus

References

1. Cacciatore B, Tiitinen A, Sterman U, *et al*. Normal early pregnancy: serum βhCG levels and vaginal ultrasonography findings. *Br J Obstet Gynaecol* 1990; 97:899–903

2. Bernaschek G, Rudelstorfer R, Csaicsich P. Vaginal sonography versus serum human chorionic gonadotropin in early detection of pregnancy. *Am J Obstet Gynecol* 1988;158:608–12

3. Fleischer AC, Kepple DM. Transvaginal sonography in normal and abnormal early pregnancy. In Winfield AC, Wentz AC, eds. *Diagnostic Imaging in Infertility*. Baltimore: Williams & Wilkins, 1992:269

4. Nyberg DA, Laing FC, Filly RA, *et al*. Ultrasonographic differentiation of the gestational sac of early intrauterine pregnancy from the pseudogestational sac of ectopic pregnancy. *Radiology* 1983; 146:755–9

5. Nyberg DA, Mack LA, Laing FC, *et al*. Distinguishing normal from abnormal gestational sac growth in early pregnancy. *J Ultrasound Med* 1987;6:23–7

6. Dudson MG. Early pregnancy. In Dudson MG, ed. *Transvaginal Ultrasound*, New York: Churchill Livingstone, 1991:165–201

7. Nyberg DA, Mack LA, Harvey D, *et al*. Value of the yolk sac in evaluating early pregnancy. *J Ultrasound Med* 1988;7:129–35

8. Kurtz AB, Needleman L, Pennel RG, *et al*. Can detection of the yolk sac in the first trimester be used to predict the outcome of pregnancy? *Am J Radiol* 1992;158:843–6

9. Lindsay DJ, Lovett IS, Lyons EA, *et al*. Yolk sac diameter and shape at endovaginal US: Predictors of pregnancy outcome in the first trimester. *Radiology* 1992;183:115–18

10. Holzgreve W, Westendorp J, Tercanli S. First trimester ultrasound. In Evans MI, ed. *Reproductive Risks and Prenatal Diagnosis*. East Norwalk: Appleton & Lange, 1992:121–9

11. Schats R, Jansen AM, Wladimiroff JW. Embryonic heart activity: appearance and development in early human pregnancy. *Br J Obstet Gynaecol* 1990;97: 989–94

12. Levi CS, Lyons EA, Zheng XH, *et al*. Endovaginal US: demonstration of cardiac activity in embryos of less than 5.0 mm in crown-rump length. *Radiology* 1990;176:71–4

13. Robinson HP, Fleming JEE. A critical evaluation of sonar 'crown-rump length' measurements. *Br J Obstet Gynaecol* 1975;82:702–10

14. Evans J. Fetal crown-rump length values in the first trimester based upon ovulation timing using the luteinizing hormone surge. *Br J Obstet Gynaecol* 1991;98:48–51

15. Kopta MM, May RR, Crane JP. A comparison of the reliability of the estimated date of confinement predicted by crown-rump length and biparietal diameter. *Am J Obstet Gynecol* 1983;145:562–5

16. Drumm JE, Clinch J, MacKinzie G. The ultrasonic measurement of fetal crown-rump length as a method of assessing gestational age. *Br J Obstet*

Gynaecol 1976;83:417–21

17. Goldstein SR. Embryonic ultrasonographic measurements: Crown-rump length revisited. *Am J Obstet Gynecol* 1991;165:497–501

18. Timor-Tritsch IE, Peisner DB, Raju S. Sonoembryology: an organ-oriented approach using a high-frequency vaginal probe. *J Clin Ultrasound* 1990; 18:286–90

19. Timor-Tritsch IE, Farine D, Rosen MG. A close look at early embryonic development with the high-frequency transvaginal transducer. *Am J Obstet Gynecol* 1988;159:676–81

20. O'Rahilly R, Müller F. The cardiovascular and lymphatic system. In O'Rahilly R, Müller F, eds. *Human Embryology and Teratology.* New York: Wiley-Liss, 1992:107–38

21. O'Rahilly R, Müller F. The nervous system. In O'Rahilly R, Müller F, eds. *Human Embryology and Teratology.* New York: Wiley-Liss, 1992:253–92

22. Nyberg DA, Laing FC, Filly RA. Threatened abortion: sonographic distinction of normal and abnormal gestational sacs. *Radiology* 1986;158: 397–400

23. Simpson JL. Fetal wastage. In Gabbe SG, Niebyl JR, Simpson JL, eds. *Obstetrics: Normal and Problem Pregnancies.* New York: Churchill Livingstone, 1986: 651–73

24. Bernard KG, Cooperberg PL. Sonographic differentiation between blighted ovum and early viable pregnancy. *Am J Radiol* 1985;144:597–602

25. Avrech OM, Jaffe R, Zabow PH, *et al.* Triploidy, partial hydatiform mole. *The Fetus* 1991;1:3

26. Cartwright PS. Incidence, epidemiology, risk factors, and etiology. In Stovall TG, Ling FW, eds. *Extrauterine Pregnancy – Clinical Diagnosis and Management.* New York: McGraw-Hill, 1993:27–63

27. Fleischer A, Cartwright P, Pennel R, *et al.* Sonography of ectopic pregnancy with trans-abdominal and transvaginal scanning. In Fleischer A, Romero R, Manning F, Jeanty P, eds. *The Principles and Practice of Ultrasonography in Obstetrics and Gynecology,* 4th edn. East Norwalk: Appleton & Lange, 1991:57–72

28. Kurtz A, Middleton W, eds. Ectopic pregnancy. In *Ultrasound, The Requisites.* St Louis: Mosby Year Book, 1996:415–28

29. Kadar N, DeVore G, Romero R. Discriminatory hCG zone: its use in the sonographic evaluation for ectopic pregnancy. *Obstet Gynecol* 1981;58:156–61

30. Brown D, Doubilet P. Transvaginal sonography for diagnosing ectopic pregnancy. *J Ultrasound Med* 1994;13:259–66

31. Laing F. Ectopic pregnancy. In Ferruci J, ed. *Diagnostic Imaging.* Philadelphia: 1988:1–11

32. Bonilla-Musoles F, Ballester M, Tarin J, *et al.* Does transvaginal color Doppler sonography differentiate between developing and involuting ectopic pregnancies? *J Ultrasound Med* 1995;14:175–81

33. Ylostalo P, Cacciatore B, Sjoberg J, *et al.* Expectant management of ectopic pregnancy. *Obstet Gynecol* 1992;80:345–8

34. Landy HJ, Keith L, Keith D. The vanishing twin. *Acta Genet Med Gamellot* 1982;31:179–81

Sonoembryology

John M. G. van Vugt

High-frequency ultrasonography, especially through transvaginal application, allows visualization of the normal and abnormal early pregnancy. Because of the increased image resolution embryonic and extra-embryonic structures are easily detectable. Various authors have described the embryonic structures seen by transvaginal ultrasonography, which has led to possibilities for a new diagnostic field in early pregnancy[1-5]. High-frequency transvaginal ultrasonography allows early detection of fetal anomalies[6-10]. However, detailed knowledge about early development of the embryo and fetus is a prerequisite for evaluation of the pregnancy at risk for genetic diseases of the fetus, or when abnormal development of the embryo or fetus is suspected[11]. This chapter presents an overview on normal first trimester development and corresponding ultrasonographic images of the various organs of the embryo and fetus.

THE HEART

On the 22nd day after conception, as blood begins to circulate, the cardiovascular system is the first system that starts to function in the embryo. Development of the heart starts with the formation of the cardiogenic cords at day 18 or 19 of gestation. At day 20 or 21 canalization and fusion of the cardiogenic cords takes place. One day later a single heart tube has formed[12]. The heart starts to beat, resulting in a one-directional blood flow through the tube at day 27 or 28. The crown–rump length (CRL), when heart activity begins at day 21, is about 2.0 mm. High-frequency transvaginal ultrasonography enables the detection of fetal heart beats at 5 weeks and 3 days menstrual age (day 24)[4]. There is a progressive rise in fetal heart rate from a mean of 70 bpm at 22 days to a mean of 170 bpm at the 10th week of pregnancy, thereafter decreasing to a mean of 120 bpm[13]. As the heart tube grows, it bends upon itself to the right. The atrio-ventricular canal begins its partitioning into four chambers in the 4th week and is completed in the 7th week of pregnancy.

During this period the aorta and the pulmonary trunk are formed out of the truncus arteriosus. The basic adult aortic arch pattern is formed during the 6th–8th week[12].

Several reports have been published on normal cardiac anatomy and cardiac dimensions in the first trimester[4,14-20]. By transvaginal echocardiography a linear increase of cardiac dimensions with gestational age between 11 and 17 weeks was shown[15]. The heart covers about 50% of the transverse thoracic area. At 10 weeks of gestation the moving valves and the interventricular septum can already be identified[20]. In the majority of fetuses the four-chamber view can be visualized by transvaginal ultrasound in the 12th week of gestation (Figure 1). The transverse diameter of the heart is then about 5 mm[16]. Normative data on detailed cardiac anatomy between 10 and 14 weeks of gestation were provided by Dolkart and Reimers[16] using a 7.5 MHz transvaginal probe. Blaas and colleagues[20] have given detailed

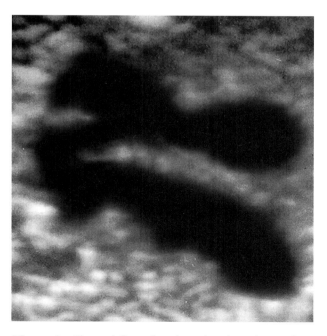

Figure 1 Normal four-chamber view in a fetus of 12 weeks gestation

normative data from 7 to 12 weeks of gestation. The mean heart diameter increased linearly from 1.9 mm at 7 weeks to 6.9 mm at 12 weeks of gestation. The earliest cardiac structures visible were the mitral and tricuspid valves. The complete four-chamber view could be visualized by week 12 of gestation in 90% of the cases. At week 13 and 14 of gestation visualization was possible in 100% of the cases. The aorta and the pulmonary trunk was demonstrated in approximately 40% of the cases.

Gembruch and colleagues[18], combining color Doppler with two-dimensional ultrasound, reported a success rate of 100% in obtaining full cardiac anatomy at week 13 and 14 of gestation. Identifying the origin and crossing of the great vessels in particular was simplified by using the combined technique. Similar results were reported by Achiron and colleagues[19].

THE CENTRAL NERVOUS SYSTEM

The normal spine

Development of the central nervous system (CNS) begins at day 18 from conception with formation of the neural plate. Soon thereafter the lateral edges of the plate become elevated, thus forming the neural folds. The depressed region between the neural folds is known as the neural groove. The neural folds elevate further, approach each other at the midline and finally fuse; the neural tube is formed[4].

In normally developing embryos the spine can be recognized from week 8 of gestation onwards by its parallel lines representing the not yet ossified vertebrae[21] (Figure 2). Primary ossification of the vertebrae starts at week 10 to 11 of gestation. The process starts in the cervical spine and gradually migrates caudally. Complete mineralization of the vertebrae is achieved between week 12 to 14 of gestation[21] (Figure 3). Because of the curled position of the embryo in the first trimester, evaluation of the spine requires consecutive scanning planes to visualize the entire neural tube[4,22].

The normal brain

At week 5, three primary brain vesicles are formed at the cephalic part of the neural tube: forebrain (prosencephalon), midbrain (mesencephalon) and hindbrain (rhombencephalon). At this stage no clear CNS is detectable by ultrasound. One week later

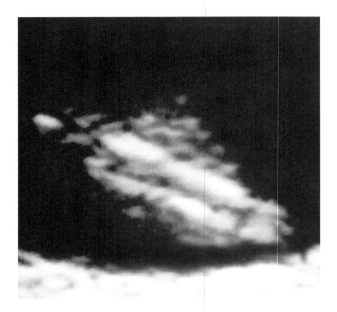

Figure 2 The spine visible as two parallel lines in a fetus of 8 weeks gestation

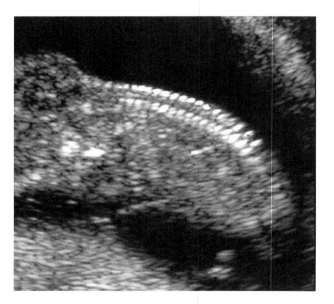

Figure 3 Complete mineralization of the vertebrae in a fetus of 15 weeks gestation

the secondary brain vesicles are formed. The prosencephalon differentiates into the telencephalon and diencephalon and the rhombencephalon divides into the metencephalon and myeloencephalon. The embryonic cephalic pole is clearly visible and distinguishable from the embryonic torso[22].

The cavity of the rhombencephalon is one of the first structures in the developing CNS that can be recognized by transvaginal ultrasonography[21,23] (Figure 4). The rhombencephalic cavity is no longer visible after 10 to 12 weeks of gestation (Table 1). Measurement of the mean cavity diameter showed a slow increase to a maximum at 9 weeks of approximately 32 mm[21]. Blaas and colleagues showed that what initially was the largest cavity in the cranial pole represented later the fourth ventricle[24].

The hyperechogenic cerebellar hemispheres are clearly distinguishable after 10 to 11 weeks of gestation. Before that time it is not always possible to recognize the cerebellum[24]. The width of the cerebellum increases from 4.8 mm at 9 weeks to 8.1 mm at 12 weeks of gestation[24] (Figure 5). The bilateral choroid plexus of the fourth ventricle is always visible after 10 to 11 weeks of gestation (Figures 6 and 7).

During week 7 of gestation the cavities of the hemispheres can be demonstrated anteriorly to the rhombencephalic cavity. After week 9 in all embryos it is possible to measure the hemispheres. At the end of the first trimester the thickness is about 1 mm[11]. The choroid plexus of the lateral ventricles are visible after week 10.

The diencephalon, especially its cavity, later the third ventricle, can be recognized from week 7 onwards. Gradually the width of this cavity decreases and therefore its measurement after 9 to 10 weeks of gestation is difficult.

The cavity of the mesencephalon or midbrain, later the aquaeducts Sylvii, has a mean diameter of

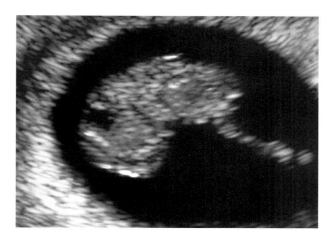

Figure 4 The cavity of the rhombencephalon in a fetus of 8 weeks gestation

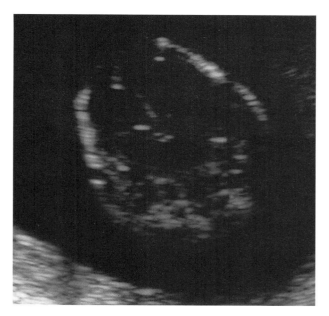

Figure 5 The hyperechogenic cerebellar hemispheres in a fetus of 14 weeks gestation

Table 1 Sequential appearance of central nervous system (CNS) development by transvaginal ultrasound

CNS development	*Weeks of gestation*							
	5	6	7	8	9	10	11	12
(Cavity of) hemispheres	S	S	A	A	A	A	A	A
(Cavity of) diencephalon		S	A	A	A	A	A	A
(Cavity of) mesencephalon	S	A	A	A	A	A	A	A
(Cavity of) rhombencephalon	S	A	A	A	A	A	A	A
Choroid plexus				S	A	A	A	A
Cerebellum			S	S	S	A	A	A
Spine			S	S	S	S	A	A
Vertebrae						S	S	A

S, not in all cases; A, in all cases

2.3 mm at about 10 weeks of gestation. It is initially situated in the anterior part of the embryonic head. By deflection of the embryonic head this cavity is found later in the middle of the head.

From week 12, the head and the brain of the fetus assume the appearance of those of the early second trimester fetus.

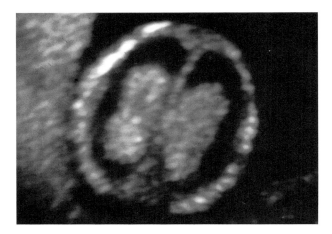

Figure 6   The bilateral choroid plexus in a fetus of 12 weeks gestation

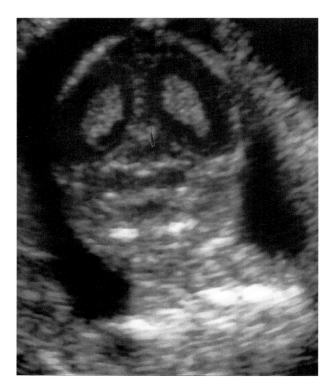

Figure 7   Coronal view of the bilateral choroid plexus in a fetus of 12 weeks gestation

THE SKELETAL SYSTEM

Most bones of the skeletal system are preformed in hyaline cartilage. Gradually they develop from a soft tissue model by the process of osteogenesis. Osteogenesis starts centrally in the 'bone' and spreads to the edges until the whole skeletal element is ossified[25]. High frequency transvaginal ultrasound allows an early recognition of the ossification centers, in general 1 to 2 weeks earlier than abdominal scanning (Table 2).

The limbs

The upper limbs start to develop at the end of week 6 of gestation, followed by the lower limbs. At week 8 to 9 of gestation complete embryonic upper and lower limbs are visible by ultrasound (Figure 8). One week later it is possible to recognize the early ossification centers of the humerus, ulna, radius, fibula and tibia. The ossification centers are small and slightly more echogenic than the surrounding tissue. From week 10 to 11 of gestation satisfactory measurement of the long bones can be made. The iliac bones are visible from week 11 onwards[27], as are the terminal phalanges of the fingers (Figure 9) and toes (Figure 10)[28,29].

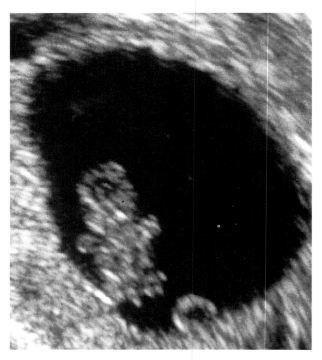

Figure 8   An embryo of 8 weeks gestation with clearly visible limb buds

Table 2 The appearance of skeletal structures as observed by transabdominal (TA) and transvaginal (TV) ultrasound

| | Weeks of gestation | | | | | |
	9	10	11	12	13	14
Mandibula	TV	TA				
Clavicula	TV		TA			
Maxilla		TV	TA			
Humerus		TV/TA				
Ulna/radius		TV/TA				
Femur		TV/TA				
Tibia/fibula		TV/TA				
Os occipitale		TV	TA			
Terminal phalanges			TV	TA		
Os ilium			TV/TA			
Scapula			TV	TA		
Ribs	TV				TA	
Vertebra			TV		TA	
Phalanges (hand)				TV	TA	
Metacarpals				TV	TA	
Metatarsals					TV	TA
Skull				TV		TA

Adapted with persmission[26]

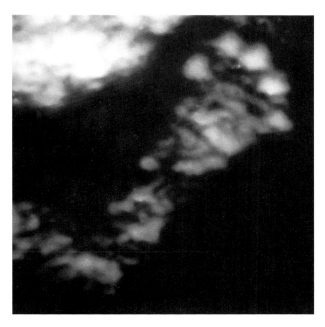

Figure 9 The hand of a fetus at 12 weeks gestation

The facial bones/skull

The first structure of the face to be observed is the mandibula. The ossification starts at week 9 of gestation. One week later it is followed by the

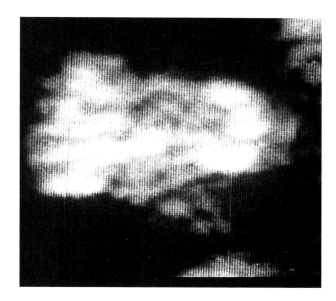

Figure 10 The foot of a fetus at 11 weeks gestation

maxilla (Figure 11). In week 8 of gestation the faint outline of the skull can be recognized. The occipital bone is the first recognizable ossified part of the skull. The ossification goes gradually on and in the following 2 to 3 weeks the entire skull becomes more echogenic. At week 14 complete ossification of the skull is achieved.

The spine

Ossification of the spine starts in the cervical region. The cervical vertebrae are recognizable at week 11 of gestation. One week later the thoracic and lumbosacral parts are ossified. The complete ossified spine can be visualized at week 13[6] (Figure 3).

The clavicula/ribs

The clavicula is one of the first ossified structures to be observed by transvaginal ultrasound. At week 9 of gestation complete ossification of the clavicula has taken place (Figure 12). Two weeks later the ossification of the ribs has taken place and they are recognizable with transvaginal ultrasound[27].

THE URINARY TRACT

The first two stages of kidney development involve the formation of the pronephros and mesonephros during week 5 to 7 of pregnancy. The mesonephros

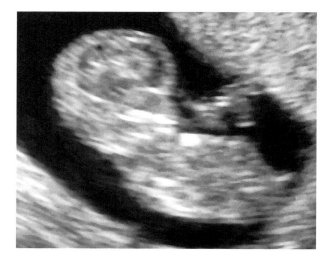

Figure 11 A fetus of 11 weeks gestation with the mandibula and maxilla clearly visible

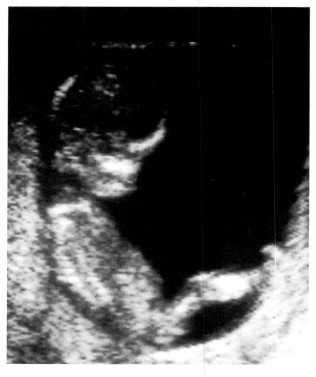

Figure 12 A fetus of 12 weeks gestation with clearly visible clavicula

becomes excretory at the 11th week. At the 7th week of pregnancy the Wolffian duct develops caudally and encounters the nephrogenic cord; the definitive kidney is formed (metanephros). Further differentiation of the kidney is achieved at the 12th to 14th week of pregnancy; the renal pelvis and major calices are formed. The fetal urinary bladder is partially formed from the mesonephric ducts and from the cloaca. From the 11th week of pregnancy onwards the bladder can be visualized using transvaginal ultrasound. It can be sonographically identified as a spherical hypo-echogenic mass within the fetal pelvis[30,31] (Figure 13). The fetal kidneys can be first recognized at 9 to 10 weeks of gestation with high frequency transvaginal ultrasonography because of their hyperechogenic aspect (Figure 14). The kidney has an oval appearance with a hypoechogenic area centrally, representing the renal pelvis. From week 12 onwards it is possible to recognize the kidney and differentiate it from the hypoechogenic adrenals[32]. Also during that time the kidneys have reached their adult position and are located at each side of the fetal spine. Bronshtein and colleagues[33] published nomograms of the normal fetal kidneys from week 12 to 14 of pregnancy. The anteroposterior and transverse diameter increased from about 4 mm (12 weeks) to 6 mm (14 weeks). The longitudinal diameter increased from 6 to 9 mm.

THE GASTROINTESTINAL SYSTEM

The primitive gastrointestinal tract develops during the 8th week of pregnancy. The three parts of the primitive gut, the foregut, midgut and hindgut, develop eventually to be the organs of the gastrointestinal system. A part of the foregut forms the liver, gallbladder and biliary ducts. Simultaneous expansion of the liver and the kidneys fills much of the abdominal cavity. The abdominal cavity becomes temporarily too small and the intestinal loops protrude in the extraembryonic coelom in the umbilical cord[12]. The physiologic midgut herniation is formed, which exists from week 7 to 11 of pregnancy[34] (Figure 15 and Color plate 5). The herniation starts as a thickening of the cord, ultrasonographically recognizable as a slight echogenic area at the abdominal insertion[20]. In the 11th week the intestines are retracted into the abdominal cavity. This is possible because of the decrease in relative size of the liver and enlargement of the abdominal cavity. After 11 weeks of gestation fetuses do not demonstrate any sign of herniation[34].

The stomach is formed during the 6th week of pregnancy and can easily be recognized from week

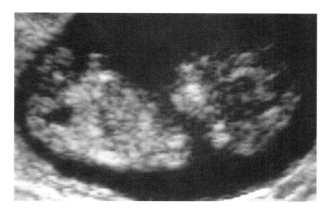

Figure 13 A fetus of 11 weeks gestation with visible bladder

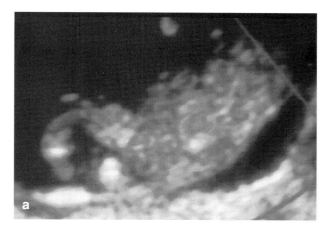

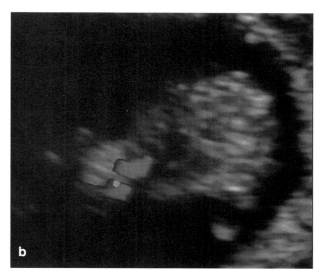

Figure 15 Physiological midgut herniation in a 10 week fetus. (**a**) Sagittal plane. (**b**) Transverse plane. See also Color plates 5a and b

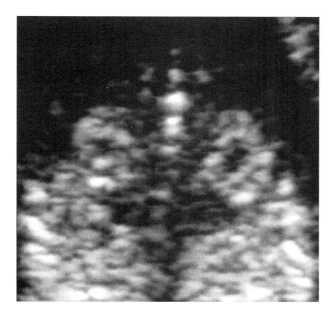

Figure 14 Fetal kidneys at 13 weeks gestation

10 onwards as an anechogenic structure in the left side of the abdomen[4,35,36]. Blaas and colleagues described a location of a small hypoechogenic area thought to be the stomach on the left side of the upper abdomen below the heart during the 8th week of gestation[20]. With increasing gestational age they could confirm this to be the developing stomach.

The jejunum, ileum, cecum, appendix, much of the colon and the distal part of the duodenum are formed from the midgut. The hindgut forms the later distal part of the colon, the rectum and the anal canal. Ultrasound in the first trimester can not identify the intestinal parts distinctly.

THE GENITALIA

The external male and female genitalia do not differ at week 6 of gestation. Between week 6 and 11 differentiation occurs and the penial part is formed[12]. In only 80% of cases can a correct identification of the fetal sex be made at 12 weeks. Correct prediction rates from 13 weeks of gestation onward depend on the experience of the observer[37].

The female gender is ultrasonographically recognized by the presence of 2 to 4 parallel lines in the genital area. The female clitoris is always directed caudally. The male gender can be recognized by a cranially directed phallus. It is assumed that the corpora cavernosum is in a permanently congested state in early pregnancy and therefore the penis is in a constant erect state.

CONCLUSIONS

The introduction of transvaginal ultrasonography in obstetrics has raised the quality of images of the embryo in early pregnancy and provides us with a powerful tool to study embryonic development. With the use of 7.5 MHz transvaginal transducers more detailed information on embryonic structures is gained compared to the use of abdominal transducers. Improving ultrasound techniques in the (near) future, especially the use of 3D imaging, will enable a still better view of the developing embryo. An understanding of normal embryonic development is important for the recognition of early fetal anomalies.

References

1. Timor-Tritsch IE, Farine D, Rosen MG. A close look at early embryonic development with the high frequency transvaginal transducer. *Am J Obstet Gynecol* 1988;159:676–81

2. Cullen MT, Green JJ, Reece E, *et al*. A comparison of transvaginal and abdominal ultrasound in visualizing the first trimester conceptus. *J Ultrasound Med* 1989;8:565–9

3. Bree RL, Marn CS. Transvaginal ultrasonography in the first trimester: embryology, anatomy and HCG correlation. *Semin Ultrasound, CT MR* 1990;11:12–21

4. Timor-Tritsch IE, Peisner DB, Raju R. Sonoembryology: an organ-oriented approach using a high-frequency vaginal probe. *J Clin Ultrasound* 1990;18:286–98

5. Bronshtein M, Yoffe N, Zimmer EZ. Transvaginal sonography at 5 to 14 weeks' gestation: fetal stomach, abnormal cord insertion and yolk sac. *Am J Perinatol* 1992;9:344–7

6. Rottem S, Bronshtein M, Thaler I, *et al*. First trimester transvaginal sonographic diagnosis of fetal anomalies. *Lancet* 1989;1:444–5

7. Cullen MT, Green J, Whetham J, *et al*. Transvaginal ultrasonographic detection of congenital anomalies in the first trimester. *Am J Obstet Gynecol* 1990;163:466–76

8. Rottem S, Bronshtein M. Transvaginal sonographic diagnosis of congenital anomalies between 9 weeks and 16 weeks menstrual age. *J Clin Ultrasound* 1990;18:307–14

9. Rottem S. First trimester transvaginal ultrasonographic screening: incidence of structural anomalies. *Am J Obstet Gynecol* 1990;164:933

10. Achiron R, Tadmor O. Screening for fetal anomalies during the first trimester of pregnancy: transvaginal versus transabdominal sonography. *Ultrasound Obstet Gynecol* 1991;1:186–91

11. Blaas HG, Eik-Nes SH, Kiserud T, *et al*. Early development of the forebrain and midbrain: a longitudinal ultrasound study from 7–12 weeks of gestation. *Ultrasound Obstet Gynecol* 1994;4:183–92

12. Moore KL. *The Developing Human*, 2nd edn. New York: WB Saunders, 1982:259–300

13. Schats R, Jansen CAM, Wladimiroff JW. Embryonic heart activity: appearance and development in early pregnancy. *Br J Obstet Gynaecol* 1990;97:330–3

14. D'Amelio R, Giorlandino G, Masala L, *et al*. Fetal echocardiography using transvaginal and transabdominal probes during the first period of pregnancy: a comparative study. *Prenat Diagn* 1991;11:69–75

15. Bronshtein M, Siegler E, Escholi Z, *et al*. Transvaginal ultrasound measurements of the fetal heart rate at 11 to 17 weeks of gestation. *Am J Perinatol* 1992;9:38–42

16. Dolkart LA, Reimers FT. Transvaginal fetal echocardiography in early pregnancy: normative data. *Am J Obstet Gynecol* 1991;165:688–91

17. Johnson P, Sharland G, Maxwell D, *et al*. The role of transvaginal sonography in the early detection of congenital heart disease. *Ultrasound Obstet Gynecol* 1992;2:248–51

18. Gembruch U, Knopfle G, Bald R, *et al*. Early diagnosis of fetal congenital heart disease by transvaginal echocardiography. *Ultrasound Obstet Gynecol* 1993;3:310–17

19. Achiron R, Weissman A, Rotstein Z, *et al*. Transvaginal echocardiographic examination of the fetal heart between 13 and 15 weeks' gestation in a low risk population. *J Ultrasound Med* 1994;13:783–9

20. Blaas HG, Eik-Nes SH, Kiserud T, *et al*. Early development of the abdominal wall, stomach and heart from 7 to 12 weeks of gestation: a longitudinal study. *Ultrasound Obstet Gynecol* 1995;6:240–9

21. van Zalen-Sprock RM, van Vugt JMG, van Geijn HP. First and early trimester diagnosis of anomalies of the central nervous system. *J Ultrasound Med* 1995;14:603–10

22. Achiron R, Achiron A. Transvaginal ultrasonic assessment of the early fetal brain. *Ultrasound Obstet Gynecol* 1991;1:336–44

23. Cyr DR, Mack LA, Nyberg DA, *et al*. Fetal rhomben-cephalon: normal US findings. *Radiology* 1988;166:691–2

24. Blaas HG, Eik-Nes SH, Kiserud T, *et al*. Early development of the hindbrain: a longitudinal ultrasound study from 7 to 12 weeks of gestation. *Ultrasound Obstet Gynecol* 1995;5:151–60

25. Cragsma B. Gray's Anatomy: Human skeletal morphology. In Williams P, Warwich K, eds. *Gray's Anatomy*, 35th edn. Edinburgh: Churchill Livingstone, 1973:206–10

26. van Geijn HP. Normale anatomie van de foetus. In Stoutenbeek PL, van Vugt JMG, Wladimiroff JW, eds. *Echoscopie in de Gynaecologie en Obstetrie*. Utrecht: Wetenschappelijke uitgeverij Bunge, 1997:60–76

27. Van Zalen-Sprock RM, Brons JTJ, van Vugt JMG, *et al*. Ultrasonographic and radiologic aspects of the developing embryonic skeleton. *Ultrasound Obstet Gynecol* 1997;9:392–7

28. Mahoney BS, Filly RA. High resolution sonographic assessment of the fetal extremities. *J Ultrasound Med* 1984;3:489–98

29. Zorzoli A, Kustermann E, Caravelli E, *et al*. Measurements of fetal limb bones in early pregnancy. *Ultrasound Obstet Gynecol* 1994;4:29–33

30. Bronshtein M, Yoffe N, Brandes JM, *et al*. First and early second trimester diagnosis of fetal urinary tract anomalies using transvaginal sonography. *Prenat Diagn* 1990;10:653–66

31. Rosati P, Guariglia L. Transvaginal sonographic assessment of the fetal urinary tract in early pregnancy. *Ultrasound Obstet Gynecol* 1996;7:95–100

32. Grannum P, Bracken M, Silverman R, *et al*. Assessment of fetal kidney size in normal gestation by comparison of ratio of kidney circumference to abdominal circumference. *Am J Obstet Gynecol* 1980; 136:249–54

33. Bronshtein M, Kushnir O, Ben-Rafael Z, *et al*. Transvaginal measurements of fetal kidneys in the first trimester of pregnancy. *J Clin Ultrasound* 1990; 18:299–301

34. Van Zalen-Sprock RM, van Vugt JMG, van Geijn HP. First trimester sonography of physiologic mid-gut herniation and early diagnosis of omphalocele. *Prenat Diagn* 1997;17:511–18

35. Neiman HL. Sonoembryography. In Nyberg DA, Hill LM, Bîhm-VÇlez M, Mendelson EB, eds. *Transvaginal Ultrasound*. St Louis: Mosby Year Book, 1992:133–45

36. Green JJ, Hobbins JC. Abdominal ultrasound examination of the first-trimester fetus. *Am J Obstet Gynecol* 1988;159:165–75

37. Bronshtein M, Rottem S, Yoffe N, *et al*. Early determination of fetal sex using transvaginal sonography: technique and pitfalls. *J Clin Ultrasound* 1990;18: 302–6

Fetal biometry and gestational age estimation 4

Bobbi Stebbins and Richard Jaffe

Accurate gestational age (GA) assignment is of particular importance with the increasing number of tests which rely on such dating for their own accuracy such as amniocentesis, chorionic villous sampling (CVS), and maternal serum alpha-fetoprotein (AFP) testing. The most reliable method to determine gestational age is by use of a combination of ultrasound parameters. Ultrasonography has been shown to be superior to an optimal menstrual history in predicting the date of delivery[1].

Since fetal growth may vary considerably in the third trimester due to intrinsic factors (genetic growth potential) and varying growth support received from the placenta and mother, fetuses of similar gestational ages may have markedly different sizes. Early pregnancy dating can therefore enhance overall pregnancy care and delivery planning and is equally important when elective termination, cervical cerclage or elective cesarean section is planned.

FIRST TRIMESTER

The most accurate GA determination is performed prior to 20 weeks. This is because normal early fetal growth is spontaneous and not affected by secondary factors as is growth in the second and third trimesters. Dating established at this time is used as reference for all later gestational age and percentile determinations.

Gestational sac

The first ultrasonographic sign of pregnancy is the gestational sac (GS) (Figure 1). The decidual reaction around the GS may create a 'double sac sign' seen as a fluid collection surrounded by a bilayered (decidua capsularis and decidual parietalis) echogenic rim. The GS can be seen as early as four weeks gestation when its greatest diameter is only 2 mm in length[2]. Mean gestational sac diameter growth has a linear relationship with GA, and increases 1.0 to 1.2 mm/day[3]. It should be

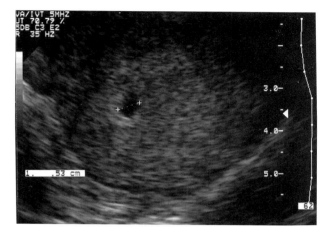

Figure 1 Early intrauterine gestational sac seen on transvaginal scan

measured in three dimensions with an average diameter obtained. The gestational sac may not be visualized when human chorionic gonadotropin levels are low and the presence of a GS does not in itself confirm a viable intrauterine pregnancy.

Yolk sac

The secondary yolk sac (YS) may be ultrasonographically visible at 4.5 to 5 weeks menstrual age and may persist up to 15 weeks gestation. It has a characteristic ultrasonographic appearance of a round hypoechogenic structure within the gestational sac, and may measure 3–7 mm[4] (Figure 2). The yolk sac serves as a useful landmark in the detection of embryonic cardiac pulsations that may be detected at 5 weeks gestation.

Visualization of a yolk sac is reliable evidence for a true gestational sac prior to detection of an embryo[5]. Normal yolk sac size and shape are associated with good pregnancy outcome whereas abnormal yolk sac size and shape are often a first sign of abnormal embryonic development[6]. Absence of a yolk sac in the presence of a visible embryo is abnormal and associated with subsequent embryonic death.

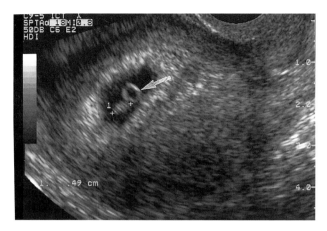

Figure 2 Six week gestation demonstrating embryo (between calipers) and normal yolk sac (arrow)

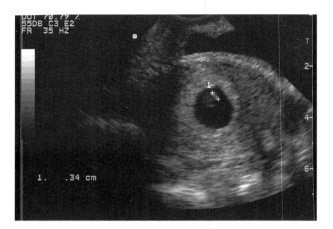

Figure 3 Five week gestation demonstrating early embryonic size measurement

Crown–rump length

The American Institute of Ultrasound in Medicine (AIUM) Guidelines for performance of antepartum obstetrical ultrasound examination recommend the use of the crown–rump length (CRL) measurement throughout the first trimester[7]. The CRL is easy to measure, there is a rapid increase in its size from week to week, a linear relationship exists between early CRL measurements and gestational age, and little biological variation occurs in early pregnancy.

True landmarks for an actual 'crown–rump' measurement appear at 8 weeks gestation. Prior to this, it is suggested that the longest linear measurement is taken and it has appropriately been termed 'early embryonic size'[8] (Figure 3). Later in the first trimester, CRL measurement should be performed once the fetus has assumed its natural curvature (Figure 4), as fetal flexion may decrease true CRL by 5%[9]. The CRL grows approximately 10 mm per week from week 8 to 12 and ranges from 10 mm at 7 weeks to 40 mm at 11 weeks. A simple calculation of GA in weeks can be made by adding 6.5 to the CRL (cm).

As a result of the introduction of transvaginal ultrasonography into early pregnancy management a new approach to dating before 8 weeks gestation was necessary. Transvaginal scanning has eliminated the need to rely on the GS as an indicator of normal pregnancy, as objective evidence such as the yolk sac and embryo can be visualized at an earlier stage. Embryonic heartbeat can be documented when the GS is as small as 2 cm and body movements seen when the GS reaches 3 cm. These findings can be used to evaluate the well being of

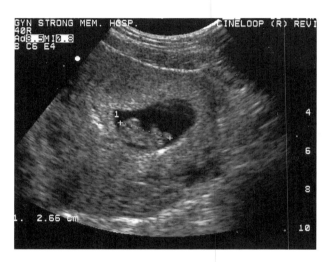

Figure 4 Nine week gestation demonstrating crown–rump length measurement

an early pregnancy and serve as markers of normal embryo growth[10,11]. The time of appearance of sonographically visible structures may determine gestational age better than any measurement performed at that age[12] (Table 1).

SECOND AND THIRD TRIMESTER

In the second and third trimesters, parameters for measurement are selected in accordance with the estimated gestational age at which they are used. At this time it is helpful to create a fetal growth profile that would include measurements of head size, trunk size, soft tissue mass, length, weight and proportionality of parameters. The AIUM

Table 1 Transvaginal ultrasonographic findings of early embryonic development

Menstrual age (week)	Crown–rump length (mm)	Ultrasonographic landmark
3–4	–	Decidual reaction
4 (+2 days)	–	Gestational sac, double sac sign
5	1–2	Yolk sac and embryonic pole, amniotic cavity
5–6	5–6	Cardiac activity
6–7	10	Single ventricle, early embryonic size
7–8	18–20	Limb buds, physiologic bowel herniation
8–9	20–25	Falx, choroid plexus, cranial and caudal poles seen, embryonic movements
9–10	30–35	Fingers, jaw and limb movements
12	40	Midgut herniation resolved, yolk sac absorbed, stomach visible

recommends assessment of gestational age using the biparietal diameter (BPD) and femur length (FL) in the 2nd and 3rd trimester, and in the 3rd trimester fetal growth and weight assessment are performed using the BPD, FL and abdominal circumference (AC).

Fetal growth profile

Biparietal diameter

The BPD is measured in the transaxial plane at the widest portion of the skull at the level of the thalami. Calipers are placed from leading edge to leading edge (outer to inner skull table) (Figure 5). Other structures that should be visible at the level of the BPD include the cavum septum pellucidum and the falx cerebri. Coronal biparietal diameters are taken at the same level as the traditional BPD.

The BPD is maximally accurate from 12 to 20 weeks gestational age. After this, it becomes less reliable for gestational dating due to changes in shape, growth disturbances, and individual variation. Confidence intervals range from ± 1 week between 12 and 22 weeks, to ± 3 to 4 weeks between 32 weeks and term. The BPD demonstrates linear growth of 3 mm per week from week

14 through 29, with continued mean growth until term of approximately 2 mm per week[13,14].

The examiner must be aware of some of the disadvantages of this measurement. Accuracy decreases as pregnancy progresses and changes in head shape due to conditions such as premature rupture of membranes, breech position, or multiple pregnancy, or deviations from normal growth may cause under- or overestimation of true GA[15]. If measurement error is suspected, the examiner should review accuracy of caliper placement and scan plane landmarks, and any suspected genetic variation or specific fetal condition should be considered as they relate to the accuracy of the BPD measurement.

Occipito-frontal diameter (OFD)

The occipito-frontal diameter (OFD) (Figure 5) is measured in the same plane as the BPD with the calipers placed on the outer skull table. This parameter is used in conjunction with BPD to calculate the head circumference (HC) and the cephalic index (CI) and is important in gestational age assessment when accurate BPD measurements are not obtainable.

Cephalic index

Changes in skull shape, such as flattening or rounding can be identified by the cephalic index. This ratio compares the BPD to the OFD to identify brachycephalic (CI ≥ 0.83) or dolichocephalic (CI ≤ 0.74) conditions. A cephalic index outside of the normal range may be associated with a significant alteration in the BPD measurement. Therefore, these thresholds are used to maximize identification of misleading BPDs due to altered head shape[16,17].

Head circumference

The HC grows approximately 1.4 cm per week between 14 and 17 weeks, slowing to 0.5 cm per week by 38 weeks. The BPD and OFD can be used to calculate the circumference. Manual calculation of this circumference [HC = 1.57 (BPD + OFD)] is unnecessary when utilizing modern equipment which can create an ellipse or trace the outline of the fetal head. HC is directly measured around the perimeter of the skull at the same level as the BPD

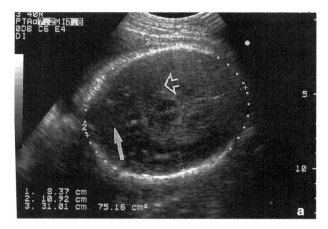

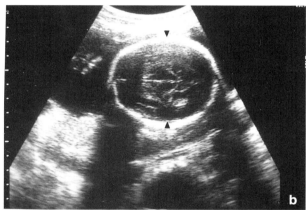

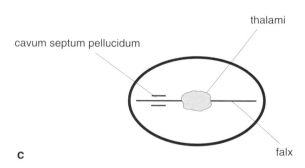

thalami

cavum septum pellucidum

falx

c

leading edge to leading edge

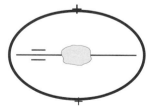

d

Figure 5 (**a**) Plane of biparietal diameter (BPD) (open arrow) and occipito-frontal diameter (arrow) measurement. (**b**) Proper placements of calipers for BPD measurement. (**c**, **d**) Schematic drawings of BPD landmarks and caliper placement

(Figure 6). Correction factors based upon the BPD/OFD ratio have been applied to the formula for a circle in an attempt to improve the accuracy of HC correlation with gestational age[18].

Abdominal circumference

The AC demonstrates linear growth with a mean of 1.1–1.2 cm per week throughout the entire pregnancy and correlates strongly with overall fetal size. Optimal use of the AC is during the third trimester and it should not be singularly used to predict GA, as it can be difficult to accurately reproduce.

The AC can be calculated using measurements of the transverse abdominal diameter (TAD) and the antero-posterior abdominal diameter (APAD) [AC = 1.57 (APAD + TAD)], similar to the calculation of HC. The stomach and the junction of the umbilical vein and portal sinus should be

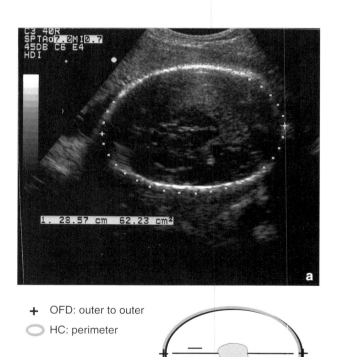

+ OFD: outer to outer

◯ HC: perimeter

HC = 1.57 (BPD + OFD)

Figure 6 (**a**) Measurement of head circumference. (**b**) Schematic drawing of caliper placement for head circumference measurement. BPD, biparietal diameter; HC, head circumference; OFD, occipito-frontal diameter

visible in the correct measurement plane[7]. When using an ellipse or trace function, the AC is measured around the extreme perimeter of the fetal abdomen (Figure 7). This parameter is used for estimation of fetal weight and is an integral part of many ratios used to assess fetal growth.

Soft tissue parameters

Abnormal fetal growth often results in modified amounts of adipose tissue and muscle mass, and soft tissue parameters have been investigated in attempts to correlate them with fetal nutritional state. Thigh circumference has been used as an index of amount of soft tissue to estimate fetal growth[19]. Cheek to cheek measurements obtained on the ultrasonographic coronal view of the face at the level of the nostrils and lips (Figure 8) have been used to calculate a ratio with the BPD which is independent of gestational age[20]. Other investigated parameters are less reliable, as the degree of overlap in subcutaneous tissue thickness between normal fetuses and those with known growth disturbances is such that tissue thickness measurements do not reliably predict macrosomia or intrauterine growth restriction (IUGR)[21].

Femur length

Due to early ossification of the fetal femur, this bone can be measured as early as 10 weeks[22] and should always be included in fetal biometric assessment from early second trimester onwards. FL growth is 0.3 cm per week from 14–27 weeks and slows down to 0.1 cm per week in the third trimester. The FL is measured along the long axis of the femur from outer to outer margin (Figure 9). One must be careful to measure only ossified diaphysis, excluding the epiphyses. There are discrepancies in the variability of this parameter, and reported accuracies range from ± 1 week in the second trimester to ± 3 to 4 weeks at term.

Ultrasonographically determined femoral length is strongly correlated with actual crown–heel length of newborn fetuses[23–25], and this parameter should be included in a sonographic growth profile designed to detect abnormal fetal growth patterns. It is also a more stable (compared to BPD) estimator of GA when fetal growth deviates from normal because it is less affected by intrauterine growth abnormalities or fetal presentation[26,27].

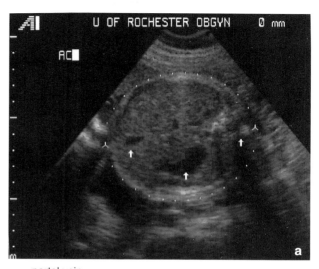

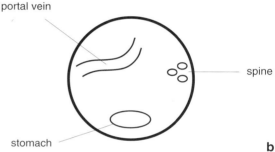

Figure 7 (a) Ultrasound demonstrating abdominal circumference (AC) measurement with appropriate landmarks (arrows from left to right – portal vein, stomach and spine). (b) Schematic drawing demonstrating appropriate landmarks in place for AC measurement

Fetal weight estimation

The human embryo weighs approximately 2 g at 7 to 9 weeks gestation and grows to a mean weight of 3240 g at 40 weeks. Ninety-five per cent of fetal weight gain occurs in the second half of the gestation[28]. Reliability of ultrasonic prediction of estimated fetal weight (EFW) depends to a great extent on the technique and skill of the examiner. An experienced operator and properly calibrated scanner are at least as important as the formula used for calculation. At least two of the three major biometric parameters (BPD and AC, or AC and FL) should be obtained, with EFW prediction most accurate when BPD, AC and FL measurements are combined. Knowledge of the correct gestational age is needed for growth correlation and necessary

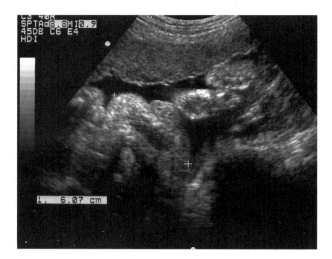

Figure 8 Cheek-to-cheek measurement

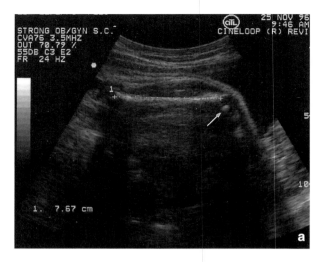

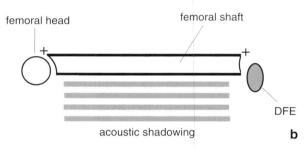

Figure 9 (**a**) Ultrasound measurement of femur avoiding inclusion of distal femoral epiphysis (arrow). (**b**) Schematic drawing of appropriate caliper placement for femur measurement

for percentile determination. Birthweight prediction is similar whether one or multiple sonographic examinations are performed in the third trimester[29] with a reported accuracy of ± 15%. FL should always be included when predicting estimated fetal weight, as fetal length can significantly alter fetal weight estimations. Models that include FL have the smallest error at the upper end of the weight scale[30].

The greatest error in fetal weight estimation is seen with fetuses that are small or large for gestational age. Formulas using FL and AC with or without BPD tend to overestimate weight in a small for gestational age (SGA) fetus, and underestimate in a large for gestational age (LGA) fetus[31,32]. A fetus with an EFW of 1 kg will have an error of ± 150 g, while one with an EFW of 4 kg will have an error of ± 600 g. There is also a tendency to over-identify those fetuses less than the 10th percentile and to under-identify fetuses greater than the 90th percentile[33]. Accuracy of weight prediction decreases in the presence of maternal conditions such as diabetes or severe growth restriction with oligohydramnios[34].

Growth parameter ratios

Ratios comparing growth of different parameters can alert the examiner to a variety of fetal conditions ranging from IUGR due to reduced placental perfusion to genetic disorders affecting fetal growth[35]. The range for ratios of measurements is wide because, throughout gestation, the increase in size of different body parts is not synchronous. Some authors have reported that several ratios (such as HC/AC, and FL/AC) can be utilized without knowledge of gestational age since these ratios remain constant after 20 weeks gestation[36]; however, not all agree[37].

The HC/AC ratio can be employed between 15 and 42 weeks. This ratio is, under normal growth conditions, greater than 1 : 1 until 36 weeks. After this, AC becomes the larger of the two circumferences. This ratio can help us to distinguish between different types of IUGR. With symmetric IUGR (often caused by genetic abnormalities) the HC/AC ratio remains normal. This ratio is more useful in cases of non-symmetric IUGR, which is often caused by placental insufficiency. In these fetuses the 'brain sparing effect' becomes evident and the HC/AC ratio increases.

Another important ratio is FL/AC ratio. This ratio remains constant after 24 weeks at 0.22 ± 0.02. Growth restriction is suspected if the value is greater than 0.235 and macrosomia may be present if it is less than 0.205[37]. As a rule, AC should not be used in fetal gestational age assessment when the FL/AC ratio is less than 0.20 or greater than 0.24

The normal range for FL/BPD ratio is 79 ± 8%[38]. Values greater than this could indicate microcephaly. If the ratio is abnormally high, one should reassess FL measurements to make sure epiphyses were not included in the measurement. With unexpectedly low values, skeletal dysplasias and head anomalies must be excluded. The FL/BPD ratio is a good indicator of skeletal dysplasia, as there is little chance that normal fetuses will fall outside – 4 SD[38].

Thoracic length and circumference, measured at the level of the four chamber view of the heart, grow linearly throughout gestation. The ratio of thoracic circumference (TC) to AC remains constant throughout pregnancy. It is suggested that a low TC/AC (0.89 ± 0.06) ratio can predict pulmonary hypoplasia in patients with oligo-hydramnios, ruptured membranes or skeletal dysplasias[39].

Miscellaneous parameters

Ultrasonographic visualization of fetal organs has improved significantly over recent years, with optimal visualization occurring at 21–23 weeks gestation[40]. Transvaginal imaging makes it possible to visualize anatomic detail in the first trimester, with most major fetal structures visible as soon as 13 weeks gestation[41].

A curvilinear relation exists between the transverse cerebellar diameter (TCD) (Figure 10) and gestational age and is independent of shape of the head. The ratio of TCD to AC remains constant throughout pregnancy with respect to gestational age and can be useful in the early detection of fetal growth abnormalities[42]. While this measurement may be used satisfactorily to predict gestational age in fetuses with asymmetric growth retardation it is not so useful in cases of symmetric growth retardation, and the use of TCD for evaluation of SGA fetuses is debated[43,44].

Another parameter with good gestational age correlation is the orbital diameter (Figure 11). This is measured from outer orbital wall to outer orbital wall, inside the bone table. Binocular measurements have been suggested for use when fetal

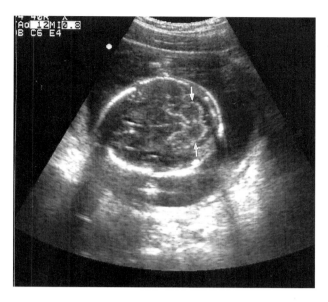

Figure 10   Cerebellar measurement

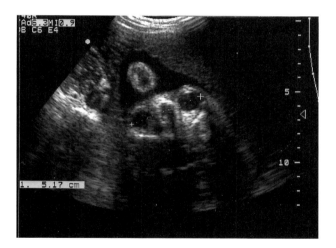

Figure 11   Biorbital distance as measured by ultrasound

occipital position prevents accurate transaxial BPD measurement. Growth of the binocular distance is non-linear. Variability associated with predicting menstrual age between 14 and 27 weeks is ± 14 days, increasing to ± 24 days between 29 and 40 weeks.

Several nomograms have been developed for fetal bony structures. The humerus can be used when the femur length is not obtainable or as an adjunct to other gestational age predictors. Other long bone measurements are useful for detection of severe skeletal abnormalities.

Assumptions can be made about gestational age based upon visualization of single or combinations of ossification centers (epiphyses). Since BPD and FL lengths in the third trimester have a 2 to 3 week deviation in either direction, ossification center visualization can help to narrow down possible gestational age range. Ultrasonographically, ossification centers appear as hyperechoic, egg-shaped areas in close proximity to the ends of long bones and the timing of their appearance is associated with gestational age. The distal femoral epiphysis (DFE) is seen in 94.5% of fetuses from 34 weeks but is not visualized prior to 28 weeks. Visualization may be affected by IUGR, resulting in delayed appearance or smaller than normal measurements. The smaller proximal tibial epiphysis (PTE) appears from 34–37 weeks and is seen in approximately 87% of normal fetuses from 37 weeks until term.

Clavicular and scapular measurements may be applied as additional growth parameters in fetuses with normal growth. These structures are consistently identifiable and demonstrate relatively linear growth throughout the second and third trimesters[45,46]. Measurements of the fetal spine and foot have also demonstrated good correlation with FL and BPD respectively. Both have also been shown to relate well to gestational age[47–49]. Iliac bone width and growth can also be used in identification of abnormal fetal growth as it correlates well with gestational age and femur length[50,51] (Figure 12).

Fetal kidneys are consistently recognizable on transabdominal scans after 15 weeks gestation. Measurements (AP, length and diameter) demonstrate a relatively good relation to gestational age. Renal to abdominal ratios in the second and third trimester have also been evaluated[52].

A four chamber view of the heart can be reliably visualized in early second trimester. Measurements of heart circumference taken at the level of this view demonstrate a good correlation to gestational age in normally growing fetuses[53]. Aortic and pulmonary artery diameters taken from inner wall to inner wall at the level of the semilunar valves are also closely related to fetal age, and thus may be useful predictors of gestational age when growth restriction is suspected[54,55]. Growth disturbances have an inconsistent effect on fetal heart size and it should not be used for determination of IUGR or macrosomia.

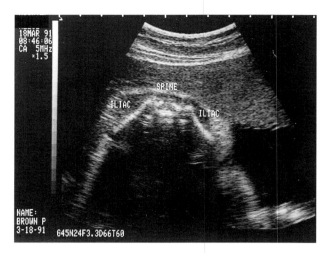

Figure 12   Measurement of iliac bone size in transverse plane

GESTATIONAL AGE ESTIMATION

Ultrasonographic measurements of early pregnancy provide the most accurate estimate of gestational age from which an EDC can be derived. It is important that the gestational age determined at the time of the first examination is maintained throughout pregnancy and EDC should in most cases not be revised when serial ultrasonographic examinations provide conflicting data.

Overall, ultrasonographically determined gestational age tolerance widens from ± 7 days for ultrasonographic examinations performed before 16 weeks to ± 21 days after 28 weeks gestation[56]. The ultrasonographic composite age is used for gestational age assignment after the first trimester. Table 2 summarizes the most accurate measurement parameters for different gestational age groups. The examiner should obtain measurements of as many parameters as possible, as the arithmetic average of gestational age predicted by several parameters is most accurate.

Most formulae used for gestational age determination underestimate true GA when used between 38 and 42 weeks. Suggested formulae which compensate for this underestimation still present wide 95% confidence intervals of ± 3 weeks as a result of biologic variability[57]. Most commonly used parameters report confidence ranges of ± 14 days or less until late pregnancy, thus complete sets of measurements (including EFW) should be performed at intervals greater than two weeks.

Table 2 Accuracy of ultrasound measurements for different gestational age groups

Ultrasound parameter	Accuracy
Gestational sac diameter	± 7 days
Crown–rump length	± 3 to 5 days
BPD second trimester	± 1 to 1.5 weeks
BPD third trimester	± 2 to 4 weeks
FL second trimester	± 1 to 1.5 weeks
FL third trimester	± 3 to 3.5 weeks
Multiple parameters (Second trimester)	± 1.5 weeks
Multiple parameters (Late third trimester)	± 2.5 weeks

BPD, biparietal diameter; FL, femur length

MULTIPLE GESTATION

Accurate dating and growth assessment is essential in multiple gestation because increased risks common to all varieties of twins result from the high frequency of prematurity and low birth weights. While tables for the size of fetal body parts as a function of gestational age are well established for singleton pregnancy, most authors agree that the literature is confusing about whether measurement tables for singletons are accurate for use in twin pregnancies. The majority of evidence, however, seems to support the idea that there are no differences in the second trimester BPD measurement, yet there is progressive fall off in the third trimester. Femur lengths show very little difference in the third trimester. For these reasons most authors agree that the tables used for singleton pregnancies should be employed in multiple gestations as well (see chapter 15).

It is important that the examiners not only include an assessment of each fetus individually, but also a comparison of the two fetuses. Monochorionic twins may show growth discrepancy which could be indicative of twin to twin transfusion syndrome or genetic abnormality of one fetus. Weight differences of 25% or greater[58], or an abdominal circumference difference of at least 20 mm[59] are generally accepted definitions of twin growth discordance. Any discrepancy of growth in conjunction with decreased amniotic fluid volume increases the likelihood of clinical significance.

With triplets, mean BPD lags up to 2.5 weeks behind singletons from 25th to 36th week gestation. HC/AC ratios do not differ from those of singleton pregnancies. Triplets tend to demonstrate a 1 to 3 week delay compared to singletons, and as much as a 2 week delay when compared with normal twin pregnancies.

COMMON ERRORS

Measurement errors must be avoided if accurate growth assessment and gestational age assignment are to be performed. The following guidelines may be helpful:

(1) Examiners must be certain that measurements are obtained in the correct scan plane and calipers correctly placed.

(2) Each measurement should be obtained twice, as the accuracy of the average of two measurements is generally greater than any single measurement.

(3) Gestational ages must be calculated using nomograms which were created using the same landmarks and caliper placements.

(4) Any changes in a parameter caused by a positional/pathological variant must be recognized.

(5) Ultrasound laboratories should employ regular phantom and caliper testing and have a quality assurance program.

(6) Do not revise an ultrasonographically assigned due date even if serially performed scans provide conflicting data.

CONCLUSIONS

Measurements obtained using sophisticated real-time scanners are surprisingly similar to those obtained with static scanners. Thus, biometric charts have changed little over the last 20 years[60,61]. Modern technology, however, has made it much easier to identify and therefore measure fetal anatomy in hopes of obtaining more clinically useful information about the unborn child. Certainly, ultrasonographic assessment has grown in its ability to accurately assess fetal growth over the last two decades. We, as users of this technology, have similarly improved our ability to interpret and utilize the information obtained.

Some investigators have questioned the value of routine ultrasonographic screening in low-risk populations. It is our opinion that information provided by thorough, competently performed ultrasonographic examinations increases the amount of knowledge the provider has regarding the patient. Thus both patient and provider are offered a more educated approach to prenatal management.

References

1. Campbell S, Warsof SL, Little D, *et al*. Routine ultrasound screening for the prediction of gestational age. *Obstet Gynecol* 1985;65:613–20
2. Platt L. First trimester ultrasound. Syllabus from Current practice and controversies in obstetrical ultrasound. Tufts University School of Medicine, 1993
3. Daya S, Woods S, Ward S, *et al*. Early pregnancy assessment with transvaginal ultrasound scanning. *Can Med Assoc J* 1991;144:441–6
4. Manton M, Pederson JF. Ultrasound visualization of the human yolk sac. *J Clin Ultrasound* 1979;7:459
5. Nyberg DA, Mack LA, Harvey D, *et al*. Value of the yolk sac in evaluating early pregnancies. *J Ultrasound Med* 1988;7:129–35
6. Lindsay DJ, Lovett IS, Lyons EA, *et al*. Yolk sac diameter and shape at endovaginal US: predictors of pregnancy outcome in the first trimester. *Radiology* 1992;183:115–8
7. American Institute of Ultrasound in Medicine. *Guidelines for Performance of the Antepartum Obstetrical Ultrasound Examination*. Boston: AIUM, 1991
8. Goldstein SR, Wolfson R. Endovaginal ultrasonic measurement of early embryonic size as a means of assessing gestational age. *J Ultrasound Med* 1994;13:27–31
9. Wilson RD. Prenatal evaluation of growth by ultrasound. *Growth: Genetics and Hormones* 1993;9:1–3
10. Goldstein SR, Subramanyam BR, Snyder JR. Ratio of gestational sac volume to crown-rump length in early pregnancy. *J Reprod Med* 1986;31:320–1
11. Goldstein I, Zimmer EA, Tamir A, *et al*. Evaluation of normal gestational sac growth: appearance of embryonic heartbeat and embryo body movements using the transvaginal technique. *Obstet Gynecol* 1991;77:885–8
12. Warran WB, Timor-Tritsch I, Peisner DB, *et al*. Dating the early pregnancy by sequential appearance of embryonic structures. *Am J Obstet Gynecol* 1989;161:747–53
13. Deter RL, Harrist RB. Growth standards for anatomic measurements and growth rates derived from longitudinal studies of normal fetal growth. *J Clin Ultrasound* 1992;20:381–8
14. Crang-Svalenius E, Jorgensen C, Mariscal UB. Intrauterine growth of the fetus at term: a prospective and longitudinal study with real-time ultrasound. *J Ultrasound Med* 1990;9:35–8
15. Graham D, Sanders RC. Assessment of gestational age in the second and third trimesters. In Sanders RC, James AE, eds. *The Principles and Practice of Ultrasonography in Obstetrics and Gynecology*. Norwalk, CT: Appleton-Century-Crofts, 1985:147–55
16. Gray DL, Songster GS, Parvin CA, *et al*. Cephalic index: a gestational age dependent biometric parameter. *Obstet Gynecol* 1989;74:600–3
17. Hadlock FP, Deter RL, Carpenter RJ, *et al*. Estimating fetal age: effect of head shape on BPD. *Am J Radiol* 1981;137:83
18. Kurtz AB, Kurtz RJ. The ideal fetal head circumference calculation. *J Ultrasound Med* 1989;8:25–9
19. Vintzileos AM, Neckles A, Campbell WA, *et al*. Ultrasound fetal thigh-calf circumference and gestational age-independent fetal ratios in normal pregnancy. *J Ultrasound Med* 1987;4:287–92
20. Abramowicz JS, Sherer DM, Bar-Tov E, *et al*. The cheek-to-cheek diameter in the ultrasonographic assessment of fetal growth. *Am J Obstet Gynecol* 1991;165:846–52
21. Hill LM, Guzick D, Boyles D, *et al*. Subcutaneous tissue thickness cannot be used to distinguish abnormalities of fetal growth. *Obstet Gynecol* 1992;80:268–71
22. Jeanty P. Fetal limb biometry [Letter]. *Radiology* 1983;147:602
23. Hadlock FP, Harrist FP, Deter RL, *et al*. Ultrasonically measured fetal femur length as a predictor of menstrual age. *Am J Radiol* 1982;138:875–8
24. Deter RL, Rossavik IK, Hill RB, *et al*. Longitudinal studies of femur growth in normal fetuses. *J Clin Ultrasound* 1987;15:299–305
25. Kurniawan YS, Deter RL, Visser GH, *et al*. Prediction of the neonatal crown-heel length from femur diaphysis length measurements. *J Clin Ultrasound* 1994;22:245–52
26. Wolfson RN, Peisner DB, Chik LL, *et al*. Comparison of biparietal diameter and femur length in the third trimester: effects of gestational age and variation in fetal growth. *J Ultrasound Med* 1986;5:145–9
27. Abramowicz JS, Jaffe R, Warsof SL. Ultrasonographic measurement of fetal femur length in growth disturbances. *Am J Obstet Gynecol* 1989;161:1137–40
28. Vorheer A. Factors influencing fetal growth. *Am J Obstet Gynecol* 1982;142:577–88

29. Hedriana HL, Moore TR. A comparison of single versus multiple growth ultrasonographic examinations in predicting birth weight. *Am J Obstet Gynecol* 1994;170:1600–5

30. Simon NV, Levisky JS, Sherer DM, *et al*. Influence of fetal growth patterns on sonographic estimation of fetal weight. *J Clin Ultrasound* 1987;15:376–83

31. Larsen T, Peterson S, Freisen G, *et al*. Normal fetal growth evaluated by longitudinal ultrasound examinations. *Early Hum Dev* 1990;24:36–45

32. Miller JM, Kissling GA, Brown HL, *et al*. Estimated fetal weight: applicability to small- and large-for-gestational-age fetus. *J Clin Ultrasound* 1988;16:95–7

33. Benaceraf BR, Gelman R, Frigoletto FD. Sono-graphically estimated fetal weights: accuracy and limitation. *Am J Obstet Gynecol* 1988;159:1118–21

34. Tamura RK, Sabbagha RE, Dooley SE, *et al*. Real-time ultrasound estimations of weight in fetuses of diabetic gravid women. *Am J Obstet Gynecol* 1985; 153:57–60

35. Crang-Svalenius E, Jorgensen C. Normal ultrasonic fetal growth ratios evaluated in cases of fetal disproportion. *J Ultrasound Med* 1991;10:89–92

36. Snijders RJM, Nicolaides KH. Fetal biometry at 14–40 weeks gestation. *Ultrasound Obstet Gynecol* 1994;4:34–48

37. Hadlock FP, Harrist RB, Fearneyhough TC, *et al*. Use of femur length/abdominal circumference ratio in detecting the marcosomic fetus. *Radiology* 1985; 154:503

38. Hohler CW, Quetel TA. Comparison of ultrasound femur length and biparietal diameter in late pregnancy. *Am J Obstet Gynecol* 1981;141:759

39. Chikara U, Rosenberg J, Chevernak FA, *et al*. Prenatal sonographic assessment of the fetal thorax: normal values. *Am J Obstet Gynecol* 1987;156: 1069–74

40. Wolfe HM, Zador IE, Bottoms MC, *et al*. Trends in sonographic fetal organ visualization. *Ultrasound Obstet Gynecol* 1993;3:97–9

41. Quashie C, Weiner S, Bolognese R. Efficacy of first trimester transvaginal sonography in detecting normal fetal development. *Am J Perinatol* 1992;9: 202–13

42. Meyer WJ, Gauthier DW, Goldenberg B, *et al*. The fetal transverse cerebellar diameter/abdominal circumference ratio: a gestational age-independent method of assessing fetal size. *J Ultrasound Med* 1993;12:379–82

43. Co E, Raju TN, Aldana O. Cerebellar dimensions in assessment of gestational age in neonates. *Radiology* 1991;181:581–5

44. Hill LM, Guzick D, Rivello D, *et al*. The transverse cerebellar diameter cannot be used to assess gestational age in the small for gestational age fetus. *Obstet Gynecol* 1990;75:329–33

45. Goldstein I, Lockwood C, Belanger K, *et al*. Ultrasonographic assessment of gestational age with distal femoral and proximal tibial ossification centers. I The third trimester. *Am J Obstet Gynecol* 1988;158:127–30

46. Yarkoni S, Schmidt W, Jeanty P, *et al*. Clavicular measurements. A new biometric parameter for fetal evaluation. *J Ultrasound Med* 1985;4:467–70

47. Sherer DM, Plessinger MA, Allen TA. Fetal scapular length in the ultrasonographic assessment of gestational age. *J Ultrasound Med* 1994;13:523–8

48. Sherer DM, Abramowicz JS, Plessinger MA, *et al*. Fetal sacral length in the ultrasonographic assessment of gestational age. *Am J Obstet Gynecol* 1993; 168:626–33

49. Shalev E, Weiner E, Zuckerman H, *et al*. Reliability of sonographic measurement of the fetal foot. *J Ultrasound Med* 1989;8:259–62

50. Jaffe R, Santolaya J, Warsof SL. Sonographic measurement of the fetal iliac bone: growth and relation to femur length in assessment of gestational age. *Am J Perinatol* 1993;10:105–8

51. Hata T, Deter RL. A review of fetal organ measurements obtained with ultrasound: normal growth. *J Clin Ultrasound* 1992;20:155–74

52. Grannum P, Bracken M, Silverman R, *et al*. Assessment of fetal kidney size in normal gestation by comparison of ratio of kidney circumference to abdominal circumference. *Am J Obstet Gynecol* 1980; 136:249–70

53. Shultz SM, Pretorious DH, Budorick NE. Four-chamber view of the fetal heart: demonstration related to menstrual age. *J Ultrasound Med* 1994;13: 285–9

54. Cartier M, Doubilet PM. Fetal aortic and pulmonary artery diameters: sonographic measurements in growth retarded fetuses. *Am J Radiol* 1988;151: 991–3

55. Comstock CH, Riggs T, Lee W, *et al*. Pulmonary to aorta diameter ratio in the normal and abnormal fetal heart. *Am J Obstet Gynecol* 1991;165:1038–44

56. Doubilet PM. Fetal measurements. Syllabus. 'Ultrasound 1990'. Harvard Medical School

57. Doubilet PM, Benson CB. Improved prediction of gestational age in the late third trimester. *J Ultrasound Med* 1993;12:647–53

58. Erkkola R, Ala-Mello S, Pirroinen O, *et al*. Growth discordance in twin pregnancies: a risk factor not detected by measurements of biparietal diameter. *Obstet Gynecol* 1987;66:203–6

59. Brown CEL, Guzick DS, Leveno KJ, *et al*. Prediction of discordant twin using ultrasound measurement of biparietal diameter and abdominal perimeter. *Obstet Gynecol* 1987;70:677–81

60. Harrington K, Campbell S. Fetal size and growth. *Curr Opin Obstet Gynecol* 1993;5:186–94

61. Geirsson RT. Ultrasound instead of the last menstrual period as the basis of gestational age assignment. *Ultrasound Obstet Gynecol* 1991;1:212–9

Intrauterine growth restriction

5

John J. Anthony and Patricia A. Smith

Intrauterine growth restriction (IUGR) arises in consequence of miscellaneous abnormalities and defies precise antenatal definition. The development of IUGR is of clinical significance because it may be a harbinger of preterm delivery, underlying fetal disease and possible long term morbidity and mortality[1-6].

Normal intrauterine development depends upon the interaction between genetically programmed growth and a permissive environment. Growth restriction may occur because of intrinsic fetal abnormalities or may follow substrate deprivation. In the latter event, growth restriction is part of an adaptive fetal response to environmental deprivation. Growth restriction arising because of intrinsic fetal disease is associated with an abnormal maternal adaptive response to pregnancy.

Our current views of IUGR are limited by a fragmented understanding of the pathophysiology and an inability to dissect out those abnormalities attributable to genetic, environmental or compensatory mechanisms.

This chapter will review the definition, pathophysiology, diagnosis, management and consequences of IUGR.

DEFINITION

The definition of IUGR is imprecise and arbitrary for at least three reasons. Firstly, it is often a retrospective diagnosis made after delivery; secondly it is usually diagnosed by measuring the growth of an individual fetus against (arbitrary) population-based centile charts rather than the genetic potential of a specific fetus; and finally, depending on the choice of growth parameters, impaired 'growth' may reflect fetal growth restriction, fetal wasting or both[7].

Weight-for-gestational age was originally conceived as a measure of risk but is frequently used to define growth retarded infants; the arbitrary identification of infants less than the 10th or third centile as affected infants fails to recognize that some babies will be constitutionally small and therefore appropriately grown although less than the 10th centile. This definition also fails to recognize that infants with a birthweight above the 10th centile may have failed to attain their genetic potential despite being born within 'normal' weight criteria for a given population.

Because of these problems pertaining to definition, numerous other ways of identifying growth restricted infants have been proposed: ponderal index[8], skinfold thickness[9], the use of Rossavik growth models, and individualized birthweight ratios have all been utilized[10,11]. These methods all attempt to identify the abnormally grown infant on the basis of characterizing those aspects of morphometry that most appropriately define the neonate likely to suffer from an adverse perinatal outcome (low apgar score, abnormal cardiotocograph, acidosis). Recent attempts to define the abnormally grown fetus have been derived from the examination of multiple morphometric variables in the form of a neonatal growth profile consisting of weight, head, arm and thigh circumference as well as crown–heel length. This profile has been further refined by using Rossavik growth models derived from second trimester ultrasound measurements to predict individualized measurements for the specific neonate rather than using cross-sectional population based data. Deter and colleagues have used these data to construct a growth potential realization index which is the ratio of the actual to predicted growth of the neonate; they have further refined this measurement by combining the growth potential realization indices for the different components of the neonatal growth profile into a 'neonatal growth assessment score'[12,13]. While methodology of this nature adds precision to the process of correctly identifying the affected infant, such measurements are not sufficiently robust for routine clinical use. Furthermore, they are concerned with the fundamental (albeit important) issue of identifying an abnormal outcome rather than the antenatal detection of the compromised infant. However, until the endpoint that defines abnormal growth is itself clearly recognized, the process of defining IUGR will be unsatisfactory.

With these difficulties concerning endpoints in mind, the process of antenatal fetal assessment is better served by examining growth rather than size itself[7]. Unfortunately most charts used to plot ultrasound morphometrics represent cross-sectional data although a few growth velocity charts have been designed[14–16]. The validity of these charts as an investigational tool is yet to be assessed with respect to the predictive value that might be derived from each chart. This should not rest upon the arbitrary utilization of a 10th centile cut-off point but should be derived from seeking the greatest probability of correctly predicting growth restriction from receiver operating characteristic curves generated for different centile values (measured against a pre-defined endpoint).

PATHOPHYSIOLOGY

Abnormal growth arises either because of fetal disease or because of environmental abnormalities.

Fetal disorders

Chromosomal disorders

Chromosomal abnormalities have been estimated to occur in 6% of conceptions[17]. The majority of these conceptions end in abortion. Although the overall reported incidence in live births is much lower (0.6%)[18], chromosomal abnormalities remain an important cause of intrauterine growth restriction. The majority of these fetuses (> 90%) will have structural abnormalities and the risk of an associated chromosomal abnormality has been reported to rise from 7% with a single anomaly to 31% in the presence of multiple anomalies[19,20]. Severe early growth restriction is most commonly associated with triploidy whereas growth restriction manifesting in later gestation (> 26 weeks) has been linked to autosomal aberrations (commonly trisomy 18 – Edwards' syndrome)[20].

Placental mosaicism

Confined placental mosaicism has been recently identified following the introduction of chorion villous biopsy; a retrospective survey of 11 775 chorion villous biopsies identified 73 such cases among whom there was an increased risk of low or high birthweight in the absence of any other adverse outcome. Isolated IUGR has been linked to confined placental mosaicism in 6% of cases with the commonest abnormalities being trisomy 9 and deletion of the short arm of chromosome 13[21].

Non-genetic anomalies

Fetal anomalies unassociated with chromosomal abnormalities (anencephaly, gastrointestinal abnormalities such as gastroschisis and omphalocele as well as renal agenesis) have all be identified as causes of IUGR[22].

Infections

Fetal infections linked to growth restriction are mainly viral in origin. Despite this, certain bacterial infections occur commonly; syphilis remains a prevalent (and preventable) condition in developing countries and is a recognized cause of both growth restriction and perinatal mortality[22]. Primary viral infection with rubella, cytomegalovirus, varicella-zoster and parvovirus may all lead to growth restriction and reproductive failure. Although recurrent infection with the herpes group of viruses may lead to fetal infection, the virus is less likely to affect the fetus adversely because of maternal antibody production.

Parasitic infections such as malaria lead to growth restriction in about one-fifth of affected mothers[23]. The mechanism of growth restriction is linked to placental pathology, anemia and maternal parasitemia rather than fetal infection. Toxoplasmosis is associated with a high risk of fetal damage if the infection develops in the mother during the first trimester.

Environmental factors

Environmentally linked causes of IUGR may be considered in two broad categories: those disorders arising from pregnancy maladaptation (uteroplacental insufficiency, pre-eclampsia) and secondly those extrinsic to the pregnancy itself (nutritional factors, the effects of drugs and superimposed diseases).

Pregnancy maladaption

Physiological changes   The maternal adaptation to normal pregnancy is a well-documented incremental process of immunological, metabolic, endocrine, cardiorespiratory and renal change designed to accommodate the metabolic needs of the growing conceptus. In broad detail, two fundamental changes may be considered central events in pregnancy adaptation: the first is endocrinologically mediated and leads to augmentation of the renin–angiotensin–aldosterone system resulting in massive sodium and water retention. The maternal cardiovascular system adapts to plasma volume expansion by reducing peripheral vascular resistance through augmented production of prostacyclin and nitric oxide[24]. The extent of the vasodilatation is such that despite a compensatory 40% increase in cardiac output, blood pressure decreases[25]. These events augment tissue substrate delivery to the point where substrate delivery per unit time exceeds the extra requirements attributable to pregnancy. In the case of oxygen delivery and consumption, the arteriovenous oxygen difference falls during pregnancy despite increased metabolic demands. The second important maternal adaptation occurs just prior to mid-pregnancy; this involves the remodeling of the terminal maternal arterial blood supply to the placenta. The spiral arteries, which are branches of the radial arteries, show extensive medial changes resulting from destruction of the smooth muscle in the vessel wall and dilatation of these vessels within the decidua and sub-decidual myometrium. The transformed and dilated vessels are presumed to conduct a far greater volume of blood to the placental bed than would have occurred through morphologically normal (narrow) arteries[26]. These transformed terminal arteries are also incapable of vasoconstriction. These vascular changes are associated with trophoblast invasion into the spiral arteries and surrounding myometrium; the co-incidence of these two events has led to the presumption that they are linked. The process of this second wave of trophoblast invasion between the 16th and 20th week of pregnancy is ill-understood but almost certainly dependent on the normal expression of cell surface adhesion molecules that facilitate intercellular binding.

These two key changes – increased cardiovascular rate of substrate delivery and vascular remodeling – secure an adequate blood supply to the growing fetus. Of these adaptations, the most vulnerable to failure are those linked to perfusion of the choriodecidual space.

Maternal maladaptation In the absence of any other extrinsic pathology, normal adaptation may fail to occur. This is characterized by suboptimal plasma volume expansion, smaller increments in cardiac output and failure of vascular remodeling which is associated with deficient trophoblast infiltration of the decidual bed. These changes in maternal volume homeostasis may be manifest within the first trimester and may be a consequence rather than a cause of growth restriction[27].

In patients who develop pre-eclampsia, not only is there a failure of physiological transformation in the spiral arteries but additional pathological changes are evident. The vessels show evidence of lipid deposition in myointimal cells giving rise to the lesion of acute atherosis which is analogous to atherosclerotic vascular damage in older non-pregnant patients. This may cause luminal obstruction of the spiral arteries as well as increasing the risk of thrombotic occlusion in the vessel[28].

The consequences of these changes are manifest in both the fetoplacental unit and the mother. The most obvious abnormality lies in the development of placental ischemia leading to discrete areas of infarction in the placenta as well as other histological changes (such as basal membrane calcification and syncytial knotting[29]) consistent with global placental ischemia[29]. Endocrinopathy develops simultaneously in patients with underlying hypertensive disease in the form of altered placental prostanoid metabolism (thromboxane dominance) and augmented placental vascular nitric oxide production[30]. In the case of pre-eclampsia this placental process disseminates to the systemic vasculature giving rise to evidence of disturbed endothelial function, platelet consumption and elevated peripheral vascular resistance with overt hypertension[31,32]. Patients with idiopathic growth restriction may have placental and placental bed pathology characteristic of pre-eclampsia without the maternal syndrome of hypertension and multiorgan disease.

The fetus responds to choriodecidual ischemia by restricting growth. The extent of IUGR may be related to the cumulative number and severity of placental lesions reflecting abnormal uteroplacental or fetoplacental blood flow. A restricted pattern of fetal growth is mediated by decreased elaboration of growth factors and through the redistribution of fetal cardiac output (see below).

Factors extrinsic to pregnancy: malnutrition and disease

Calorie restricted diets may have an effect on birth weight. This has been clearly demonstrated in the Dutch famine of 1944 when the average reduction in birthweight was measured to be about 300 g[33]. The effects of malnutrition are measurable when calorie deprivation occurs in the latter half of pregnancy but have little effect during the first trimester. It is important to draw a distinction between babies born light for gestational age due to maternal malnutrition and those born small and light for gestational age because of substrate deprivation arising from uteroplacental insufficiency. The one circumstance may be appropriately corrected by calorie supplementation whereas in the latter case calorie supplementation will not correct abnormal growth and may result in accelerated fetal anaerobic metabolism with resultant fetal acidosis[34].

Immunological disorders   Collagen vascular disorders, such as systemic lupus erythematosis, may affect fetal growth because of vascular disease or because of antibody production. Humeral events in these patients may give rise to antibodies that affect the fetus directly by crossing the placenta (e.g. Ro and La antibodies) or by indirect vascular damage and thrombosis in the uteroplacental circulation. The specific antibodies present may be identified by their effects on tests of coagulation which show evidence of uncorrectable prolongation (partial thromboplastin time, kaolin-cephalin clotting time, russel viper venom time). These abnormalities identified *in vitro* denote the presence of a lupus anticoagulant[35]. Antibodies may, however, be present without any functional derangement of coagulation. The antiphospholipid antibodies associated with the presence of a lupus anticoagulant include the anticardiolipin antibody (occasionally giving rise to false positive syphilis serology), antiphosphotidylserine, antiphosphotidylethnanolamine, antiphosphotidylglycerol, antiphosphotidylinositol, antiphosphatidic acid and anticephalin antibodies[36]. Of the antiphospholipid antibodies the anticardiolipin antibodies are most clearly linked to reproductive failure[37–39]. The presence of these antibodies is not necessarily associated with underlying systemic lupus erythematosis and may occur in normal patients as well as more frequently in patients with pre-eclampsia. The presence of these antibodies in pre-eclamptic patients increases the risk of growth restriction developing in the affected pregnancy. The mechanism of action of the antiphospholipid antibodies is not well established but may be related to inhibition of prostacyclin production leading to *in vivo* fibrin deposition.

Cardiovascular disease   Both hypertension and cardiac disease may have an influence on growth and reproduction. Underlying maternal hypertensive disease (as distinct from pre-eclampsia)

may lead to IUGR although the risk and extent of growth restriction seen is less than that associated with pre-eclampsia[40]. Likewise, the risk of perinatal mortality in chronically hypertensive pregnancies is far lower than in pregnancies complicated by pre-eclampsia. The mechanisms underlying growth restriction in these pregnancies are probably related to changes in the placental bed vasculature, which may be distinguished from the pathology characterizing pre-eclampsia by an absence of acute atherosis although other vascular pathology is present (including deficient physiologic transformation, medial hyperplasia, endothelial vacuolation and fibrin deposition)[28].

Globally impaired substrate delivery may occur in mothers with cardiac disease. The nature of the cardiac disease may vary from severe acquired valvular lesions to congenital cyanotic heart disease. The effects of these disorders on reproduction are related to the severity of the underlying disease; typically mothers with more severe grades of symptomatic impairment (New York Heart Association Grade II and IV) are more likely to have growth restricted babies[41].

Dyslipidemia influences the extent and nature of vascular disease in non-pregnant patients. The same might be true of pregnancy. No adequate data addressing this issue yet exist. Isolated case reports, however, have drawn attention to the possible association between dyslipidemia and vasculopathy-dependent growth restriction[42].

Hematological disorders   Anemia may contribute to the development of growth restriction although the dominance of plasma volume expansion and increased cardiac output as a mechanism for securing adequate substrate delivery to the fetus (see above) are such that mild degrees of anemia are unlikely to affect fetal oxygenation directly. Anemia may develop for different reasons; anemia occurring on a nutritional basis may be associated with the delivery of light for gestational age infants because of calorie restriction. Other important causes of anemia include those due to the hemoglobinopathies, especially sickle cell disease. Sickle cell disease causes uteroplacental insufficiency by precipitating intravascular thrombosis in the uteroplacental circulation and not through the development of anemia itself[43].

Thrombophilia may also compromise choriodecidual perfusion. Pregnancy, being a procoagulant state, is a susceptible period during which thrombophilia may find clinical expression. The causes of thrombophilia range from autoimmune conditions (cardiolipin syndrome, discussed above) to deficiency syndromes affecting proteins C and S, antithrombin III and factor V deficiency (Leiden mutation). Again, data are lacking but all these conditions have the potential to influence fetal growth.

Effect of drugs Socially accepted drugs include tobacco and alcohol. Both are associated with significant adverse reproductive effects. Smoking may affect uteroplacental perfusion in a variety of ways including the generation of carboxy-hemoglobin and through the vasospastic effects of nicotine. Recent studies indicate that the effects of smoking are most evident during the third trimester of pregnancy and those who cease smoking before the latter half of pregnancy may escape the consequences of their actions[44,45]. Alcohol consumption in pregnancy gives rise to the neonatal condition recognized as the fetal alcohol syndrome[46]. This syndrome consists of restricted intrauterine growth, mental retardation and characteristic facial dysmorphology. The reasons for these effects may be related to the drug itself or its principal metabolite, acetaldehyde. Coexistent drug use and nutritional deprivation may all play a role. The fetal alcohol syndrome may result in persistent growth and intellectual impairment.

Narcotic drug addiction is also clearly linked to the development of IUGR. Cocaine use during pregnancy is associated with asymmetrical growth retardation and a proportionately greater reduction in head circumference than birthweight (similar to the pattern seen with alcohol abuse)[47].

Epilepsy is a condition associated with an increased risk of poor perinatal outcome. Drug usage in the treatment of epilepsy correlates with aspects of abnormal growth. Neonatal head circumferences have shown significantly greater chance of falling below the 10th centile for gestational age with increasing polypharmacy during the first trimester of pregnancy[48].

FETAL ADAPTATION TO INTRAUTERINE GROWTH RESTRICTION

The fetal adaptation to substrate deprivation is complex, incompletely understood and involves both vascular and metabolic changes.

Vascular adaptation

The vascular changes have been studied by means of Doppler ultrasound, by measurement of regulatory peptides obtained from percutaneous umbilical blood sampling and finally by means of immunohistochemistry of the placental vasculature.

Doppler ultrasound examination of the umbilical artery flow velocity waveform shows that the anticipated fall in placental vascular resistance which normally occurs with advancing gestational age is not seen in pregnancies complicated by uteroplacenta insufficiency. A rising fetoplacental vascular resistance with advancing gestational age results in changes in the umbilical artery flow velocity waveform that are characterized by diminishing flow during fetal diastole. In severe cases of growth retardation absent or even reverse flow occurs within the artery during fetal diastole[49,50]. The reason for these observed changes in umbilical artery blood flow were initially ascribed to selective obliterative loss of small stem villous arteries in the diameter range of 20 to 90 μm[51]. This view was reinforced by experimental animal work showing that microsphere embolization of the fetoplacental circulation brought about the anticipated changes in both resistance and the umbilical artery flow velocity waveform[52]. These ideas have been challenged; two publications have failed to identify any reduction in the number of vessels per stem villous, nor any reduction in mean villous vessel diameter between placentae from growth restricted pregnancies and those of controls[53,54]. One study (using monoclonal antibodies) has identified smooth muscle actin positive cells in the stroma of non-muscularized intermediate and terminal placental villi of growth restricted babies. These changes were not observed in controls[54]. Alterations in the endo-, para- and autocrine mechanisms governing vascular tone may also change the placental vascular resistance[55]. The endocrine profile of the growth retarded fetus is one in which elevated levels of certain vasoconstrictors are identifiable. Both angiotensin II (vasoconstrictor) and vasoactive intestinal peptide (vasodilator) have been shown to be elevated in the cord blood obtained by percutaneous sampling[56,57]. Endothelin I has also been identified in increased concentrations in fetuses with abnormal umbilical artery flow velocity waveforms whereas both atrial natriuretic peptide and aldosterone have shown concentrations appropriate to the clinical circumstance of the fetus (with respect to pH)[58,59].

Endothelin may be a particularly important peptide because it is also a recognized smooth muscle mitogen that may account for the presence of myofibroblasts in the peripheral villous vessels of some growth retarded babies[54,55].

The immunohistochemical studies of the placenta further confound the possible evidence of vasoconstrictor dominance in the placental vasculature; the constitutive form of endothelial cell nitric oxide synthase enzyme has been identified in increased concentrations in the villous vascular endothelium of patients with both pre-eclampsia and IUGR without pre-eclampsia[30]. The role of nitric oxide in the terminal placental stem villous vessels may be that of a vasodilator as well as an antioxidant effective against free radicals. Nitric oxide interacts with superoxide anions giving rise to peroxynitrite anions which in turn react with tyrosine residues in the tissues. Nitrotyrosine residues form identifiable tissue markers of the pro-oxidant effects of peroxynitrite; they are absent from villous tissue of normal pregnancy but present in significantly increased concentrations both in the endothelium and the smooth muscle of villous vascular tissues taken from pre-eclamptic pregnancies and those characterized by IUGR[30].

The emerging picture is difficult to interpret and any concept of placental vascular change must therefore be speculative. It seems likely that placental vascular changes, and their mediating mechanisms, will be regionalized and dependent on the adequacy of regional maternal spiral arteriolar perfusion. Increased fetoplacental vascular resistance may increase perfusion through more adequately oxygenated villi much in the same way that pulmonary ventilation–perfusion mismatches are regulated through selective vasoconstriction. Evidence of rising placental vascular resistance with advancing gestational age has also been coupled to increasing centralization of fetal blood flow (to the brain stem in particular) – see below.

Metabolic adaptation

Energy utilization

Glucose, as a metabolic substrate, is present in lower concentrations in the fetal serum of growth retarded infants with an increased maternal–fetal gradient[60]. The reason for fetal hypoglycemia may be related to diminished placental surface area because glucose transporter protein 1 is abundantly present in the syncytiotrophoblast without any difference in receptor density between growth retarded placentae and normal controls[61].

Insulin levels that normally rise with increasing gestational age are lower in growth retarded infants. Lower insulin levels are appropriately adapted to the lower glucose concentration but may also reflect pancreatic beta cell dysfunction[62]. The latter view is supported by the slow and delayed response of the growth retarded fetus to intravenous glucose tolerance testing[63]. By contrast, levels of counter-regulatory hormones are elevated. Alpha pancreatic cell production of glucagon is augmented in growth retarded infants[64].

Growth retarded babies have elevated levels of triglycerides, probably reflecting lower utilization rates of lipids as well as decreased fat deposition after the 24th week of gestation[65].

Anabolic metabolism

Fetal amino acid levels are usually higher than maternal values, reflecting active transport to the fetus. Fetal growth retardation leads to rising maternal amino acid levels with falling fetal levels of essential amino acids[65,66]. These changes reflect decreased placental transfer and the pattern of falling essential to non-essential amino acids in the growth retarded fetus mirror the biochemistry seen in children with protein–calorie malnutrition. Serum levels of ferritin, another essential co-factor for dividing cells, also fall in growth retarded babies[67].

Fetal growth is normally mediated by a number of growth factors of which insulin-like growth factor and epidermal growth factor are likely to be the most important. Insulin-like growth factor 1 normally increases with increasing gestational age. Insulin-like growth factors 1 and 2 as well as insulin-like growth factor binding protein 3 are all markedly depressed in fetal blood obtained from growth retarded babies[68–71]. Epidermal growth factor has been studied in the urine and plasma of neonates. Growth retarded babies show lower levels of epidermal growth factor than controls; unlike the controls, fetal plasma levels are also lower than maternal values[72,73].

Other endocrine changes

Fetal thyroid function usually improves with increasing gestational age giving rise to increasing levels of thyroid stimulating hormone (TSH), T4 and T3. Growth retarded infants have high TSH levels although T4 and T3 levels are both low. These changes in thyroid function are proportional to the degree of hypoxia present in the growth retarded fetus. Falling levels of thyroxine may be an adaptive response to slow the rate of cellular metabolism in the face of substrate deficit[74].

Fetal adrenal function shows elevated cortisol levels in affected infants. The degree of elevation in the cortisol is inversely proportional to the blood glucose level, suggesting an intrauterine counter-regulatory function for insulin[75]. These findings have been disputed, with contradictory results reported suggesting that cortisol levels in growth retarded babies show little change (compared to controls), but that both adrenocorticotropic hormone and corticotropin releasing hormone levels are elevated, presumably as part of a fetal stress response[76].

Erythropoietin levels rise *in utero* and may precede the development of erythroblastosis[77]. Growth hormone and prolactin levels are both elevated in growth retarded fetuses.

Fetal cerebral changes

IUGR is associated with abnormal neurological outcome (see below). The reasons for abnormal outcome may be related to overt fetal hypoxia although most cases of cerebral palsy are not related to a discrete intrapartum event[78]. Growth restriction due to substrate deficiency is associated with centralization of cerebral blood flow which has a protective effect against the effects of global hypoxia. Growth retarded fetuses are also hypoglycemic; a possible compensatory mechanism may exist in the form of increased brain lactate levels which have been demonstrated in the brains of human preterm IUGR infants[79].

The occurrence of oxidative stress in hypoxic fetuses as a mechanism of cerebral vascular damage has been studied in animal models. The rat and pig models have demonstrated an association between cerebral oxidative stress and hypoxia in growth restricted fetuses along with depletion of certain naturally occurring antioxidant substances (such as glutathione peroxidase)[80,81]. Lipid peroxidation may directly damage cells and may also trigger apoptotic changes[82].

The clinical scenario, following a 'honeymoon period', of evolving cerebral injury 24 to 48 hours after birth may be due to a reperfusion injury through the release into the circulation of reactive species from previously ischemic tissue. Apoptosis (triggered cell death) may be stimulated by the presence of oxidants and free radicals; apoptotic change may be further enhanced by zinc deficiency (more frequent in IUGR fetuses) and estrogen withdrawal.

MANAGEMENT

The management of IUGR depends upon accurate diagnosis and accurate assessment of fetal well-being because few (if any) antenatal interventions have made any difference in the pathogenesis of fetal growth restriction. Iatrogenic preterm delivery can only be justified if it diminishes the risk of reproductive failure.

Growth retardation due to substrate deficiency sets in train a sequence of events that begins with abnormal placentation, then enters a phase of fetal adaptation that may ultimately end in failure, decompensation and intrauterine death. Delivery must take place at the time of decompensation (if not before). It may be more appropriate to deliver the fetus before it decompensates. However, the necessary data addressing this question are yet to be provided although randomized studies are currently underway [Growth Restriction Intervention Trial (GRIT) study].

This section will examine the question of diagnosis, the use of ultrasound and some of the antenatal interventions used in the management of IUGR.

Antenatal diagnosis

Clinical assessment and symphysis fundal height measurements

The uncertainties of accurate diagnosis have necessitated the use of risk factor analysis to define a subset of patients at high risk of delivering a growth restricted baby. These risk factors are self-evident and related to the etiology of IUGR. Abdominal palpation is an inadequate adjunct to history for the detection of the growth restricted baby (sensitivity 43.9%, specificity 87.8% and positive predictive value 28.7%)[83]. Intra- and interobserver variability is high with factors such as maternal obesity and uncertain dates increasing the inaccuracy.

Because of the inadequacies of clinical diagnosis, weighted risk factor scoring systems that incorporate measurements of abdominal girth and fundal height (Table 1) have been formulated[84]. Wennergren and colleagues[85], in an unselected small series of 611 patients, showed that such scoring systems may improve sensitivity to 100% and specificity to 95.5%.

The measurement of symphysis fundal height has provoked interest since the late 1970s because of improved detection rates over simple clinical palpation[86–88]. Wide variations in sensitivity (46–86%, mean 67%) and specificity (79–89.5%)[7] have nevertheless been reported[89]. The reliability of the method with respect to interobserver variability is considered (by some) to be too great to consider fundal height measurement as a valid screening tool[90].

The controversy surrounding symphysis fundal height measurements serves to open a debate that is generic to the broader issue of assessing any biological variable measured antenatally as a surrogate or direct measure of IUGR; statisticians construct arguments concerned with mathematical precision that may be unattainable in complex biological systems associated with numerous and pervasive confounding variables. In the case of symphysis fundal height measurements, the acceptability of the measurement has been rejected because of the likelihood of interobserver variability producing a false positive or negative result. This argument has been derived by assuming that the extreme confidence limits of interobserver variability are applicable to any given measurement; by making this assumption, even normal values may be converted to data above and below the 5th and 95th centile of normal population-based cross-sectional data. This is a statistically sound but clinically improbable argument because the mean interobserver variability (and not the extremes of interobserver variability) is likely to apply in most cases.

Precision in biological studies is often part of a spectrum. Clinical assessment remains an imprecise but essential adjunct to management and all methods of detecting growth retardation are inadequate to some degree. Symphysis fundal height may be the least inadequate of these methods. Similar statistical rigor has not been extracted from studies examining clinical palpation.

The role of ultrasound in the diagnosis of intrauterine growth restriction

Repeated ultrasound assessments are not feasible for all pregnant women; therefore the identification

Table 1 Wennergren risk scoring system[176]

Variable	Weighted value
Previous IUGR/SB/NND	1
BP 140/90 after 34 weeks	1
Renal disease/ UTI in pregnancy	1
Smoking	2
Bleeding/preterm labor	1
Inadequate weight gain	1
Decrease (or no gain) in abdominal girth	1
Decrease (or no gain) in fundal height	3

Score of ± 4: at risk of intrauterine growth restriction (IUGR)

of the growth restricted fetus begins with the clinical selection of high-risk pregnancies. These patients need early, accurate dating scans (if menstrual dates are uncertain) as well as serial follow-up sonography to evaluate interval fetal growth and to assess the state of fetal wellbeing.

Biparietal diameter measurements Biparietal diameter (BPD) measurements correlate poorly with the development of IUGR. Sensitivity rates range from 43.8% to 100% with most values between 50% and 60%. A wide range of positive predictive values are also noted (6–86%)[91–98]. There are a number of reasons for these wide discrepancies: firstly sensitivity improves with gestational age because of the increasing difference between the appropriately grown fetus and the affected infant as gestation progresses. This is reflected in studies that show an improvement in positive predictive value from 41% in the early third trimester to 61% at term[99]. The second reason for the poor performance of BPD measurements in the detection of growth restricted babies lies in the pattern of growth retardation studied. Symmetrically small babies will have small heads; an overall sensitivity of 67%, separated into symmetrical and asymmetrical groups, show respective sensitivities of 94% and 42%[100].

Head circumference measurements may be preferable to BPD measurements because the latter are influenced by the fetal lie and position as well as the normal variations that occur in fetal head shape during pregnancy. Warsof et al.[101] analyzed the scans of 3616 pregnancies and showed that among 450 IUGR fetuses the BPD had a sensitivity of 89% (positive predictive value 68%) compared to head circumference measurements with a sensitivity of 63% (positive predictive value of 75%). This led to the conclusion that head circumference may be the preferable measurement because of a better positive predictive value.

Femur length The growth of the femur is similar to that of the biparietal diameter[102]. It is affected early in symmetrical IUGR but late in asymmetrical growth restriction. It has a linear relationship to crown–heel length in the neonatal period and hence has been shown to be a better predictor of symmetrical growth restriction[103]. O'Brien and Queenan[103] showed a reduced femur length (FL) in 60% of IUGR fetuses, the vast majority having symmetrical IUGR.

Chinn and colleagues[104] have demonstrated that the presence of distal femoral and proximal tibial ossification centers correlates with a gestational age of greater than 35 weeks. This is a useful sonographic feature when scanning patients whose gestational age is unknown because of unreliable menstrual dates.

Abdominal circumference As a single measure, the abdominal circumference (AC) has a better correlation with growth restriction than either BPD or FL[92,98,101,105]. AC measurements reflect hepatic size (and to a lesser degree the amount of subcutaneous fat). Hepatic size decreases with nutritional deprivation and experimental animal work suggests that the AC is the first fetal parameter to show diminished growth[106].

AC measurements less than the 25th centile, have a sensitivity of 83–86% and a specificity of 79–80% in the detection of IUGR[107,108]. They are better predictors of low birthweight than either ponderal index or morphometric ratios although less sensitive in detecting symmetrical IUGR[107].

The choice of percentile used to define abnormal AC measurements influences the predictive value of the test. Decreasing the centile value to the 10th centile decreases the sensitivity of the test but improves the specificity.

Gestational age may also influence the predictive value of the test: Warsof *et al.*[109] showed a maximum sensitivity of 70% at 34 weeks gestation and suggested that this was the optimum gestational age for screening. Ferrazzi[99] noted a sensitivity of 41% at 29 to 31 weeks but this improved to 88% at term.

The direct measurement of liver size to predict growth retardation has been disappointing; sensitivity varies between 46 and 100%, depending on gestational age at the time of measurement and the cut-off values used[89,110].

Morphometric ratios Head circumference (HC) to AC ratios and FL to AC ratios have been evaluated. In normal pregnancies, the HC/AC ratio falls linearly from 16 to 40 weeks gestation. At 34 to 36 weeks the HC equals the AC after which the AC becomes larger. Campbell and Thoms[111] have shown that a HC/AC ratio more than two standard deviations from the mean has a sensitivity of 70% to detect the growth restricted fetus. Others have shown similarly high sensitivities[92,112]. In growth restriction of mixed etiology, HC/AC ratios are less accurate (sensitivity of 36% with a true positive rate 67% and a specificity of 70%)[113]. FL to AC ratios have similar utility but are less sensitive[113,114].

Despite the reasonable sensitivity of these tests, the high false positive rates makes them a poor screening test for IUGR.

Ponderal index The ponderal index (PDI) of birthweight/crown–heel length[3] is used to identify the growth restricted, underweight for height neonate. It correlates well with the complications of birth asphyxia and neonatal hypoglycemia seen in these infants[107,116]. Consequently intrauterine measurements of a modified PDI have been examined as a diagnostic test for IUGR. The formula of AC/FL has been used because FL is reasonably well preserved in growth retarded babies and correlates with neonatal crown–heel length. AC is a reflection of soft tissue mass and neonatal weight. On theoretical grounds, the index is likely to perform poorly in symmetrically growth restricted babies but should show good correlation with asymmetrical growth restriction.

Normally the antenatal PDI increases with gestational age, being approximately 1.6 in the early third trimester and approaching 3 by term[116]. Contrary to theoretical considerations, clinical studies show a poor correlation between PDI and birth weight with sensitivities between 56 and 77% and specificities ranging from 82 to 84%[117,118]. The ability of the antenatal PDI to predict the neonatal PDI appears even worse with a sensitivity of 52% and specificity of 77%[107]. This may be due to significant interobserver variability noted in the measurements of the AC and FL in late pregnancy.

Estimated fetal weight The estimated fetal weight (EFW) is most commonly used to diagnose IUGR; it is the most accurate predictor of birthweight. It is demonstrably superior to AC, BPD, HC, FL/AC ratio, amniotic fluid index and Doppler velocimetry in the prediction of low birthweight[98,113,119,120].

BPD, HC, AC and FL are the commonly used parameters from which EFW is calculated. Various formulae exist for estimating the fetal weight; most rely heavily on the AC measurement for their accuracy. Using AC alone to calculate fetal weight has a 1 SD variability of 11.1 to 13.7%[121]. Formulae that incorporate both BPD and AC have an average variability of approximately 9%. Combined used of BPD, AC and FL has the least error for diagnosing the growth restricted baby[122-125].

Babies with EFW less than the 10th centile for weight are commonly regarded as small for gestational age. Using this criterion, EFW measurements have sensitivities for diagnosing IUGR that range from 87 to 90% with specificities of 80 to 87%[113,119]. Reducing the number of false positives may be achieved by using the fifth or even the third centiles.

Despite the apparent success of EFW in identifying abnormally grown babies it only separates small for gestational age fetuses from the majority of normally grown babies; it does not distinguish the constitutionally small baby from the functionally impaired fetus. Nor does it identify the large but growth restricted fetus.

Fetal growth velocity Growth is a functional measure of the fetal condition and hence a better determinant of fetal status than pure biometry. Growth is also independent of gestational age and an important factor when fetal age is unknown.

Numerous ultrasound centile charts exist that reflect cross-sectional population data. Menstrual dates are usually used as the dependent variable. There are numerous problems applying these models to the pattern of growth in individual fetuses. For example, growth patterns may vary significantly between populations due to ethnic variation, geographical location, socio-economic status, sex of the fetus and the maternal parity. Data collection methods, selection criteria and measurement techniques may also vary.

Longitudinally constructed growth charts are similar to those derived from cross-sectional studies but the confidence intervals are narrower[126]. Growth velocity may also be derived for a particular fetus by using the Deter and Rossavik model that predicts individual growth patterns from specific biometric measurements in the second trimester[127,128]. This approach is promising but needs further clinical evaluation.

Having elected to use a particular set of centile charts, the definition of 'poor' or abnormal growth velocity is also difficult. Because of intra- and inter-observer variability, measurements should be taken at a minimum of two-weekly intervals. The obvious absence of growth or very minimal growth is abnormal even if the growth curve is above the 10th centile. However, quantifying the limits of normal variation is more difficult.

Various measurements have been used to assess growth velocity; BPD and HC both reflect brain size; FL correlates with skeletal size; AC reflects growth of the liver and somatic tissues while EFW the overall size of the fetus. AC and EFW appear to be the most accurate in detecting growth restriction[129].

Growth of the fetal abdomen is linear from 16 weeks gestation, thus providing an age-independent parameter to assess fetal growth. Divon[129] showed a mean growth rate of 6.0 mm (SD 4.9 mm)/14 days in 40 IUGR fetuses compared to 14.7 mm (SD 7.1 mm)/14 days in 50 normal fetuses. Growth in AC of less than 10 mm in 14 days had a sensitivity of 85% and a specificity of 74% for detecting low birthweight.

Growth velocity measurements in respect of the BPD are less predictive of IUGR than the AC. This is due to 'head sparing' in asymmetrical IUGR with a late decline in head growth measurements. There is also significant physiological variability in the BPD and head shape within the third trimester giving rise to a broad pattern of normal variation.

Amniotic fluid volume With centralization of blood flow in the growth restricted fetus reduced renal perfusion leads to a diminution in urine output. Oligohydramnios develops because fetal urine is the major component of liquor volume after 20 weeks gestation. Amniotic fluid volume therefore reflects the functional status of the fetus. The development of oligohydramnios may occur, however, under other circumstances, namely fetal renal agenesis, preterm rupture of membranes and in post-dates pregnancies.

The measurement of the amniotic fluid volume should occur in a reproducible, semi-quantitative manner. Manning *et al.*[130], defining oligohydramnios as the largest pool of liquor being less than 1 cm in diameter, was able to predict IUGR in 26 of 29 infants from a group of 120 high-risk cases (sensitivity 90%, specificity 93.4%). Subsequent studies have not been able to replicate this data: Hoddick *et al.*[131] using the same definition only predicted 5 of 125 small-for-gestational age (SGA) individuals. Others, using a less strict definition (largest vertical pocket less than 2 cm) showed a sensitivity of 16%, with specificity of 98% and a positive predictive value of 78%[113].

Philipson et al.[132] suggested a three tiered diagnosis of oligohydramnios ranging from 'obvious lack of amniotic fluid' to 'poor fluid–fetal interface' and in the most severe cases 'marked crowding of the fetal small parts'. With this he was able to predict IUGR with a sensitivity of 40% and a specificity of 92%. Patterson et al.[133] measured and averaged the vertical and two perpendicular horizontal diameters of the largest pocket of fluid that was free of cord or fetal parts and showed that an average diameter of 10 mm had a poor sensitivity of 27% but that increasing this to 32 mm gave a sensitivity of 40% and a specificity of 91%.

More work needs to be done on the best method of assessing amniotic fluid volume in order to use it more precisely in defining IUGR.

Placental changes　Grannum et al.[134] first described a placental grading of grade 0 to 3 in 1979. In early pregnancy the placenta was homogenous and lacked calcification (grade 0). With maturation it developed extensive calcification with indentations from the chorionic plate to the basal layer (grade 3). By 40 weeks gestation 30% of fetuses have grade 3 placentae[135]. Kazzi et al.[136,137] showed that early mutation of the placenta correlated well with the diagnosis of IUGR.

Placental grading, however, remains subjective with a high false-negative rate and dependence on gestational age.

Because IUGR is also associated with decreased placental weight, placental size has been examined as a predictor of IUGR. This has been approached by performing serial sonograms at 1 to 2 cm intervals in transverse and longitudinal directions[138,139]. This is a time consuming test to perform with wide interobserver variability and poor reproducibility. It has little role in clinical practice.

Total intrauterine volume　Total intrauterine volume represents the combined fetal and placental mass plus the liquor volume. Theoretically, any reduction in growth would be reflected in a reduction in the intrauterine volume. Gohari et al.[140] derived a method for calculating total intrauterine volume using the sonographic measurements of longitudinal, transverse and anterior–posterior measurements of the uterus. Using this method 75% of the IUGR fetuses were identified. The accuracy of this

measurement has not been replicated in other studies which have only shown a 41% accuracy in predicting IUGR[141]. Kurtz et al.[142] modified the measurement by developing the total uterine volume. Neither this measurement nor the total intrauterine volume have become routinely used for the detection of IUGR.

Transverse cerebellar diameter　Conflicting evidence exists regarding the value of transverse cerebellar diameter (TCD) in the detection of IUGR. It has been suggested that it is unaffected by growth restriction and hence is a good indicator of gestational age[139,143]. Cabbard found the TCD within the normal range for gestational age in IUGR fetuses. Discordance between TCD and the EFW predicted IUGR with a 96% sensitivity and specificity[144].

Animal experimental models of IUGR have, however, shown a significant reduction in cerebellar brain tissue growth. These findings have been confirmed by a series examining 44 SGA fetuses between 27 and 43 weeks which showed that TCD values more than 2 SD below the mean were present in 59.1% of the fetuses. A further 13.6% were 1–2 SD. below the mean and only 27.3% of cases fell within the normal range[145].

Two factors contribute to this conflicting evidence: first, the broad variance of normal values in the third trimester for measurements of the transverse cerebellar diameter and second, the measurement may only be of comparative use in asymmetrical growth restriction.

Other measurements　Researchers have looked at subcutaneous tissue thickness over the mid-calf and thigh as well as over the abdomen, but have not been able to find a significant difference between growth restricted and normal fetuses[146]. Calf and thigh circumference have been compared to femur and tibial length (reflecting both muscle mass and subcutaneous fat). Using these measurements Jeanty was able to calculate fetal limb volume which correlated with gestational age[148]. Femur length to thigh circumference and tibial length to calf circumference are relatively constant at different gestational ages. Vintzileos was able to detect 83.3% of IUGR fetuses using these ratios[149]. Hill et al.[150] showed, however, that an abnormal thigh circumference to FL ratio had a sensitivity of only 40.7% with a specificity of 95%. When Hill used only thigh circumference he was able to show that measures less than 2 SD below the mean were associated with a sensitivity of 78% and a specificity of 75% in suspected IUGR.

The value of limb circumference to length ratios would be poor in detecting symmetrical IUGR but of greater value in asymmetrical IUGR.

ANTENATAL MANAGEMENT AND ASSESSMENT OF FETAL WELLBEING

Few interventions have been attempted or shown to be of benefit in managing the growth restricted fetus. Two interventions deserve mention: maternal plasma volume expansion and hyperoxygenation have both been attempted[151,152]. Unfortunately, despite promising results reported with each of these interventions, the number of cases reported in each series is small and no clear conclusions can be reached.

Currently, the most important aspect of management therefore concerns the correct assessment of whether an affected fetus requires premature delivery.

Ultrasound plays a key role in this decision: Doppler velocimetry, and assessment of biophysical profile findings and cordocentesis have all contributed to more precise management of IUGR.

Doppler velocimetry

Doppler ultrasound flow velocity waveform analysis has added precision to the identification of growth restricted fetuses most at risk of perinatal mortality[153,154]. Umbilical artery Doppler velocimetry is, however, a poor screening test for intrauterine growth restriction in a low-risk population[155]. The reported sensitivity of velocimetry in the detection of IUGR ranges from 22 to 100% (specificity 73 to 95% and positive predictive value 9 to 71%). Compared to fetal biometry, Doppler velocimetry is a less sensitive test for the identification of the affected fetus[156–159]. This is true for growth restriction defined by weight criteria, PDI, skinfold thickness and mid-arm circumference/HC ratio[160]. Abnormal umbilical artery Doppler findings occur most commonly in those fetuses where growth restriction occurs because of uteroplacental vascular disease. Growth restriction associated with normal umbilical artery Doppler velocimetry may indicate the need to consider other etiological possibilities such as chromosomal and structural anomalies as well as congenital infections.

Abnormal umbilical artery velocimetry has long been recognized as a marker of increased perinatal mortality[161]. Nicolaides has shown that absent end diastolic flow is a marker of acidosis and hypoxia in 46 and 80% of fetuses respectively. Fetuses with either absent or reversed diastolic umbilical artery blood flow are more likely to be delivered by cesarean section for fetal distress, are more likely to be asphyxiated at delivery and have a higher incidence of neonatal complications such as hypoglycemia, cerebral hemorrhage and necotising enterocolitis. They are also more likely to require neonatal admission to intensive care[89,162,163]. Absent or reverse end-diastolic umbilical artery blood flow also correlates with poorer long-term neurological outcome.

Meta-analysis of randomized controlled trials examining the role of Doppler velocimetry in clinical management has shown that when clinicians are aware of Doppler findings there has been a statistically significant reduction in perinatal mortality[164]. As a clinical tool, it is an important adjunct to cardiotocography and some data would suggest that it may surpass cardiotocography by eliminating false positive tests. One such study showed that a Doppler ultrasound monitored group had fewer hospital admissions, fewer inductions of labor and fewer cesarean sections done for fetal distress than a comparable group of patients monitored by cardiotocography alone. This reduction in intervention was not associated with any change in substantive measures of perinatal outcome[165].

Despite the evidence accumulating in favor of widespread utilization of Doppler umbilical artery velocimetry, it should also be noted that normal velocimetry does not guarantee a normal outcome[166,167].

Umbilical artery versus multi-vessel flow velocity waveform analysis

The growth restricted fetus adapts to substrate deprivation in a number of ways (see above). Part of that adaptive mechanism depends on a redistribution of fetal blood flow ('centralization'). This manifests as increasing impedance to flow in the descending thoracic aorta matched to decreasing resistance in the distribution of the middle cerebral artery. These changes have been shown to be associated with falling umbilical venous pH and oxygen concentration[168]. Centralization may lead to discordant blood flow in the brachial blood supply to the left and right arms as well as decreased blood flow velocity in the venous system with increased pulsatility in the ductus venosus and inferior vena cava[168,169]. The fetal venous system is affected once centralization has occurred because rising peripheral resistance increases ventricular afterload leading to elevated end-diastolic pressure. This in turn increases atrial contractility with resultant pulsatility in the ductus venosus waveform.

Although the umbilical artery velocimetry is most frequently measured, flow velocity waveform analysis of the middle cerebral and thoracic aorta is also of value. The ratio of middle cerebral artery to aortic or middle cerebral artery to umbilical artery pulsatility index measured in growth restricted fetuses exhibits greater deviation from normal values than the velocimetry of any single vessel. It is also noteworthy that hemodynamic changes reflecting centralization may take place before any change is evident in the Doppler waveform of the umbilical artery[170].

The use of Doppler parameters other than the umbilical artery velocimetry as an adjunct to clinical management should be approached with caution because no adequately sized randomized studies exist yet to justify the use of these measurements in clinical practice. Preterm delivery based upon concern about abnormal velocimetry (other than umbilical artery findings) may lead to unjustifiable neonatal complications. Establishing the clinical utility of these measurements should take place within the confines of a properly monitored and designed randomized study.

Intraplacental villous vessel Doppler ultrasound

Arborization of the vascular tree leads to a progressively increasing surface area with descending order of vessel size. Consequently small changes in peripheral vessel diameter have a large influence on proximal impedance.

The presence or absence of intraplacental villous artery Doppler flow signals may be a further marker of severe disease in growth restricted fetuses. Villous flow is usually present even if the umbilical artery velocimetry is abnormal. Absent villous flow has been associated with a significantly greater risk of fetal distress[171].

Uterine artery Doppler

A low resistance circulation is established within the placenta as it invades the myometrium in the first half of pregnancy. Failure to achieve this has been associated with pre-eclampsia and/or IUGR. Assessing the uterine artery waveform with color flow Doppler has been used to describe abnormal placentation prior to the development of fetal or maternal disease.

In normal pregnancy there is a progressive increase in the diastolic flow in the uterine vessels reflected by a fall in resistance index, and gradual attenuation of the notching noted in the waveform from early pregnancy.

An abnormal resistance index alone (or as part of an averaged resistance index) has poor sensitivity for detecting IUGR (15%) but is associated with a 9.8 times higher risk of developing severe complications. This predictive value increases with gestational age but sensitivity remains low (36%)[172]. The persistence of uterine artery notching has better sensitivity (70%) but the specificity remains low[173].

The role of cordocentesis

Cordocentesis is used to exclude aneuploidy and fetal infection in growth restricted infants[174]. It also allows blood gas analysis in affected infants. The use of cordocentesis for the latter purpose should be restricted to babies with abnormal umbilical artery velocimetry since growth restricted fetuses with normal cardiotocography and normal velocimetry are unlikely to be acidotic or hypoxic[175]. The probability of identifying an acidotic, hypoxic fetus increases with increasingly abnormal tests of fetal wellbeing[175]. Hence babies that have abnormal fetal heart rate patterns combined with abnormal flow velocity waveform analysis are more likely to be acidotic than those with abnormal velocimetry alone. Although the degree of acidemia may be correlated with the extent of the changes seen in the arterial and venous systems of the fetus, only cross-sectional data exist at present and interpolation of fetal blood gas status from the Doppler findings is not yet possible.

Cordocentesis may also play a role in identifying hypoxic fetuses where other forms of fetal monitoring have indicated that the baby may be compromised. Abnormal biophysical profiles are uniformly associated with acidosis where the profile is scored at 0 out of 10 and uniformly associated with normal values where the score is 10 out of 10[176]. Between these extremes, cordocentesis may help to limit iatrogenic preterm delivery by excluding hypoxia and allowing continuation of the pregnancy.

Cordocentesis is associated with a risk of intrauterine death. The neonatal prognosis of babies delivered greater than 1500 grams in weight is probably sufficiently good to preclude cordocentesis as a diagnostic procedure carried out in preference to delivery of the baby[174].

The role of biophysical profile

The use of ultrasound examination to generate a biophysical profile of fetal movement, tone and fetal breathing movement has been advocated since the 1980s. The addition of an accumulative number of variables to the biophysical profile has been associated with an improved predictive value for the detection of abnormal perinatal outcome[177].

Highly abnormal tests are unequivocally associated with fetal acidosis as well as perinatal morbidity and mortality[149,176]. Regrettably, little randomized data exist despite the longevity of this test of fetal wellbeing. Those which are available compares biophysical profile monitoring to the use of cardiotocography alone and fails to confirm the clinical utility of the test. No improvement in perinatal outcome accrues from the use of biophysical profile monitoring compared to the cardiotocography alone[148]. Further, larger randomized studies are justified to confirm or refute these findings.

THE DECOMPENSATED FETUS AND LONG TERM SEQUELAE OF IUGR

Neonatal death as well as many other short-term neonatal complications (respiratory distress syndrome, hypoglycemia, transient neurological signs) occur more frequently in growth restricted infants[1,2]. The frequency of abnormal outcome is directly related to the severity of the underlying IUGR. The risk of cerebral palsy is likewise increased in IUGR babies.

Nutritional deprivation augments hypoxic damage; growth restricted babies have diminished levels of essential amino acids that are known to be required for normal brain development and which have been associated with experimentally induced visual and cognitive impairment periventricular hemorrhage[177]. Renal changes have also been linked to IUGR: growth restriction induced in rats by both ischemia and protein deficient diets ends in the delivery of offspring that have significantly fewer nephrons in direct correlation to the birthweight of the growth retarded animals[178]. These data find clinical expression in reporting of renal damage *in utero* as well as persistently abnormal renal blood flow occurring in growth restricted infants during their neonatal period[179,180].

Recent work has drawn attention to the possibility that intrauterine events may result in adult disease. This has been referred to as the fetal origins hypothesis. Hypertension has been associated with prior intrauterine growth restriction in several studies[4,5]. A fetal origin has also been linked to the occurrence of coronary heart disease with the notion arising that fetal endocrine adaptation to a hostile environment 'imprints' for life leading to the evolution of cardiovascular disease in adulthood[181,182]. The problem with these theories lies not in the association between intrauterine events and adult disease rather than our inability to distinguish between the effects of nature and nurture. In essence, the genes that cause hypertension in the mother may be present in the offspring; is later hypertensive disease then the consequence of the inherited genes or the associated growth restriction that occurred in the pregnancy because the mother was hypertensive?

CONCLUSION

Intrauterine growth restriction is a complex miscellany of conditions. Ultrasound is the cornerstone of accurate diagnosis as well as the key to successful monitoring. Ultrasound has given us (and continues to do so) a far better understanding of fetal pathophysiology. What remains to be established is which tests of fetal wellbeing are likely to provide the best clinical precision with respect to preterm delivery.

Acknowledgement

The authors would like to thank Professor David Woods for his help in the preparation of the script.

References

1. Piper JM, Xenakis EM, McFarland M, *et al*. Do growth retarded premature infants have different rates of perinatal morbidity and mortality than appropriately grown premature infants? *Obstet Gynecol* 1996;87:169–74

2. Spinillo A, Capuzzo E, Egbe TO, *et al*. Pregnancies complicated by idiopathic intrauterine growth retardation. Severity of growth failure, neonatal morbidity and 2 year infant neurodevelopmental outcome. *J Reprod Med* 1995;40:209–15

3. Barker DJ, Gluckman PD, Godfrey KM, *et al*. Fetal nutrition and cardiovascular disease in adult life. *Lancet* 1993;341:938–41

4. Barker DJ. Fetal origins of adult hypertension. *J Hypertens* 1992;10(Suppl.):S39–44

5. Williams S, St George IM, Silva PA. Intrauterine growth retardation and blood pressure at age 7 and 18. *J Clin Epidemiol* 1992;45:1257–63

6. Uvebrant P, Hagberg G. Intrauterine growth in children with cerebral palsy. *Acta Paediatr* 1992;81:407–12

7. Mahadevan N, Pearce M, Steer P. The proper measure of intrauterine growth retardation is function, not size. *Br J Obstet Gynaecol* 1994;101:1032–5

8. Georgiff MK, Sasanow SR, Mammel MC, *et al*. Mid arm circumference/head circumference ratios for identification of symptomatic LGA, AGA and SGA newborn infant death syndrome. *Paediatr Path* 1996;13:333–43

9. Oakley JR, Parsons RJ, Whitelaw AGL. Standards for skinfold thickness in British newborn infants. *Arch Dis Child* 1977;52:287–90

10. Deter RL, Rossavik IK. A simplified method for determining individual growth curb standards. *Obstet Gynecol* 1977;70:101–5

11. Wilcox MA, Johnson I, Maynard PV, *et al*. The individualised birthweight ratio: a more logical outcome measure of pregnancy than birthweight alone. *Br J Obstet Gynaecol* 1993;100:342–7

12. Deter RL, Harrist RB, Hill RM. Neonatal growth assessment score: a new approach to the detection of intrauterine growth retardation in the newborn. *Am J Obstet Gynecol* 1990;162:1030–6

13. Deter RL, Nazar R, Milner LL. Modified neonatal growth assessment score: a multivariate approach to the detection of intrauterine growth retardation in the neonate. *Ultrasound Obstet Gynecol* 1995;6:400–10

14. Altman DJ, Chitty LS. Charts of fetal size. 1. Methodology. *Br J Obstet Gynaecol* 1994;101:29–34

15. Deter RL, Harrist RB, Hadlock FP, *et al*. Longitudinal studies of fetal growth which use dynamic image ultrasonography. *Am J Obstet Gynecol* 1992;143:545–54

16. Gallivan S, Robson SC, Chang TC, *et al*. An investigation of fetal growth using serial ultrasound data. *Ultrasound Obstet Gynecol* 1993;3:109–14

17. Right EV. Chromosomes and human fetal development. In Roberts DF, Tomson AM, eds. *The Biology of Human Fetal Growth*. London: Taylor and Francis, 1976:237–52

18. Hook EB. Prevalence of chromosome abnormalities during human gestation and implications for studies of environmental mutigens. *Lancet* 1991;2:169–72

19. den Hollander NS, Cohen-Overbeek TE, Heydanus R, *et al*. Cordocentesis for rapid karyotyping in fetuses with congenital anomalies or severe IUGR. *Eur J Obstet Gynecol Reprod Biol* 1994;53:183–7

20. Snijders RJ, Sheerod C, Gosden CM, *et al*. Fetal growth retardation associated malformations and chromosomal abnormalities. *Am J Obstet Gynecol* 1993;168:547–55

21. Wolstenholme J, Rooney DE, Davison EV. Confined placental mosaicism, IUGR, and adverse pregnancy outcome: a controlled retrospective UK collaborative survey. *Prenat Diag* 1994;14:345–61

22. Keirse MJNC. Epidemiology and aetiology of the growth retarded baby. *Clin Obstet Gynecol* 1984;11:415–36

23. Meuris S, Piko VV, Eerens P, *et al*. Gestational malaria: assessment of its consequences on fetal growth. *Am J Trop Med Hyg* 1993;48:603–9

24. Myatt L. Nitric oxide. Presented at the 10th World Congress of the International Society for the Study of Hypertension in Pregnancy. Seattle, 1996

25. Longo LD. Maternal blood volume and cardiac output during pregnancy: a hypothesis of endocrinologic control. *Am J Physiol* 1983;245:720–5

26. Brosens I, Robertson WB, Dixon HG. The physiological response of the vessels of the placental bed to normal pregnancy. *J Path Bact* 1967;93:569–79

27. Duvekot JJ, Cheriex EC, Pieters FA, *et al*. Maternal volume homeostasis in early pregnancy in relation to fetal growth restriction. *Obstet Gynecol* 1995;85:361–7

28. Pijnenborg R, Anthony J, Davey DA, *et al*. Placental bed spiral arteries in the hypertensive disorders of pregnancy. *Br J Obstet Gynaecol* 1991;98:648–55

29. Salafia CM, Vogel CA, Bhantham KF, *et al*. Preterm delivery: correlations of fetal growth and placental pathology. *Am J Perinatol* 1992;9:190–3

30. Nasiell J, Blanck A, Lunell NO, *et al*. Altered mRNA expression of placental nitric oxide synthase in pregnancies complicated by pre-eclampsia and or intrauterine growth retardation. Presented at the 10th World Congress of the International Society for the Study of Hypertension in Pregnancy. Seattle, 1996

31. Rodgers GM, Taylor RN, Roberts JM. Pre-eclampsia is associated with a serum factor cytotoxic to human endothelial cells. *Am J Obstet Gynecol* 1988;159:908–14

32. Lyall F, Greer JA. Pre-eclampsia: a multifaceted vascular disorder of pregnancy. *J Hypertens* 1994;12: 1339–45

33. Stein Z, Susser M. The Dutch Famine 1944–1945, and the reproductive process. I. Effects on six indices at birth. *Pediatr Res* 1975;9:70

34. Nicolini U, Hubinont C, Santolaya J, *et al*. Effects of fetal intravenous glucose challenge in normal and growth retarded fetuses. *Horm Metab Res* 1990;22: 426–30

35. Lockwood CJ, Rand JH. The immunobiology and obstetrical consequences of antiphospholipid antibodies. *Obstet Gynecol Surv* 1994;49:432–41

36. Gilman-Sachs A, Lubinski J, Beer AE, *et al*. Patterns of anti-phospholipids antibodies specificities. *J Clin Lab Immunol* 1991;35:83–8

37. Bocciolone L, Meroni P, Parazzini F, *et al*. Anti-phospholipids antibodies and risk of intrauterine late fetal death. *Acta Obstet Gynecol Scand* 1994;73: 389–92

38. Ruiz JE, Cubillos, Mendoza JC, *et al*. Aorta antibodies to phospholipids and nuclear antigens in non pregnant and pregnant Colombian women with recurrent spontaneous abortions. *J Reprod Immunol* 1995;28: 41–51

39. Lynch A, Marlar R, Murphy J, *et al*. Antiphospholipid antibodies in predicting adverse pregnancy outcome. A prospective study. *Ann Intern Med* 1994;120:470–5

40. Brown MA, Buddle MC. The importance of non-proteinuric hypertension in pregnancy. *Hyperten Preg* 1995;14:57–65

41. Sermer M. Congenital Heart Disease in Pregnancy. Presented at the Combined meeting of the Obstetric Medicine Groups (Society of Obstetric Medicine, McDonald Club, Obstetric Medicine Group of Australia, South African Obstetric Medicine Group). Seattle, August 1996

42. Berg K, Roald B, Sande H. High Lp (a) lypho protein level in maternal serum may interfere with placental circulation and cause fetal growth retardation. *Clin Genet* 1994;46:52–6

43. Tuck SM, Studd JWW, White JM. Pregnancy in sickle cell disease in the UK. *Br J Obstet Gynaecol* 1983;90:112–17

44. Lieberman E, Gremy I, Lang JM, *et al*. Low birth weight at term and the timing of fetal exposure to maternal smoking. *Am J Public Health* 1994;84: 1127–31

45. Pirani BBK. Smoking during pregnancy. *Obstet Gynecol Surv* 1978;33:1–13

46. Rosett HL, Weiner L, Lee A, *et al*. Patterns of alcohol consumption and fetal development. *Obstet Gynecol* 1983;61:539–46

47. Little BB, Snell LM. Brain growth among fetuses exposed to cocaine *in utero*. Asymmetrical growth retardation. *Obstet Gynecol* 1991;77:361–4

48. Battino D, Granata T, Binelli S, *et al*. Intrauterine growth in the offspring of epileptic mothers. *Acta Neurol Scand* 1992;86:555–7

49. Berar HS, Platt LD. Reverse endiastolic flow velocity on umbilical artery velocimetry in high risk pregnancies: an ominous finding with adverse pregnancy outcome. *Am J Obstet Gynecol* 1988;159: 559

50. Rochelson B, Schulman H, Farmakides G, *et al*. The significance of absent endiastolic velocity in umbilical artery waveforms. *Am J Obstet Gynecol* 1987;156:1213–8

51. Giles WB, Trudinger VJ, Baird PJ. Fetal umbilical artery flow velocity waveforms and placenta resistance: pathological correlations. *Br J Obstet Gynaecol* 1985;92:31–8

52. Copel JA, Schlafer D, Wentworth R, *et al*. Does the umbilical artery systolic/diastolic ratio reflect flow or acidosis? An umbilical artery Doppler study of fetal sheep. *Am J Obstet Gynecol* 1990;163:751–6

53. Jackson MR, Walsh AJ, Morrow RJ, *et al*. Reduced placental villous tree elaboration in small for gestational age pregnancies: relationship with umbilical artery Doppler waveforms. *Am J Obstet Gynecol* 1995;172:518–25

54. Macara L, Kingdom JCP, Kohnen G, *et al*. Elaboration of stem villous vessels in growth restricted pregnancies with abnormal umbilical artery Doppler waveforms. *Br J Obstet Gynaecol* 1995;102:807–12

55. McQueen J, Kingdom JC, Connell JM, *et al*. Fetal endothelin levels and placental vascular endo-thelin receptors in intrauterine growth retard-ation. *Obstet Gynecol* 1993;82:992–8

56. Kingdom JC, McQueen J, Connell JM, *et al*. Fetal angiotensin II levels and vascular (type I) angiotensin receptors in pregnancies complicated by intrauterine growth retardation. *Br J Obstet Gynaecol* 1983;100:476–82

57. Rizzo G, Montuschi P, Capponi A, *et al*. Blood levels of vasoactive intestinal polypeptide in normal and growth retarded fetuses: relationship with acid-base and haemodynamic status. *Early Hum Dev* 1995;41:69–77

58. Ville Y, Proudler A, Kuhn P, *et al*. Aldosterone concentration in normal, growth retarded, anaemic, and hydropic fetuses. *Obstet Gynecol* 1994;84:511–4

59. Ville Y, Proudler A, Abbas A, et al. Atrial natriuretic factor concentration in normal, growth retarded, anaemic and hydropic fetuses. Am J Obstet Gynecol 1994;171:777–83

60. Marconi AM, Paolini C, Puscaglia M, et al. The impact of gestational age in fetal growth and the maternal–fetal glucose concentration difference. Obstet Gynecol 1996;87:937–42

61. Jansson T, Wennergren M, Illsley NP. Glucose transporter protein expression in human placenta throughout gestation and in intrauterine growth retardation. J Clin Endocrinol Metab 1993;77:1554–62

62. Economides DL, Proudler A, Nicolaides KH. Plasma insulin in appropriate and small for gestational age fetuses. Am J Obstet Gynecol 1989;160:1091–4

63. Nicolini U, Huvinont J, Santolaya J, et al. Effects of fetal intravenous glucose challenge in normal and growth retarded fetuses. Horm Metab Res 1990;22:426–30

64. Hubinont C, Nicolini U, Fisk NM, et al. Endocrine pancreatic function in growth retarded fetuses. Obstet Gynecol 1991;77:541–4

65. Soothill PW, Ajayi RA, Nicolaides KH. Fetal biochemistry in growth retardation. Early Hum Dev 1992;29:91–7

66. Cetin I, Corbetta C, Serenio LP, et al. Umbilical aminoacid concentration in normal and growth retarded fetuses sampled in utero by cordocentesis. Am J Obstet Gynecol 1990;162:253–61

67. Bernardini I, Evans MI, Nicolaides KH, et al. The fetal concentrating index has a gestational age independent measure of placental dysfunction in intrauterine growth retardation. Am J Obstet Gynecol 1991;164:1481–90

68. Whitehead RG. Rapid determination of some plasma amino acids in sub-clinical kwashiorkor. Lancet 1964;1:250–2

69. Arosio M, Cortelazzi D, Persani L, et al. Circulating levels of growth hormone insulin-like growth factor-I and prolactin in normal, growth retarded and enencephalic human fetuses. J Endocrinol Invest 1995;18:346–53

70. Nieto-Diaz A, Villar J, Matorras-Weinig R, et al. Intrauterine growth retardation at term: association between anthropometric and endocrine parameters. Acta Obstet Gynecol Scand 1996;75:127–31

71. Giudice LC, De Zegher F, Gargosky SE, et al. Insulin like growth factors and their binding proteins in the term and preterm human fetus and neonate with normal and extremes of intrauterine growth. J Clin Endocrinol Metab 1995;80:1548–55

72. Kamei Y, Tsutsumi O, Cuwabara Y, et al. Intrauterine growth retardation and fetal loses are caused by epidermal growth factor deficiency in mice. Am J Physiol 1993;264:597

73. Shigeta K, Hiramatsu T, Eguchi K, Seikba K. Urinary and plasma epidermal growth factor levels are decreased in neonates with intrauterine growth retardation and in their mothers. Biol Neonate 1992;62:76–82

74. Thorpe-Beeston JG, Nicolaides KH, Felton CV, et al. Thyroid function in small for gestational age fetuses. Obstet Gynecol 1991;77:701–6

75. Economides DL, Nicolaides KH, Linton EA, et al. Plasma cortisol and ACTH in appropriate and small for gestational age fetuses. Fetal Ther 1989;3:158–64

76. Goland RS, Jozak S, Warren WB, et al. Elevated levels of umbilical cord plasma corticotrophin-releasing hormone in growth retarded fetuses. J Clin Endocrinol Metab 1993;77:1174–9

77. Snijders RJ, Abbas A, Melby O, et al. Fetal plasma erythropoietin concentration in severe growth retardation. Am J Obstet Gynecol 1993;168:615–9

78. Uvebrant P, Hagberg G. Intrauterine growth in children with cerebral palsy. Acta Paediatr 1992;81:407–12

79. Leth H, Toft PB, Pryds O, et al. Brain lactate in preterm and growth retarded neonates. Acta Paediatr 1995;84:495–9

80. Barth A, Bauer R, Kluge H, et al. Brain peroxidative and glutathione status after moderate hypoxia in normal weight and intrauterine growth restricted newborn piglets. Exp Toxicol Pathol 1995;47:139–47

81. Thordstein M, Lilsson UA. Cerebral lipid perioxidation in the growth retarded rat fetus under normoxia and hypoxia. J Perinat Med 1992;20:15–23

82. Steller H. Mechanisms and genes of cellular suicide. Sciences 1995;267:1445–9

83. Hall MH, Chng PK, MacGillivray I. Is routine antenatal care worthwhile? Lancet 1980;2:78

84. Simpson GF, Creasy RK. Obstetric management of the growth retarded baby. Clin Obstet Gynecol 1994;11:481–97

85. Wennergren M, Karisson K, Olsson T. A scoring system for antenatal identification of fetal growth retardation. Br J Obstet Gynaecol 1982;89:320–4

86. Rosenberg K, Grant JM, Aitchison T. Measurement of fundal height as a screening test for fetal growth retardation. Br J Obstet Gynaecol 1992;89:447–50

87. Persson B, Stangenberg M, Lunell NO, et al. Prediction of size of infants at birth by measurement of symphysis fundus height. Br J Obstet Gynaecol 1996;93:206–11

88. Lindhard A, Nielsen PV, Mouritsen LA, et al. Implications of introducing the symphyseal–fundal height measurement. A prospective randomised controlled trial. Br J Obstet Gynaecol 1990;97:675–80

89. Sabrina D, Craigo. The role of ultrasound in the diagnosis and management of intrauterine growth retardation. Semin Perinatol 1994;18:292–304

90. Bailey SM, Grant JM. Clinical detection of the small fetus: requiem for the symphysis fundal height. In Studd J, ed. *The Yearbook of the Royal College of Obstetricians and Gynaecologists, 1995*. London: RCOG Press, 1995:231–8

91. Lee JN, Chard T. Determination of biparietal diameter in the second trimester as a predictor of intrauterine growth retardation. *Int J Gynaecol Obstet* 1983;21:213–5

92. Kurjak A, Kirkinen P, Latin V. Biometric and dynamic ultrasound assessment of small-for-dates infants: report of 260 cases. *Obstet Gynecol* 1980;56:281–4

93. Hughey MJ. Routine ultrasound for detection and management of the small-for-gestational-age fetus. *Obstet Gynecol* 1984;64:101–7

94. Sabbagha RE. Intrauterine growth retardation. Antenatal diagnosis by ultrasound. *Obstet Gynecol* 1978;52:252–6

95. Hohler CW, Lea J, Collins H. Screening for intrauterine growth retardation using the ultrasound biparietal diameter. *J Clin Ultrasound* 1976;4:187–91

96. Crane JP, Kopta MM, Welt SI, et al. Abnormal fetal growth patterns. Ultrasonic diagnosis and management. *Obstet Gynecol* 1977;50:205–11

97. Queenan JT, Kubarych SF, Cook LN, et al. Diagnostic ultrasound for detection of intrauterine growth retardation. *Am J Obstet Gynecol* 1976;124:865–73

98. Batra A, Chellani HK, Mahajan J, et al. Ultrasonic variables in the diagnosis of intrauterine growth retardation. *Indian J Med Res* 1990;92:399–403

99. Ferrazzi E, Nicolini U, Kustermann A, et al. Routine obstetric ultrasound: effectiveness of cross-sectional screening for fetal growth retardation. *J Clin Ultrasound* 1986;14:17–22

100. Fescini RH, Martell M, Martinez G, et al. Small for dates: evaluation of different diagnostic methods. *Acta Obstet Gynecol Scand* 1987;66:221

101. Warsof SL, Cooper DJ, Little D, et al. *Obstet Gynecol* 1986;67:33–9

102. Woo J, Wan CW, Fang A, et al. Is fetal femur length a better indicator of gestational age in the growth-retarded fetus as compared with biparietal diameter? *J Ultrasound Med* 1985;4:132

103. O'Brien GD, Queenan JT. Ultrasound fetal femur length in relation to intrauterine growth retardation. Part II. *Am J Obstet Gynecol* 1982;144:35–9

104. Chinn DH, Bolding DB, Callen PW, et al. Ultrasonographic identification of fetal lower extremity epiphyseal ossification centers. *Radiology* 1983;147:185–8

105. Weiner CP, Robinson D. Sonographic diagnosis of intrauterine growth retardation using the postnatal ponderal index and the crown-heel length as standards of diagnosis. *Am J Perinatol* 1989;6:380–3

106. Barbera A, Jones OW 3rd, Zerbe GO, et al. Early ultrasonographic detection of fetal growth retardation in an ovine model of placental insufficiency. *Am J Obstet Gynecol* 1995;173:1071–4

107. Sarmandal P, Grant GM. Effectiveness of ultrasound determination of fetal abdominal circumference and fetal ponderal index in the diagnosis of asymmetrical growth retardation. *Br J Obstet Gynaecol* 1990;97:118–23

108. Pearce JM, Campbell S. A comparison of symphysis-fundal height and ultrasound as screening tests for light for-gestational age infants. *Br J Obstet Gynaecol* 1987;94:100–4

109. Warsof SI, Cooper DJ, Little D, et al. Routine ultrasound screening for antenatal detection of intrauterine growth retardation. *Obstet Gynecol* 1986;67:33–9

110. Murao F, Takamiya O, Yamamoto K, et al. Detection of intrauterine growth retardation based on measurements of size of the liver. *Gynecol Obstet Invest* 1990;29:26–31

111. Campbell S, Thoms A. Ultrasound measurement of the fetal head to abdomen circumference ratio in the assessment of growth retardation. *Br J Obstet Gynaecol* 1977;84:165–74

112. Crane JP, Kopta MM. Prediction of intrauterine growth retardation via ultrasonically measured head/abdominal circumference ratio. *Obstet Gynecol* 1979;54:597–601

113. Divon MY, Guidetti DA, Braverman JJ, et al. Intrauterine growth retardation – a prospective study of the diagnostic value of real-time sonography combined with umbilical artery flow velocimetry. *Obstet Gynecol* 1988;72:611–4

114. Hadlock FP, Deter RL, Harrist RB, et al. A date-independent predictor of intrauterine growth retardation: femur length/abdominal circumference ratio. *Am J Obstet Gynecol* 1983;141:979–84

115. Varma TR, Taylor H, Bridges C. Ultrasound assessment of fetal growth. *Br J Obstet Gynaecol* 1979;86:623–32

116. Gross W, Michele W, Seewald HJ, et al. Synchronous cardiotocographic registration of fetal body and respiratory movements in placenta insufficiency. *Zentralbl Gynakol* 1989;111:433–43

117. Chellani HK, Mahajan J, Batra A, et al. Fetal ponderal index in predicting growth. *Indian J Med Res* 1990;92:163–6

118. Vintzileos AM, Lodeiro JG, Feinstein SJ, et al. Value of fetal ponderal index in predicting growth retardation. *Obstet Gynecol* 1986;67:584–8

119. Dudley NJ, Lamb MP, Hatfield JA, et al. Estimated fetal weight in the detection of the small-for-menstrual-age fetus. *J Clin Ultrasound* 1990;18:387–93

120. Laurin J, Persson PH. Ultrasound screening for detection of intra-uterine growth retardation. *Acta Obstet Gynecol Scand* 1987;66:493–500

121. Mintz M, Landon M. Sonographic diagnosis of fetal growth disorders. *Clin Obstet Gynecol* 1988; 31:44–52

122. Hadlock FP, Harrist RB, Carpenter RJ, *et al.* Sonographic estimation of fetal weight. The value of femur length in addition to head and abdomen measurements. *Radiology* 1984;150:535–40

123. Guidetti DA, Divon MY, Braverman JJ, *et al.* Sonographic estimates of fetal weight in the intrauterine growth retardation population. *Am J Perinatol* 1990;7:5–7

124. Woo JS, Wan MC. An evaluation of fetal weight prediction using a simple equation containing the fetal femur length. *J Ultrasound Med* 1986;5:453–7

125. Hadlock FP, Harrist RB, Sharman RS, *et al.* Estimation of fetal weight with the use of head, body and femur measurements – a prospective study. *Am J Obstet Gynecol* 1985;151:333–7

126. Deter RL, Harrist RB, Hadlock FP, *et al.* Longitudinal studies of fetal growth with the use of dynamic image ultrasonography. *Am J Obstet Gynecol* 1982;143:545–54

127. Rossavik IK, Deter RL. Mathematical modeling of fetal growth: I. Basic principles. *J Clin Ultrasound* 1984;12:329–33

128. Deter RL, Rossavik IK, Harrist RB, *et al.* Mathematic modeling of fetal growth: development of individual growth curve standards. *Obstet Gynecol* 1986;67:156–61

129. Divon MY, Chamberlain PF, Sipos L, *et al.* Identification of the small for gestational age fetus with the use of gestational age-independent indices of fetal growth. *Am J Obstet Gynecol* 1986;155:1197–201

130. Manning FA, Hill LM, Platt LD. Qualitative amniotic fluid volume determination by ultrasound: antepartum detection of intrauterine growth retardation. *Am J Obstet Gynecol* 1981;139: 254–8

131. Hoddick WK, Callen PW, Filly RA, *et al.* Ultrasonographic determination of qualitative amniotic fluid volume in intrauterine growth retardation: reassessment of the 1cm rule. *Am J Obstet Gynecol* 1984;149:758–62

132. Philipson EH, Sokol RJ, Williams T. Oligohydramnios: clinical associations and predictive value for intrauterine growth retardation. *Am J Obstet Gynecol* 1983;146:271–8

133. Patterson RM, Phrihoda TJ, Poulliot MR. Sonographic amniotic fluid measurement and fetal growth retardation: a reappraisal. *Am J Obstet Gynecol* 1987;157:1406–10

134. Grannum PA, Berkowitz RL, Hobbins JC. The ultrasonic changes in the maturing placenta and their relation to fetal pulmonic maturity. *Am J Obstet Gynecol* 133:915–22

135. Kazzi GM, Gross TL, Sokol RJ. Fetal biparietal diameter and placental grade: predictors of intrauterine growth retardation. *Obstet Gynecol* 1983;62:755

136. Kazzi GM, Gross TL, Sokol RJ. Fetal biparietal diameter and placental grade: predictors of intrauterine growth retardation. *Obstet Gynecol* 1983;62:755–9

137. Kazzi GM, Gross TL, Sokoi RJ, *et al.* Detection of intrauterine growth retardation: a new use for sonographic placental grading. *Am J Obstet Gynecol* 1983;145:733–7

138. Hoogland HJ, de Haan J, Martin CB Jr. Placental size during early pregnancy and fetal outcome: a preliminary report of a sequential ultrasonographic study. *Am J Obstet Gynecol* 1980;138:441–3

139. Wolf H, Oosting H, Treffers PE. Second-trimester placental volume measurement by ultrasound: prediction of fetal outcome. *Am J Obstet Gynecol* 1989;160:121–6

140. Gohari P, Berkowitz RL, Hobbins JC. Prediction of intrauterine volume. 1977;127:255–60

141. Chinn DH, Filly RA, Callen PW. Prediction of intrauterine growth retardation by sonographic estimation of total intrauterine volume. *J Clin Ultrasound* 1981;9:175–9

142. Kurtz AB, Shaw WM, Kurtz RJ, *et al.* The inaccuracy of total uterine volume measurements: sources of error and a proposed solution. *J Ultrasound Med* 1984;3:289–97

143. Reece EA, Goldstein I, Pilu G, *et al.* Fetal cerebellar growth unaffected by intrauterine growth retardation: a new parameter for prenatal diagnosis. *Am J Obstet Gynecol* 1987;157:632–8

144. Cabbad M, Kofinas A, Simon N, *et al.* Fetal weight–cerebellar diameter discordance as an indicator of asymmetrical fetal growth impairment. *J Reprod Med* 1992;37:794–8

145. Hill LM, Guzick D, Riveilo D, *et al.* The transverse cerebellar diameter cannot be used to assess gestational age in the small for gestational age fetus. *Obstet Gynecol* 1990;75:329–33

146. Hill LM, Guzick D, Boyles D, *et al.* Subcutaneous tissue thickness cannot be used to distinguish abnormalities of fetal growth. *Obstet Gynecol* 1992; 80:268–71

147. Santolaya-Forgas J, Meyer WJ, Gauthier DW, *et al.* Intrapartum fetal subcutaneous tissue/femur length ratio: an ultrasonographic clue to fetal macrosomia. *Am J Obstet Gynecol* 1994;171:1072–5

148. Neilson JP, Alfirevic Z. Biophysical profile for antepartum fetal assessment. In Keirse MJNC, Renfrew MJ, Neilson JP, Crowther C, eds. Pregnancy and Childbirth Module in the Cochrane Pregnancy and Childbirth database; The Cochrane Collaboration, Issue 2. Oxford: Update Software, 1995. Available from BMJ Publishing Group, London

149. Manning FA, Harman CR, Morrison I, *et al.* Fetal assessment based on fetal biophysical profile scoring. III. Positive predictive accuracy of the very abnormal test (biophysical profile score = 0). *Am J Obstet Gynecol* 1990;162:398–402

150. Hill LM, Guzick D, Thomas ML, *et al*. Thigh circumference in the detection of intrauterine growth retardation. *Am J Perinatol* 1989;6:349–52

151. Karstorp VH, van Vugt JM, Dekker GA, *et al*. Reappearance of endiastolic velocities in the umbilical artery following maternal volume expansion. A preliminary study. *Obstet Gynecol* 1992;80:679–83

152. Battaglia C, Artimi PG, D-Ambrogio G, *et al*. Maternal hyperoxygenation in the treatment of intrauterine growth retardation. *Am J Obstet Gynecol* 1992;167:430–5

153. Karstorb VH, van Vugt JM, van Geijn HP, *et al*. Clinical significance of absent or reverse endiastolic velocity waveforms in umbilical artery. *Lancet* 1994;344:1664–8

154. Steiner H, Staudach A, Spitzer D, *et al*. Growth deficient fetuses with absent or reversed umbilical artery endiastolic flow of metabolically compromised. *Early Hum Dev* 1995;41:1–9

155. Atkinson MW, Maher JE, Owen J, *et al*. The predictive value of umbilical artery Doppler studies for pre-eclampsia or fetal growth retardation in a pre-eclampsia prevention trial. *Obstet Gynecol* 1994;83:609–12

156. Chang TC, Cheng HH. Recent advances in the use of Doppler waveform indices in the antenatal assessment of intrauterine growth retardation. *Aust NZ J Obstet Gynaecol* 1994;34:8–13

157. Kay HH, Carroll BB, Dahmus M, *et al*. Sonographic measurement with umbilical and uterine artery Doppler analysis in suspected intrauterine growth retardation. *J Reprod Med* 1991;36:65–8

158. Chang TC, Robson SC, Spencer JA, *et al*. Identification of fetal growth retardation: comparison of Doppler waveform indices and serial ultrasound measurements of abdominal circumference and fetal weight. *Obstet Gynecol* 1993;82:230–6

159. Chambers SE, Hoskins PR, Haddad NG, *et al*. A comparison of fetal abdominal circumference measurements and Doppler ultrasound in the prediction of small-for-dates babies and fetal compromise. *Br J Obstet Gynaecol* 1989;96:803–8

160. Beatti RB, Dornan. Antenatal screening for intrauterine growth retardation with umbilical artery Doppler ultrasonography. *Br Med J* 1989;298:631–5

161. Karsdorp VHM, van Vugt JMG, van Geijn HP, *et al*. Clinical significance of absent or reversed end diastolic velocity waveforms in umbilical artery. *Lancet* 1994;344:1664–8

162. Bruinse HW, Sijmons EA, Reuwer PJ. Clinical value of screening for fetal growth retardation by Doppler ultrasound. *J Ultrasound Med* 1989;8:207–9

163. Weiss E, Ulrich S, Berle P. Condition at birth of infants with previously absent for reverse umbilical artery end-diastolic low velocities. *Arch Gynecol Obstet* 1992;252:37–43

164. Neilson JP. Doppler ultrasound (all trials). In The Cochrane Pregnancy and Childbirth database, The Cochrane Collaboration, Issue 2. Oxford: Update Software, 1995. Available from BMJ Publishing Group, London

165. Almstrom H, Axelsson O, Cnattingius S, *et al*. Comparison of umbilical artery velocimetry and cardiotocography for surveillance of small for gestational age fetuses. *Lancet* 1992;340:936–40

166. Gaziano EP, Knox H, Ferrera B, *et al*. Is it time to reassess the risk for the growth retarded fetus with normal Doppler velocimetry of the umbilical artery? *Am J Obstet Gynecol* 1994;170:1734–41

167. Craigo SD. The role of ultrasound in the diagnosis and management of intrauterine growth retardation. *Semin Perinatol* 1994;18:292–304

168. Hecher K, Snijders R, Campbell S, *et al*. Fetal venous, intracardiac, and arterial blood flow measurements in intrauterine growth retardation: relationship with fetal blood gases. *Am J Obstet Gynecol* 1995;173:10–15

169. Sepulveda W, Bower S, Nicolaidis P, *et al*. Discordant blood flow velocity waveforms in left and right brachial arteries in growth retarded fetuses. *Obstet Gynecol* 1995;86:734–8

170. Harrington K, Carpenter RG, Nguyen M, *et al*. Changes observed in Doppler studies in the fetal circulation in pregnancies complicated by pre-eclampsia or the delivery of a small for gestational age baby. 1. Cross sectional analysis. *Ultrasound Obstet Gynaecol* 1995;6:19–28

171. Rotmensch S, Liberati M, Luo JS, *et al*. Colour Doppler flow patterns and flow velocity waveforms of the intraplacental fetal circulation in growth retarded fetuses. *Am J Obstet Gynecol* 1994;171:1257–64

172. Bewley S, Cooper D, Campbell S. Doppler investigation of uteroplacental blood resistance in the second trimester: a screening study for pre-eclampsia and intrauterine growth retardation. *Br J Obstet Gynaecol* 1991;98:871–9

173. Bower S, Bewley S, Campbell S. Improved prediction of pre-eclampsia by two stage screening for uterine arteries using the early diastolic notch and colour Doppler imaging. *Obstet Gynecol* 1993;82:78–83

174. Shalev E, Blondheim O, Peleg D. Use of cordocentesis in the management of preterm or growth-restricted fetuses with abnormal monitoring. *Obstet Gynecol Surv* 1995;50:839–44

175. Pardi G, Cetin I, Marconi AM, *et al*. Diagnostic value of blood sampling in fetuses with growth retardation. *N Engl J Med* 1993;328:692–6

176. Manning FA, Snijders R, Harman CR, *et al*. Fetal biophysical profile score. VI. Correlation with antepartum umbilical venous fetal pH. *Am J Obstet Gynecol* 1993;169:755–63

177. Crawford MA, Doyle W, Leaf A, *et al*. Nutrition and neurodevelopmental disorders. *Nutr Health* 1993; 9:81–97

178. Merlet-Benichou C, Gilbert T, Muffat-Joly M, *et al*. Intrauterine growth retardation leads to permanent nephron deficit in the rat. *Pediatr Nephrol* 1994;8:175–80

179. Patchi A, Lubrano R, Maggi E, *et al*. Renal tubular damage in fetuses with intrauterine growth retardation. *Fetal Diagn Ther* 1993;8:109–13

180. Kempley ST, Gamsu HR, Nicolaides KH. Renal artery blood flow velocity in very low birthweight infants with intrauterine growth retardation. *Arch Dis Child* 1993;68:588–90

181. Barker DJP. Fetal origins of coronary heart disease. *Br Med J* 1995;311:171–4

182. Barker DJ, Gluckman PD, Godfrey KM, *et al*. Fetal nutrition and cardiovascular disease in adult life. *Lancet* 1993;141:41

Macrosomia

6

Edward J. Coetzee

The reason for wanting to identify the macrosomic infant is based on the alleged relationship between excessive size of the newborn and adverse perinatal and maternal outcome. This chapter will explore the validity of the high-risk nature of macrosomic births, then look at the pathophysiology of macrosomia, methods for identifying macrosomic infants and finally whether obstetric interventions can alter macrosomia and its sequelae.

DEFINITION

If the definition of IUGR is imprecise and arbitrary then that of macrosomia is even more so. Macrosomia has been defined as a birth weight greater than or equal to 4000 g, $\geq$ 4200 g and $\geq$ 4500 g. More correctly it should be defined according to population-based centile charts where once again the 90th, 95th or 97th centile can be used. It will, therefore, be used interchangeably with the term 'large for gestational age' (LGA).

However, as with IUGR, all these definitions fail to differentiate between the infant who is genetically programmed to be large and the infant who is overgrown, because of various pathophysiological processes. The prevalence of macrosomia varies depending on the definition used and varies between population groups but on average is 5–10% for newborns over 4000 g and 1–2% for those weighing over 4500 g. This prevalence is increased dramatically where the mother has diabetes.

RISKS ASSOCIATED WITH MACROSOMIA

Perinatal mortality and morbidity are said to be increased when compared to neonates who are appropriate for gestational age. These risks include shoulder dystocia, Erb's palsy, fractures and other trauma to the skeletal system and birth asphyxia. Protracted labor and delay in the second stage may occur leading to greater birth canal injury and postpartum hemorrhage.

In reviewing the literature there appears to be a difference in the prevalence of these results depending on the pathophysiology causing the macrosomia.

McFarland and colleagues[1] reported on 210 974 births in the state of Washington, USA, from 1980–1982. The incidence of Erb's palsy was 50.2 cases per 100 000 live births. In a univariable and multivariable analysis of the 106 study cases compared to 386 case controls, birthweight was shown to be a significant risk factor. A newborn weighing between 4000 and 4500 g had 2.5 times the risk of having a brachial plexus injury compared with the normal sized infant. The risk for infants greater than 4500 g increased another 10-fold [odds ratio (OR) = 21.0]. Delivery by cesarean section was associated with a significant protective effect compared with instrumental vaginal delivery (OR = 0.5).

In a retrospective study in Los Angeles the records were reviewed for the whole of 1991 and 277 infants with birthweight of at least 4500 g were identified[2]. Of these, 35 (15.4%) had elective cesarean sections while in 192 (84.6%) vaginal delivery was attempted. In 18.2% the attempt failed and an intrapartum cesarean section was done. Vaginal delivery was achieved in 157 patients, but in 29 cases shoulder dystocia occurred resulting in 15 fetal injuries (51.7%). Of interest is that there were 10 fetal injuries (7.8%) among patients who reputedly did not have shoulder dystocia. These included 5 Erb's palsies and 5 clavicular fractures. Thus 25% (or 1 in 4 patients) who had an attempted vaginal delivery had a problem associated with labor.

In addition, maternal lacerations requiring repair (including 3rd and 4th degree tears) increased dramatically when vaginal delivery was complicated by shoulder dystocia [relative risk (RR) 5.4]. Fifteen per cent of all vaginal deliveries had 3rd or 4th degree tears and this increased to 66% where shoulder dystocia was encountered. There was apparently no difference in hospital stay between women who had a vaginal delivery compared with women who had cesarean sections.

However, women who had a cesarean section after attempted vaginal delivery had significantly increased infectious morbidity compared to those who had an elective cesarean section or a vaginal delivery (RR 7.1 and 5.4, respectively).

Because there was no apparent residual pathology in the infants who had suffered fractures and Erb's palsy at the 2 months' follow-up visit the authors concluded that vaginal delivery was a reasonable alternative to elective cesarean section for infants with an estimated birthweight of at least 4500 g. No details are given about the mothers' urinary, anal or perineal functions at follow-up visits.

Their data showed a marked difference in the risk of developing shoulder dystocia between infants of diabetic and non-diabetic macrosomic infants, i.e. 50% for diabetic mothers and 13.3% for non-diabetic mothers, and they urge extra caution in the former group.

Langer et al.[3] searched the obstetric computer data base of the University of Texas Health Center at San Antonio for the years 1970–1985. A total of 75 979 women delivered vaginally during this period. Defining macrosomia as ≥ 4000 g they found the incidence to be 7.6% among non-diabetic mothers and 20.6% among diabetic mothers. The overall incidence of shoulder dystocia was 3.1% for diabetic mothers and 0.5% for non-diabetic mothers. Once again, they showed clearly that the diabetic mother was at greater risk for shoulder dystocia even when her infant weighed less than 4000 g, i.e. 2.6-fold increase and 3.6-fold increase for higher birthweights.

Lazer and colleagues[4] reviewed 525 infants who weighed > 4500 g. The incidence of shoulder dystocia was 18.5% (control group 0.2%) and the mothers in the macrosomic group had increased oxytocin augmentation, postpartum hemorrhage, birth canal damage and puerperal fever.

Fetal outcome was also very much poorer, with a 2.3% perinatal mortality (against 0.4% in the controls). Low Apgar scores were more prevalent. Erb's palsy occurred in 5.7% (0.2% in controls) and the clavicle was fractured in 4.0% (0.0% in controls). All these increases in the maternal and neonatal morbidity mentioned were statistically significant. In addition, three horror stories of stuck babies dying intrapartum vividly bring home the final consequences of making a wrong decision.

Finally, in a large study including 574 macrosomic infants, Spellacy and colleagues[5] identified the typical maternal characteristics – obesity, postdatism plus diabetes, and confirmed the high perinatal morbidity, that was prevented by elective cesarean section.

PATHOPHYSIOLOGY

The fetal genome will programme certain infants to be large for gestational age as judged by population centile charts. However, many factors, such as available nutrients and the transfer of such nutrients across the placenta, modulate the genetically programmed growth pattern.

It is, therefore, appropriate to study the epidemiological evidence to identify associations with high birthweight. In a study of 2082 infants with birth weights > 4000 g born in Washington State from 1984 and 1986, Brunskill and colleagues[6] compared the former to a random sample of 4440 live births with weights of 2.5–4.0 kg.

Both established and gestational diabetes were associated with a higher risk of macrosomia, i.e. OR of 6.4 + 3.2 respectively. Other associations were male sex of the infant (OR 2.4), parity and length of gestation. Prolonged pregnancy had an OR 3.3.

Other risk factors that have been identified are maternal height and weight (at the beginning of the pregnancy), total weight increase during the pregnancy and a previous history of an infant with high birthweight[7]. In mothers with pregravid body mass index ≥ 95th centile the odds of delivering a macrosomic infant (> 4000 g) were 2.2 times higher after adjustment for factors known to be important predictors for birthweight[8].

It is not quite clear why heavier mothers have heavier children. This could be genetic or because of the altered nutrient mixture presented to the placental exchange system in these mothers. The increased risk of macrosomia in postdatism seems a logical conclusion as the fetus obviously continues to grow after term where placental function is not reduced.

The mechanism of the excessive fetal growth in diabetes is the high maternal glucose concentrations presented to the placental exchange surface. The rate by which glucose and other nutrients are transferred to the fetus is influenced strongly by the concentration gradient across the placenta. Maternal hyperglycemia, therefore, leads to fetal hyperglycemia. Under normal circumstances the fetal pancreatic beta cells do not have to respond to fluctuations in fetal glycemic levels, as this is done for the fetus by the mother who has a normal carbohydrate metabolism. However, in the poorly controlled diabetic mother the fetal beta cells are confronted with high blood glucose concentrations.

Because they have normal function they will be activated and secrete insulin to lower the blood glucose concentration. In the absence of the maternal blood glucose being lowered as well this will result in an increased glucose concentration gradient with a further influx of glucose to the fetus.

The fetus is, therefore, not only supplied with an excessive supply of nutrients, but its beta cells are also constantly stimulated to produce further insulin in an attempt to create euglycemia in the fetus.

This hypothesis was first proposed by Pedersen[9]. The hyperinsulinism specifically affects insulin-sensitive tissues and this results in selective organomegaly such as of the heart and liver.

There are also increases in both fat and muscle tissue. Collectively, all these areas contribute to a disproportionate increase in the size of the trunk and shoulders. Brain growth is not affected and the BPD and HC usually remain within normal limits[10]. It is this specific change to fetal morphometry that is labelled diabetic fetopathy and it results in the very much increased risk of shoulder dystocia already referred to.

It is too simplistic to assume that glucose is solely responsible for the changes in the fetus of a diabetic mother. Other metabolic alterations inherent to the diabetic also play a role, such as increased serum levels of free fatty acids, triglycerides and certain amino acids. These nutrients may also contribute to fetal hyperinsulinemia[11].

Evidence from amniotic fluid and cord blood insulin and c-peptide levels has provided further corroboration for the Pederen theory[12,13].

It is by understanding the pathophysiology (at least in diabetic pregnancies) that we can find mechanisms to intervene in the process, resulting in a reduction of birthweight of the newborn. In turn this should lead to a decline in morbidity.

If we, therefore, can deliver a normal nutrient mix to the placental exchange surface, it should be possible to prevent hyperinsulinism and thus diabetic fetopathy. Such normalization of the metabolic fuels can be achieved by dietary manipulation and expert use of new insulin regimens. Although metabolic normalization has long been proven to improve perinatal mortality in infants of diabetic mothers, the medical fraternity has been slow in accepting proof that birthweight can be altered by such regimens.

The Diabetes in Early Pregnancy Study has now provided compelling evidence that strict control of postprandial glucose levels can reduce the prevalence of macrosomia[14].

However, it is impossible to create complete metabolic normalization with any of the currently available regimens. Even multiple insulin injection regimens do not emulate the carefully regulated release of insulin into the portal venous system by the normal healthy pancreas. Our method of checking the success of our regimens (i.e. a single blood glucose estimation 1 or 2 hours after a meal) is also crude, as it does not check all the metabolic nutrients. It seems likely that the area under the curve of the various nutrients can still vary tremendously, resulting in an excess of calories being delivered across the placental exchange system. It seems plausible that this will then not cause hyperinsulinism (as the fetus no longer has to respond to high glucose values) but that the fetus may still be large because of a surfeit of calories.

DETECTION OF THE MACROSOMIC INFANT

In the light of the above, we should make every attempt at detecting the macrosomic infant, and because of the increased risks to the infant with diabetic fetopathy, special emphasis should be placed on identifying it and managing it appropriately.

Such detection starts with identifying the antecedent risk factors for macrosomia, especially the obese mother, postdatism, and diabetes. It is important to realize that gestational diabetes and unrecognized non-insulin dependent diabetes also have a potent influence on birthweight and that a detection program for macrosomia must include a detection program for occult diabetes.

Careful clinical examination of the pregnant abdomen including symphysis fundal height[15] remains a useful way of identifying a large infant. However, as many of the mothers are obese this will limit its usefulness. Sonographic detection of macrosomia, therefore, seems likely to offer the most value. However, not all investigators believe that sonographic detection is worthwhile.

Traditionally, fetal size has been related to three structures:

(1) BPD or HC, reflecting brain size;

(2) AC, reflecting the nutritional state of the fetus; and

(3) FL, reflecting height or length of the fetus.

These three basic measurements have been combined in various ways and used to estimate fetal weight.

Two commonly used equations for estimated fetal weight are the Shepard formula[16] (BPD + AC) and the Hadlock formula[17] using the AC + FL.

Because weight seems seductively simple, easy to understand and fits in with our definition of macrosomia, it is tempting to use sonographic estimations of fetal weight to influence clinical decision-making.

It must however be remembered that the infant of a diabetic mother (i.e. the ones most at risk), has a body morphometry that sets it apart from the general fetal population. Benson and colleagues[18] tested several formulae in diabetic pregnancies, including the Shepard and Hadlock formulae, and even tried to devise customized diabetic formulae. In 160 infants, they found their relative error (error as a percentage of birthweight) had standard deviations of 12.2 to 13.1%, with no statistically significant difference among formulae. When they tried to customize the formulae their best attempt yielded a standard deviation of 11%. Clinically, this means that if the estimated weight is > 4000 g then only 77% of newborns will actually weigh > 4000 g.

These large standard deviations in mean differences of actual versus estimated fetal weight imply that the use of the sonographic EFW alone is not clinically defensible. However, using EFW plus morphometry could improve detection of a macrosomic infant in a diabetic mother. Tamura and colleagues[19] reached a similar conclusion about EFW but found that when AC + EFW exceeded the 90th centile, macrosomia was correctly diagnosed in 88.8%.

Hadlock and colleagues[20], evaluating their FL/AC, ratio, found that in a small subset ($n = 9$) of infants of diabetic mothers this ratio correctly identified 89% of LGA fetuses compared to 63% in non-diabetic fetuses. Landon and colleagues[10] evolved the morphometric approach further by studying fetal abdominal growth patterns during the third trimester. At least three readings of HC, AC + FL were measured in the third trimester and growth in centimeters for these parameters was calculated.

They found no statistical difference between LGA and AGA fetuses in HC + FL growth, but AC growth was clearly accelerated from 32 weeks in the LGA group. Using a receiver operator characteristic curve they calculated that a growth of ≥ 1.2 cm per week was the optimal cut-off point for detecting LGA infants. At this cut-off point they had a sensitivity of 83.8%, a specificity of 85.4%, a positive predictive value of 78.7% and a negative predictive value of 89%. It is not always possible to have serial measurements and in the same study an AC of greater than 2 SD performed almost as well in identifying the LGA infant.

Lastly, especially in the developing world, gestational age is not always known and although the Hadlock FL/AC ratio[20] performed less well, because it is gestational age-independent, it is very useful in identifying at-risk infants. Landon and colleagues[10] used a ratio of < 21% as a cut-off for macrosomia whereas Hadlock and colleagues suggested 20.5%. HC/AC ratios can also be used to detect excessive fetal abdominal girth, but this is gestational age-dependent and an accurate gestational age is, therefore, required. If accurate gestational age is available, it is best to plot the readings on accurate growth/size charts to determine in which percentile each reading lies.

Detection of macrosomia without altered morphometry is still problematic as here we have to rely on EFW calculations and this can lead to poor clinical decision-making[21]. In Levine's study, the incorrect sonographic diagnosis of an LGA fetus had a statistically significant effect on both the diagnosis of labor abnormalities and the incidence of elective cesarean section.

These data were confirmed by Weeks and colleagues[22] who found a cesarean section rate of 52% in a group of patients where macrosomia was predicted before delivery compared to 30% where it was not. All infants in the study weighed 4200 g or more. There was no significant difference in fetal morbidity or shoulder dystocia between the two groups.

In an effort to improve the predictive value of sonographic detection, clinical investigators have directed their attention to a variety of soft tissue thickness measurements.

Sood and colleagues[23] evaluated humeral soft tissue thickness while Abramowicz and colleagues[24] measured cheek-to-cheek diameter in fetal growth disturbances. Santolaya-Forgas[25] measured fetal subcutaneous tissue at the level of the femoral diaphysis and suggested using a tissue/FL ratio. All these new techniques were able to identify the macrosomic infant, but did not add to the accuracy of previously described tests.

MANAGEMENT STRATEGIES

Macrosomia still represents a substantial risk to the newborn and accurate programs for detection are needed. Unfortunately, such programs are not available. Risk factors for macrosomia should be identified and ultrasound evaluation should be confined to mothers who are diabetic, obese or postdates. However, the clinician must realize that sonographic EFW has a relatively poor positive predictive value, i.e. 64%[26]. Virtually all EFW formulae systematically over-estimate birthweight.

Clinicians are, therefore, in danger of over-reacting to false information and thereby increasing the cesarean section rate. There is no reason for inducing labor in a postdates pregnancy just because of macrosomia[21].

However, in the diabetic mother a sonographic EFW of over 4200 g with morphometric changes of an increased AC in comparison to other growth parameters (HC + FL) should persuade the clinician to do an elective cesarean section. Such a policy will have only a very small effect on cesarean section rates but have a large beneficial effect on preventing shoulder dystocia and its morbidity.

In addition, the above pattern strongly predicts multiple further problems associated with diabetic fetopathy that may lie ahead for the newborn, such as hypoglycemia, polycythemia and jaundice.

References

1. MacFarland LV, Raskin M, Daling JR, *et al.* Erb/Duchenne's palsy: a consequence of fetal macrosomia and method of delivery. *Obstet Gynecol* 1986;68:784–8

2. Lipscomb KR, Gregory K, Shaw K. The outcome of macrosomic infants weighing at least 4500 grams: Los Angeles County and University of Southern California Experience. *Obstet Gynecol* 1995;85:558–64

3. Langer O, Berkus MD, Huff RW, *et al.* Shoulder dystocia: should the fetus weighing > 4000 grams be delivered by cesarean section? *Am J Obstet Gynecol* 1991;165:831–7

4. Lazer S, Biale Y, Mazor M, *et al.* Complications associated with the macrosomic fetus. *J Reprod Med* 1986;31:501–5

5. Spellacy WN, Miller S, Winegar A, *et al.* Macrosomia–maternal characteristics and infant complications. *Obstet Gynecol* 1985;66:158

6. Brunskill AJ, Rossing MA, Connell FA, *et al.* Antecedents of macrosomia. *Paediatr Perinat Epidemiol* 1991;5:392–401

7. Wikstrom I, Axelsson O, Bergstrom R. Maternal factors associated with high birth weight. *Acta Obstet Gynecol Scand* 1991;70:55–61

8. Larsen CE, Serdula MK, Sullivan KM. Macrosomia: influence of maternal overweight among a low-income population. *Am J Obstet Gynecol* 1990;162:490–4

9. Pedersen J. Hyperglycaemia – hyperinsulinism theory and birth weight. In Pedersen J, ed. *The Pregnant Diabetic and her Newborn.* Baltimore: Williams & Wilkins, 1977:211–20

10. Landon MB, Marshall C, Mintz, *et al.* Sonographic evaluation of fetal abdominal growth: predictor of the large-for-gestational-age infant in pregnancies complicated by diabetes mellitus. *Am J Obstet Gynecol* 1990;160:115-21

11. Freinkel N. Banting Lecture: of pregnancy and progeny. *Diabetes* 1980;29:1023–35

12. Weiss PAM. Gestational diabetes and screening during pregnancy. *Obstet Gynecol* 1985;63:534

13. Sosenko IR, Kitzmiller JL, Loo SW, *et al.* The infant of the diabetic mother: correlation of increased cord C-peptide levels with macrosomia and hypoglycemia. *N Engl J Med* 1979;301:859–62

14. Jovanovic-Peterson L, Peterson CM, Reed GF, *et al.* Maternal postprandial glucose levels and infant birth weight: the diabetes in early pregnancy study. *Am J Obstet Gynecol* 1991;164:103–11

15. Wikstrom I, Bergstrom R, Bakketeig L, *et al.* Prediction of high birthweight from maternal characteristics, symphysis fundal height and ultrasound biometry. *Gynecol Obstet Invest* 1993;35:27–33

16. Shephard MJ. An evaluation of two equations for predicting fetal weight by ultrasound. *Am J Obstet Gynecol* 1982;142:47

17. Hadlock FP, Harrist RB, Carpenter RJ, *et al.* Sonographic estimation of fetal weight. The value of femur length in addition to head and abdomen measurements. *Radiology* 1984;150:535–40

18. Benson CB, Doubilet PM, Saltzman DH. Sonographic determination of fetal weights in diabetic pregnancies. *Am J Obstet Gynecol* 1987;156:441–4

19. Tamura RK, Sabbaha RE, Depp R, *et al.* Diabetic macrosomia: accuracy of third trimester ultrasound. *Obstet Gynecol* 1986;67:828

20. Hadlock FP, Harrist RB, Fearneyhough TC, *et al.* Use of femur length/abdominal circumference ratio

in detecting the macrosomic fetus. *Radiology* 1985;154:503–5

21. Levine AB, Lockwood CJ, Brown B, *et al*. Sonographic diagnosis of the large for gestational age fetus at term: does it make a difference? *Obstet Gynecol* 1992;79:55–8

22. Weeks JW, Pitman T, Spinnato JA. Fetal macrosomia: does antenatal prediction affect delivery route and birth outcome? *Am J Obstet Gynecol* 1995;173:1215–9

23. Sood AK, Yancey M, Richards D. Prediction of fetal macrosomia using humeral soft tissue thickness. *Obstet Gynecol* 1995;85:937–40

24. Abramowicz JS, Sherer DM, Woods JR. Ultrasonographic measurement of cheek-to-cheek diameter in fetal growth disturbances. *Am J Obstet Gynecol* 1993;169:405–8

25. Santolaya-Forgas J, Meyer WJ, Gauthier DW, *et al*. Intrapartum fetal subcutaneous tissue/femur length ratio: an ultrasonographic clue to fetal macrosomia. *Am J Obstet Gynecol* 1994;171:1072–5

26. Pollack RN, Hauer-Pollack G, Divon MY. Macrosomia in postdates pregnancies: the accuracy of routine ultrasonographic screening. *Am J Obstet Gynecol* 1992;167:7–11

Placenta, umbilical cord and amniotic fluid

7

Moshe D. Fejgin, Ron Tepper and Dvora Kidron

PLACENTA

In recent years the placenta has been receiving increasing attention during assessment of fetal wellbeing. With abnormal pregnancy outcome examination of placenta by an expert pathologist may solve some of the mysteries regarding cause and timetable of an adverse outcome. Therefore, the placenta has been referred to as the 'black box' of the pregnancy. Since changes in the placenta may precede events in the fetus, the ultrasonographer can use placental appearance as an early warning system.

In this chapter we outline common pathologic conditions of the placenta, umbilical cord and amniotic fluid. Some of the ultrasonographic pictures are shown next to the pictures of relevant pathology/histology specimens.

Ultrasonographic evaluation of the placenta

Every obstetrical ultrasonographic examination should include evaluation of the placenta. The evaluation should include the following parameters:

(1) Location (anterior, posterior, fundal etc.). Whenever the placenta has a low implantation, placenta previa should be ruled out;
(2) Maturity grading (I to III);
(3) Presence of intraplacental lesions;
(4) Signs of separation (abruption) or abnormal implantation (accreta).

Normal ultrasonographic appearance

The placenta can be identified at 6 to 7 weeks gestation using a transvaginal approach and at 7 to 8 weeks gestation by the abdominal approach. At this stage the villi opposite the site of implantation regress while the definitive placenta appears as a thickened area representing the decidua basalis and the chorion frondosum. At approximately 12 weeks gestation the placenta develops a granular pattern with a typical recognizable ultrasonographic appearance. This ultrasonographic appearance is due to the echoes arising from the villous tree which is bathed in maternal blood. In the second half of pregnancy the echogenic picture gradually changes with the development of septations, echo-free areas and hyperechogenic spots representing calcium deposits. These calcium deposits may be found along the basal plate, the septations and in fibrin collections in the intervillous space.

Placental grading

Placental echogenic changes occur with the progression of gestational age and have been used for placental grading. This grading has been related to fetal lung maturity[1] as well as associated with intrauterine growth retardation and toxemia of pregnancy[2].

Grade 0: A uniform granular appearance with minimal echogenic spots.

Grade I: Early indentation of the chorionic plate and some calcium deposits.

Grade II: Incomplete separation of the placental parenchyma and obvious calcifications of the basal plate (Figure 1).

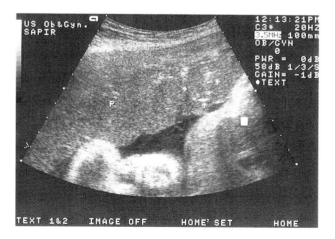

Figure 1 A grade II placenta

Grade III: Complete septation with calcium deposits in combination of echo-free venous lakes (Figure 2).

A new grading system was developed to improve the predictability of pulmonary maturity and neonatal outcome. This system classifies the placenta into:

Immature: Grade 0 to 2 with no grade 3.
Intermediate: Some placental parts graded 3.
Mature: Entire placenta grade 3.

The main difference between the two classifications is that in the modified system only placentas that demonstrate grade 3 throughout the whole placenta are considered mature. Initial studies have shown that no neonates developed respiratory distress syndrome when placenta had been classified as mature.

Placental abnormalities

Abnormalities of implantation

Site of placental attachment   The placental attachment site becomes apparent as early as 6–8 weeks gestation with the utilization of transvaginal ultrasonography. The placenta will, in most cases, implant in the upper uterine segment, and specifically on anterior and posterior walls of the upper segment. Lower segment implantations are rare but responsible for severe pregnancy complications. Placenta previa is frequently diagnosed in mid-trimester (20%). However, with the phenomenon of placental migration[3] that occurs with the development of the lower segment in the third trimester, 90% of asymptomatic second trimester diagnosed placenta previas will resolve[4] and the incidence of placental previa at term is estimated to be only 1 in 250 live births[5].

Placenta previa is a situation in which placental implantation is over the internal cervical opening. It may present in three variations: complete, partial and marginal.

In complete placenta previa the internal cervical os is covered entirely by the placenta, while in partial placenta previa the internal os is only partially covered. The edge of the marginal placenta previa reaches the internal os but does not cover it. Sometimes the term low-lying placenta is also used when the tip of the placenta is implanted in the lower segment close to the internal os, but does not

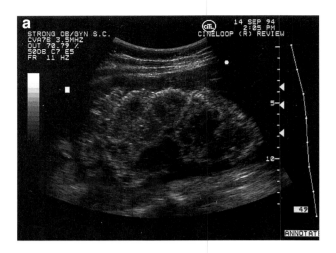

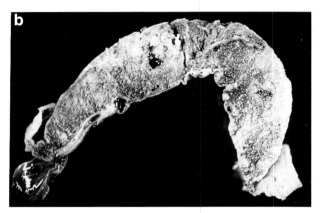

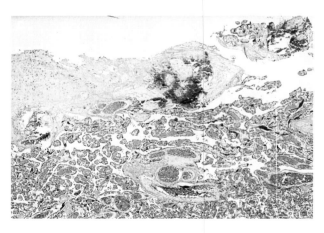

Figure 2   (**a**) Grade III placenta at 40 weeks gestation demonstrating widespread calcifications. (**b**) A cut section of placenta at 40 weeks gestation. The fine granular, spongy appearance is created by the fully developed villous tree which is soaked in maternal blood. (**c**) Calcifications of the basal plate, term placenta (H&E, × 40) (see also Color plate 6)

reach it. The diagnosis of a complete placenta previa at term is of utmost significance, since it disallows vaginal delivery. Ultrasonographic diagnosis using an abdominal approach may be problematic, especially when the placenta has a posterior attachment, since it is sometimes difficult to identify the internal os precisely. A full bladder can result in a false positive diagnosis of placenta previa because of compression of the lower uterine segment. Farine and colleagues[6] demonstrated that careful use of a transvaginal probe is both safe and accurate in the diagnosis of placenta previa. The combination of the abdominal and vaginal approaches increases the accuracy of the diagnosis of the degree of placenta previa and thus eliminates the need for a digital examination. The utilization of a transperineal scan has also been suggested.

Type of implantation Placenta extrachorialis is formed when fetal membranes do not extend to the edges of the placenta. A flat attachment of fetal membranes to the chorionic plate forms a placenta circummarginata. In placenta circumvallata this attachment is folded (Figure 3). This last type may be associated with chronic vaginal and intra-amniotic bleeding and preterm labor. Ultrasonographic evaluation in these cases demonstrates an unusual placental margin with upturned edge and hypoechogenic areas representing subchorionic fibrin and hemorrhage.

Abnormalities of adherence

Trophoblastic cells have the ability to invade the myometrial tissue. When the placenta develops in an area of scant or absent decidual layer, the risk of such invasion, which may lead to the development of placenta accreta, is significant. There are three recognized degrees of invasion: placenta accreta, which is minimal invasion of the myometrium by villi; placenta increta, involving significant invasion of the myometrium but not the serosa; and placenta percreta, when villi invade the myometrium throughout, including the serosa, and sometimes beyond the serosa into nearby organs (Figure 4).

The clinical picture depends on the extent of invasion. It may vary from placental adherence leading to postpartum hemorrhage which may be controlled by sharp curettage, to postpartum hypogastric artery ligation, hysterectomy and even angiographic embolization. Maternal death due to blood loss can happen if the condition is unrecognized before surgery. Ideally this condition should be recognized antenatally, especially in situations prone to it, such as in the presence of a low-lying anterior placenta in a uterus with prior scars[7,8]. The ultrasonographic diagnosis is based on the absence, or significant thinning (<1 mm), of the retroplacental hypoechogenic space which can usually be seen in the second half of the pregnancy, and cystic fluid-filled areas within the placenta. The diagnosis may also be confirmed by magnetic resonance imaging[9].

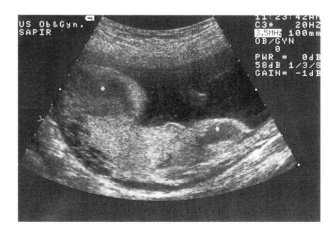

Figure 3 Circumvallate placenta: transverse scan at 27 weeks of the marginal zone of the placenta demonstrating multiple sub-amniotic echo-free areas of various sizes and shapes (*)

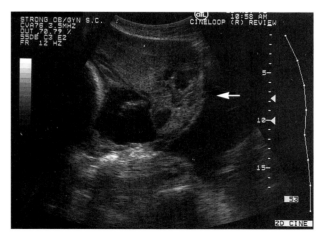

Figure 4 Placenta percreta. Scan of patient with placenta percreta that invaded myometrium and bladder. Note cystic areas within placenta and disruption of serosal lining where bladder invasion occurred (arrow)

Intraplacental abnormalities

Placental infarcts   Although placental infarcts may be found in 25% of the placentas of normal pregnancies, they are more common in pregnancies complicated by toxemia, hypertension and lupus anticoagulant positive mothers. They result from interruption in the maternal blood supply leading to coagulation necrosis of villi at the placental base. While small infarcts may be insignificant, extensive infarcts require evaluation of the mother for the presence of lupus anticoagulant or other vascular or collagen disease. Since such lesions consist of both hyperechogenic (increased cellularity) and hypoechogenic (fibrin deposits) conditions, they can be difficult to diagnose ultrasonographically unless one of the two is dominant. Fresh infarcts may be more echogenic due to their hypercellularity, while old ones with ample fibrin deposits are mainly hypoechogenic (Figure 5).

Hemorrhage   Hemorrhage is basically an obvious clinical diagnosis.

Fibrin deposits   Isolated or multiple sonolucent subchorionic lesions may be seen in 10–15% of placentas. They represent subchorionic fibrin deposits. They are probably the result of pooling of blood and subsequent formation of fibrin thrombi in the intervillous space beneath the chorion. A large lesion may reflect the presence of a freshly formed hematoma. The clinical picture is of utmost importance (Figure 6, Color plates 8–10).

Calcifications   The development of calcium deposits in the placenta is a normal physiological process in the progression of pregnancy. These deposits may be found in the basal plate, the septa and in the subchorionic plate. They can be detected by ultrasonography as early as the beginning of the third trimester, and are present in 50% of scans at 33 weeks gestation[10]. Although used in placenta maturity grading, they probably have minimal clinical significance.

Thickness   This may vary with gestational age, with grade I mean measurement of 3.8 cm, grade II of 3.6 cm and grade III of 3.4 cm[11]. Thick placentas (hyperplacentosis) over 4 cm, have been observed in conditions like diabetes mellitus, perinatal infections and hydrops fetalis (both immune and non-immune). Histologic examination of such placentas reveals mainly villous edema (Figure 8).

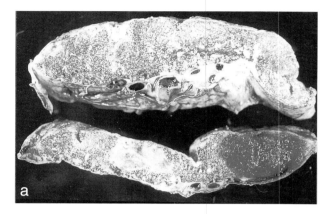

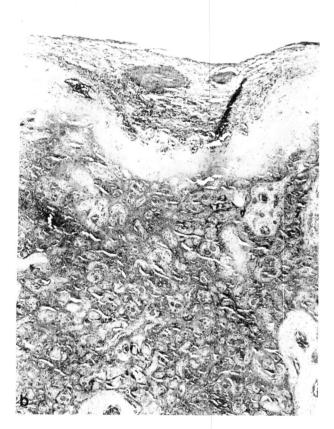

Figure 5   (**a**) Multiple infarcts of placenta, 36 weeks gestation, recent pre-eclamptic toxemia. Several small old infarcts involve the basal aspect of the cut sections. A large recent infarct is seen on the right hand side of the lower slice (see also Color plate 7). (**b**) Histologic section of a recent infarct: the chorionic villi are clumped together and have lost their trophoblast. Occluding thrombi in two decidual vessels are seen in the maternal floor (H&E, × 40)

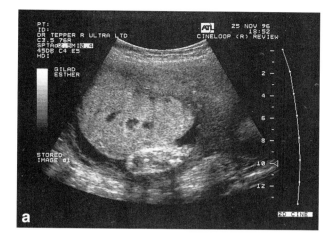

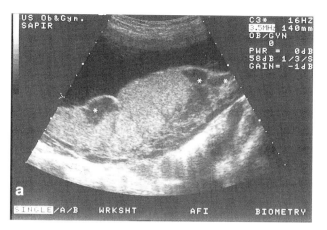

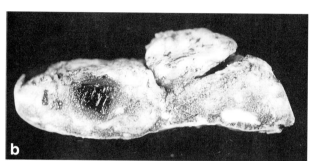

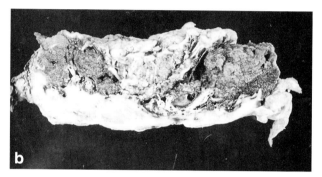

Figure 7 (**a**) Subchorionic fibrin deposition. A posterior placenta at 20 weeks showing prominent hypoechoic subchorionic lesions (*), which correlated with subchorionic fibrin deposition at delivery. (**b**) Massive subchorionic fibrin deposits of the placenta at 33 weeks gestation. The mother had cardiomyopathy due to doxorubicine cardiotoxicity (see also Color plate 10)

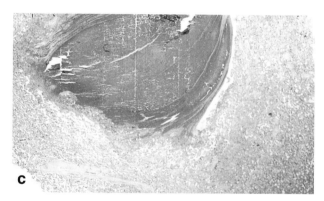

Figure 6 (**a**) Scan at 22 weeks gestation demonstrates an intra-placental sonolucent lesion representing an area of villi surrounded by fibrin. (**b**) Intervillous hematoma measuring 2 cm in diameter (see also Color plate 8). (**c**) Histologic section of an intervillous hematoma surrounded by normal appearing chorionic villi (see also Color plate 9) (H&E, × 10)

Intrauterine infection Intrauterine infection by different agents such as listeria, parvovirus, syphilis, cytomegalovirus, toxoplasma, or human immunodeficiency virus may cause placental thickening and villitis (Figure 9).

Hydatiform change The presence of multiple sonolucent lesions in the placenta should raise the suspicion of hydatiform disease. Several entities exist:

(1) Complete hydatiform mole: villi edema and absence of embryo. Genetic evaluation reveals diploid karyotype. In a twin pregnancy a viable fetus with a normal placenta may be present adjacently (Figure 10, Color plates 11 and 12).

(2) Partial mole: coexistence of hydatiform and normal placenta (Figure 11) or the presence of a fetus. The karyotype of these pregnancies is usually triploidy. Other placental conditions associated with abnormal karyotypes are listed in Table 1.

(3) Pseudo mole: multiple echo-free lesions in abnormal-appearing placenta with a normal blood flow by Doppler ultrasonography and a normal appearing fetus with a normal karyotype (Figure 12).

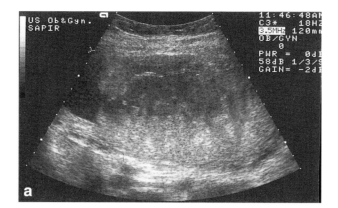

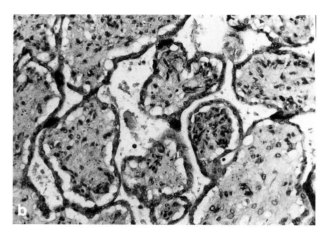

Figure 8 (**a**) Non-immune hydrops at 32 weeks gestation secondary to fetal cardiac anomaly. Hyper-placentosis is noted. (**b**) Villous edema. The trophoblast is separated from the villous stroma by fluid accumulation. Non-immune fetal hydrops and antepartum fetal death at 33 weeks gestation (H&E, × 250)

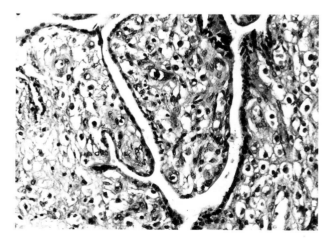

Figure 9 Chronic villitis caused by cytomegalovirus (CMV). The villi are large and infiltrated by lymphocytes and plasma cells. Nuclear debris is also seen. A typical intranuclear CMV inclusion body is seen at the central villus (H&E, × 250)

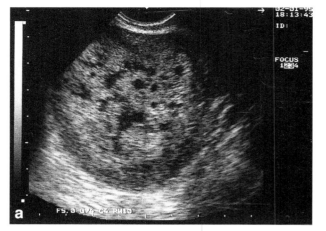

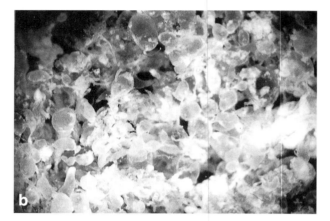

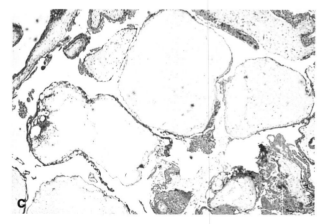

Figure 10 (**a**) Ultrasonography of hydatidiform mole showing vesicular pattern. (**b**) Gross appearance of complete mole: the entire villous tree is converted into numerous vesicles of 0.5 cm in average diameter (see also Color plate 11). (**c**) Histologic section of a partial mole: some villi are markedly distended, show cystic degeneration in the center and focal trophoblastic proliferation to various degrees (H&E, × 40) (see also Color plate 12)

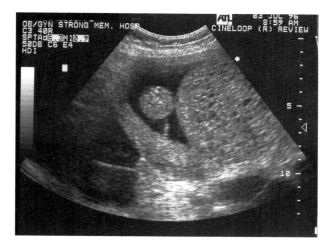

Figure 11 Partial mole demonstrating hydropic placenta and a fetus

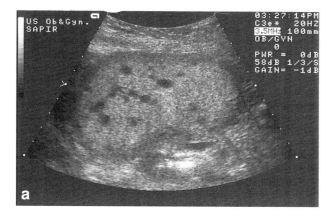

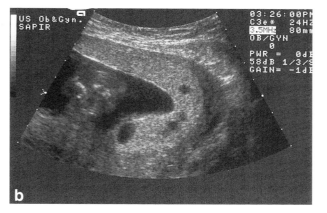

Figure 12 (**a**) Transverse scan at 17 weeks gestation showing large placenta containing multiple echo-free spaces. (**b**) Longitudinal scan demonstrating pseudo-molar placenta. Karyotype of amniotic fluid cells and placenta was normal

Table 1 Placenta in chromosomal abnormalities

Chromosomal abnormality	Placenta and cord findings
Triploidy	Partial mole
Trisomy 13	Small placenta, single umbilical artery, dysmature villi, hypovascular villi
Trisomy 18	High resistance to flow, syncytial knots, villous cellularity, cisternae in villi
Trisomy 21	Villous dysmaturity and hypovascularity

Hydropic degeneration may be mis-diagnosed as a molar pregnancy. It can be part of the picture of missed abortion (Figure 13, Color plate 13).

Neoplasms Chorioangioma is the most common neoplasm of the placenta. Although generally small (a few centimeters in diameter) it may be found in up to 1% of pregnancies with no clinical significance. Large chorioangiomas may be ultrasonographically diagnosed as well-circumscribed intraplacental lesions with complex echo patterns. Such large diffuse lesions may be associated with fetal hydrops, DIC, umbilical vein thrombosis and fetal death[12]. Color Doppler imaging will enable differentiation between vascular and non-vascular tumors (Figure 14, Color plate 14).

Abnormalities of basal plate

Abruption Increased uterine tone accompanied by vaginal bleeding often leads to the diagnosis of placental abruption. The area of separation can frequently be seen as an elevation of the tip of the placenta or the membranes. When the possibility of concealed placental abruption is entertained due to uterine irritability without evidence of vaginal bleeding, ultrasonography may assist in confirming the diagnosis. However, a clear picture of retroplacental hematoma can be seen only in the minority of the cases and only when this separation is significant (Figure 15, Color plate 15).

Maternal vasculopathy Maternal vasculopathy in pre-eclampsia and related conditions, e.g. thrombosis, acute atherosis.

Other placental abnormalities associated with specific maternal conditions are listed in Table 2.

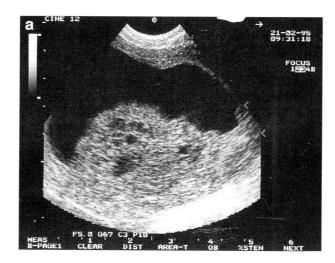

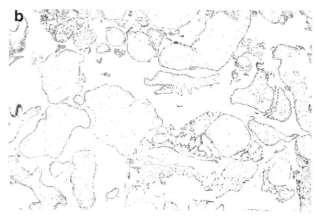

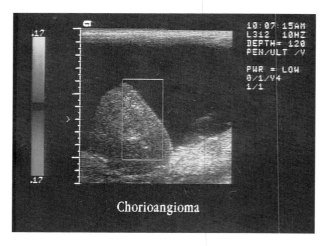

Figure 14   Color Doppler flow demonstrating some vascularity of a chorioangioma (see also Color plate 14)

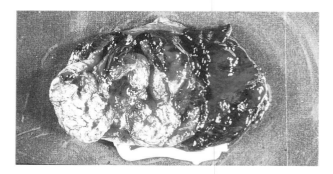

Figure 15   Abruptio placenta at 33 weeks gestation. A large retroplacental hematoma, on the right side, is firmly attached to the maternal (basal) floor, covering approximately 30% of its surface (see also Color plate 15)

Figure 13   (**a**) Cystic hydropic degeneration of placenta: sagittal scan of a 14 weeks missed abortion showing hypoechoic collections within placenta. (**b**) Histologic section of hydropic degeneration. The chorionic villi are markedly distended but lack the cystic formation and the trophoblastic proliferation of molar change. Missed abortion at 14 weeks (H&E, × 40) (see also Color plate 13)

The presence of a lambda shaped structure at the base of the inter-ovular membrane (also referred to as the twin-peak sign) usually indicates dichorionicity of the pregnancy (see Chapter 15).

Membranes in multiple gestations

Dizygotic twins are dichorionic, and all dichorionic gestations are diamniotic. When a membrane is seen, its thickness provides a reasonable prediction to differentiation between monochorionic and diamniotic twins[13] (see Chapter 15).

The membrane of dichorionic, diamniotic twins is composed of four layers, whereas the membrane of monochorionic, diamniotic twins is composed of only two layers of amnion. Mahony and colleagues[14] found that lack of membrane visualization is not sufficient to establish a diagnosis of monoamniotic gestation.

UMBILICAL CORD

In the normal umbilical cord there are two arteries and a single relatively large umbilical vein. The umbilical cord is formed in the early weeks of embryogenesis from fusion between the yolk stalk and the body stalk. During this process, the two veins fuse to form a single vessel. The cord is covered by a mixed cuboidal and squamous epithelium and is firmly adherent to the Wharton's jelly, which is the underlying connective tissue. The Wharton jelly is derived from mesoderm and contains myofibroblasts and smooth muscle stromal

Table 2   Placenta in selected maternal conditions

Maternal conditions	Placenta
Diabetes mellitus	Large, thick, congested
SLE	Infarcts, abruption, placental vasculopathy, accelerated maturation
Implantation site fibroid	Abruption, placenta accreta
Malignant neoplasm	Metastasis (rare)
Alcohol ingestion	Abruption, IUGR, advanced maturation
Cocaine and smoking	Abruption, IUGR, advanced maturation, vasoconstriction of vessels
Hematologic, hydrops	Thick and large

SLE, systemic lupus erythematosus; IUGR, intrauterine growth restriction

cells within a ground substance rich in hyaluronic acid and chondritin sulfate. The quantity of jelly tends to decrease with gestation age. There are no lymphatic vessels in the cord. The arteries have elastic tissue within their media without true longitudinal or circular layers. The cord vessels are arranged in a helicoidal fashion along the cord. The arteries arise from the hypogastric arteries and carry deoxygenated blood from the fetus to the placenta. The umbilical vein proceeds into the left branch of the portal vein and then into the ductus venosus.

Cord helices are well established by 9 weeks, with an average number of 11 cord helices. The absence of spiraling of the cord has been associated with fetal abnormalities and especially those causing restriction of fetal movements (Figure 16). Excessive coiling has been associated with maternal cocaine use and with premature delivery. The mean length of umbilical cord at term is 55 cm, with a mean diameter of 3.6 cm. The length of the cord appears to be affected by genetic factors and by fetal movements[15]. Short and long cords are associated with other cord complications. Fetal movements induce forceful stretching and tension on the cord. Short cords are defined as length less than 40 cm at term and are found in less than 1% of term pregnancies. Short cords are either due to decreased fetal movement related to the fetus or to intrauterine constraints such as uterine anomalies, oligohydramnios, amniotic bands. Short umbilical cords have been associated with a higher incidence of rupture, hematoma, stricture, fetal malpresentations, prolonged second stage of labor, placental abruption, and uterine inversion. Long cords are associated with higher incidence of entanglements, torsion and thrombosis, true knots and cord

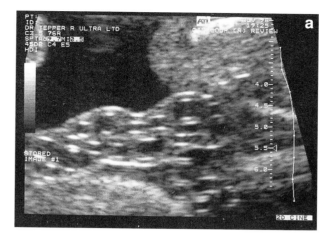

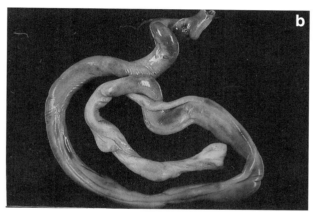

Figure 16   (a) Long axis of umbilical cord in a 21 week pregnancy demonstrating spiraling of umbilical arteries. (b) Reduced twisting of umbilical cord. One artery with very few spirals can be traced throughout the cord

prolapse (Figure 17). Cord length can not be accurately assessed by prenatal ultrasonography.

Measurement of the transverse diameter of the umbilical vein may predict severity of iso-immunization even though idiopathic enlargement of umbilical vein diameter may be seen in normal pregnancies.

Cord stricture

Focal deficiency of Wharton's jelly with or without vascular involvement is termed cord stricture. This focal deficiency usually occurs at the fetal end of the cord and is often associated with torsion. Sometimes multiple coarctations along the umbilical cord are seen. This finding has been reported in association with other anomalies such as anencephaly, cleft lip, fetal edema, polyhydramnios and tracheo-esophageal fistula.

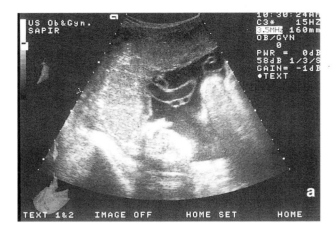

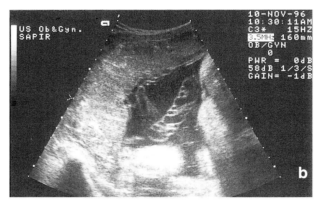

Figure 17 (**a**) Insertion of cord into placenta. (**b**) Long axis of umbilical cord in 19 week pregnancy demonstrating spiral course of umbilical arteries

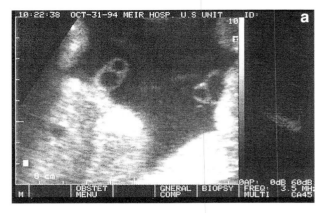

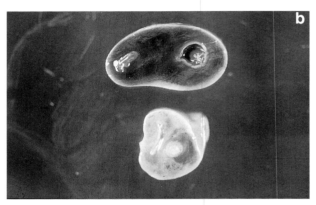

Figure 18 (**a**) Single umbilical artery: a cross-section of the umbilical cord at 32 weeks gestation. (**b**) Two cut sections of umbilical cord at 40 weeks gestation demonstrating single umbilical artery (see also Color plate 16)

Single umbilical artery

Single umbilical artery (SUA) is the result of either agenesis or atrophy of one umbilical artery (Figure 18) or failure of division of the premordial umbilical artery which derives from the single allantoic artery. Ultrasonographic diagnosis involves identification of two blood vessels in transverse section of the umbilical cord. SUA is the most common intrinsic malformation of the cord. The condition is present in 0.6% to 1% of singleton deliveries, and is four times more common in dizygotic twins (5%). Two-vessel cords are also more prevalent with advanced maternal age, high parity, intrauterine growth restriction (IUGR) and diabetes. Twenty per cent of fetuses with SUA have associated morphologic abnormalities, in addition to an increased risk for chromosomal abnormalities, prenatal mortality, premature delivery and IUGR[16,17]. In twins, the known correlation of SUA with fetal anomalies is smaller than in singleton pregnancies.

Useful views of umbilical arteries can be obtained by tracing their course caudally as they separate to straddle the bladder and join the hypogastric arteries (Figure 19, Color plates 17 and 18). With an excessive number of twists of the cord the picture may be confusing, and SUA may be mistakenly diagnosed.

Fetal malformations associated with SUA are:

(1) Urogenital tract: renal agenesis or dysplasia, hydroureter or hydronephrosis, horseshoe kidney, malformed genitalia;

(2) Cardiac: ventricular and atrial septal defects, patent ductus arteriosus;

(3) Musculoskeletal: cleft lip and palate, talipes, finger or toe anomalies, vertebral anomalies;

(4) Gastrointestinal: omphalocele, tracheoesophageal fistula with atresia or stenosis, imperforated anus;

(5) Central nervous system: anencephaly, spina bifida, hydrocephaly, holoprosencephaly;

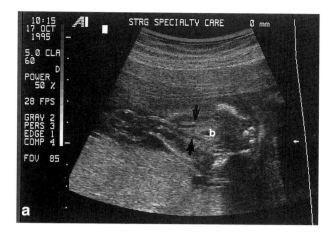

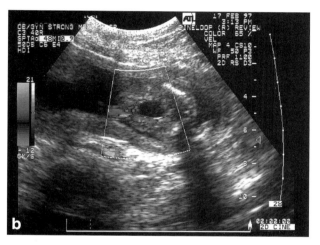

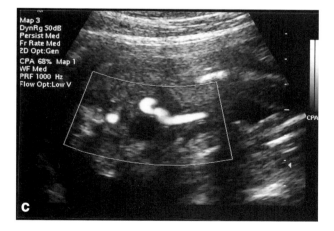

Figure 19 (a) Two umbilical arteries (arrows) seen as they join the hypogastric arteries on each side of the bladder (b). (b) Color Doppler demonstrating two umbilical arteries entering umbilical cord (see also Color plate 17). (c) Power Doppler demonstrating single umbilical artery around bladder (see also Color plate 18)

(6) Other: diaphragmatic hernia, pulmonary hypoplasia, sacrococcygeal teratoma.

Management of pregnancies with SUA involves:

(1) Detailed ultrasonographic survey including fetal echocardiography;
(2) Fetal karyotyping;
(3) Periodic evaluation of fetal wellbeing.

Supernumerary cord vessels

This is a very rare event, and is associated with increased risk of malformations, with no specific organ or system involvement.

Persistent right umbilical vein is a rare prenatal diagnosis. The vein sweeps in a cephalic direction to the fetal gall bladder. More than half of the cases with persistent right umbilical vein have additional anomalies.

Umbilical edema

With the diagnosis of a cord mass the main concern is fetal circulation. Edema or swelling of cord can be classified as localized or general (Table 3). General cord edema may be found in up to 10% of all deliveries and is related to fetal death, placental abruption, pre-eclampsia, Rh incompatibility, diabetes mellitus, chorioamnionitis, prematurity and delivery by elective cesarean section.

Uncommon cord masses

Cystic masses of umbilical cord may be of either allantoic (Figure 20) or omphalomesenteric origin. These cystic masses are distinguishable only by histology. The cysts are usually small and represent remnants of the allantois or the umbilical vesicle. The presence of such cysts usually does not carry any risk and does not jeopardize fetal circulation.

The omphalomesenteric cyst is a dilatation of a segment of the omphalomesenteric duct lined by epithelium of gastrointestinal origin (Figure 21). The allantoic cyst has its origin in fetal adnexal tissue (amnion, chorion, yolk sac, and allantoid).

The differential diagnosis of cystic umbilical cord structures also includes old hematomas of umbilical cord. These are mostly a result of traumatic insult causing extravasation of blood into the Wharton's jelly. The umbilical vein is frequently involved, with the most common site

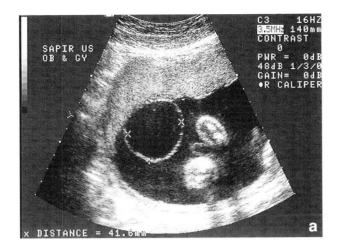

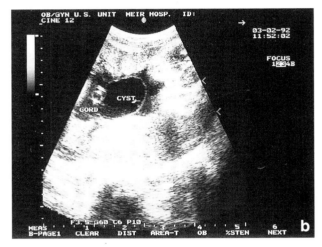

Figure 20 (**a**) Allantoic cyst: large cystic structure (x – x) of umbilical cord representing an allantoic cyst. (**b**) Large cyst within cord

Table 3   The cord in different clinical conditions

Narrow cord	Localized edema	Generalized edema
Intrauterine growth restriction	Aneuploidy	Prematurity
Fetal malformation	Hemangioma	Abruption
Cord prolapse	Omphalocele	Pre-eclampsia
Twin to twin transfusion	Patent urachus	Rh incompatibility
		Diabetes mellitus
		Chorioamnionitis
		Fetal death

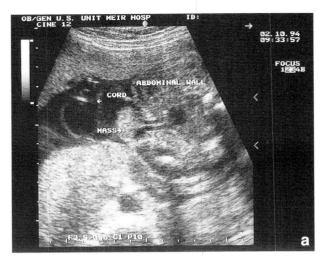

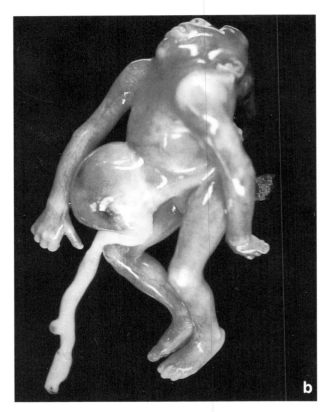

Figure 21 (**a**) Omphalocele: transverse section of the fetal trunk showing a small omphalocele (mass). The umbilical cord is implanted at the apex of the mass (arrow) also demonstrating a cystic structure. Corresponding section of the cord at the cystic structure confirmed the diagnosis of omphalomesenteric cyst. (**b**) Omphalocele at 20 weeks gestation. The omphalocele sac contains liver and loops of small intestine. Cranio-cervico-thoracal rachischisis and iniencephaly are also seen

located near the fetal insertion. The ultrasonographic appearance is that of an irregular mass rather than a cystic lesion. The nature of the mass can be related to the duration of the existence of the clot. An old clot is usually hypoechogenic in appearance while a fresh clot is commonly hyperechogenic. Increased perinatal and fetal mortality has been reported in this condition probably due to compression of the vessels.

Hemangioma of umbilical cord (Figure 22) is a tumor which originally arises from the endothelial cells of the vessels of the umbilical cord. Ultrasonography of the umbilical cord may demonstrate localized edema with or without a solid component. Cord hemangiomas are associated with elevated serum alpha-fetoprotein levels. Similar to placental chorangiomas, umbilical cord hemangiomas may be associated with fetal hydrops.

Thrombosis of the umbilical vessels is usually the result of needle puncture of the cord. The incidence of cord thrombosis as a primary event is higher in infants born to diabetic mothers. Thrombosis of cord has also been associated with non-immune hydrops.

Amniotic band

Amniotic bands are considered to be a result of vascular damage and disruption or rupture of the amnion in early pregnancy which leads to entrapment of fetal structures by mesodermic bands from the chorionic side of the amnion. Amniotic band syndrome is a group of congenital fetal malformations ranging from minor constriction rings and digital edema to severe structural abnormalities such as cleft lip and palate and limb amputation (Figure 23).

AMNIOTIC FLUID

The amniotic cavity first appears at 4 weeks after the last menstrual period. Prior to the 12th week of pregnancy the amniotic fluid is mainly a transudate across the placental membranes and represents a filtrate of maternal plasma. Later in pregnancy the composition of the amniotic fluid changes due to the development of multiple fluid exchange pathways between fetus and amniotic fluid. By the 20th week of pregnancy fetal urine accounts for the majority of amniotic fluid. Fluid is removed from the amniotic space largely by fetal swallowing and absorption from the gastrointestinal tract. The overall amount of fluid present depends on the balance of fetal swallowing and micturition. Other less significant contributions to changes in amniotic fluid volume are fetal breathing movements and leakage through the fetal skin.

Near term approximately 95% of the total amniotic fluid volume is replaced every day. Amniotic fluid volume rises progressively from approximately 250 ml at 16 weeks to a mean of 800 ml in the third trimester with a reduction post-term.

Amniotic fluid plays an important role in temperature control, pulmonary development, fetal movement and fetal growth. Normal amniotic fluid volume is thus thought to be a reflection of normal fetal–maternal exchange. A variety of abnormal conditions are associated with abnormalities of amniotic fluid volume.

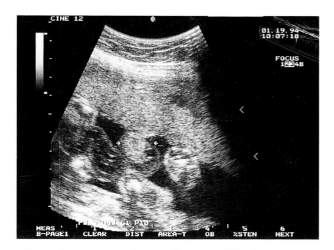

Figure 22 Hemangioma of the umbilical cord. The echogenic lesion (arrows) of the fetal cord did not change in size during the course of pregnancy. Intensive Doppler flow monitoring throughout pregnancy showed no evidence of fetal compromise

Methods of measurement of amniotic fluid

The earliest amniotic fluid estimations were performed in the 18th century. An early clinical approach used three diameters of the uterus to calculate its volume. A variety of methods have been introduced for ultrasonographic estimation of amniotic fluid volume[18].

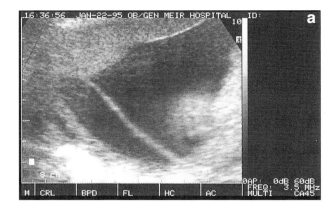

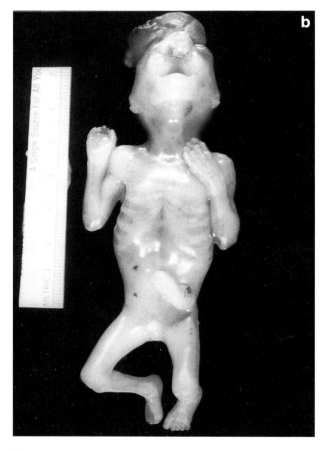

Figure 23 (a) Transverse image at 28 weeks gestation showing amniotic band. (b) Amniotic band syndrome at 15 weeks gestation. Multiple irregular facial clefts, amputated fingers and a delicate amniotic band between right hand and head are seen

Subjective criteria

The user integrates the size and the number of amniotic fluid pockets from several plains into a unified impression of an overall amniotic fluid volume. Research has shown that a fairly accurate estimation can be obtained when the observer is experienced.

One centimeter rule (qualitative amniotic fluid volume)

This method involves measurement of the vertical depth of the largest pocket of amniotic fluid found at the time of scanning. The depth of the pocket is measured at a right angle to the uterine contour. The presence of at least one pocket of fluid with vertical depth of 1 cm and more led to determining the amniotic fluid volume as normal[19]. However, according to Sepulveda et al.[20], there is poor correlation between the deepest pocket measurements and amniotic fluid volume. Therefore this method is considered to be insufficient for determination of normal and abnormal amniotic fluid volume.

Amniotic Fluid Index method

This four-quadrant technique was first reported by Phelan et al. in 1987[21]. The Amniotic Fluid Index (AFI) technique involves dividing the uterine cavity into four quadrants. The largest vertical dimension of amniotic fluid is identified in each quadrant. The four largest vertical dimensions are measured and their summation is the AFI. Oligohydramnios is defined as an AFI which is smaller than the 5 percentile for gestational age of pregnancy, while polyhydramnios is the summation of AFI which is larger than 95%. Normal values of the AFI for each gestation age have been developed[22].

The dye dilution technique

The dye dilution technique is currently considered to be the most accurate way to determine amniotic fluid volume. However, being an invasive method, it involves a higher risk of complications, and it is not applied as a routine procedure. In this technique a needle is inserted into the amniotic cavity and a solution with known concentration is injected. The solution and amniotic fluid are allowed to mix for 30 minutes and a small sample of amniotic fluid is aspirated. The new concentration determines the total amniotic fluid volume.

Table 4 Fetal states associated with oligohydramnios

Syndromes
Beckwith–Wiedemann
Branchio-oto-renal
Herrmann–Opitz
Holzgreve–Wagner–Rehder
Larsen
Lowry hyperkeratosis
Meckel
Neu–Laxova
Roberts
Smith–Lemli–Opitz
Weyers

Central nervous system abnormalities
Cerebroventricular hemorrhage
Encephalocele
Holoprosencephaly
Microcephaly
Microcephaly micrognathia
Intrauterine growth restriction
VATER association

Chromosomal aberration
XXX
Deletion chromosome 14q
Trisomy 21
Duplication, partial chromosome 1q mosaicism
Inversion, duplication chromosome 1
Monosomy 4p/partial trisomy 20p
Triploidy
Trisomy 13
Trisomy 14q
Trisomy 16 mosaicism
Trisomy 18
45, X

Twins: conjoined twins; twin-to-twin transfusion

Neck anomalies
Cystic hygroma

Cardiac anomalies
Endocardial fibroelastosis
Tetralogy of Fallot

Gastrointestinal abnormalities
Gastroschisis
Mesenchymal hamartoma of the liver
Megacystis-microcolon-intestinal hypoperistalsis
Persistent cloaca

Genitourinary abnormalities
Polycystic kidney disease (autosomal dominant and recessive)
Potter type 2A
Renal dyplasia
Renal agenesis
Renal tubular dysgenesis
Uretero-vesical junction obstruction
Urethral obstruction malformation
Urorectal septum malformation sequence

Skeletal abnormalities
Limb/pelvis-hypoplasia/aplasia
Short rib-polydactyly
Sirenomalia

Metabolic/endocrine anomalies
Hypothyroidism
Hypophosphatasia (infantile form)

Placental abnormalities
Molar pregnancy
Single umbilical artery

Other
Fetal demise
Intrauterine growth restriction
Lupus erythematosus
Parvovirus infection

Table 5 Conditions associated with polyhydramnios

Cardiac anomalies
Acardia
Aortic valve atresia
Aortic valve stenosis
Atrial flutter

Skeletal anomalies
Achondrogenesis type 1 & 2
Agnathia-microstomia-synotia
Arthrogryposis
Asphyxiating thoracic dystrophy

Syndromes
Aminopterin syndrome

Bartter syndrome
Beckwith-Wiederman syndrome

Placental abnormalities
Amniotic band disruption sequence (amniotic band syndrome)

Central nervous system anomalies
Anencephaly
Arachnoid cyst

Gastrointestinal
Annular pancreas

Oligohydramnios

Oligohydramnios is associated with a variety of anomalous fetal states, as listed in Table 4.

Polyhydramnios

Polyhydramnios may be present in the conditions listed in Table 5.

CONCLUSIONS

The placenta is the essential connection between mother and fetus. During pregnancy it performs the functions of many organs and normal placental development is crucial for fetal growth and development. As we have seen, many adverse conditions affecting the developing fetus demonstrate ultrasonographic signs that often are the initial or only signs of abnormal development or growth. Ultrasonographic assessment of the placenta and amniotic fluid should be performed on every examination to improve detection of abnormal fetal development and enhance prenatal care of mother and fetus.

References

1. Grannum PAT, Berkowitz RL, Hobbins JC. The ultrasonic changes in maturing placenta and their relation to fetal pulmonic maturity. *Am J Obstet Gynecol* 1979;133:915–22
2. Patterson RM, Hayashi RH, Cavazos D. Ultrasonographically observed early placental maturation and perinatal outcome. *Am J Obstet Gynecol* 1983;147:773–7
3. Lavery JP. Placenta previa. *Clin Obstet Gynecol* 1990; 33:414–21
4. Wexler P, Gottesfeld KR. Early diagnosis of placenta previa. *Obstet Gynecol* 1979;54:231–4
5. Cotton DB, Read JA, Paul RH, *et al*. The conservative aggressive management of placenta previa. *Am J Obstet Gynecol* 1980;137:687–95
6. Farine D, Peisner DB, Timor-Tritsch IE. Placenta previa – is the traditional diagnostic approach satisfactory? *J Clin Ultrasound* 1990;18:328–31
7. Clark SL, Koonings PP, Phelan JP. Placent previa/accreta and prior cesarean section. *Obstet Gynecol* 1985;66:89–92
8. Jaffe R, DuBeshter B, Sherer DM, *et al*. Failure of methotrexate for term placenta percreta. *Am J Obstet Gynecol* 1994;171:558–9
9. Fejgin M, Rosen D, Ben-Nun I, *et al*. Ultrasonic and magnetic resonance imaging diagnosis of placenta accreta managed conservatively. *J Perinat Med* 1993; 21:165–8
10. Spirt BA, Cohen WN, Weinstein HM. The incidence of placental calcification in normal pregnancy. *Radiology* 1982;142:707–11
11. Grannum PAT, Hobbins JC. The placenta. *Radiol Clin North Am* 1982;20:353–65
12. Jaffe R, Siegal A, Rat L, *et al*. Placental chorioangiomatosis – a high risk pregnancy. *Postgrad Med J* 1985;61:453–5
13. Townsend RR, Simpson GF, Filly RA. Membrane thickness in ultrasound prediction of chorionicity of twin gestations. *J Ultrasound Med* 1988;7:327–32
14. Mahony BS, Filly RA, Callen PW. Amnionicity and chorionicity in twin pregnancies: prediction using ultrasound. *Radiology* 1985;155:205–9
15. Mills JL, Harley EE, Moessinger AC. Standards for measuring umbilical cord length. *Placenta* 1983;4: 423–6
16. Nyberg DA, Mahony BS, Luthy D, *et al*. Single umbilical artery. Prenatal detection of concurrent anomalies. *J Ultrasound Med* 1991;10:247–53
17. Heifetz SA. Single umbilical artery: a statistical analysis of 237 autopsy cases and review of the literature. *Perspect Pediatr Pathol* 1984;8:345–78
18. Williams K. Amniotic fluid assessment. *Obstet Gynecol Surv* 1993;48:12
19. Chamberlin P. Amniotic fluid volume: ultrasound assessment and clinical significance. *Semin Perinatol* 1985;9:163–7
20. Sepulveda W, Flack NJ, Fisk NM. Direct volume measurement at midtrimester amnioinfusion in relation to ultrasonographic index of amniotic fluid volume. *Am J Obstet Gynecol* 1994;170:1160–3
21. Phelan JP, Smith CV, Broussard P, *et al*. Amniotic fluid assessment with the four-quadrant technique at 36–42 weeks gestation. *J Reprod Med* 1987;32:540–2
22. Moore TR, Cayle SE. The amniotic fluid index in normal pregnancy. *Am J Obstet Gynecol* 1990;162: 1168–73

Fetal face and central nervous system

Ana Monteagudo and Ilan E. Timor-Tritsch

8

Scanning for the location of the fetal head is usually how most ultrasound studies begin. Biometric measurements such as biparietal diameter, head circumference, occipito-frontal diameter and the measurement of the fetal lateral ventricles are routinely obtained in every scan. Traditionally these measurements as well as detailed anatomical studies of the brain are performed using transabdominal sonography (TAS).

TAS allows the fetal brain to be imaged in the axial plane as well as in the coronal planes. Sagittal sections are seldom possible unless the fetus is in a non-vertex presentation. By adding transvaginal sonography (TVS) to the transabdominal scan the sagittal plane can be added. Therefore, in cases of a known anomaly, or in a patient in which an anomaly is suspected, both scanning modalities, i.e. the transabdominal and the transvaginal, should be used to image the fetal head (Figure 1).

In this chapter we will concentrate on the TVS appearance of the fetal brain. Most imaging textbooks dealing with the subject of fetal anomalies have vast numbers of pictures detailing the transabdominal images of central nervous system pathology. Therefore, we will not duplicate this material but will introduce the reader to imaging several fetal brain anomalies using TVS.

In 1991, we reported on our preliminary study of 70 normal fetuses scanned by the transvaginal technique described in this chapter[2]. In our initial study we documented that there is a learning curve to master the transvaginal technique; however, we were able to image all planes in approximately 75% of the fetuses. The first attempts to perform TVS of the brain may either be very rewarding or somewhat frustrating, but, as with any new technique, with time the ability to capture the desired structures improves. Therefore, as experience is gained, fewer and fewer cases will result in non-visualization of the planes.

The use of TVS to scan the fetus throughout pregnancy has become widely accepted among sonographers, sonologists and most importantly among patients. Scanning the fetal brain during the second and third trimesters using TVS is chiefly

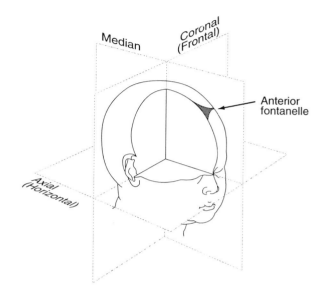

Figure 1 The three classic planes through the fetal head. Multiple coronal (frontal) sections are possible. Only one median section is feasible in the sagittal direction. Every section on each side of the median is a paramedian or simply a sagittal section. Many axial (horizontal) sections are possible. Reproduced with permission[1]

done through the relatively large anterior fontanelle of the fetus. Other fontanelles as well as sutures can be used to provide an acoustic window into the fetal brain. The technique of TVS of the fetal brain is comparable to neonatal brain imaging. In both cases the scanning is performed through the anterior fontanelle and the sections obtained are basically in the coronal and sagittal planes. Some of the advantages of scanning the fetal brain using the transvaginal/transfontanelle route are: both hemispheres can be clearly imaged since the fetal cranial bones do not obscure the image; imaging artifacts encountered by TAS are avoided; maternal obesity does not preclude sonographic exam; and lastly the sections obtained by TVS can be correlated with neonatal imaging studies.

SCANNING TECHNIQUE

TVS can be easily and safely performed any time during the pregnancy. The scanning technique is relatively simple, but requires a different approach for fetuses up to 12 weeks. These first trimester embryos/fetuses can be scanned with a transvaginal probe regardless of their position. However, after 12 weeks, it is important to have the fetus in a vertex presentation. However, at this gestational age this is easily accomplished by very slightly maneuvering the fetus using the abdominal hand and/or the vaginal probe. Up to 16 weeks, in the case of singleton pregnancies, the transvaginal approach should be the first line approach to fetal neuroscanning. Beyond 16–17 weeks, the transabdominal and the transvaginal approaches should be used individually or in combination as required by fetal position. It should always be remembered that if the fetus is in the vertex presentation, the transvaginal approach yields pictures of better quality and resolution.

The ideal probe to perform TVS of the fetal brain with is an end-firing 5.0–7.5 MHz transvaginal probe. Off-axis probes do not allow easy application of their active flat surface to the round fetal head. In addition, rotating off-axis probes within the vagina result in discomfort and decreased tolerance of the procedure. The probe should be advanced under real-time sonography until a clear image of the fetal brain is obtained. The best images are procured when the probe has been aligned with the anterior fontanelle or any other fontanelles or sutures of the fetal head (Figure 2). This can be achieved by either angling the probe anteriorly or posteriorly, moving it up or down or sweeping it side to side over the head until a clear image appears. A helpful maneuver is to place the free hand over the maternal abdomen just above the symphysis pubis and gently manipulate the head through the abdomen into a desired position.

Orientation: scanning sections

The scanning sections obtained by TVS actually 'radiate' in a fan shape from the single point originating from the anterior fontanelle. Hence most of the scanning sections obtained are not parallel to each other. Due to this peculiar way of imaging the fetal (as well as the neonatal) brain we described a new nomenclature to deal with the sections which are obtained in the 'sagittal' and in the 'coronal' planes[2]. The 'new' proposed 'coronal' scanning

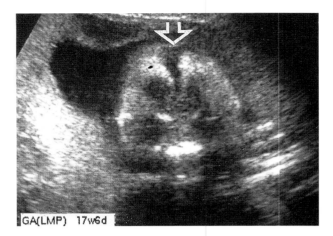

Figure 2   An anterior coronal section showing the anterior fontanelle (open arrow). Reproduced with permission[3]

sections are divided into the frontal, mid-coronal and occipital group. Each group is subsequently further divided into two or three specific sections. Similarly in the 'sagittal' plane the median and two oblique sections (both on the right and left side) were described.

Normal anatomy

Before describing the normal anatomy there are several helpful hints that are useful to keep in mind when scanning.

The fetal brain is a symmetric organ. Hence, the left hemisphere should be comparable in size to the right hemisphere. Therefore, any obvious deviation of this symmetry should trigger a careful evaluation and search for possible abnormalities. Several exceptions come to mind: there seems to be an asymmetry of the fetal brain regarding the body of the lateral ventricles; the left lateral ventricle has been found to be larger than the right[4,5]; and another exception is that gyri and sulci are not perfectly symmetric.

The brain has several highly echogenic structures which may help in orientation. These echogenic structures can be easily identified. They include: the fetal skull and facial bones, the choroid plexus (starting at 9 weeks), the soft membranous covers of the brain (pia mater and arachnoid also known as leptomeninges), the internal linings of the ventricles and last but not least the cerebellum. The cerebellum has the numerous deep gyri and sulci; therefore the cerebellum appears as an extremely bright, echogenic structure located in the posterior fossa.

Coronal sections (Figure 3)

The frontal-1 and -2 are sections anterior to the corpus callosum. The interhemispheric fissure is seen as a bright midline echo between the brain parenchyma of the frontal lobes. During the second trimester this fissure appears relatively straight, but with advancing gestational age and the rapid growth of the brain and the newly formed gyri and sulci the interhemispheric fissure becomes progressively irregular. In the frontal-2 the anterior horn of the lateral ventricle can be seen up to approximately the 14th week of gestation. Beyond 14 weeks of gestation if the anterior horn of the lateral ventricle is detected in this section, ventriculomegaly or hydrocephalus has to be suspected.

The falx cerebri is seen in the midline arising from the inferior surface of the superior sagittal sinus, traverses the subarachnoid space, and continues through the interhemispheric fissure.

The mid-coronal-1 and -2 sections pass through the body of the lateral ventricle (Figures 3 and 4). The mid-coronal-3 passes through the atrium of the lateral ventricle. At the base of the interhemispheric fissure and at right angles to it the hypoechoic corpus callosum can be seen crossing the midline. In the midline below the corpus callosum two sheets of tissue are seen flanking a space: these are the cavum septi pellucidi. Below and to the right and left side of the corpus callosum the lateral ventricles appear as bilateral fluid-filled structures which are concave laterally. As the

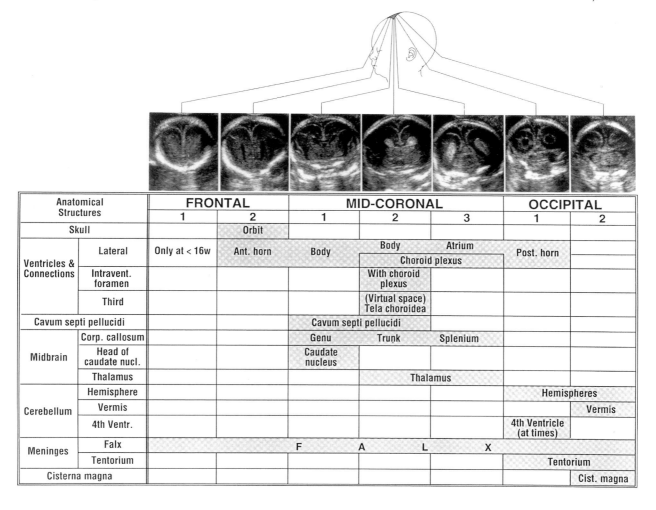

Anatomical Structures		FRONTAL		MID-CORONAL			OCCIPITAL	
		1	2	1	2	3	1	2
Skull			Orbit					
Ventricles & Connections	Lateral	Only at < 16w	Ant. horn	Body	Body	Atrium	Post. horn	
					Choroid plexus			
	Intravent. foramen				With choroid plexus			
	Third				(Virtual space) Tela choroidea			
Cavum septi pellucidi				Cavum septi pellucidi				
Midbrain	Corp. callosum			Genu	Trunk	Splenium		
	Head of caudate nucl.			Caudate nucleus				
	Thalamus				Thalamus			
Cerebellum	Hemisphere						Hemispheres	
	Vermis							Vermis
	4th Ventr.						4th Ventricle (at times)	
Meninges	Falx			F	A	L X		
	Tentorium						Tentorium	
Cisterna magna								Cist. magna

Figure 3 Structures seen on serial coronal sections of the fetal brain after 20 postmenstrual weeks, from anterior to posterior. The table indicates the different and specific structures seen across each of these sections. The combination of these structures renders each section its unique appearance. Reproduced with permission[1]

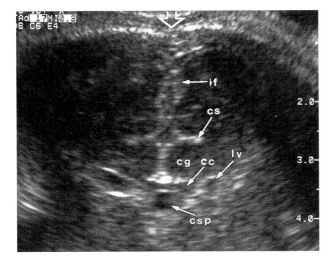

Figure 4 A mid-coronal-2 section of a fetus at 31 postmenstrual weeks of gestation. The white open arrow points to the anterior fontanelle. The midline structures shown are: the interhemisphere fissure (if), the cingulate sulcus (cs), the cingulate gyrus (cg), the hypoechoic corpus callosum (cc) at the base of the interhemispheric fissure, the body of the lateral ventricles (lv) and the midline sonolucent cavum septi pellucidi (csp)

fetus matures the lateral ventricles in these sections become progressively narrower. The echogenic choroid plexus may be seen as a bright echo lining the most inferior wall of the lateral ventricle. Medially, the bilateral choroid plexus slips through the left and right interventricular foramen (of Monroe) into the third ventricle. Eventually, as term nears, the anterior horns become slit-like and at sometimes difficult to image. Between the thalami in the midline the third ventricle is occasionally imaged. This lack of visualization of the third ventricle is due to its normal but small transverse diameter. Posterior and adjacent to the ventricles, in the mid-coronal-1 section the caudate nucleus of the basal ganglia can be imaged.

In the occipital-1 section the posterior horns of the lateral ventricles as well as the structures of the posterior fossa can be seen. On this section the occipital horns appear as rounded sonolucent structures. In the posterior fossa the cerebellum is imaged between two sonolucent structures: above the fourth ventricle and below the cisterna magna. Between the thalami in the midline the third ventricle is occasionally imaged. This lack of visualization of the third ventricle is due to its normal but small transverse diameter. The occipital-2 section is the most posterior coronal section which cannot always be imaged. It contains the occipital lobes, the tentorium of the cerebellum, the cerebellum, the vermis of the cerebellum and the cerebello-medullary cistern (cisterna magna).

Sagittal sections (Figure 5)

The median section reveals the corpus callosum and the sonolucent cavum septi pellucidi. The corpus callosum is a centrally located hypoechoic, semilunar midline structure located above the sonolucent cavum septi pellucidi. The corpus callosum becomes sonographically obvious by 18–20 weeks and is fully developed by 22–28 weeks gestation. The corpus callosum is composed of three parts: genu (anterior), trunk (middle) and the splenium (posterior). The cingulate gyrus is evident above the corpus callosum (Figure 6). The cerebellum appears in the posterior fossa, below the tentorium of the cerebellum, as a hyperechoic structure indented by the sonolucent fourth ventricle. The cisterna magna is another sonolucent structure located below the cerebellum in the posterior fossa.

The left and right oblique-1 sections reveal portions of the anterior horn and body of the lateral ventricles which appears as the mirror image of the letter C, the open end of which points towards the fetal face. This seems to be the clinically most revealing section.

The oblique-2 sections are lateral to the oblique-1 sections. In this section the insula and the lateral sulcus (Sylvian fissure) are imaged. In addition, within the insula the pulsating middle cerebral artery can be appreciated. At times it is virtually impossible to obtain this section. Reasons for this include the limited mobility of the probe within the vagina, the less than perfect positioning of the fetal head, and the constant fetal movements. The most important goal, however, is to try to keep the tip of the probe opposite the fontanelle, otherwise a blurred image or no image at all can be created on the screen.

The gyri, sulci and fissures can also be imaged. However, it is important to remember that during the second trimester the surface of the brain is smooth, due to the lack of well developed gyri and sulci. Between 28–30 weeks of gestation a fetal brain growth spurt occurs and many new gyri and sulci develop[6–8]. The sonographic appearance of the cortex after 28–30 weeks changes from a smooth

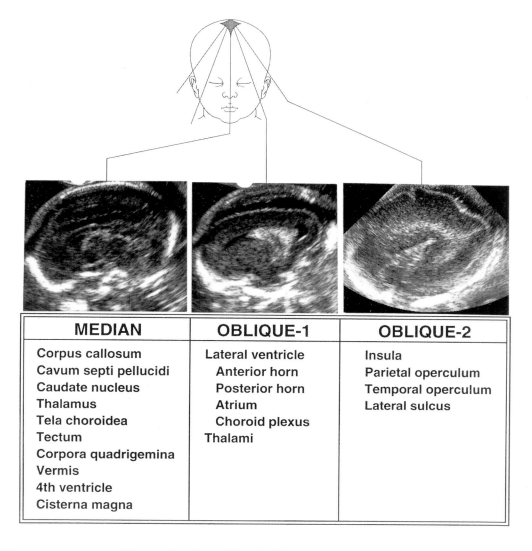

MEDIAN	OBLIQUE-1	OBLIQUE-2
Corpus callosum	Lateral ventricle	Insula
Cavum septi pellucidi	Anterior horn	Parietal operculum
Caudate nucleus	Posterior horn	Temporal operculum
Thalamus	Atrium	Lateral sulcus
Tela choroidea	Choroid plexus	
Tectum	Thalami	
Corpora quadrigemina		
Vermis		
4th ventricle		
Cisterna magna		

Figure 5 Structures seen on serial sagittal sections of the fetal brain after 20 postmenstrual weeks. The table indicates the different and specific structures for that section. Reproduced with permission[1]

surface to one with an increasingly complex pattern of echodense lines covering the cerebral surfaces. Gyri, sulci and fissures can be imaged using the following sections: (1) a median section when the flat interhemispheric surface is tangentially scanned; (2) in the mid-coronal-1; and (3) oblique-2 section[6–8].

FETAL BRAIN ANOMALIES

Timing is a very important factor when looking for a congenital anomaly. For example in a patient at risk for agenesis of the corpus callosum a brain scan at 14 weeks will miss the anomaly. This is due to the well known fact that the corpus callosum does not start to become sonographically apparent until 18–20 weeks and does not acquire its final form until 28–30 weeks of gestation. Kohlenberg and colleagues[9] performed a population-based study of 55 226 pregnancies in Victoria, Australia. There were 143 central nervous system (CNS) defects reported during the study period, of which 85 (60%) had a scan between 16–20 weeks gestation. In 64 (75%) the diagnosis of a CNS defect was made, in 17 (20%) the diagnosis was not made and in 4 (5%) the diagnosis was questionable. Their conclusion was that poor timing of the examination rather than poor sensitivity was the most important factor in the detection of CNS defects.

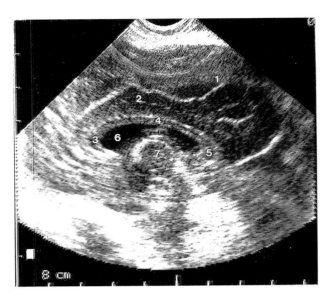

Figure 6 Median section of a fetus at 32 postmenstrual weeks showing the cingulate sulcus (1), cingulate gyrus (2), the genu (3), trunk (4), and splenium (5) of the corpus callosum, the cavum septi pellucidi (6) and the thalamus (7). Note that the fetus is facing down and the forehead is on the left and the occiput is to the right

Neural tube defects: exencephaly, anencephaly, iniencephaly, cephalocele, spinal dysraphism

The neural groove begins to close at about 22 days postconception in an area near the junction between the future brain and spine. Closure of the groove proceeds simultaneously in rostral and caudal fashion[10]. Failure of the rostral neuropore to close during day 24–26 of gestation results in an abnormal development of the cranium and malformation of the brain and meninges. When the cranial defect is large, the resulting forebrain develops partially and then degenerates (acrania, exencephaly, anencephaly)[11]. If the cranial defect is small, it results in varying degrees of herniation of the brain or the meninges (cephalocele).

Exencephaly

Exencephaly (acrania) refers to an anomaly in which there is absence of the entire or a substantial portion of the cranium in the presence of varying amount of brain tissue. This condition is theorized to be the embryologic predecessor of anencephaly in man[10–15]. Further proof that exencephaly is the predecessor of anencephaly has been derived by the detection of exencephalic fetuses by sono-graphy[16] and histologic studies of the cells present in the amniotic fluid[17].

Anencephaly

Anencephaly is the partial or total absence of the brain in conjunction with a missing calvaria. Anencephaly is the most common of the neural tube defects occurring in about 1 per 1000 births[12,18,19]. Anencephaly is a lethal condition with about 75% of the fetuses being stillborn and the rest dying shortly after birth. Polyhydramnios is present in up to 50% of the cases during the second and third trimester due to decreased fetal swallowing[11,20–22]. The sonographic findings of an anencephalic fetus is the absence of the cranium above the prominent orbits with varying degree of brain tissue; there is preservation of the base of the skull and facial features[23]. In the oblique view the fetal profile is seen, but beyond the orbital ridges the forehead and calvarium are missing. In approximately 10% of the anencephalic fetuses an open spinal defect (craniorachischisis) is present[22] (Figure 7).

Iniencephaly

Iniencephaly is a rare and lethal anomaly which results from a developmental arrest of the embryo during the third week of gestation resulting in persistence of the embryonic cervical retroflexion which leads to failure of the neural groove to close in the area of the cervical spine or upper thorax[25–34]. The three main features of iniencephaly are: a defect in the occiput involving the foramen magnum; retroflexion of the entire spine which forces the fetus to look upwards with its head directly on to the lumbar region; and open spinal defects of variable degrees[25–28]. Iniencephaly associated with a cephalocele is referred to as iniencephalus apertus and that without it as iniencephaly clausus[30]. In up to 84% of the fetuses with iniencephaly multiple anomalies such as hydrocephalus, microcephalus, ventricular atresia, holoprosencephaly, polymicrogyria, agenesis of the cerebellar vermis, occipital encephalocele, diaphragmatic hernia, thoracic cage deformities, urinary tract anomalies, cleft lip and palate and omphalocele are present[25–29,31,35]. Typical sonographic findings include retroflexion of the fetal head with short neck and trunk and open cervical and thoracic spinal defects (rachischisis). Polyhydramnois was found to be associated with

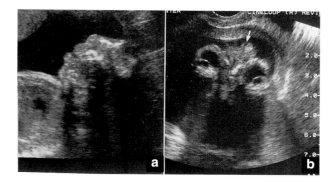

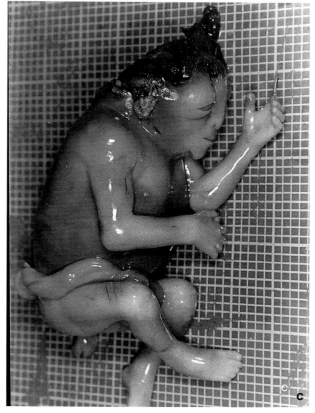

Figure 7 Seventeen week fetus with anencephaly. (**a**) and (**b**) are transvaginal sonographic images. In (**a**) the profile is seen and beyond the orbits, the cranium is missing. (**b**) A coronal section showing the orbits, lenses and some remnant brain tissue (arrow). (**c**) The specimen which shows the remnant brain tissue seen in ultrasound. (**a**) and (**b**) reproduced with permission[24]

iniencephaly apertus. The short neck and trunk may lead to a very early size/dates discrepancy.

Cephalocele

Cephalocele is a midline cranial defect through which the brain and/or meninges are herniating.

Cephalocele may occur in the occipital, frontal parietal, orbital, nasal or nasopharyngeal region of the head. The reported incidence ranges from 1/3500 to 1/5000 live births[36]. The prevalence of the different types of cephalocele show geographical variation, with 80% of those occurring in the West being occipital cephalocele (Figure 8) and the other 20% being equally divided among the frontal and parietal cephalocele. In the East frontal cephalocele are more common[19,21,23,37–40] (Figure 9). The majority of cephalocele are isolated lesions, but a small number may be associated with syndromes. Of these, Meckel syndrome (or Meckel–Gruber) is the most significant. Meckel syndrome is an autosomal recessive condition. The syndrome is characterized by occipital cephalocele (present in 80%), bilateral polycystic kidneys and post-axial polydactyly[38,40]. Sonographic findings of cephalocele include a defect in the bony skull with a protruding sac-like structure, the contents of which may be cystic, containing cerebrospinal fluid, or solid with obvious brain tissue or a combination of both[23,41,42] Other associated brain abnormalities in non-syndromic cephalocele include hydrocephalus (85–95%), agenesis of the corpus callosum and Dandy–Walker syndrome[21,43]. Microcephaly may also be present in cases of cephalocele.

Spinal dysraphism

Spinal dysraphism is characterized by an open spine with protrusion of the spinal contents through the bony defect. The incidence of myelomeningocele in the United States is 0.2 to 0.4 per 1000 live births[44]. The development of myelomeningocele starts probably around the fourth week of gestation at the time of closure of the posterior neural tube. Myelocele and myelomeningocele develop similarly, but the term myelocele refers to a midline plaque of neural tissue (neural placode) that is flush with the surface, and is not covered by skin. In contrast the myelomeningocele is a bulging defect in which the elevated neural plate and meninges are contiguous laterally with the subcutaneous tissue. Ten to 15% of spinal dysraphic defects are closed and normal skin covers the bony defect. Approximately 80% of the lesions occur in the lumbar, thoraco-lumbar, or lumbo-sacral areas of the spine and the balance in the cervical and sacral areas[45].

The diagnostic sensitivities for the prenatal sonographic detection of myelomeningocele are

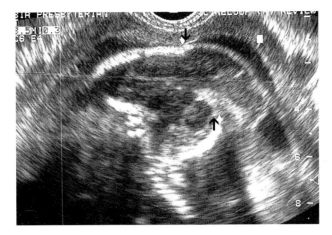

Figure 8 Median section obtained transvaginally of a 28 weeks fetus with an occipital cephalocele. The skull defect through which the sac is herniating is marked with black arrows

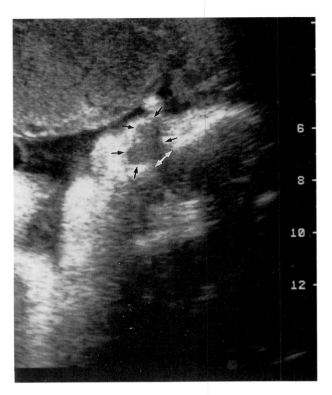

Figure 9 Paramedian section showing the profile of a 36 weeks fetus. The anterior cephalocele is marked by black arrows. The defect in the ethmoid bone through which the cephalocele sac is herniated is highlighted by white arrows. Reproduced with permission[24]

reported to be between 80 and 90% and even higher prior to the knowledge of the maternal serum alpha-fetoprotein results[46–48]. On the sagittal view there are irregularities of the bony spine, a bulging within the posterior contour of the fetal back or obvious disruption of the fetal skin contours. On transverse sections the open spine has a U-shape and in the coronal section the affected bony segment shows a divergent configuration replacing the normal parallel lines of the normal vertebral arches (Figure 10). Determining the site and the extent of the spinal lesion is important because it correlates with the neurologic outcome of the fetus. The higher and the larger the lesion, the more severe the neurologic dysfunction of the neonate.

During the second trimester there are well established intracranial sonographic findings that can enhance the detection of spina bifida, namely 'the lemon sign', 'the banana sign', and hydrocephaly (Figures 11 and 12). The 'lemon sign' refers to deformity of the frontal bone and the 'banana sign' refers to an abnormal shape of the flattened cerebellum which obliterates the cisterna magna. Blumenfeld and colleagues[49] reported on the diagnosis of neural tube defects between 12–17 weeks by using the 'banana' and the 'lemon' signs. They found that the earliest appearance of the 'lemon' and 'banana' signs is at 14 weeks. Therefore, from the early second trimester these indirect cranial findings may be used to enhance the detection of open neural tube defects. Since these findings may be subtle at 14 to 15 weeks a follow-up scan later in the second trimester may be indicated in cases at risk. The 'lemon sign' is present in virtually all cases between 16 to 24 postmenstrual weeks, but after 24 weeks of gestation the 'lemon sign' is a less reliable marker and is present in only 13–50% of the fetuses with spinal defects[50–53]. Cerebellar abnormalities with obliteration of the cisterna magna is present all through gestation in 95–100% of the cases of spinal dysraphism, although after 24 weeks cerebellar absence is more commonly seen than the 'banana sign'[50,53–55]. These indirect cranial findings in conjunction with a spinal defect are termed the Arnold–Chiari type II malformation.

The Arnold–Chiari II malformation is present in almost every case of thoracolumbar, lumbar and lumbosacral myelomeningocele (Figures 10 and 12). The hydrocephalus probably results from either the hindbrain malformation that blocks the flow of cerebrospinal fluid through the fourth ventricle or posterior fossa or from aqueductal stenosis that may be present in 40 to 75% of the cases[56].

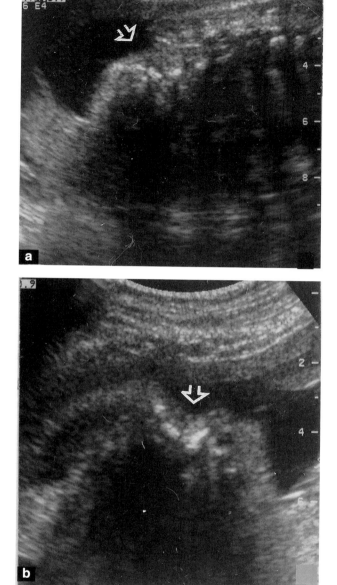

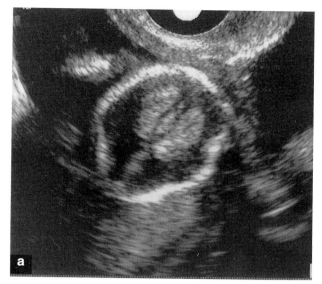

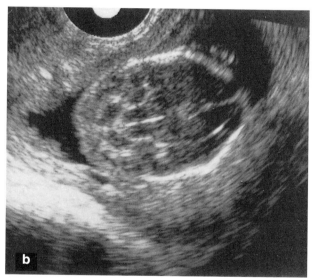

Figure 10 Spina bifida. (**a**) A median section. (**b**) A transverse section depicting the open spinal lesion (open arrowhead). There is loss of the skin contours at the level of the defect and the U-shaped vertebra and the open spinal defect freely communicates with the amniotic fluid

Figure 11 The lemon and banana sign in a fetus at 15 postmenstrual weeks of gestation. (**a**) The depression of the frontal bones termed the lemon sign. (**b**) The cerebellum has herniated through the foramen magnum and has become banana shaped. Reproduced with permission[24]

Midline anomalies: holoprosencephaly, agenesis of the corpus callosum, agenesis of the septi pellucidi, Dandy–Walker malformation

Holoprosencephaly

Holoprosencephaly is a malformation sequence which results from failure of the prosencephalon to differentiate into the cerebral hemispheres and lateral ventricles between the fourth to eighth

Associated brain abnormalities seen with myelomeningocele include hydrocephalus, relative microcephaly, agenesis of the corpus callosum, and diastematomyelia. Other non-CNS anomalies include congenital scoliosis or kyphosis and hip deformities[53,57].

week of gestation. Three types are described: alobar, semilobar, and lobar holoprosencephaly, depending on the degree of failed differentiation. In addition, variable degrees of facial dysmorphism such as cyclopia (single eye or partially divided eye in a single orbit), ethmocephaly (orbital hypotelorism, but separate orbits), cebocephaly (ocular hypotelorism and blind-ended, single nostril nose), hypotelorism (orbits too close together) and other midline facial defects may be present[19,58–61]. Microcephaly may be present in all three types of

holoprosencephalies[61]. The incidence in abortuses has been reported to be 0.4 per 1000 with a lower incidence in live births of 0.06 per 1000[19].

Alobar holoprosencephaly is the most severe of the three types of holoprosencephalies. The anomaly consists of a single ventricle, small cerebrum, fused thalami, agenesis of the corpus callosum and falx cerebri[41]. Sonographic findings of alobar holoprosencephaly include absence of midline structures (falx cerebri, interhemispheric fissure, absence of the corpus callosum), monoventricular cavity with communicating dorsal cyst, fused thalami and facial dysmorphism (Figure 13). The most severe facial dysmorphism, cyclopia, ethmocephaly and cebocephaly, are usually present with alobar holoprosencephaly[61] (Figure 14).

In semilobar holoprosencephaly, some cleavage of the brain has occurred, the ventricles and the cerebral hemispheres are partially separated posteriorly, there is incomplete separation of the thalami, but anteriorly there is still a mono-ventricular cavity[41].

Lobar holoprosencephaly is the most subtle of the three types of holoprosencephalies. The sonographic findings include the presence of the interhemispheric fissure, the fused frontal horns have a flat roof and communicate freely with the third ventricle, the septum pellucidum is always absent, the corpus callosum may be absent, hypoplastic or normal, and there may be midline fusion of the cingulate gyrus. Pilu and colleagues[62] have described an echogenic linear structure running within the third ventricle as a specific sign

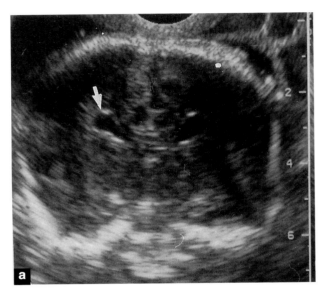

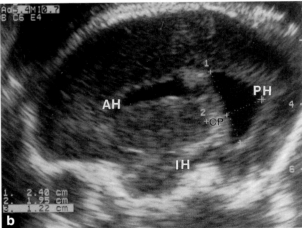

Figure 12 Same fetus as in Figure 10. (**a**) A mid-coronal-2 section showing the dilated bodies of the lateral ventricles (arrow). (**b**) An oblique-1 section showing the dilated lateral ventricle. In this section all three parts of the lateral ventricles are imaged. The choroid plexus (CP) is thin and appears compressed by the increasing cerebrospinal fluid pressure. AH, anterior horn; PH, posterior horn; IH, inferior horn

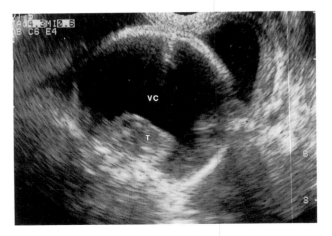

Figure 13 Alobar holoprosencephaly. Note the missing midline structures: interhemispheric fissure, corpus callosum, cavum septi pellucidi. In addition, a single monoventricular cavity (VC) is seen and the thalami are fused (T)

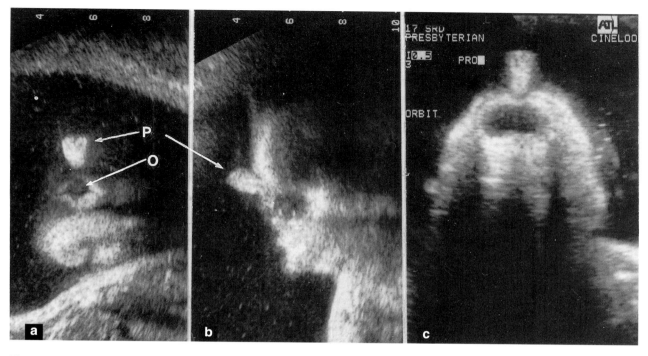

Figure 14   Three views of the face of a fetus with alobar holoprosencephaly. (**a**) A coronal section showing a proboscis (P), single orbit (O) and eye and the lips. (**b**) The profile; note the proboscis (arrow) above the single orbit. (**c**) A close-up view of the single orbit below the proboscis (PRO)

of fetal lobar holoprosencephaly. In the mid-coronal plane, this structure appears as a small, round, solid structure approximately in the mid-portion of the third ventricle. It is believed this structure demonstrates the abnormally fused fornices in the midline[60,62]. In the semilobar and the lobar holoprosencephaly the face may show ocular hypotelorism or hypertelorism, unilateral or bilateral cleft lip or other mild facial dysmorphic features[60].

Agenesis of the corpus callosum and absence of the septi pellucidi

Agenesis of the corpus callosum can be complete or partial, depending on the stage of development at which growth was arrested. The corpus callosum begins to develop anterior to the interventricular foramina (of Monroe) at about 12 weeks of gestation[63]. Then it grows upwards and backwards, in a C shape, as the primitive cerebral hemispheres grow laterally and then poste-riorly[64,65]. By 18 to 20 weeks gestation the corpus callosum can be sonographically appreciated. The total or partial lack of this structure can occur as an isolated anomaly, but 80% of the cases have other

associated malformations[63,64,66,67]. Partial agenesis of the corpus callosum usually involves the posterior portion, since embryologically it develops in a cranial–caudal fashion and may also be associated with other malformations[68]. Most cases of agenesis of the corpus callosum are sporadic, but several genetic disorders as well as chromosomal disorders have been associated with its absence[68]. Using TVS the corpus callosum can be easily imaged on a median section[67,69–73]. In agenesis of the corpus callosum the gyri and sulci appear to be radiating in a perpendicular fashion from the dilated third ventricle in a 'sunburst' pattern[64,67,74]. On an oblique section the frontal horns appear narrow and laterally displaced, and the atria and occipital horns appear slightly dilated[67]. The coronal section demonstrates a wide interhemispheric fissure within which the falx cerebri is present, the lateral ventricles are widely separated and have a distinctive configuration similar to a 'Viking helmet', and lastly the thalami are widely separated due to the dilated third ventricle[75] (Figure 15). The cavum septum pellucidum in most cases of complete agenesis of the corpus callosum is absent or severely distorted[74,76].

Absence of the septi pellucidi may occur as an isolated abnormality or associated with other brain malformations such as septo-optic dysplasia (de Morsier syndrome), holoprosencephaly, Chiari type II malformation, and abnormalities of the corpus callosum[77,78]. Sonographic findings of absent septi pellucidi on the coronal section are the lateral ventricles forming a contiguous hypoechoic area just below the thalami[78] (Figure 16).

Dandy–Walker malformations

In Dandy–Walker malformation (DWM) there is a retro-cerebellar cyst which communicates with the fourth ventricle through a complete or partial defect of the cerebellar vermis[79]. The incidence of DWM has been estimated to be 1 in 30 000 births[80].

Hydrocephalus is frequently found in association with DWM and accounts for up to 12% of cases of congenital hydrocephalus[81–87]. A recent classification of DWM has been introduced based on postnatal neuroimaging study. In this classification DWM is separated into the classic malformation, the Dandy–Walker variant (small defect in the cerebellar vermis without dilatation of the cisterna magna) and mega-cisterna magna (large cisterna magna without cerebellar abnormalities)[79,88]. Sonographic findings of the coronal and the median sagittal planes include a large posterior fossa cyst contiguous with the fourth ventricle, an elevated tentorium, and dilatation of the third and lateral ventricles[89] (Figure 17). Dandy–Walker may occur as part of a Mendelian disorder (i.e. Meckel syndrome), can be associated with chromosomal aneuploidy (i.e. 45, X, triploidy), can result from

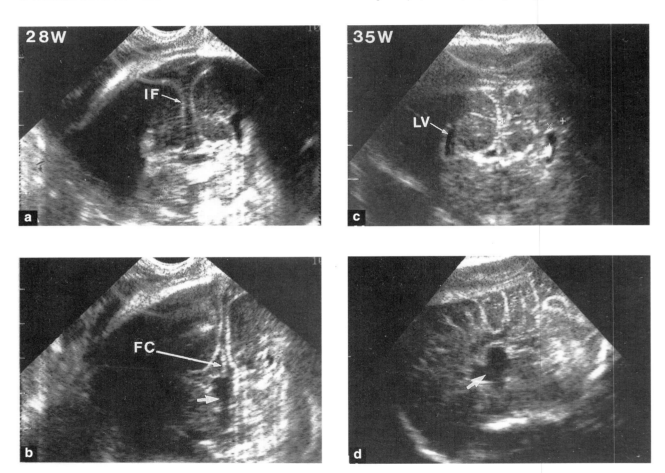

Figure 15 Fetus at 28 weeks and at 35 weeks gestation with agenesis of the corpus callosum. (**a**), (**b**) and (**c**) are mid-coronal-1 and -2 sections showing the interhemispheric fissure (IF) is wide and the falx cerebri (FC) can be seen within. The lateral ventricles (LV) are widely separated and pointing upward similar to a 'viking helmet'. In (**b**) the thalami are separated due to the dilated third ventricle (arrow). (**d**) A median section showing the gyri and sulci which appear to be radiating in a perpendicular fashion from the dilated third ventricle (arrow) in a 'sunburst' pattern

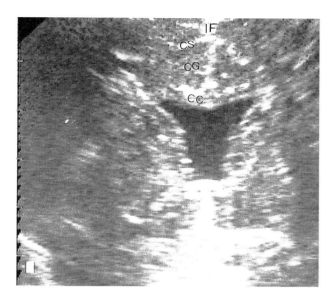

Figure 16 Mid-coronal-1 section of a newborn infant with septo-optic dysplasia. The interhemispheric fissure (IF), cingulate sulcus (CS) and gyrus (CG), and the corpus callosum (CC) are present. The cavum septi pellucidi is missing. The lateral ventricles and the third ventricle freely communicate with each other forming a midline box-like sonolucent structure

environmental exposures (i.e. rubella, alcohol), multifactorial (i.e. congenital heart defect, neural tube defects) and lastly as a sporadic defect (i.e. holoprosencephaly)[79]. Differentiation between a DWM and an arachnoid cyst of the posterior fossa relies on the demonstration of a hypoplastic vermis and connection of the cyst with the fourth ventricle[67].

Congenital hydrocephalus: aqueductal stenosis, communicating hydrocephalus

Hydrocephalus or ventriculomegaly is defined as dilatation of the ventricular system with or without enlargement of the cranium not secondary to atrophy of the brain. In ventriculomegaly, the ventricular dilatation is in the presence of normal fetal intraventricular pressures. In contrast, in hydrocephalus the dilatation of the fetal lateral ventricle results from an increased amount of cerebrospinal fluid and subsequent increase in intraventricular pressures. The overall incidence of congenital hydrocephalus has been estimated to be between 0.5 and 3 per 1000 live births and the incidence of isolated hydrocephalus between 0.39 and 0.87 per 1000 live births[90]. Hydrocephalus can

be grouped into two general types, namely non-communicating and communicating. Non-communicating hydrocephalus refers to the fact that there is an intraventricular obstruction leading to hydrocephalus. In communicating hydrocephalus there are extraventricular causes for the hydrocephalus[91]. Aqueductal stenosis is the most common form of non-communicating hydrocephalus; it can be the result of genetic diseases, infections or exposures to teratogen and accounts for 43% of the cases of hydrocephalus. DWM accounts for 13% of the non-communicating cases of hydrocephalus and was discussed above under midline anomalies. Communicating hydrocephalus, which accounts for 38% of hydrocephalus, is the second most common cause of hydrocephalus. In this general group Arnold–Chiari malformation, encephalocele and congenital absence of the arachnoid granulations are among the causes of hydrocephalus[91]. Other causes which account for about 6% of all cases include agenesis of the corpus callosum, arachnoid cysts and aneurysm of the vein of Galen[86]. Polyhydramnios is present in 30% of the cases[92].

When assessing the lateral ventricles for the presence of ventriculomegaly and/or hydrocephalus either quantitative or qualitative ultrasound methods can be employed[93–97]. Qualitatively one can look for: (1) rounding and bulging of the superior and lateral angles of the frontal horns with inferior pointing in the coronal sections; and (2) dilatation of the occipital horns of the lateral ventricles with thinning and distortion of the choroid plexus on the oblique plane[98–100] (Figures 12, 17 and 18). The qualitative methods however are subjective and dependent on the expertise of the sonographer or sonologist. On the other hand, the quantitative methods are objective and allow different and subsequent examiners to assess if there has been any change in the degree of dilatation. Many published nomograms are available. Most of these nomograms have been generated using TAS[100–105]. In 1993, we reported on nine nomograms generated using TVS. The nomograms were developed using 347 fetuses between 14 and 40 weeks gestation[106,107]. Our results demonstrated that all parts of the lateral ventricles increase with increasing ventriculomegaly, apart from the thickness of the choroid plexus which decreases[107]. The normal choroid plexus appears fluffy and usually fills the antrum of the lateral ventricle totally. In cases of ventriculomegaly the choroid plexus becomes

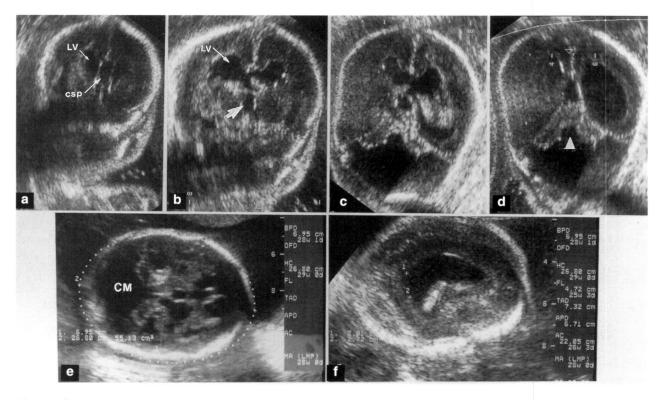

Figure 17 Fetus at 28 postmenstrual weeks of gestation with a Dandy–Walker malformation (**a**) to (**d**) are serial coronal sections. (**a**) A frontal-2 section showing the prominent lateral ventricles (LV), and cavum septi pellucidi (csp). (**b**) A mid-coronal-2 section demonstrating the dilatation of the lateral ventricles (LV) and the third ventricle (arrow). (**c**) and (**d**) are occipital-1 and 2 respectively. The cerebellar hemispheres are splayed, the fourth ventricle (arrowhead) communicates with the large cisterna magna. (**e**) An axial section showing the cisterna magna cyst (cm). (**f**) An oblique-1 section showing the dilatation of the lateral ventricle and the thin and dysmorphic choroid plexus

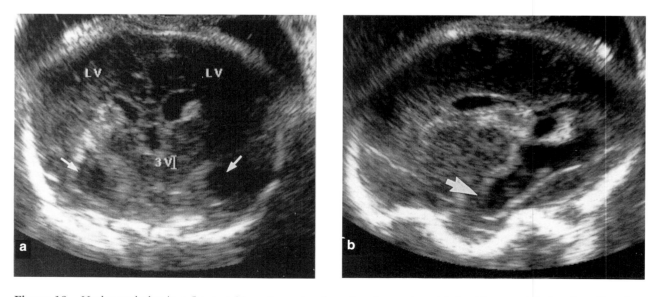

Figure 18 Hydrocephalus in a fetus at 31 postmenstrual weeks of gestation. (**a**) A mid-coronal-2 showing dilatation of the anterior horn (LV), third ventricle (3V) and the inferior horn (arrow) of the lateral ventricle. (**b**) An oblique-1 showing dilatation of all three parts of the lateral ventricle and the dysmorphic and thin choroid plexus (arrow: inferior horn). Reproduced with permission[3]

thin, and floats within the dilated ventricle ('dangling choroid plexus sign')[108].

Ventriculomegaly and/or hydrocephalus first develops in the occipital horns of the lateral ventricles in the up and down direction. This is the direction of least resistance to the increasing pressures of the cerebrospinal fluid. Subsequently, there is compression of the choroid plexus as the cerebrospinal fluid pressure increases[94,95,107–111].

CYSTIC LESIONS OF THE BRAIN

Choroid plexus cysts

Choroid plexus cysts are among the most common intracranial sonographic findings detected during routine second trimester sonography. Choroid plexus cysts may be present in up to 2.5% of fetuses during the second trimester. The pathogenesis of the choroid plexus cysts is not clear but is thought to be due to filling of the neuroepithelial folds with cerebrospinal fluid[112]. Sonographic appearance of the usual choroid plexus cyst is a unilateral, small, round, sonolucent structure measuring less than 1 cm in size, but, at times, the choroid plexus cyst may be bilateral and contain multiple cysts within[113–118] (Figure 19). Choroid plexus cysts may be an isolated and transient finding associated with normal fetal karyotype[114,118–121]. However, in the presence of other structural anomalies, choroid plexus cysts may be associated with chromosomal aneuploidy, especially trisomy 18 and 21[114,118–124].

Arachnoid cysts

Arachnoid cysts, like the choroid plexus cysts, are collections of cerebrospinal fluid within the layers of the arachnoid membrane, which may or may not communicate with the subarachnoid space[59]. Arachnoid cysts account for 1% of all intracranial cystic structures during childhood[125,126]. The arachnoid cysts can be an isolated lesion or associated with other brain malformations such as agenesis of the corpus callosum, absent cavum septi pellucidi, deficient cerebellar lobulation, and Chiari type I malformation[127–129]. The cysts may be located on the surface of the brain, commonly at the level of the cerebral fissures and within the anterior, middle, and posterior fossa. A large cyst can cause hydrocephalus as a result of a mass effect, causing obstruction of flow of the cerebrospinal fluid[125,126]. Sonographic findings include an anechoic cystic

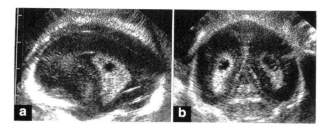

Figure 19 Transvaginal scan of a 19 weeks fetus showing a bilateral choroid plexus cyst. (**a**) An oblique-1 section showing a sonolucent round choroid plexus cyst within the echogenic choroid plexus. (**b**) Almost an occipital-1 section showing the bilateral choroid plexus cyst

mass with thin smooth walls lying adjacent to the cerebral hemispheres, cerebellum or brain stem[21]. The arachnoid cyst does not communicate with the lateral ventricles, and at times can cause a mass effect[127] (Figure 20). No color Doppler flow or Doppler signal is imaged within the cyst. The differential diagnosis of cystic brain lesions includes porencephalic cyst, supratentorial arachnoid cyst, cystic tumors and aneurysm of the vein of Galen[127,128].

Aneurysms of the vein of Galen

The vein of Galen is a median structure which drains the blood from the inferior sagittal sinus and continues into the straight sinus. Aneurysms of the vein of Galen are rare arteriovenous malformations of the brain. The aneurysm of the vein of Galen may cause obstruction of the ventricular system (aqueduct of Silvius), resulting in hydrocephalus[130]. The sonographic appearance of the aneurysm in the mid-sagittal plane is that of a large, well defined, supratentorial, non-pulsatile structure running from the splenium of the corpus callosum above the cerebellum all the way to the bony cranium. In the coronal plane the aneurysm appears as a round centrally located structure (Figure 21a). Using color Doppler sonography the structure fills up with bright color due to the turbulent flow within the dilated cavity[131–133] (Figure 21b, Color plate 19). Other sonographic findings include hydrops secondary to high output congestive heart failure and polyhydramnios. The prognosis for the fetus/neonate depends upon the severity and time of presentation of the cardiovascular symptomatology. Development of high output failure *in utero* or before 3 months of

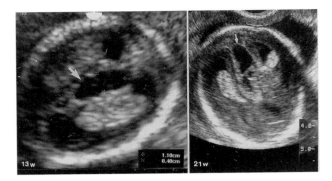

Figure 20 Transvaginal scan at 13 and 21 postmenstrual weeks gestation of fetus with arachnoid cyst (arrow)

life is usually lethal despite medical and surgical treatments[134–136].

THE FETAL FACE

No fetal brain scan is complete without imaging the fetal face. In 1964, DeMyer and colleagues[61] reported on the importance of the facial anomalies when faced with children with holoprosencephaly. They stated that the face predicts the anatomy of the brain. Hence, the children with the most dysmorphic facial features also had the most severe type of holoprosencephaly, namely alobar holoprosencephaly.

The fetal face begins to resemble that of a 'baby' by the end of the embryonic period. Development of the face occurs mostly between the 4th and 8th weeks postconception or 6–10 postmenstrual weeks. During this period there is transformation of the brachial apparatus into the tongue, face, lips, jaws, palate, pharynx and neck, eventually resulting in the typical human facies[11].

Scanning the fetal face

The face similarly to the fetal brain can and should be imaged in all three planes (coronal, axial and sagittal)[137]. In the median plane the profile is obtained. The profile demonstrates the forehead, nasal bridge, upper and lower lip and the jaw. In addition, the position of the tongue and opening and closing of the mouth can be seen (Figure 22a,b). Coronal plane from the very anterior to a more posterior allows visualization of the lips, nose, orbits, lenses and soft tissues of the face (Figure 22c,d). Developmentally a continuous upper lip is formed by 8 weeks when the medial

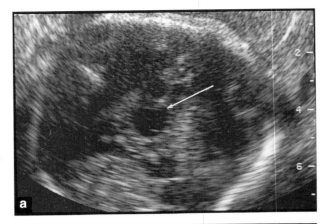

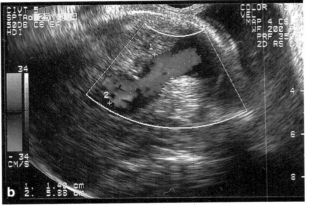

Figure 21 Thirty-two and a half weeks fetus with a vein of Galen aneurysm. (**a**) A coronal section showing a round, midline sonolucent structure (arrow). (**b**) An oblique-1 section in which color Doppler has been applied and shows the turbulent flow within the aneurysm of the vein of Galen (see Color plate 19)

nasal and maxillary processes fuse. Failure of fusion of the medial nasal and maxillary processes will result in a cleft lip affecting one or both sides[10,11]. The palate develops from the primary and secondary palate. Its development starts at 7 weeks, but is not complete until the 14th week of gestation[11] (Figure 23).

The axial section slightly below the level of the biparietal diameter allows visualization of both orbits and lenses. In this section ocular biometry (binocular, interocular and ocular diameter) should be performed. Conditions such as hyper- and hypotelorism, anophthalmia and microphthalmia have been diagnosed from 12–16 weeks gestation by measuring the interocular distance, ocular diameter and binocular distance[138,139]. All of these measurements can be made in a single transverse section at the plane of the orbits[139,140]. The

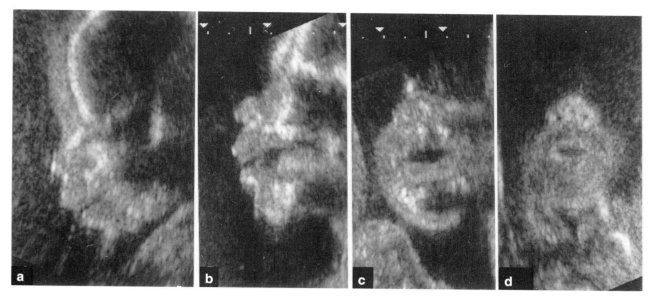

Figure 22 Nineteen weeks fetus: (**a**) and (**b**) show the profile of the fetal face; (**c**) and (**d**) are anterior coronal sections showing the nose and the lips

fetal lens can be imaged consistently from the 12th week of gestation[140]. The sonographic appearance of the normal lens is that of a hyperechogenic ring with a sonolucent core located within the fetal orbits. The lens is best viewed in an anterior coronal section of the face. The hyaloid artery can be seen posterior to the lens as a thin echogenic line between the lens and the posterior aspect of the lens[140]. The hyaloid artery is best imaged in a paramedian section through the orbits. Ideally the artery should be scanned at a right angle to the incoming sound waves.

Facial anomalies

Facial malformations are rare, and the true prevalence of many specific malformations is unknown[141]. Facial anomalies may be an isolated lesion, but are commonly seen in fetuses with multiple congenital anomalies or as a feature of a variety of chromosomal and non-chromosomal syndromes[142-145]. When a facial anomaly is imaged, a targeted scan of the fetus as well as genetic counseling and testing is indicated. Among the chromosomal syndromes associated with facial anomalies are trisomy 21, 18 and 13. Syndromes such as Meckel–Gruber, holoprosencephaly, Beckwith–Wiedemann, Treacher Collins, and Pierre Robin all have specific facial anomalies.

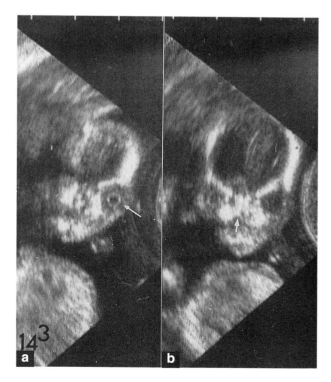

Figure 23 Two anterior coronal sections of a fetus at 14 weeks and 3 days; (**a**) and (**b**) show the orbits and the lenses within. The palate (arrow) is seen and appears intact

The eye

Ocular anomalies affecting the developing fetus have been reported during 12–18 weeks gestation using TVS[140]. Isolated anomalies affecting the developing fetal eye are rare, and in most cases anomalies are associated with other malformations, especially those of the developing brain (alobar holoprosencephaly) as well as with chromosomal aneuploidy (trisomy 13) and non-chromosomal syndromes[139,140]. Stoll and colleagues[138] found a prevalence of congenital eye malformations in the population which they studied to be 7.5 per 10 000 live births. Approximately 54% of the cases had other associated malformations. Included in this group of anomalies were clubfeet, microcephaly, hydrocephaly and facial dysmorphism.

Fetal cataracts or opacification of the lens has been diagnosed in utero[140,146–148]. The lens affected with cataracts no longer has its typical sonographic appearance of a single hyperechogenic ring with a clear center, but it has a variety of appearances such as thick, irregular or crenated border, two concentric rings, dense homogenous echogenic center or with clusters of hyperechogenic material[146] (Figures 23 and 24). Using these sonographic appearances congenital cataract has been diagnosed from 14 weeks of gestation[146]. Congenital cataracts are commonly inherited in an autosomal dominant fashion, but are also the result of in utero infections especially rubella during the 6th to 9th weeks of gestation[11,34,146].

Cleft lip and palate

Cleft lip and palate are not only the most common facial anomalies, but are also among the most common anomalies affecting the developing fetus with a reported incidence of 1 per 1000 live births[10,11]. Up to 80% of cleft lip cases are unilateral rather than bilateral and most of the affected fetuses are male. Unilateral cleft lip is more commonly located on the left side[10]. Cleft palate with or without cleft lip has a reported incidence of 1 in 2500 live births and more commonly affects female fetuses[10,11]. Cleft palate results from failure of the mesenchymal masses of the lateral palatine processes to fuse. Clefts may be unilateral or bilateral. Cleft lip and palate have been diagnosed in utero as early as the 13–14th week of gestation[149,150].

There are several sonographic markers that aid in the detection of this anomaly. One such marker is the paranasal echogenic mass which actually is the premaxillary protrusion made up of soft tissue, osseous as well as dental structures[151]. This mass can be imaged either in the sagittal or in the

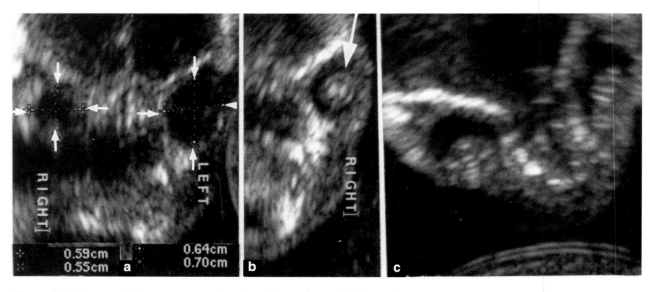

Figure 24 Fetus at 19 postmenstrual weeks of gestation with bilateral cataracts. (**a**) A coronal section of the orbits (arrows) is measured and shows the right orbit to be smaller than the left. (**b**) Another coronal section showing the right orbit and lens. The lens is not sonolucent, but contains a hyperechogenic core (arrow). (**c**) An axial section showing the right orbit and lens with cataract

coronal plane and can be especially useful in the second trimester to detect this anomaly. Using this marker, cleft lip and palate have been diagnosed as early as the 17th week[151]. A second sonographic marker is pseudo-prognathism[149,150]. Pseudo-prognathism or prolabium refers to a relative protrusion of the maxilla as compared to the mandible imaged on the sagittal or paramedian section which passes through the cleft lip and palate. Using this sign cleft lip and palate have been diagnosed as early as the 13–14th week[149,150] (Figure 25). In summary, at 13–14 weeks using coronal and sagittal views of the fetal face, cleft lip and palate can be reliably diagnosed. When this anomaly is imaged genetic counseling as well as a search for other anomalies must be undertaken.

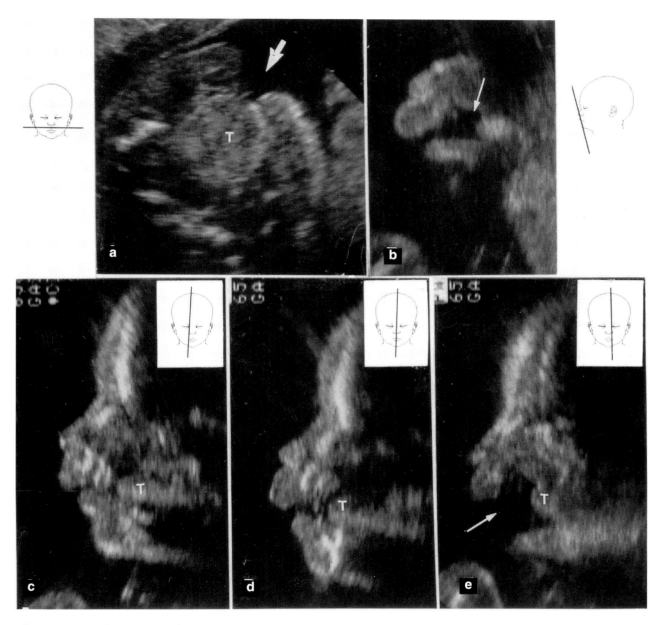

Figure 25 Median, paramedian, axial and coronal sections showing unilateral cleft lip and palate. (**a**) Axial section showing the cleft lip. (**b**) A coronal section showing the cleft lip at the arrow. (**c**) A right paramedian section showing a relatively normal fetal profile. (**d**) The upper lip appears to be protruding; this has been termed pseudo-prognathism or prolabium. (**e**) A left paramedian section showing the defect (arrow)

The mandible

Anomalies of the mandible result from abnormalities of the first branchial arch. It is believed that the origin for these malformations is a deficiency of migration of the neural crest cells during the fourth week of development[10,11,141]. The first arch syndrome is a term used to describe a collection of congenital anomalies affecting the face, upper lip, palate and ear. Since the neural cells also contribute to the formation of the aortic and pulmonary arteries, first arch syndrome is commonly associated with congenital heart defects[10,141,152]. Fetal micrognathia may be present in many syndromes such as Treacher Collins (mandibulofacial dysostosis), Pierre Robin, Goldenhar (hemifacial microsomia) and lethal multiple pterygium syndrome to name a few. In addition, fetuses with autosomal trisomies such as trisomy 18 and trisomy 13 may also show micrognathia[33,152-155] (Figure 26).

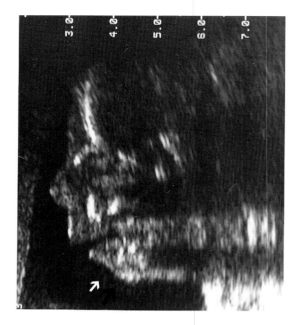

Figure 26 Profile of a 32 postmenstrual weeks fetus with trisomy 18. The white arrow points to the micrognathia

CONCLUSIONS

In this section we have attempted to introduce the reader to the advantages of TVS in examining the fetal central nervous system, and to make the reader more aware of the importance of closely imaging the fetal face. During a targeted scan of the fetal brain the face including the profile, orbits, lenses, and ocular biometry should precede the brain scan. This part of the study may be abdominal or transvaginal depending on the gestational age of the fetus. After the fetus has been examined transabdominally, by switching to TVS the coronal and sagittal planes can be obtained. Although the coronal and sagittal planes can be obtained with TAS, often the planes are technically difficult to image due to maternal or fetal factors precluding adequate imaging.

This chapter has described the basic fetal neuro-anatomy in the coronal and sagittal planes. The anatomy described is by no means complete, but provides a basis upon which a more detailed knowledge of fetal neuro-anatomy can be built. We have described simple-to-recognize anomalies that are usually encountered during scanning.

In conclusion, transvaginal/transfontanelle imaging of the fetal brain should become part of the imaging armamentarium of the sonologist or sonographer who is dedicated to prenatal diagnosis of congenital anomalies.

References

1. Timor-Tritsch IE, Monteagudo A. Transvaginal fetal neurosonography: standardization of the planes and sections used by anatomic landmarks. *Ultrasound Obstet Gynecol* 1996;8:42–7
2. Monteagudo A, Reuss ML, Timor-Tritsch IE. Imaging the fetal brain in the second and third trimesters using transvaginal sonography. *Obstet Gynecol* 1991;77:27–32
3. Monteagudo A, Timor-Tritsch IE. New dimension in fetal neuroscanning. In Chervenak FA, Kurjak A, eds. *The Fetus as a Patient*. New York: Parthenon Publishing, 1996:159–84

4. Cohen M, Slabaugh R, Smith J, *et al*. Neurosono-graphic identification of ventricular asymmetry in premature infants. *Clin Radiol* 1984;35:29–31

5. Horbar J, Leahy K, Lucey J. Ultrasound identi-fication of lateral ventricular asymmetry in the human neonate. *J Clin Ultrasound* 1983;11:67–9

6. Chi JG, Dooling EC, Gilles FH. Gyral development of the human brain. *Ann Neurol* 1977;1:86–93

7. Dorovini-Zis K, Dolman CL. Gestational develop-ment of the brain. *Arch Pathol Lab Med* 1977;101: 192–5

8. Monteagudo A, Timor-Tritsch IE. Sonographic evaluation of fetal cortical maturation. *J Ultrasound Med* 1996;15:S69

9. Kohlenberg C, Lumley J, Yates J, *et al*. A prospective population-based study of CNS abnormality detection at 16 to 20 weeks by ultrasonography. *J Ultrasound Med* 1996;15:S29

10. O'Rahilly R, Muller F. *Human Embryology and Teratology*. New York: Wiley-Liss Inc., 1992

11. Moore K. *Clinically Oriented Embryology*. Philadelphia: WB Saunders Company, 1988

12. Limb CJ, Holmes LB. Anencephaly: changes in prenatal detection and birth status, 1972 through 1990. *Am J Obstet Gynecol* 1994;170:1333–8

13. Vergani P, Ghidini A, Sirtori M, *et al*. Antenatal diagnosis of fetal acrania. *J Ultrasound Med* 1987;6: 715–7

14. Cox GG, Rosenthal SJ, Holsapple JW. Exencephaly: sonographic findings and radiologic-pathologic correlation. *Radiology* 1985;155:755–6

15. Ganchrow D, Ornoy A. A pathological anatomy and histology. Possible evidence for secondary degeneration of central nervous system in the pathogenesis of anencephaly and brain dysraphia. A study in young human fetuses. *Virchows Archives*, 1979;384:285–94

16. Bronshtein M, Ornoy A. Acrania: anencephaly resulting from secondary degeneration of a closed neural tube: two cases in the same family. *J Clin Ultrasound* 1991;19:230–4

17. Timor-Tritsch I, Greenebaum E, Monteagudo A, *et al*. Exencephaly-anencephaly sequence: proof by ultrasound imaging and amniotic fluid cytology. *J Matern Fetal Med* 1996;5:182–5

18. Cunningham ME, Walls WJ. Ultrasound in the evaluation of anencephaly. *Radiology* 1976;118: 165–7

19. Icenogle DA, Kaplan AM. A review of congenital neurologic malformations. *Clin Ped* 1981;20: 565–76

20. Johnson A, Losure TA, Weiner S. Early diagnosis of fetal anencephaly. *J Clin Ultrasound* 1985;13:503–5

21. Pretorius DH, Russ PD, Rumack CM, *et al*. Diagnosis of brain neuropathology in utero. *Neuroradiology* 1986;28:386–97

22. Salamanca A, Gonzalez-Gomez F, Padilla M. Prenatal ultrasound semiography of anencephaly: sonographic-pathological correlations. *Ultrasound Obstet Gynecol* 1992;2:95–100

23. Hidalgo H, Bowie J, Rosenberg ER, *et al*. In utero sonographic diagnosis of fetal cerebral anomalies. *Am J Roentgenol* 1982;139:143–8

24. Monteagudo A, Timor-Tritsch IE. Fetal neuro-sonography of congenital brain anomalies. In Timor-Tritsch IE, Monteagudo A, Cohen HL, eds. *Ultrasonography of the Prenatal and Neonatal Brain*. Stamford: Appleton & Lange, 1996:147–219

25. Foderaro AE, Abu-Yousef MM, Benda JA, *et al*. Antenatal ultrasound diagnosis of iniencephaly. *J Clin Ultrasound* 1987;15:550–4

26. Shoham Z, Caspi B, Chemke J, *et al*. Iniencephaly: prenatal ultrasonographic diagnosis – a case report. *J Perinat Med* 1988;16:139–43

27. Lemire R, Beckwith J, Shepard T. Iniencephaly and anencephaly with spinal retroflexion. A comparative study of eight human specimens. *Birth Defects* 1987;23:225

28. Rodriguez MM, Reik RA, Carreno TD, *et al*. Cluster of iniencephaly in Miami. *Pediatr Pathol* 1991;11:211–21

29. Nishimura H, Okamoto N. Iniencephaly. In Vinken P, Bruyn G, eds. *Handbook of Clinical Neurology*. Vol. 30. Amsterdam: Elsevier-North Holland, 1976:257–68

30. Aleksic SN, Budzilovich GN. Iniencephaly. In Myrianthopoulos N, ed. *Handbook of Clinical Neurology*. Amsterdam: Elsevier Science, 1987;6:129–36

31. Romero R, Pilu G, Jeanty P, *et al*. *Prenatal Diagnosis of Congenital Anomalies*, 1st edn. Norwalk: Appleton & Lange, 1988

32. Naidich TP, Grant JL, Altman N, *et al*. The developing cerebral surface.Preliminary report on the patterns of sulcal and gyral maturation – anatomy, ultrasound, and magnetic resonance imaging. *Neuroimag Clin N Am* 1994;4:201–40

33. Aleksic S, Budzilovich G, Greco MA, *et al*. Inience-phaly: a neuropathologic study. *Clin Neuropathol* 1983;2:55–61

34. Jones K. *Smith's Recognizable Patterns of Human Malformations*. Fourth edn. Philadelphia: WB Saunders Company, 1988

35. David TJ, Nixon A. Congenital malformations associated with anencephaly and iniencephaly. *J Med Genet* 1976;13:263–5

36. Harley EH. Pediatric congenital nasal masses. *Ear Nose Throat J* 1991;70:28–32

37. Chervenak FA, Isaacson G, Mahoney MJ, *et al*. Diagnosis and management of fetal cephalocele. *Obstet Gynecol* 1984;64:86–91

38. Naidich TP, Altman NR, Braffman BH, *et al*. Cephaloceles and related malformations. *Am J Neuroradiol* 1992;13:655–90

39. McLaurin RL. Encephalocele and cranium bifidum. In Myrianthopoulos N, ed. *Handbook of*

Clinical Neurology. New York: Elsevier Science, 1987;6:97–111

40. Monteagudo A. Cephalocele: Anterior. *Fetus* 1992; 2:1–4

41. Nyberg D, Pretorius D. Cerebral malformations. In Nyberg D, Mahoney B, Pretorius D, eds. *Diagnostic Ultrasound of Fetal Anomalies. Text and Atlas*. 1st edn. Chicago: Year Book Medical Publishers, 1990: 83–202

42. Fiske CE, Filly FA. Ultrasound evaluation of the normal and abnormal fetal neural axis. *Radiol Clin N Am* 1982;20:285–96

43. Fiske CE, Filly FA. Ultrasound evaluation of the normal and abnormal fetal neural axis. *Radiol Clin N Am* 1982;20:285–96

44. Yen IH, Khoury MJ, Erickson JD, *et al*. The changing epidemiology of neural tube defects. United States, 1968–1989. *Am J Dis Child* 1992;146:857–61

45. Welch K, Winston K. Spina bifida. In Myrianthopoulos N, ed. *Handbook of Clinical Neurology*. Amsterdam: Elsevier, 1987;6:477–508

46. Main DM, Mennuti MT. Neural tube defects: issues in prenatal diagnosis and counseling. *Obstet Gynecol* 1986;67:1–16

47. Thornton JG, Lilford RJ, Newcombe RG. Tables for estimation of individual risks of fetal neural tube and ventral wall defects, incorporating prior probability, maternal serum alpha-fetoprotein levels, and ultrasonographic examination results [see comments]. *Am J Obstet Gynecol* 1991;164: 154–60

48. Hogge WA, Thiagarajah S, Ferguson JED, *et al*. The role of ultrasonography and amniocentesis in the evaluation of pregnancies at risk for neural tube defects [see comments]. *Am J Obstet Gynecol* 1989;161:520–3, discussion 3–4

49. Blumenfeld Z, Siegler E, Bronshtein M. The early diagnosis of neural tube defects. *Prenat Diagn* 1993;13:863–71

50. Thiagarajah S, Henke J, Hogge WA, *et al*. Early diagnosis of spina bifida: the value of cranial ultrasound markers. *Obstet Gynecol* 1990;76:54–7

51. Nyberg DA, Mack LA, Hirsch J, *et al*. Abnormalities of fetal cranial contour in sonographic detection of spina bifida: evaluation of the 'lemon' sign. *Radiology* 1988;167:387–92

52. Penso C, Redline RW, Benacerraf BR. A sonographic sign which predicts which fetuses with hydrocephalus have an associated neural tube defect. *J Ultrasound Med* 1987;6:307–11

53. Van den Hof MC, Nicolaides KH, Campbell J, *et al*. Evaluation of the lemon and banana signs in one hundred thirty fetuses with open spina bifida. *Am J Obstet Gynecol* 1990;162:322–7

54. Goldstein RB, Podrasky AE, Filly RA, *et al*. Effacement of the fetal cisterna magna in association with myelomeningocele [see comments]. *Radiology* 1989;172:409–13

55. Pilu G, Romero R, Reece EA, *et al*. Subnormal cerebellum in fetuses with spina bifida. *Am J Obstet Gynecol* 1988;158:1052–6

56. Volpe J. Neuronal proliferation, migration, organization and myelination. In *Neurology of the Newborn*, 3rd edn. Philadelphia: WB Saunders, 1995:3–42

57. Osborn A. Normal anatomy and congenital anomalies of the spine and spinal cord. In *Diagnostic Neuroradiology*. St. Louis: Mosby-Year Book, 1994:799–807

58. Filly RA, Chinn DH, Callen PW. Alobar holoprosencephaly: ultrasonographic prenatal diagnosis. *Radiology* 1984;151:455–9

59. Babcock DS. Sonography of congenital malformations of the brain. *Neuroradiology* 1986;28: 428–39

60. Cohen MM Jr, Sulik KK. Perspectives on holoprosencephaly: Part II. Central nervous system, craniofacial anatomy, syndrome commentary, diagnostic approach, and experimental studies. *J Genet Dev Biol* 1992;12:196–244

61. DeMyer W, Zeman W, Palmer CG. The face predicts the brain: diagnostic significance of medial facial anomalies for holoprosencephaly (arrhinencephaly). *Pediatrics* 1964;34:256–62

62. Pilu G, Ambrosetto P, Sandri F, *et al*. Intraventricular fused fornices: a specific sign of fetal lobar holoprosencephaly. *Ultrasound Obstet Gynecol* 1994;4:65–7

63. Kendall BE. Dysgenesis of the corpus callosum. *Neuroradiology* 1983;25:239–56

64. Hernanz-Schulman M, Dohan FC Jr, Jones T, *et al*. Sonographic appearance of callosal agenesis: correlation with radiologic pathologic findings. *Am J Neuroradiol* 1985;6:361–8

65. Babcock DS. The normal, absent, and abnormal corpus callosum: sonographic findings. *Radiology* 1984;151:449–53

66. Barkovich AJ, Normal D. Anomalies of the corpus callosum: correlation with further anomalies of the brain. *Am J Roentgenol* 1988;151:171–9

67. Atlas SW, Shkolnik A, Naidich TP. Sonographic recognition of agenesis of the corpus callosum. *Am J Roentgenol* 1985;145:167–73

68. Bertino RE, Nyberg DA, Cyr DR, *et al*. Prenatal diagnosis of agenesis of the corpus callosum. *J Ultrasound Med* 1988;7:251–60

69. Hilpert PL, Kurtz AB. Prenatal diagnosis of agenesis of the corpus callosum using endovaginal ultrasound. *J Ultrasound Med* 1990;9:363–5

70. Gebarski SS, Gebarski KS, Bowerman RA, *et al*. Agenesis of the corpus callosum: sonographic features. *Radiology* 1984;151:443–8

71. Lockwood CJ, Ghidini A, Aggarwal R, *et al*. Antenatal diagnosis of partial agenesis of the corpus callosum: a benign cause of ventriculomegaly. *Am J Obstet Gynecol* 1988;159:184–6

72. Vergani P, Ghidini A, Mariani S, *et al*. Antenatal sonographic findings of agenesis of corpus callosum. *Am J Perinatol* 1988;5:105–8

73. Meizner I, Barki Y, Hertzanu Y. Prenatal sonographic diagnosis of agenesis of corpus callosum. *J Clin Ultrasound* 1987;15:262–4

74. Pilu G, Sandri A, Perolo A, *et al*. Sonography of fetal agenesis of the corpus callosum: a survey of 35 cases. *Ultrasound Obstet Gynecol* 1993;3:318–29

75. Poe L, Coleman L, Mahmud F. Congenital central nervous system anomalies. *Radiographics* 1989;9: 801–26

76. Leech RW, Shuman RM. Holoprosencephaly and related midline cerebral anomalies: a review. *J Child Neurol* 1986;1:3–18

77. Barkovich AJ, Norman D. Absence of the septum pellucidum: a useful sign in the diagnosis of congenital brain malformations. *Am J Roentgenol* 1989;152:353–60

78. Kuhn MJ, Swenson LC, Youssef HT. Absence of the septum pellucidum and related disorders. *Comput Med Imag Graphics* 1993;17:137–47

79. Pilu G, Perolo A, David C. Midline anomalies of the brain. In Timor-Tritsch I. Monteagudo A, Cohen H, eds. *Ultrasonography of the Prenatal and Neonatal Brain*, 1st edn. Stamford: Appleton & Lange, 1996: 241–58

80. Osenbach R, Menezes A. Diagnosis and management of the Dandy–Walker malformation: 30 years of experience. *Peds Neurosurg* 1991;18:179

81. Russ PD, Pretorius DH, Johnson MJ. Dandy–Walker syndrome: a review of fifteen cases evaluated by prenatal sonography. *Am J Obstet Gynecol* 1989;161:401–6

82. Hirsch JF, Pierre-Kahn A, Renier D, *et al*. The Dandy–Walker malformation. A review of 40 cases. *J Neurosurg* 1984;61:515–22

83. Nyberg DA, Cyr DR, Mack LA, *et al*. The Dandy–Walker malformation prenatal sonographic diagnosis and its clinical significance. *J Ultrasound Med* 1988;7:65–71

84. Taylor GA, Sander RC. Dandy–Walker syndrome: recognition by sonography. *Am J Neuroradiol* 1983; 4:1203

85. Kirkinen P, Jouppila P, Valkeakari T, *et al*. Ultrasonic evaluation of the Dandy–Walker syndrome. *Obstet Gynecol* 1982;59:18S–21S

86. Fileni A, Colosimo C Jr, Mirk P, *et al*. Dandy–Walker syndrome: diagnosis *in utero* by means of ultrasound and CT correlations. *Neuroradiology* 1983;24:233–5

87. Burton BK. Recurrence risks for congenital hydrocephalus. *Clin Genet* 1979;16:47–53

88. Barkovich AJ, Kjos BO, Norman D, *et al*. Revised classification of posterior fossa cysts and cystlike malformations based on the results of multiplanar MR imaging. *Am J Roentgenol* 1989;153:1289–300

89. Pilu G, Goldstein I, Reece E, *et al*. Sonography of fetal Dandy–Walker malformations: a reappraisal. *Ultrasound Obstet Gynecol* 1992;2:151–7

90. Habib Z. Genetics and genetic counseling in neonatal hydrocephalus. *Obstet Gynecol Surv* 1981; 36:529–34

91. Milhorat R. Hydrocephaly. In Myrianthopoulos N, ed. *Handbook of Clinical Neurology*. Amsterdam: Elsevier, 1987;6:285–300

92. Vintzileos AM, Ingardia CJ, Nochimson DJ. Congenital hydrocephalus: a review of protocol for perinatal management. *Obstet Gynecol* 1983;62: 539–49

93. London DA, Carroll BA, Enzmann DR. Sonography of ventricular size and germinal matrix hemorrhage in premature infants. *Am J Roentgenol* 1980;135:559–64

94. Sauerbrei EE, Digney M, Harrison PB, *et al*. Ultrasonic evaluation of neonatal intracranial hemorrhage and its complications. *Radiology* 1981;139: 677–85

95. Poland RL, Slovis TL, Shankaran S. Normal values for ventricular size as determined by real time sonographic techniques. *Pediatric Radiol* 1985;15:12–14

96. Rumack CM, Johnson ML. Real-time ultrasound evaluation of the neonatal brain. *Clin Diagn Ultrasound* 1982;10:179

97. Shackelford GD. Neurosonography of hydrocephalus in infants. *Neuroradiology* 1986;28: 452–62

98. Naidich TP, Schott LH, Baron RL. Computed tomography in evaluation of hydrocephalus. *Radiol Clin N Am* 1982;20:143–67

99. Naidich TP, Epstein F, Lin JP, *et al*. Evaluation of pediatric hydrocephalus by computed tomography. *Radiology* 1976;119:337–45

100. Edwards MK, Brown DL, Muller J, *et al*. Cribside neurosonography: real-time sonography for intracranial investigation of the neonate. *Am J Roentgenol* 1981;136:271–5

101. Goldstein I, Reece E, Pilu G, *et al*. Sonographic evaluation of the normal developmental anatomy of the fetal cerebral ventricles. IV: The posterior horn. *Am J Perinatol* 1990;7:29–83

102. Johnson M, Dunne M, Mack L, *et al*. Evaluation of fetal intracranial anatomy by static and real time ultrasound. *J Clin Ultrasound* 1980;8:311–8

103. Goldstein I, Reece E, Pilu G, *et al*. Sonographic evaluation of the normal developmental anatomy of the fetal cerebral ventricles. I: The frontal horn. *Obstet Gynecol* 1988;72:588–92

104. Cardoza JD, Goldstein RB, Filly RA. Exclusion of fetal ventriculomegaly with a single measurement: the width of the lateral ventricular atrium. *Radiology* 1988;169:711–4

105. Pilu G, Reece EA, Goldstein I, *et al*. Sonographic evaluation of the normal developmental anatomy of the fetal cerebral ventricles: II. The atria. *Obstet Gynecol* 1989;73:250–6

106. Monteagudo A, Timor-Tritsch IE, Moomjy M. Nomograms of the fetal lateral ventricles using

transvaginal sonography. *J Ultrasound Med* 1993; 12:265–9

107. Monteagudo A, Timor-Tritsch IE, Moomjy M. *In utero* detection of ventriculomegaly during the second and third trimesters by transvaginal sonography. *Ultrasound Obstet Gynecol* 1994;4:193–8

108. Cardoza JD, Filly RA, Podrasky AE. The dangling choroid plexus: a sonographic observation of value in excluding ventriculomegaly. *Am J Roentgenol* 1988;151:767–70

109. Chinn DH, Callen PW, Filly RA. The lateral cerebral ventricle in early second trimester. *Radiology* 1983;148:529–31

110. Bronshtein M, Ben-Shlomo I. Choroid plexus dysmorphism detected by transvaginal sonography: the earliest sign of fetal hydrocephalus. *J Clin Ultrasound* 1991;19:547–53

111. Benacerraf BR, Birnholz JC. The diagnosis of fetal hydrocephalus prior to 22 weeks. *J Clin Ultrasound* 1987;15:531–6

112. Shuangshoti S, Netsky MG. Neuroepithelial (colloid) cysts of the nervous system. Further observations on pathogenesis, incidence, and histochemistry. *Neurology* 1966;16:887

113. Chitkara U, Cogswell C, Norton K, *et al*. Choroid plexus cysts in the fetus: a benign anatomic variant or pathologic entity? Report of 41 cases and review of the literature. *Obstet Gynecol* 198;72:185–9

114. Benacerraf BR, Harlow B, Frigoletto FD Jr. Are choroid plexus cysts an indication for second-trimester amniocentesis? [see comments]. *Am J Obstet Gynecol* 1990;162:1001–6

115. DeRoo TR, Harris RD, Sargent SK, *et al*. Fetal choroid plexus cysts: prevalence, clinical significance, and sonographic appearance. *Am J Roentgenol* 1988;151:1179–81

116. Benacerraf BR. Asymptomatic cysts of the fetal choroid plexus in the second trimester. *J Ultrasound Med* 1987;6:475–8

117. Chudleigh P, Pearce JM, Campbell S. The prenatal diagnosis of transient cysts of the fetal choroid plexus. *Prenat Diagn* 1984;4:135–7

118. Hertzberg BS, Kay HH, Bowie JD. Fetal choroid plexus lesions. Relationship of antenatal sonographic appearance to clinical outcome. *J Ultrasound Med* 1989;8:77–82

119. Farhood AI, Morris JH, Bieber FR. Transient cysts of the fetal choroid plexus: morphology and histogenesis. *Am J Med Genet* 1987;27:977–82

120. Nicolaides KH, Rodeck CH, Gosden CM. Rapid karyotyping in non-lethal fetal malformations. *Lancet* 1986;1:283–7

121. Fitzsimmons J, Wilson D, Pascoe-Mason J, *et al*. Choroid plexus cysts in fetuses with trisomy 18. *Obstet Gynecol* 1989;73:257–60

122. Gross S, Shulman L, Tolley E, *et al*. Isolated fetal choroid plexus cysts and trisomy 18: a review and meta-analysis. *Am J Obstet Gynecol* 1995;172:83–7

123. Platt LD, Carlson DE, Medearis AL. Fetal choroid plexus cysts in the second trimester of pregnancy: a cause for concern [see comments]. *Am J Obstet Gynecol* 1991;164:1652–5, discussion 5–6

124. Kupferminc M, Tamura R, Sabbagha R, *et al*. Isolated choroid plexus cyst(s): an indication for amniocentesis. *Am J Obstet Gynecol* 1994;171: 1068–71

125. Chuang S, Harwood-Nash D. Tumors and cysts. *Neuroradiology* 1986;28:463–75

126. Banna M. Arachnoid cysts on computed tomography. *Am J Roentgenol* 1976;127:979–82

127. Langer B, Haddad J, Favre R, *et al*. Fetal arachnoid cyst: report of two cases. *Ultrasound Obstet Gynecol* 1994;4:68–72

128. Galassi E, Tognetti F, Frank F, *et al*. Infratentorial arachnoid cysts. *J Neurosurg* 1985;63:210–7

129. Pascual-Castroviejo I, Roche MC, Martinez Bermejo A. Primary intracranial arachnoidal cysts. A study of 67 childhood cases. *Child Nerv Sys* 1991; 7:257–63

130. Diebler C, Dulac O, Renier D, *et al*. Aneurysms of the vein of Galen in infants aged 2 to 15 months. Diagnosis and natural evolution. *Neuroradiology* 1981;21:185–97

131. Vintzileos A, Eisenfeld L, Campbell W, *et al*. Prenatal ultrasonic diagnosis of arteriovenous malformation of the vein of Galen. *Am J Perinatol* 1986;3:209

132. Ordorica SA, Marks F, Frieden FJ. Aneurysm of the vein of Galen: a new cause for Ballantyne syndrome. *Am J Obstet Gynecol* 1990;162:1166–7

133. Rodemyer CR, Smith WL. Diagnosis of a vein of Galen aneurysm by ultrasound. *J Clin Ultrasound* 1982;10:297–8

134. Reiter AA, Huhta JC, Carpenter RJ Jr, *et al*. Prenatal diagnosis of arteriovenous malformation of the vein of Galen. *J Clin Ultrasound* 1986;14: 623–8

135. Mendelsohn DB, Hertzanu Y, Butterworth A. *In utero* diagnosis of a vein of Galen aneurysm by ultrasound. *Neuroradiology* 1984;26:417–8

136. Watson DG, Smith RR, Brann AW. Arteriovenous malformation of the vein of Galen. *Am J Dis Child* 1976;130:520

137. Benacerraf B. Ultrasound evaluation of the fetal face. In Callen P, ed. *Ultrasonography in Obstetrics and Gynecology*, 3rd edn. Philadelphia: W.B. Saunders, 1994:235–53

138. Stoll C, Alembik Y, Dott B, *et al*. Epidemiology of congenital eye malformations in 131 760 consecutive births. *Opth Paediatrics Gent* 1992;13: 179–86

139. Jeanty P, Dramaix-Wilmet M, Van Gansbeke D, *et al*. Fetal ocular biometry by ultrasound. *Radiology* 1982;143:513–6

140. Bronshtein M, Zimmer E, Gershoni-Baruch R, *et al*. First- and second-trimester diagnosis of fetal ocular defects and associated anomalies: report of eight cases. *Obstet Gynecol* 1991;77:443–9

141. Meizner I. Ultrasonography of the fetal face. In Timor-Tritsch I, Monteagudo A, Cohen H, eds. *Ultrasonography of the Prenatal and Neonatal Brain.* Stamford: Appleton & Lange, 1996:299–332

142. Pilu G, Reece EA, Romero R, *et al*. Prenatal diagnosis of craniofacial malformations with ultrasonography. *Am J Obstet Gynecol* 1986;155:45–50

143. Seeds JW, Cefalo RC. Technique of early sonographic diagnosis of bilateral cleft lip and palate. *Obstet Gynecol* 1983;62:2s–7s

144. Kraus B, Kitamura H, Ooe T. Malformations associated with cleft lip and palate in human embryos and fetuses. *Am J Obstet Gynecol* 1963; 86:321–26

145. Saltzman D, Benacerraf B, Frigoletto F. Diagnosis and management of fetal facial clefts. *Am J Obstet Gynecol* 1986;155:377–82

146. Zimmer E, Bronshtein M, Ophir E, *et al*. Sonographic diagnosis of fetal congenital cataracts. *Prenat Diagn* 1993;13:503–11

147. Gaary E, Rawnsley E, Marin-Padilla J, *et al*. *In utero* detection of fetal cataracts. *J Ultrasound Med* 1993; 4:234–6

148. Monteagudo A, Timor-Tritsch I, Friedman A, *et al*. Autosomal dominant cataracts of the fetus: early detection by transvaginal ultrasound. *Ultrasound Obstet Gynecol* 1996;8:104–8

149. Bronshtein M, Blumenfeld I, Kohn J, *et al*. Detection of cleft lip by early second-trimester transvaginal sonography. *Obstet Gynecol* 1994;84: 73–6

150. Bronshtein M, Mashiah N, Blumenfeld I, *et al*. Pseudoprognathism – an auxiliary ultrasonographic sign for transvaginal ultrasonographic diagnosis of cleft lip and palate in the early second trimester. *Am J Obstet Gynecol* 1991;165:1314–6

151. Nyberg D, Mahoney B, Kramer D. Paranasal echogenic mass: sonographic sign of bilateral complete cleft lip and palate before 20 menstrual weeks. *Radiology* 1992;184:757–59

152. McKenzie J. The first arch syndrome. *Dev Med Child Neurol* 1966;8:55–62

153. Cayea P, Bieber F, Ross M, *et al*. Sonographic findings in otocephaly (synotia). *J Ultrasound Med* 1985;4:377–9

154. Pilu G, Romero R, Reece E, *et al*. The prenatal diagnosis of Robin anomalad. *Am J Obstet Gynecol* 1986;154:630–2

155. Tamas DE, Mahoney BS, Bowie JD, *et al*. Prenatal sonographic diagnosis of hemifacial microsomia (Goldenhar-Gorlin syndrome). *J Ultrasound Med* 1986;5:461–3

Abnormalities of fetal neck and thorax 9

Oded Inbar, Reuven Achiron and Richard Jaffe

THE FETAL NECK

Current ultrasound instrumentation yields high-resolution scans that allow accurate assessment of the fetal neck. Most neck structures are normally small and barely visible, so anomalous development can be easily identified, for example, when the nuchal fold is measured in the second trimester. The abnormalities identified are differentiated with respect to their position (at the central midline or anterolateral or lateral to the midline) and ultrasonographic characteristics (solid, cystic or mixed; calcified or vascular, septated or nonseptated). Masses that can be detected antenatally include thyroid masses, teratoma, thyroglossal duct cyst, cystic hygroma, hemangioma, branchial cleft cyst[1], cystocele, myelocystocele and other developmental cystic lesions.

Cystic hygroma

Cystic hygroma is a congenital malformation of the lymphatic system resulting from failure of the communication between the jugular lymphatic canal and the internal jugular vein[2]. Its incidence is 1:6000 pregnancies[3]. The posterior cervical region is the most common site of cystic hygromas[4].

Cystic hygroma and other nuchal signs thought to indicate a very significant risk for a genetic problem detected during the first trimester may resolve and not be detected at the later abdominal scan[5]. Cystic hygroma is most often seen in the nuchal region (Figure 1) but also has been reported to exist in the mediastinum[3,6], axilla[7–10], in the parotid gland[11,12], and in the abdomen[13]. When discovered before 30 weeks of gestation it is almost always associated with chromosomal abnormalities or multiple anomalies, mainly hydrops fetalis, cardiac defects[14–16], polycystic kidneys, and bladder outlet obstruction[17]. On the contrary when appearing after the 30th week of gestation, cystic hygroma is usually an isolated malformation as when discovered during infancy or childhood. Approximately two-thirds of these 'late' cystic hygromas are

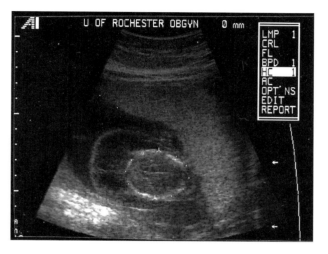

Figure 1 Nuchal cystic hygroma in an 18 week old fetus

present at birth; 90% are discovered before 2 years of age. A spontaneous regression occurs in about 15% of cases. In 70% of cases the cystic hygroma is simple without extension to the oropharynx or mediastinum and its complete surgical resection is usually easy. Extension to the oropharynx is present in about 20% of cases; there is a risk of neonatal respiratory distress and the treatment is difficult. Extension to the mediastinum is found in about 10% of the cases; respiratory distress is rare and a large surgical resection is necessary. Surgery is the primary treatment of cystic hygroma after a careful evaluation of the extension of the tumor by ultrasound, scanography or nuclear magnetic resonance imaging, and oropharyngeal endoscopy. It allows a 'macroscopically complete' resection in about 80% of cases, but a recurrence is observed in approximately one in every five cases. Following partial resection or important recurrence, treatment includes, according to the cases: new attempt of surgical resection; sclerosing therapy; and laser therapy for the oropharyngeal forms[18].

First-trimester fetuses with simple nuchal hygromas represent a population that is different from midgestation nuchal cystic hygroma in terms of chromosomal abnormalities and long-term prognosis. Cystic hygroma can be diagnosed in the first trimester using transvaginal ultrasound (32–60% of cases). Fetuses with cystic hygroma diagnosed in the first trimester have an abnormal karyotype with trisomy 21 being the most common abnormality. In 67–92% of fetuses with normal karyotype the cystic hygroma resolves spontaneously[17,19–22]. Cystic hygroma when diagnosed in the second trimester is most commonly associated with Turner's syndrome (42–73% of cases). Trisomies are found in 18% of second trimester cystic hygromas and normal karyotypes in 18%[14,23–25]. Septations are associated with an increased risk for chromosome abnormalities, hydrops fetalis, associated structural anomalies and a poor prognosis as opposed to the nonseptated variant (Figure 2). Bronshtein et al.[26] reported an aneuploidy rate of 72% in septated cystic hygroma compared with 5.7% in nonseptated cystic hygroma. However, the incidence of chromosome abnormalities was also increased (12.5%) among cases not characterized by septations[27]. Other important prognostic factors influencing the survival of fetuses with cystic hygroma are the size of the hygroma (hygromas larger than 6 cm in diameter have a grim prognosis)[28], and the presence of bilateral pleural effusions. Survival rate improves with normal karyotype (27%), unilateral pleural effusion (40%), atypical location (56%) and resolution of cystic hygroma (71%). The overall survival rate for cystic hygroma is 2–10%. If the fetus reaches 26 weeks gestation a 67% chance of survival is expected[14,25].

Dysmorphic features of the nuchal region are often markers of various syndromes such as trisomy 21[9,21,29,30], trisomy 18[9,17,30], trisomy 13[16,31–33], trisomy 4[34], duplication of the 11p region[35], Noonan syndrome[26,36–40], multiple pterygium syndrome[41–47], Fryns' syndrome[48–50], Wolf–Hirschhorn syndrome[51], Brachmann–de Lange syndrome[52], distichiasis-lymphedema syndromes[53], Langer–Saldino syndrome[54] (see chapter 18).

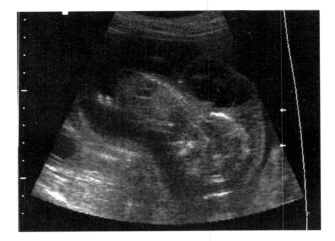

Figure 2 Extensive septated cystic hygroma in fetus with Turner's syndrome

Neck tumors

The most common mass detected prenatally in the fetal nuchal region is a cervical teratoma (Figure 3). The incidence of this tumor is 1 in 30 000 live births. The tumors tend to grow with pregnancy and can be either cystic or mostly solid. Teratomas are often associated with polyhydramnios. Due to their anterior location, in most cases, fetal and neonatal mortality is high due to respiratory obstruction and nerve compression. Surgery has been performed with some success with adequate ventilatory support immediately after delivery. The differential diagnosis includes cystic hygroma, hemangiomas and goiter (Table 1).

Cephalocele

A cephalocele is herniation of meninges with or without brain through a skull defect. The prevalence of this defect is 0.5 in 10 000 live births and is often associated with other congenital anomalies. Ultrasonographically it will appear as a

Table 1 Ultrasonographic appearance and associated anomalies of common fetal neck masses

Neck mass	Ultrasonographic appearance	Associated anomalies
Cystic hygroma	Irregular, multicystic with septations, hydrops, polyhydramnios	Turner's syndrome, other chromosomal anomalies
Nuchal edema	Follows shape of skull, hydrops	Chromosomal anomalies, fetal demise
Teratoma	Anterolateral, complex	Unknown
Encephalocele	Posterior or anterior midline, bony defect of skull, complex, microcephaly	Meckel–Gruber syndrome
Goiter	Bilateral, solid or complex	Rare

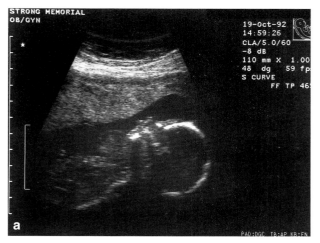

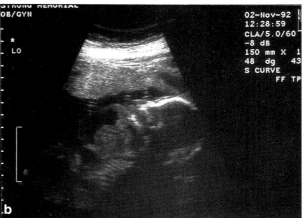

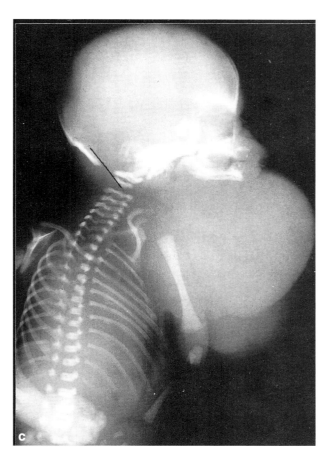

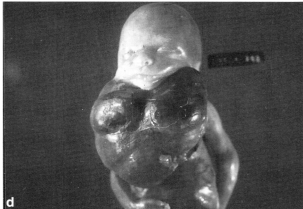

Figure 3   (**a**) Seventeen week fetus with neck teratoma. (**b**) Same fetus at 19 weeks gestation showing significant growth of tumor. (**c**) X-ray of fetus demonstrating large neck mass. (**d**) Fetus following termination of pregnancy

sac protruding from a region of the head not covered with bone (Figure 4). If brain tissue is involved the finding can be cystic and semisolid and the fetal head measurements often smaller than expected for gestational age.

With any cystic finding in the nuchal region a nuchal cord should be ruled out before final diagnosis is made. Color Doppler imaging is helpful in distinguishing between umbilical cord and a cystic mass (Figure 5, Color plate 20).

THORAX

The sonographic evaluation of the fetal thorax includes visualization of the lung parenchyma and the mediastinum. In mid-pregnancy the lungs appear moderately echogenic, slightly less than the liver. As pregnancy advances the echogenicity of the lungs increases and they become more echogenic than the liver. Attempts to correlate lung echogenicity to pulmonary maturity have been unsuccessful[55,56].

Measurement of chest circumference is obtained in a transverse view at the level in which the four-chamber view of the heart is seen. Nomograms of normal chest circumference have been reported which can aid in diagnosing abnormalities in chest

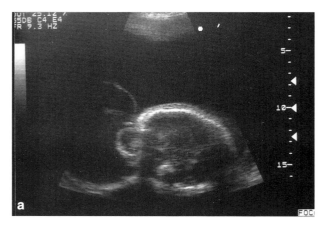

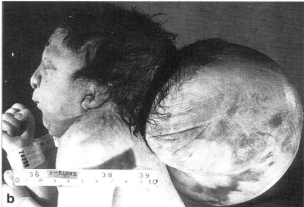

Figure 4 (**a**) Large cystocele and bony defect. (**b**) Newborn with posterior-cervical cystocele

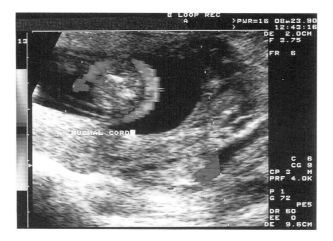

Figure 5 Demonstration of nuchal cord with color Doppler imaging (see Color plate 20)

development which exist in skeletal dysplasias[57] (Figure 6). A correlation has also been found between decreased chest circumference and pulmonary hypoplasia[58–62]. A better sensitivity is

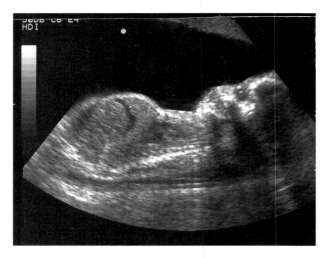

Figure 6 Small chest in fetus with thanatophoric dysplasia

reported when the thoracic/abdominal circumference (TC:AC) ratio is used[61,62]. The TC:AC ratio is greater than 0.8 in nearly all normal pregnancies after 20 weeks[61].

Anomalies of the fetal thorax constitute a major group of abnormalities currently detectable with prenatal ultrasound evaluation. Many of the abnormalities diagnosed by ultrasound are potentially life threatening by their potential to grow and cause fetal hydrops. The most common chest mass is congenital diaphragmatic hernia (CDH), followed by cystic adenomatoid malformation (CAM), pulmonary sequestration, bronchogenic cyst, and bronchial atresia (Table 2). The ultrasonographic appearance of fetal lung hyperechogenicity is most commonly associated with congenital bronchopulmonary abnormalities, such as CAM, pulmonary lobar sequestration or retention of mucus in the bronchial tree[63,64]. In a minority of fetuses CDH and CAM can not be differentiated prenatally. Color Doppler sonography is useful to rule out pulmonary sequestration; extralobar pulmonary sequestration can mimic congenital CAM in sonographic appearance[65]. Thoracic cystic hygromas appear as multilocular cystic masses.

Congenital diaphragmatic hernia

The diaphragm is formed between the 6th and 14th gestational week out of four structures: the septum transversum, pleuroperitoneal membranes, the dorsal mesentery of the esophagus, and the body wall.

Table 2 Ultrasonographic appearance and associated anomalies of fetal thoracic masses

Thoracic mass	Ultrasonographic appearance	Associated anomalies
Congenital diaphragmatic hernia (CDH)	Stomach or other abdominal organs in thorax, heart displaced to right side, polyhydramnios, hydrops	Chromosomal anomalies, cardiac defects, hydrocephaly
Pulmonary sequestration	Homogenous echogenic mass, hydrops, pleural effusion, abnormal feeding artery	Bronchogenic cysts, tracheo-esophageal fistula, cardiac
Cystic adenomatoid malformation (CAM)	Echogenic or multicystic lesions, hydrops, polyhydramnios, some regress	
Type I	Single or multiple cysts of 2–10 cm	Rare
Type II	Multiple cysts of <1 cm in diameter	Renal agenesis, tetralogy of Fallot, hydrocephaly, CDH
Type III	Microcystic and appears echogenic	Hydrothorax, pulmonary hypoplasia
Esophageal atresia	Trachea displaced anteriorly by cystic mass, absent stomach, polyhydramnios	Unknown
Bronchogenic cyst	Single intrapulmonary cyst	Rare
Hydrothorax (Pleural effusion)	Hypoechogenic finding displacing heart and lungs	CAM, CDH, hydrops, facial clefts

CAM, cystic adenomatoid malformation; CDH, congenital diaphragmatic hernia

CDH continues to be one of the most challenging problems in pediatric surgery. The frequency of CDH varies, according to the studies, between 1 in 2000 and 1 in 5000 live births[66–71]. CDH is usually unilateral (97%) and on the left (75–90%)[67,72]. Bochdalek hernias account for 90% of CDHs and are caused by the failure or incomplete closure of the posterior pleuroperitoneal membranes. These hernias classically are left-sided and posterolateral. Foramen of Morgagni hernias are the second most common type of diaphragmatic hernia. They occur in the anteromedial retrosternal portion of the diaphragm and are believed to be caused by maldevelopment of the septum transversum[73]. Complete absence of the diaphragm is rare (1–2% of diaphragmatic hernias). Associated malformations occur in 20–53%, mainly cardiac malformations (9–23%)[69,74], neural tube defects (28%), spinal defects, trisomies and various syndromes[71,75,76]. Trisomies 21 and 18 occur in 4%. The etiology of CDH is unknown but certain teratogens such as the herbicide nitrofen are known to cause CDH in experimental models in animals[77–82]. The overall mortality rate is 30–80% and death is caused by pulmonary hypoplasia, pulmonary hypertension, surfactant deficiency and decreased pulmonary compliance[75,76,83–86]. The mortality figures are higher in CDH detected antenatally than postnatally. CDH is more common on the left side but the prognosis is worse in right-sided CDH[87]. Underdevelopment of left-sided cardiac structures was found to be a helpful

prognostic factor[76]. The risk of recurrence of CDH for future sibs after one affected infant is about 2%. A multifactorial/threshold inheritance pattern with an observed high male:female sex ratio is currently favored for the rare occurrence of familial CDH, although other modes of inheritance have also been described[85,88]. CDH may be part of a lethal syndrome i.e. Fryn's syndrome, Brachmann–de Lange syndrome[49].

Many cases of CDH are currently detected before birth. The presenting symptom is usually polyhydramnios. A diagnosis is made by demonstrating abdominal contents in the thorax and the sonographic hallmark is visualization of a fluid-filled viscus in the lower chest behind the left atria and ventricle in a transverse view in which the four chambers of the heart are seen (Figure 7). Other sonographic signs suggesting CDH are lack of visualization of the stomach in the abdomen, mediastinal shift, small abdominal circumference[89,90] and polyhydramnios. In left-sided CDH, stomach, small bowel, and left lobe of the liver and occasionally the spleen or the left kidney can be seen. Occasionally, peristalsis can be seen in the chest as well[90]. Right-sided CDH is more difficult to diagnose since the part herniating into the chest cavity is liver which is similar in its echogenicity to the lungs[91], but occasionally the fluid-filled gallbladder can be seen in the right side of the chest. Bowing of the umbilical segment of the portal vein (portal sinus) to the left of midline and coursing of portal branches to the lateral segment

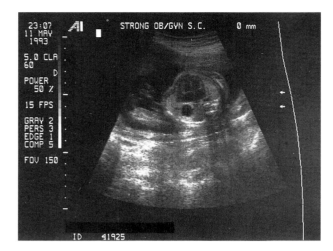

Figure 7 Fetal heart and stomach seen at same level within thorax

of the left hepatic lobe toward or above the diaphragmatic ridge are the best predictors for liver herniation into the fetal thorax. The bowel can herniate intermittently into the thorax, explaining the fact that the appearance of the CDH can change from one examination to the next one and to the fact that it is occasionally missed on sonography. The stomach position is a good predictor if observed in a posterior or midthoracic location[92]. Ultrasound visualization of an apparently intact diaphragm does not rule out CDH. Color Doppler studies can also assist in diagnosing CDH[93]. In more than 50% of cases with CDH seen prenatally, at least one or more extradiaphragmatic malformations can be detected[71]. Cardiac anomalies are seen in 9–23% of cases, and 18% of fetuses with CDH have chromosomal abnormalities, especially trisomy 18. In contrast to these findings 36% seen postnatally have associated malformations. The survival rate of fetuses with CDH and associated anomalies is poor (7%) and a 50% rate of intrauterine demise has been reported[75,94]. Other prognostic factors are the volume of the herniated contents and the stage in pregnancy when herniation occurs. It has been suggested that *in utero* repair of the defect should be performed to allow the lungs to grow and develop, in the hope of preventing fatal pulmonary insufficiency. Despite improvements in surgical techniques, the results of open fetal surgery to correct CDH have been disappointing. Hysterotomy induces preterm labour and, where there is a large volume of liver in the fetal chest, reduction of the liver into the abdomen induces immediate fetal death[95]. Survival

was only 29% in a series of 14 fetuses with CDH receiving *in utero* surgery. Five of these fetuses died intraoperatively when an incarcerated liver was reduced[96]. Less invasive techniques, using both open surgery and fetoscopy, are being developed in the hope of reducing fetal demise. These techniques include blocking the trachea and obstructing the flow of fluid from the fetal lungs, helping to expand the lungs and displace abdominal viscera from the chest, the creation of an artificial gastroschisis and induction of graft tolerance for postnatal lung transplantation[95].

Experimental fetal tracheal ligation has been shown to increase lung growth *in utero* by accelerating fetal alveolar growth[97–99] and to reduce the hernial contents in CDH[100]. Inhalation of nitric oxide as a pulmonary vasodilator has been reported to relieve hypoxemia in infants with CDH[101–103]. The mortality for potentially correctable CDH diagnosed before 24 weeks' gestation is 58%, despite optimal care presently available after birth. Infants who die *in utero* and soon after birth constitute a substantial hidden mortality[96].

The presence or absence of polyhydramnios, fetal breathing movements, mediastinal shift, thoracic position of the stomach, fetal breathing-related nasal and oropharyngeal fluid flow, ductal flow velocity modulation, and gestational age at onset and severity of ventricular disproportion may serve as markers for predicting fetal pulmonary hypoplasia[104]. In the neonate with an isolated left-sided diaphragmatic hernia, a good prognosis is to be expected if the condition was not detectable by detailed prenatal sonography in the second half of pregnancy[105]. The timing of visceral herniation into the thoracic cavity is a major indicator of the prognosis of these fetuses. Herniation that occurs after 25 weeks of gestation carries a more favorable clinical outcome[76]. However, spontaneous resolution during the third trimester of CDH diagnosed in the second trimester can occur[106]. Normal sonographic studies during the first half of pregnancy do not exclude the subsequent development of CDH. Overall survival was 42% before the introduction of extracorporeal membrane oxygenation if the CDH is localized and the patient delivers at a tertiary center and 75% afterward. There appears to have been an improvement in survival since the introduction of extracorporeal membrane oxygenation[107]. Recurrent chest infections and gastro-esophageal reflux are the most common long-term complications[87].

Congenital cystic adenomatoid malformation (CCAM)

Fetal cystic adenomatoid malformation of the lung is a rare pulmonary lesion characterized by excessive growth of terminal respiratory structures. CCAM probably occurs at less than 10 weeks gestational age[108]. Some investigators believe that CCAMs are hamartomas that form because of bronchiolar maturation arrest associated with proliferation of mesenchymal elements[109,110]. Other authors believe that CCAM results from bronchial atresia and dysplastic lung development beyond atretic segments[111]. It is usually unilateral and involves one lobe or segment. A large mass may cause mediastinal shift, hypoplasia of normal lung tissue, polyhydramnios, and cardiovascular compromise leading to fetal hydrops[112]. CCAM is occasionally associated with 'prune belly syndrome'[113–117]. Postmortem bronchography or serial microscopical examination shows segmental bronchial absence or atresia[111]. In the newborn this malformation can be responsible for respiratory distress of variable degrees with immediate or delayed onset after birth.

CCAM is now commonly diagnosed *in utero* with fetal ultrasonography[109,118–121] (Figure 8). The diagnosis can be verified by fetal lung biopsy[122]. Differential diagnoses include pulmonary sequestration, bronchogenic cyst or CDH. CCAM can be classified according to the classification proposed by Stocker as types I, II or III (Table 2). Type I lesions are characterized by large cysts measuring more than 2 cm in diameter, type II lesions typically contains cysts of a more uniform size (not exceeding 2 cm in diameter), and type III lesions contain microscopic cysts[108,123]. CCAM can also be classified by the size of the cysts as macrocystic (single or multiple cysts > 5 mm) or microcystic (cysts < 5 mm; solid appearance). Microcystic lesions are usually associated with fetal hydrops and have a poor prognosis[118].

The lesions are macrocystic in 59% and microcystic in 41% of cases. CCAM is left-sided in 51%, right-sided in 35% and bilateral in 14% of fetuses[124]. Hydrops fetalis secondary to CCAM develops in 43% and is almost invariably lethal. This poor prognosis may be attributed to the combined effects of tissue compression from the thoracic space-occupying lesion and premature delivery of a hydropic baby following rupture of the membranes in the presence of polyhydramnios[125]. Associated anomalies are present in

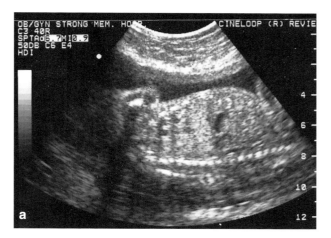
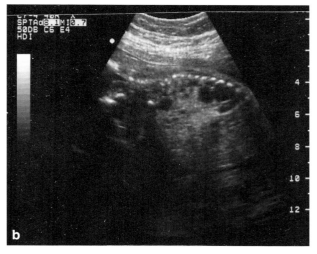

Figure 8 (**a,b**) Two fetuses with congenital cystic adenomatoid malformation demonstrating cystic appearance of one lung

11%. The prognosis is better if the CCAM is macrocystic, if there is no hydrops and if the amniotic fluid is normal or decreased[124,126]. Complete intrauterine resolution of fetal CCAM type III has been reported[127]. Current therapies for these lesions are observation, serial amniocenteses for polyhydramnios complicating CCAM[125], thoracentesis[128], thoraco-amniotic shunts[129] and fetal resection of the massively enlarged pulmonary lobe (fetal lobectomy)[130]. The outcome is usually excellent[131]. Fetal surgery in CCAM is currently reserved for only those fetuses with hydrops and a uniformly fatal outcome[132].

Pulmonary sequestration

Although the exact etiology of this abnormality is unknown, it probably represents a broncho-pulmonary foregut abnormality[133]. Sequestrations are characterized by the lack of communication with the normal bronchial tree. The lesions have been divided into extralobar and intralobar forms, and although the former is least common overall (25%), extralobar sequestration is the most common form found in neonates and nearly the only form detected prenatally[121,134–136]. The extralobar lesion consists of a mass of ectopic pulmonary tissue that is enveloped by its own pleura. This lung tissue receives its arterial blood supply ectopically, usually from the descending aorta, and its venous drainage is to systemic (inferior vena cava, azygous, or portal veins) rather than pulmonary veins[137]. Sequestrations occur most commonly on the left (90%) in the posterior and basal segments. Occasionally, sequestered lobes are found outside the thoracic cavity[138]. Subdiaphragmatic lesions (which account for 2.5% of bronchopulmonary foregut malformations) have been observed prenatally with ultrasound evaluation[139,140]. The latter association may obscure the extralobar sequestration and account for the fact that this form of sequestration has only rarely been diagnosed prenatally. Karyotype abnormalities do not seem to be increased.

Sonographically, a pulmonary sequestration appears as a well-circumscribed, uniformly echogenic mass in the fetal thorax[121,134–136] (Figure 9). Like CCAM and CDH, they too have been associated with fetal hydrops and maternal polyhydramnios that is presumed secondary to mass effect and compression of the fetal esophagus or mediastinum and heart. Although these lesions may be similar to CDH, they are distinguished by the normal intra-abdominal anatomy associated with pulmonary sequestration. In addition, color Doppler flow imaging has been used to detect the feeding systemic artery in the fetus (which has been traced from the descending aorta to lower lobe mass)[141].

Bronchogenic cysts

Bronchogenic cysts are uncommon congenital anomalies that result from an abnormal development in the budding or branching of the tracheobronchial tree, probably between the 26th and 40th day of fetal life, when the most active

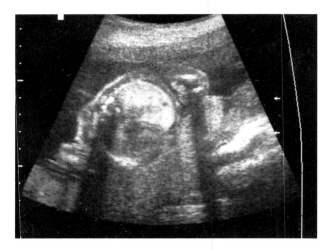

Figure 9   Ultrasonographic appearance of pulmonary sequestration

tracheobronchial development is occurring[142]. They also represent foregut abnormalities and result from abnormal budding of the ventral diverticulum of the foregut[133,142]. Posterior mediastinal neurenteric cysts occur as an anomaly of the posterior aspect of the foregut and notochord, and are associated with spinal anomalies. Abnormal development in the middle of the foregut is believed to result in esophageal duplications, and abnormal budding of the anterior diverticulum of the foregut results in bronchial cysts, most of which occur in the mediastinum, with a minority in the pulmonary parenchyma[133]. Bronchogenic cysts are not usually associated with other congenital anomalies[133,143]. They may enlarge in infancy and cause respiratory distress. Their presence in the fetus is suggested by mediastinal shift and bronchial obstruction. Very few cases have been detected antenatally, but those that have were seen as unilocular or multilocular cystic masses in the fetal chest[121]. Mediastinal cysts tend to compress the trachea.

Bronchial atresia

Congenital bronchial atresia is another unusual pulmonary anomaly that rarely has been described on prenatal sonography as an echogenic pulmonary mass lesion[144]. The cause is unknown, but the lesion is characterized by a focal obliteration of a segment of the bronchial lumen and occurs most commonly in the left upper lobe. Other relatively common sites are the right upper middle lobes. This lesion rarely occurs in the lower lobe[133] and in this way may be distinguished from extralobar pulmonary sequestration or CDH.

Tracheal/laryngeal atresia

Both fetal tracheal and laryngeal atresia have been observed prenatally. If the trachea or larynx is atretic or completely obstructed, the fluid secreted by the lungs cannot be expelled. The distended lungs appear hyperechogenic, and the bronchi become dilated by the trapped fluid. Histologically, these lungs are not hypoplastic but normal or hyperplastic. Fetal ascites is usually associated, perhaps secondary to venous compression of the mediastinal vessels and heart by the enlarged lungs. Mortality in fetuses in whom these lesions have been detected prenatally has been 100%[145,146].

Pleural effusion

Fluid in the pleural space of the fetus is abnormal at any gestational age. Pleural effusions may occur in the fetus as an isolated abnormality or in association with more serious conditions, such as the multiple causes of immune or non-immune hydrops fetalis, chest mass, or posterior urethral valves associated with urinary ascites. In cases of non-immune hydrops fetalis, prognosis is usually poor[147–149], and these serous effusions represent only a single manifestation of a more serious underlying dysfunction (cardiac anomaly, lymphangiectasia, intrauterine infection, Turner syndrome, chromosomal anomaly, and similar defects). If the fetus is believed to have immune hydrops fetalis, current therapy is directed toward intrauterine transfusion or prompt delivery, depending on the gestational age[150]. Primary pleural effusions are generally chylous and, when unassociated with hydrops, carry a much more optimistic fetal prognosis. This is generally poorer than the prognosis of the neonate whose chylous effusion is discovered after birth. Overall mortality in the fetus approaches 50%[151,152], with death after birth due to pulmonary hypoplasia, hydrops and prematurity. Bilateral effusions, diagnosis before 33 weeks, and hydrops are all associated with poorer outcome[152,153]. On the contrary, the absence of hydrops predicted 100% survival in Longaker and coworkers' series of 32 fetuses with hydrothorax. Spontaneous resolution of the pleural fluid is associated with near 100% survival[152].

Sonographically, pleural effusions appear as anechoic fluid collections in the fetal chest that usually conform to the normal chest and diaphragmatic contour but, when large enough, may be associated with bulging of the chest and flattening or inversion of the diaphragm[149] (Figure 10). Aspirated chylous fetal effusions generally show a large number of lymphocytes. Sonographic features suggestive of fetal chylothorax include the following:

(1) The pleural effusion occurs as an isolated finding;

(2) The size of the effusion is disproportionately large compared with other effusions, if present;

(3) The effusion occurs first as an isolated finding and is later followed by the development of other features associated with hydrops fetalis, such as ascites and integumentary edema.

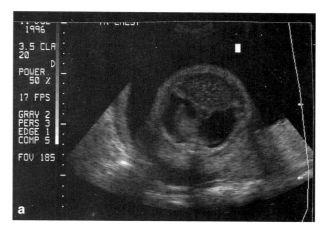

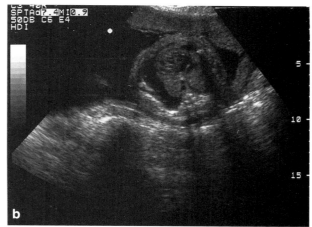

Figure 10 (a) Severe hydrothorax with fluid compressing both lungs. (b) Fetal heart and lungs seen compressed to center of thorax by bilateral hydrothorax

References

1. Suchet IB. Ultrasonography of the fetal neck in the first and second trimesters. Part 2. Anomalies of the posterior nuchal region. *J Can Assoc Radiol* 1995;46:344–52

2. Sepulveda WH, Cuiffardi I. Early sonographic diagnosis of fetal cystic hygroma colli. *J Perinat Med* 1992;20:149–52

3. Zalel Y, Shalev E, Ben-Ami M, *et al.* Ultrasonographic diagnosis of mediastinal cystic hygroma. *Prenat Diagn* 1992;12:541–4

4. Kennedy TL. Cystic hygroma-lymphangioma: a rare and still unclear entity. *Laryngoscope* 1989;99 (Suppl 49):1–10

5. Rottem S. Early detection of structural anomalies and markers of chromosomal aberrations by transvaginal ultrasonography. *Curr Opin Obstet Gynecol* 1995;7:122–5

6. Wu MP, Wu RL, Lee JS, *et al.* Spontaneous resolution of fetal mediastinal cystic hygroma. *Int J Gynaecol Obstet* 1995;48:295–8

7. Hoffman-Tretin J, Koenigsberg M, Ziprkowski M. Antenatal demonstration of axillary cystic hygroma. *J Ultrasound Med* 1988;7:233–5

8. Anderson NG, Kennedy JC. Prognosis in fetal cystic hygroma. *Aust NZ J Obstet Gynaecol* 1992;32: 36–9

9. Reichler A, Bronshtein M. Early prenatal diagnosis of axillary cystic hygroma. *J Ultrasound Med* 1995; 14:581–4

10. McCoy MC, Kuller JA, Chescheir NC, *et al.* Prenatal diagnosis and management of massive bilateral axillary cystic lymphangioma. *Obstet Gynecol* 1995;85:853–6

11. Stenson KM, Mishelle J, Toriumi DM. Cystic hygroma of the parotid gland. *Ann Otol Rhinol Laryngol* 1991;100:518–20

12. Goshen S, Ophir D. Cystic hygroma of the parotid gland. *J Laryngol Otol* 1993;107:855–7

13. Kozlowski KJ, Frazier CN, Quirk JG Jr. Prenatal diagnosis of abdominal cystic hygroma. *Prenat Diagn* 1988;8:405–9

14. Cohen MM, Schwartz S, Schwartz MF, *et al.* Antenatal detection of cystic hygroma. *Obstet Gynecol Surv* 1989;44:481–90

15. Achiron R, Rotstein Z, Lipitz S, *et al.* First trimester diagnosis of fetal congenital heart disease by transvaginal ultrasonography. *Obstet Gynecol* 1994; 84:69–72

16. Miyabara S, Sugihara H, Maehara N, *et al.* Significance of cardiovascular malformations in cystic hygroma: a new interpretation of the pathogenesis. *Am J Med Genet* 1989;34:489–501

17. Van-Zallen-Sprock RM, Van Vugt JM, Van Geijn HP. First-trimester diagnosis of cystic hygroma – course and outcome. *Am J Obstet Gynecol* 1992;167: 94–8

18. Chappuis JP. Current aspects of cystic lymphangioma of the neck. *Arch Pediatr* 1994;1:186–92

19. Cullen MT, Gabrielli S, Green JJ, *et al.* Diagnosis and significance of cystic hygroma in the first trimester. *Prenat Diagn* 1990;10:643–51

20. Shulman LP, Emerson DS, Felker RE, *et al.* High frequency of cytogenetic abnormalities in fetuses with cystic hygroma diagnosed in the first trimester. *Obstet Gynecol* 1992;80:80–2

21. Johnson MP, Johnson A, Holzgrave W, *et al.* First trimester simple hygroma: cause and outcome. *Am J Obstet Gynecol* 1993;168:156–61

22. Podobnik M, Singer Z, Podobnik-Sarkanji S, *et al.* First trimester diagnosis of cystic hygromata using transvaginal ultrasound and cytogenic evaluation. *J Perinat Med* 1995;23:283–91

23. Chervenak FA, Isaacson G, Blakemore KJ, *et al.* Fetal cystic hygroma. Cause and natural history. *N Engl J Med* 1983;309:822–5

24. Garden AS, Isaacson G, Blakemore KJ, *et al.* Fetal cystic hygroma colli: antenatal diagnosis, significance, and management. *Am J Obstet Gynecol* 1986; 154:221–5

25. Anderson NG, Kennedy JC. Prognosis in fetal cystic hygroma. *Aust NZ J Obstet Gynaecol* 1992;32: 36–9

26. Bronshtein M, Bar-Hava I, Blumenfeld I, *et al.* The difference between septated and nonseptated nuchal cystic hygroma in the early second trimester. *Obstet Gynecol* 1993;81:683–7

27. Shulman LP, Raafat NA, Mace PC, *et al.* Significance of septations in isolated fetal cystic hygroma detected in the first trimester. *Prenat Diagn* 1994;14:223–6

28. Suchet IB, van der Westhuizen NG, Labatte MF. Fetal cystic hygromas: further insights into their natural history. *J Can Assoc Radiol* 1992;43: 420–4

29. Newman DE, Cooperberg PL. Genetics of sonographically detected intrauterine fetal cystic hygromas. *J Can Assoc Radiol* 1984;35:77–9

30. Nadel A, Bromley B, Benacerraf BR. Nuchal thickening or cystic hygromas in first and early second-trimester fetuses: prognosis and outcome. *Obstet Gynecol* 1993;82:43–8

31. Greenberg F, Carpenter RJ, Ledbetter DH. Cystic hygroma and hydrops fetalis in a fetus with trisomy 13. *Clin Genet* 1983;24:389–91

32. Tannirandorn Y, Nicolini U, Nicolaidis PC, *et al.* Fetal cystic hygromata: insights gained from fetal blood sampling. *Prenat Diagn* 1990;10:189–93

33. Lehman CD, Nyberg DA, Winter TC III, *et al.* Trisomy 13 syndrome: prenatal US findings in a review of 33 cases. *Radiology* 1995;194:217–22

34. Van Allen MI, Ritchie S, Toi A, *et al.* Trisomy 4 in a fetus with cyclopia and other anomalies. *Am J Med Genet* 1993;46:193–7

35. Fryns JP, Kleczkowska A, Vandenberghe K, *et al.* Cystic hygroma and hydrops fetalis in dup(11p) syndrome. *Am J Med Genet* 1985;22:287–9

36. Zarabi M, Mieckowski GC, Mazer J. Cystic hygroma associated with Noonan's syndrome. *J Clin Ultrasound* 1983;11:398–400

37. Izquierdo L, Kushnir O, Sanchez D, *et al.* Prenatal diagnosis of Noonan's syndrome in a female infant with spontaneous resolution of cystic hygroma and hydrops. *West J Med* 1990;152:418–21

38. Donnenfeld AE, Nazir MA, Sindoni F, *et al.* Prenatal sonographic documentation of cystic hygroma regression in Noonan syndrome. *Am J Med Genet* 1991;39:461–5

39. Sonesson SE, Fouron JC, Lessard M. Intrauterine diagnosis and evolution of a cardiomyopathy in a fetus with Noonan's syndrome. *Acta Paediatr* 1992; 81:368–70

40. Daoud MS, Dahl PR, Su WP. Noonan syndrome. *Semin Dermatol* 1995;14:140–4

41. Chen H, Immken L, Lachman R, *et al.* Syndrome of multiple pterygia, camptodactyly, facial anomalies, hypoplastic lungs and heart, cystic hygroma, and skeletal anomalies: delineation of a new entity and review of lethal forms of multiple pterygium syndrome. *Am J Med Genet* 1984;17:809–26

42. Fryns JP, Vandenberghe K, Moerman P, *et al.* Cystic hygroma and multiple pterygium syndrome. *Ann Genet* 1984;27:252–3

43. Martin NJ, Hill JB, Cooper DH, *et al.* Lethal multiple pterygium syndrome: three consecutive cases in one family. *Am J Med Genet* 1986;24: 295–304

44. Zeitune M, Fejgin MD, Abramowicz J, *et al.* Prenatal diagnosis of the pterygium syndrome. *Prenat Diagn* 1988;8:145–9

45. Lockwood C, Irons M, Troiani J, *et al.* The prenatal sonographic diagnosis of lethal multiple pterygium syndrome: a heritable cause of recurrent abortion. *Am J Obstet Gynecol* 1988;159:474–6

46. Moerman P, Fryns JP, Cornelis A, *et al.* Pathogenesis of the lethal multiple pterygium syndrome. *Am J Med Genet* 1990;35:415–21

47. Spearritt DJ, Tannenberg AE, Payton DJ. Lethal multiple pterygium syndrome: report of a case with neurological anomalies. *Am J Med Genet* 1993; 47:45–9

48. Schwyzer U, Briner J, Schinzel A. Fryns syndrome in a girl born to consanguineous parents. *Acta Paediatr Scand* 1987;76:167–71

49. Bulas DI, Saal HM, Allen JF, *et al.* Cystic hygroma and congenital diaphragmatic hernia: early pre-

50. McPherson EW, Ketterer DM, Salsburey DJ. Pallister–Killian and Fryns syndromes: nosology. *Am J Med Genet* 1993;47:241–5

51. Verloes A, Schaaps JP, Herens C, *et al.* Prenatal diagnosis of cystic hygroma and chorioangioma in the Wolf–Hirschhorn syndrome. *Prenat Diagn* 1991;11:129–32

52. Dickerhoff R, Bode VU. Cyclophoshamide in non-resectable cystic hygroma [letter; comment]. *Lancet* 1990;335:1474–5

53. Edwards MJ, Graham JM Jr. Posterior nuchal cystic hygroma. *Clin Perinatol* 1990;17:611–40

54. Wenstrom KD, Williamson RA, Hoover WW, *et al.* Achondrogenesis type II (Langer–Saldino) in association with jugular lymphatic obstruction sequence. *Prenat Diagn* 1989;9:527–32

55. Fried AM, Loh FK, Umer MA, *et al.* Echogenicity of fetal lung: relation to fetal age and maturity. *Am J Roentgenol* 1985;145:591–4

56. Gayea PD, Grant DC, Doubilet PM, *et al.* Prediction of fetal lung maturity: inaccuracy of study using conventional ultrasound instruments. *Radiology* 1985;155:473

57. Chitkara U, Rosenberg J, Chervenak FA, *et al.* Prenatal sonographic assessment of the fetal thorax: normal values. *Am J Obstet Gynecol* 1987;156:1069–74

58. Nimrod C, Davies D, Iwanicki S, *et al.* Ultrasound prediction of pulmonary hypoplasia. *Obstet Gynecol* 1986;68:495–8

59. DeVore GR, Horenstein J, Platt LD. Fetal echocardiography. VI. Assessment of cardiothoracic disproportion – a new technique for the diagnosis of thoracic hypoplasia. *Am J Obstet Gynecol* 1986; 155:1066–71

60. Songster GS, Gray DL, Crane JP. Prenatal prediction of lethal pulmonary hypoplasia using ultrasonic fetal chest circumference. *Obstet Gynecol* 1989;73:261–6

61. D'Alton M, Mercer B, Riddick E, *et al.* Serial thoracic versus abdominal circumference ratios for the prediction of pulmonary hypoplasia in premature rupture of the membranes remote from term. *Am J Obstet Gynecol* 1992;166:658–63

62. Vintzileos AM, Campbell WA, Rodis JF, *et al.* Comparison of six different ultrasonographic methods for predicting lethal fetal pulmonary hypoplasia. *Am J Obstet Gynecol* 1989;161:606–12

63. Achiron R, Strauss S, Seidman DS, *et al.* Fetal lung hyperechogenicity: prenatal ultrasonographic diagnosis, natural history and neonatal outcome. *Ultrasound Obstet Gynecol* 1995;6:40–2

64. Meizner I, Rosenak D. The vanishing fetal intrathoracic mass: consider an obstructing mucous plug. *Ultrasound Obstet Gynecol* 1995;5:275–7

65. Hirose R, Suita S, Taguchi T, *et al.* Extralobar pulmonary sequestration mimicking cystic adenomatoid

malformation in prenatal sonographic appearance and histological findings. *J Pediatr Surg* 1995;30: 1390–3

66. Sarda P, Devaux P, Lefort G, *et al*. Epidemiology of diaphragmatic hernia in Languedoc–Roussillon. *Genet Couns* 1991;2:77–81

67. Schumacher RE, Farrel PM. Congenital diaphragmatic hernia: a major remaining challenge in neonatal respiratory care. *Perinat Neonatol* 1985; 9:29

68. Moore KL. Development of body cavities, primitive mesenteries, and the diaphragm. In *Clinically Oriented Embryology*, 4th edn. Philadelphia: WB Saunders, 1988

69. David TJ, Illingworth CA. Diaphragmatic hernia in the south-west of England. *J Med Genet* 1976; 13:253–62

70. Harrison MR, de Lorimer AA. Congenital diaphragmatic hernia. *Surg Clin North Am* 1981;61: 1023–35

71. Puri P, Gorman F. Lethal nonpulmonary anomalies associated with congenital diaphragmatic hernia: implications for early intrauterine surgery. *J Pediatr Surg* 1984;19:29–32

72. Goldstein RB. Ultrasound evaluation of the fetal thorax. In *Ultrasonography in Obstetrics and Gynecology*, 3rd edn. Philadelphia: WB Saunders, 1995

73. Hilpert PL, Kurtz AB. The role of transvaginal ultrasound in the second and third trimesters. *Semin Ultrasound CT Mr* 1990;11:59–70

74. Greenwood RD, Rosenthal A, Nadas AS. Cardiovascular abnormalities associated with congenital diaphragmatic hernia. *Pediatrics* 1976;57:92–7

75. Nakayama DK, Harrison MR, Chinn DH, *et al*. Prenatal diagnosis and natural history of the fetus with a congenital diaphragmatic hernia: initial clinical experience. *J Pediatr Surg* 1985;20: 118–24

76. Sharland GK, Lockhart SM, Heward AJ, *et al*. Prognosis in fetal diaphragmatic hernia. *Am J Obstet Gynecol* 1992;166:9–13

77. North AJ, Moya FR, Mysore MR, *et al*. Pulmonary endothelial nitric oxide synthase gene expression is decreased in a rat model of congenital diaphragmatic hernia. *Am J Respir Cell Mol Biol* 1995;13: 676–82

78. Alles AJ, Losty PD, Donahoe PK, *et al*. Embryonic cell death patterns associated with nitrofen-induced congenital diaphragmatic hernia. *J Pediatr Surg* 1995;30:353–8; discussion 359–60

79. Bos AP, Pattenier AM, Grobbee RE, *et al*. Etiological aspects of congenital diaphragmatic hernia: results of a case comparison study. *Hum Genet* 1994;94:445–6

80. Kluth D, Tenbrinck R, von Ekesparre M, *et al*. The natural history of congenital diaphragmatic hernia and pulmonary hypoplasia in the embryo. *J Pediatr Surg* 1993;28:456–62

81. Alfonso LF, Vilanova J, Aldazabal P, *et al*. Lung growth and maturation in the rat model of experimentally induced congenital diaphragmatic hernia. *Eur J Pediatr Surg* 1993;3:6–11

82. Wickman DS, Siebert JR, Benjamin DR. Nitrofen-induced congenital diaphragmatic defects in CD1 mice. *Teratology* 1993;47:119–25

83. Hassett MJ, Glick PL, Karamanoukian HL, *et al*. Pathophysiology of congenital diaphragmatic hernia. XVI: Elevated pulmonary collagen in the lamb model of congenital diaphragmatic hernia. *J Pediatr Surg* 1995;30:1191–4

84. Harrison MR, Adzick NS, Flake AW. Congenital diaphragmatic hernia: an unsolved problem. *Semin Pediatr Surg* 1993;2:109–12

85. Narayan H, De Chazal R, Barrow M, *et al*. Familial congenital diaphragmatic hernia: prenatal diagnosis, management, and outcome. *Prenat Diagn* 1993;13: 893–901

86. Harrison MR, Adzick NS, Nakayama DK, *et al*. Fetal diaphragmatic hernia: fatal but fixable. *Semin Perinatol* 1985;9:103–12

87. Rasheed K, Coughlan G, O'Donnell B. Congenital diaphragmatic hernia in the newborn. Outcome in 59 consecutive cases over a ten year period (1980–1989). *Ir J Med Sci* 1992;161:16–17

88. Frey P, Glanzmann R, Nars P, *et al*. Familial congenital diaphragmatic defect: transmission from father to daughter. *J Pediatr Surg* 1991;26:1396–8

89. Chinn DH, Filly RA, Callen PW, *et al*. Congenital diaphragmatic hernia diagnosed by ultrasound. *Radiology* 1983;148:119–23

90. Comstock CH. The antenatal diagnosis of diaphragmatic anomalies. *J Ultrasound Med* 1986;5: 391–6

91. Whittle MJ, Gilmore DH, McNay MB, *et al*. Diaphragmatic hernia presenting *in utero* as a unilateral hydrothorax. *Prenat Diagn* 1989;9:115–8

92. Bootstaylor BS, Filly RA, Harrison MR, *et al*. Prenatal sonographic predictors of liver herniation in congenital diaphragmatic hernia. *J Ultrasound Med* 1995;14:515–20

93. Botash RJ, Sprit BA. Color Doppler imaging aids in the prenatal diagnosis of congenital diaphragmatic hernia. *J Ultrasound Med* 1993;12:359–61

94. Adzick NS, Harrison MR, Glick PL, *et al*. Diaphragmatic hernia in the fetus: prenatal diagnosis and outcome in 94 cases. *J Pediatr Surg* 1985; 20:357–61

95. Ford WD. Fetal intervention for congenital diaphragmatic hernia. *Fetal Diagn Ther* 1994;9: 398–408

96. Harrison MR, Adzick NS, Estes JM, *et al*. A prospective study of the outcome of fetuses with diaphragmatic hernia. *J Am Med Assoc* 1994;271: 382–4

97. DiFiore JW, Fauza DO, Slavin R, *et al*. Experimental fetal tracheal ligation and congenital

diaphragmatic hernia: a pulmonary vascular morphometric analysis. *J Pediatr Surg* 1995;30:917–23

98. DiFiore JW, Fauza DO, Slavin R, *et al.* Experimental fetal tracheal ligation reverses the structural and physiological effects of pulmonary hypoplasia in congenital diaphragmatic hernia. *J Pediatr Surg* 1994;29:248–56

99. Hedrick MH, Estes JM, Sullivan KM, *et al.* Plug the lung until it grows (PLUG): a new method to treat congenital diaphragmatic hernia *in utero. J Pediatr Surg* 1994;29:612–7

100. Hashim E, Laberge JM, Chen MF, *et al.* Reversible tracheal obstruction in the fetal sheep: effects on tracheal fluid pressure and lung growth. *J Pediatr Surg* 1995;30:1172–7

101. Henneberg SW, Jepsen S, Andersen PK, *et al.* Inhalation of nitric oxide as a treatment of pulmonary hypertension in congenital diaphragmatic hernia. *J Pediatr Surg* 1995;30:853–5

102. Dillon PW, Cilley RE, Hudome SM, *et al.* Nitric oxide reversal of recurrent pulmonary hypertension and respiratory failure in an infant with CDH after successful ECMO therapy. *J Pediatr Surg* 1995;30:743–4

103. Shah N, Jacob T, Exler R, *et al.* Inhaled nitric oxide in congenital diaphragmatic hernia. *J Pediatr Surg* 1994;29:1010–4

104. Fox HE, Badalian SS. Ultrasound prediction of fetal pulmonary hypoplasia in pregnancies complicated by oligohydramnios and in cases of congenital diaphragmatic hernia: a review. *Am J Perinatol* 1994;11:104–8

105. Stringer MD, Goldstein RB, Filly RA, *et al.* Fetal diaphragmatic hernia without visceral herniation. *J Pediatr Surg* 1995;30:1264–6

106. Sherer DM, Woods JR Jr. Second trimester sonographic diagnosis of fetal congenital diaphragmatic hernia, with spontaneous resolution during the third trimester, resulting in a normal infant at delivery. *J Clin Ultrasound* 1991;19:298–302

107. Mallik K, Rodgers BM, McGahren ED. Congenital diaphragmatic hernia: experience in a single institution from 1978 through 1994. *Ann Thorac Surg* 1995;60:1331–5

108. Rosado-de-Christenson ML, Stocker JT. Congenital cystic adenomatoid malformation. *Radiographics* 1991;11:865–86

109. Johnson JA, Rumack CM, Johnson ML, *et al.* Cystic adenomatoid malformation: antenatal demonstration. *Am J Roentgenol* 1984;142:483–4

110. Miller RK, Sieber WK, Yunis EJ. Congenital adenomatoid malformation of the lung. A report of 17 cases and review of the literature. *Pathol Annu* 1980;15:387–402

111. Moerman P, Fryns JP, Vandenberghe K, *et al.* Pathogenesis of congenital cystic adenomatoid malformation of the lung. *Histopathology* 1992;21:315–21

112. Adzick NS, Harrison MR. Management of the fetus with a cystic adenomatoid malformation. *World J Surg* 1993;17:342–9

113. Kuruvilla AC, Kesler KR, Williams JW, *et al.* Congenital cystic adenomatoid malformation of the lung associated with prune belly syndrome. *J Pediatr Surg* 1987;22:370–1

114. Beluffi G, Brokensha C, Kozlowski K, *et al.* Congenital cystic adenomatoid malformation of the lung. Presentation of 16 cases. *ROFO Fortschr Geb Rontgenstr Nuklearmed* 1989;150:523–30

115. Ribet M, Pruvot FR, Dubos JP, *et al.* Congenital cystic adenomatoid malformation of the lung. *Eur J Cardiothorac Surg* 1990;4:403–5

116. Genest DR, Driscoll SG, Bieber FR. Complexities of limb anomalies: the lower extremity in the 'prune belly' phenotype. *Teratology* 1991;44:365–71

117. Ramìrez-Figueroa JL, Perez-Fernandez LF, Lûpez-Corella E, *et al.* Prune belly syndrome associated with cystic adenomatoid malformation of the lung and pulmonary sequestration. *Bol Med Hosp Infant Mex* 1993;50:336–40

118. Adzick NS, Harrison MR, Glick PL, *et al.* Fetal cystic adenomatoid malformation: prenatal diagnosis and natural history. *J Pediatr Surg* 1985;20:483–8

119. Pezzuti RT, Isler RJ. Antenatal ultrasound detection of cystic adenomatoid malformation of lung: report of a case and review of the recent literature. *J Clin Ultrasound* 1983;11:342–6

120. Graham D, Winn K, Dex W, *et al.* Prenatal diagnosis of cystic adenomatoid malformation of the lung. *J Ultrasound Med* 1982;1:9–12

121. Mayden KL, Tortora M, Chervenak FA, *et al.* The antenatal sonographic detection of lung masses. *Am J Obstet Gynecol* 1984;148:349–51

122. Murotsuki J, Uehara S, Okamura K, *et al.* Prenatal diagnosis of congenital cystic adenomatoid malformation of the lung by fetal lung biopsy. *Prenat Diagn* 1994;14:637–9

123. Stocker JT, Madewell JE, Drake RM. Congenital cystic adenomatoid malformation of the lung. Classification and morphologic spectrum. *Hum Pathol* 1977;8:155–71

124. Thorpe-Beeston JG, Nicolaides KH. Cystic adenomatoid malformation of the lung: prenatal diagnosis and outcome. *Prenat Diagn* 1994;14:677–88

125. Meagher SE, Simon DR, Hodges S, *et al.* Successful outcome, with serial amniocenteses for polyhydramnios complicating cystic adenomatoid malformation of the lung. *Aust NZ J Obstet Gynaecol* 1995;35:326–8

126. Neilson IR, Russo P, Laberge JM, *et al.* Congenital adenomatoid malformation of the lung: current management and prognosis. *J Pediatr Surg* 1991;26:975–80

127. Hsu KF, Wu MH, Chang CH, *et al.* Complete intrauterine resolution of fetal congenital cystic

adenomatoid malformation of the lung type III. *J Ultrasound Med* 1995;14:871–5

128. Nugent CE, Hayashi RH, Rubin J. Prenatal treatment of type I congenital cystic adenomatoid malformation by intrauterine fetal thoracentesis. *J Clin Ultrasound* 1989;17:675–7

129. Clark SL, Vitale DJ, Minton SD, *et al*. Successful fetal therapy for cystic adenomatoid malformation associated with second-trimester hydrops. *Am J Obstet Gynecol* 1987;157:294–5

130. Harrison MR, Adzick NS, Jennings RW, *et al*. Antenatal intervention for congenital cystic adeno-matoid malformation. *Lancet* 1990;336:965–7

131. Brown MF, Lewis D, Brouillette RM, *et al*. Successful prenatal management of hydrops, caused by congenital cystic adenomatoid malformation, using serial aspirations. *J Pediatr Surg* 1995;30: 1098–9

132. Morin L, Crombleholme TM, D'Alton ME. Prenatal diagnosis and management of fetal thoracic lesions. *Semin Perinatol* 1994;18:228–53

133. Fraser RG, Pare JAP. Pulmonary abnormalities of developmental origin. In Pare PD, Fraser RS, Genereux GP, eds. *Diagnosis of Diseases of the Chest*, 3rd edn. Philadelphia: WB Saunders, 1989:695–773

134. Thomas CS, Leopold GR, Hilton S, *et al*. Fetal hydrops associated with extralobar pulmonary sequestration. *J Ultrasound Med* 1986;5:668–71

135. Mariona F, McAlpin G, Zador I, *et al*. Sonographic detection of fetal extrathoracic pulmonary sequestration. *J Ultrasound Med* 1986;5:283–5

136. Romero R, Chervenak FA, Kotzen J, *et al*. Antenatal sonographic findings of extralobar pulmonary sequestration. *J Ultrasound Med* 1982;1: 131–2

137. Buntain WL, Woolley MM, Mahour GH, *et al*. Pulmonary sequestration in children: a twenty-five year experience. *Surgery* 1977;81:413–20

138. Savic B, Birtel FJ, Tholen W, *et al*. Lung sequestration: report of seven cases and review of 540 published cases. *Thorax* 1979;34:96–101

139. Davies RP, Ford WD, Lesquesne GW, *et al*. Ultrasonic detection of subdiaphragmatic pulmonary sequestration *in utero* and postnatal diagnosis by fine-needle aspiration biopsy. *J Ultrasound Med* 1989;8:47–9

140. Weinbaum PJ, Bors-Koefoed R, Green KW, *et al*. Antenatal sonographic findings in a case of intra-abdominal pulmonary sequestration. *Obstet Gynecol* 1989;73: 860–2

141. West MS, Donaldson JS, Shkolnik A. Pulmonary sequestration. Diagnosis by ultrasound. *J Ultrasound Med* 1989;8:125–9

142. Pare JAP, Fraser RG. *Synopsis of Diseases of the Chest*. Philadelphia: WB Saunders, 1983:239–42

143. DuMontier C, Graviss ER, Silberstein MJ, *et al*. Bronchogenic cysts in children. *Clin Radiol* 1985; 36:431–6

144. McAlister WH, Wright JR Jr, Crane JP. Main-stem bronchial atresia: intrauterine sonographic diag-nosis. *Am J Roentgenol* 1987;148:364–6

145. Dolkart LA, Reimers FT, Wertheimer IS, *et al*. Prenatal diagnosis of laryngeal atresia. *J Ultrasound Med* 1992;11:496–8

146. Watson WJ, Thorp JM Jr, Miller RC, *et al*. Prenatal diagnosis of laryngeal atresia. *Am J Obstet Gynecol* 1990;163:1456–7

147. Harrison MR, Golbus MS, Filly RA. Management of the fetus with nonimmune hydrops. In *The Unborn Patient*. Orlando, FL: Grune & Stratton, 1984: 193–216

148. Hutchinson AA, Drew JH, Yu VYH, *et al*. Non-immunologic hydrops fetalis: a review of 61 cases. *Obstet Gynecol* 1982;59:347–52

149. Mahoney BS, Filly RA, Callen PW, *et al*. Severe nonimmune hydrops fetalis: sonographic evalua-tion. *Radiology* 1984;151:757–61

150. Frigoletto FD, Greene MF, Benacerraf BR. Ultrasonographic fetal surveillance in the manage-ment of the isoimmunized pregnancy. *N Engl J Med* 1986;315:430–2

151. Weber AM, Philipson EH. Fetal pleural effusion. A review and meta-analysis for prognostic indicators. *Obstet Gynecol* 1992;79:281–6

152. Longaker MT, Laberge JM, Danserau J, *et al*. Primary fetal hydrothorax: natural history and management. *J Pediatr Surg* 1989;24:573–6

153. Estroff JA, Parad RB, Frigoletto FD Jr, *et al*. The natural history of isolated hydrothorax. *Ultrasound Obstet Gynecol* 1992;2:162

Abnormalities of fetal abdomen and pelvis

10

Richard Jaffe

The fetal abdomen includes organs of different origin and ultrasonographic identification of normal and abnormal structures is often difficult. The embryology and anatomy of normal and abnormal development of intra-abdominal and abdominal wall defects are well described in basic fetal ultrasonography books. In this chapter I will concentrate on the differential diagnosis of ultrasound findings and what constitutes proper follow-up and additional testing.

The chapter is divided into two major sections. The first evaluates normal and abnormal appearance of the gastrointestinal tract and abdominal wall and the second deals specifically with the urinary tract and the normal and abnormal appearance of its organs.

GASTROINTESTINAL SYSTEM

The abdominal wall

Abdominal wall defects are often associated with other structural or chromosomal abnormalities (Table 1). Diaphragmatic hernia is a defect in the diaphragm, the superior boundary of the abdominal cavity, and is described in chapter 9. The correct diagnosis of the abdominal wall defect is important for follow-up and appropriate counseling of the patient regarding outcome of the pregnancy and neonatal surgery. Abdominal wall defects are often diagnosed as a result of targeted scanning following an abnormally elevated maternal serum α-fetoprotein[1]. The two most common abdominal wall defects are omphalocele (Figure 1) and gastroschisis (Figure 2). The other defects that can be detected by ultrasonography are limb–body wall defect, bladder exstrophy (Figure 3), cloacal exstrophy (Figure 4) and vesicoallantoic abdominal wall defect (Figure 5) (Table 2).

With systematic scanning an accurate diagnosis of the abdominal wall defect is usually made. If the defect is localized at the level of the umbilicus it is

Table 1 Major anomalies associated with abdominal wall defects

Defect	Associated anomalies
Omphalocele	Cardiac, cloacal exstrophy, trisomies 13, 18 and 21
Gastroschisis	Intestinal atresia and obstruction, intrauterine growth restriction
Limb–body wall defect	Central nervous system (exencephaly, cephalocele), cardiac, skeletal defects, urogenital and gastrointestinal anomalies
Bladder exstrophy	Separation of pubic bones, low-set umbilicus, short penis with epispadias, skeletal and urinary tract abnormalities
Cloacal exstrophy	Omphalocele, spinal abnormalities, vertebral, urinary tract, cardiac anomalies, and single umbilical artery
Vesico-allantoic abdominal wall defect	Urogenital abnormalities

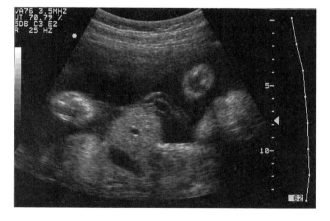

Figure 1 Longitudinal view of fetal abdomen demonstrating the omphalocele within the base of the umbilical cord

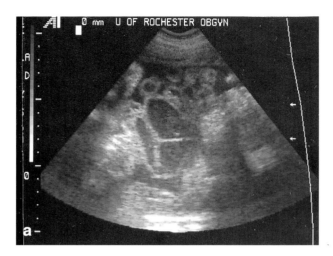

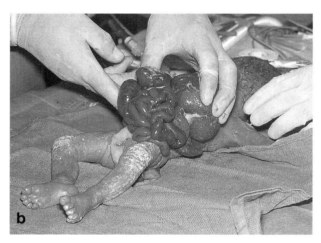

Figure 2 (**a**) Free floating bowel loops as seen in gastroschisis. (**b**) Newborn with gastroschisis

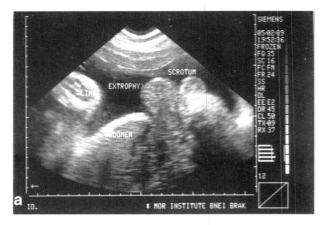

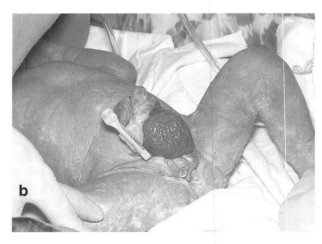

Figure 3 (**a**) Ultrasonography of bladder exstrophy demonstrating the echogenic appearance of the bladder. (**b**) Newborn with bladder exstrophy

either an omphalocele or gastroschisis. The differential diagnosis of omphalocele and gastroschisis is outlined in Table 3[2]. The most important ultrasonographic feature differentiating the two entities is localization of cord insertion. In gastroschisis the cord insertion is separate and to the left of the defect. In omphalocele the cord insertion is included in the defect and the vessels come out from the top of the defect (Figure 1). Generally speaking the omphalocele is covered by a membrane, whereas in gastroschisis free-floating bowel loops are seen within the amniotic cavity (Figure 2). In rare cases an omphalocele may rupture and bowel loops are seen floating freely in the amniotic fluid. In these cases other features should be evaluated although the correct diagnosis can not be made in all cases.

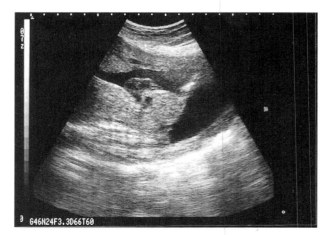

Figure 4 Large mass protruding from lower fetal abdomen in cloacal exstrophy

If the abdominal wall defect is below the cord insertion the diagnosis is most likely that of bladder or cloacal exstrophy[3]. A limb–body wall defect should be suspected when it is large and extends along a major part of the abdominal wall.

Bladder exstrophy should be suspected when normal kidneys and amniotic fluid are seen in the absence of a normal intra-abdominal filling bladder. Because the anterior wall of the bladder is absent the exstrophied bladder appears as a solid mass below the umbilicus (Figure 3). There is no obstruction to urine flow and amniotic fluid volume is normal. This anomaly may be associated with skeletal and urinary tract abnormalities. Cloacal exstrophy is more complex and difficult to accurately diagnose prenatally. The ultrasonographic features are those of a protruding mass with or without an omphalocele and cystic intra-abdominal lesions[4,5]. Cloacal exstrophy is associated with anomalies of the heart, urinary tract, skeleton and spine. Omphalocele is the only anomaly that is highly associated with chromosomal abnormalities such as trisomy 13, 18 and 21, and genetic testing should be offered to these patients[6].

Stomach

Visualization of a stomach bubble is important in ruling out several structural and functional abnormalities that may affect the fetus. When an absent stomach bubble is accompanied by polyhydramnios esophageal atresia or neuromuscular anomalies causing abnormal swallowing should be considered[7]. In the presence of an esophageal atresia with a tracheoesophageal fistula, fluid swallowed by the fetus can reach the stomach and the diagnosis can be missed. In some cases fluid is also produced by the mucosal lining of the stomach and esophageal atresia can be overlooked.

A prominent or so called 'double stomach bubble' is often associated with duodenal atresia[8] (Figure 6). This anomaly is associated with polyhydramnios and frequently present in fetuses with trisomy 21. A 'double bubble' should always be clearly distinguished from other upper abdominal cysts and prominent gallbladder. With the diagnosis of duodenal atresia genetic counseling and testing should be offered and other structural anomalies associated with trisomy 21 should be looked for.

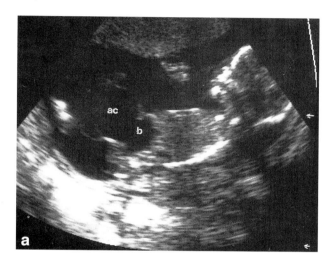

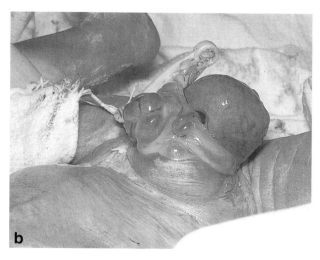

Figure 5 (**a**) A vesico-allantoic abdominal wall defect demonstrating the communication between the cyst and the bladder. ac, allantoic cyst; b, bladder. (**b**) Newborn with vesico-allantoic abdominal wall defect

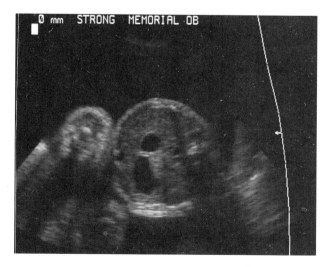

Figure 6 'Double stomach bubble' of duodenal atresia

Table 2   Abdominal wall defects, their frequency and ultrasound features

Defect	Frequency	Ultrasound features
Omphalocele	1/5000–7000	Midline defect, bowel and other intra-abdominal organs herniating into base of cord. The exteriorated organs are covered by a membrane
Gastroschisis	1/10 000–12 000	Defect lateral to cord insertion. Exteriorized organs not covered by membrane and are seen free-floating in amniotic cavity
Limb–body wall defect	1/14 000	Absent umbilical cord. Herniated organs adherent to amnion and placenta
Bladder exstrophy	1/30 000	A mass below cord insertion representing the bulging posterior wall of the bladder. No urine accumulates as the anterior bladder wall is missing. Normal fetal kidneys and amniotic fluid
Cloacal exstrophy	1/150 000	Protruding mass from abdomen, appearance similar to omphalocele, cystic intra-abdominal masses
Vesico-allantoic abdominal wall defect	Unknown	Cystic extra-abdominal mass connected to bladder. Bladder may be displaced anteriorly due to intra abdominal pressure

Table 3   Differential diagnosis of omphalocele and gastroschisis

	Omphalocele	Gastroschisis
Location	Midline	Right of cord
Cord insertion	Within defect	Separate
Covering membrane	Yes	No, free-floating bowel loops
Bowel loops	Mostly normal	Dilated, obstruction
Polyhydramnios	Rare	Common
Intrauterine growth restriction	10–20%	60–70%
Karyotype	Abnormal in 30–40%	Normal
Associated structural anomalies	Up to 70%	Rare

A missing stomach bubble in the upper fetal abdomen could indicate displacement of the gastrointestinal tract, and the fetal thorax should be carefully scanned to rule out diaphragmatic hernia (see chapter 9).

Bowel

Small bowel obstruction can be diagnosed *in utero* by identification of dilated bowel loops in association with polyhydramnios and occasionally a double stomach bubble. In rare cases Hirschsprung disease can be diagnosed late in pregnancy with the detection of dilated large bowel loops[9] (Figure 7). The exact location of the obstruction is difficult to determine, although generally speaking the more dilated loops present the lower is the obstruction.

The VACTERL syndrome is a malformation sequence with structural defects of many systems. The syndrome has been detected with increased frequency in fetuses of diabetic mothers[10]. The defects included are:

Vertebral or vascular anomalies;
Anorectal atresia;
Cardiac malformations;
Tracheoesophageal fistula or atresia;
Renal anomalies;
Limb anomalies.

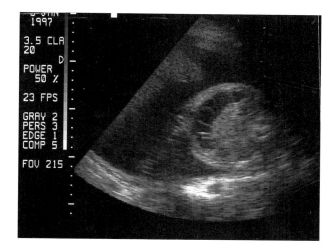

Figure 7 Dilated bowel loops seen late in gestation of fetus with Hirschsprung disease

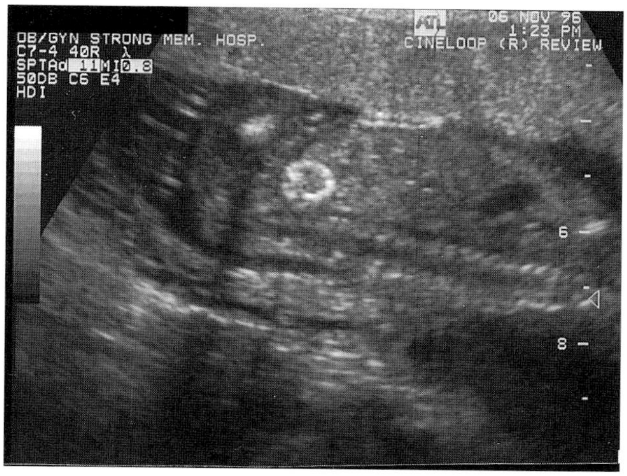

Figure 8 Echogenic bowel in fetus with trisomy 21

Echogenic appearance of fetal bowel is a common finding on routine ultrasonographic examinations. This can be a normal finding in a healthy fetus, a result of a high gain setting, or a finding associated with fetal abnormalities such as cystic fibrosis with meconium ileus[11,12] and trisomy 21[13,14] (Figure 8).

Abdominal cysts

Cystic structures within the fetal abdomen are readily detected on ultrasonography. The list of differential diagnoses is long and a systematic approach is crucial in reaching a correct diagnosis. Some of the most common cystic structures seen within the fetal abdomen are ovarian, hepatic or splenic cysts, multicystic kidney, hydronephrosis, hydroureter, enlarged bladder, persistent cloaca, and 'double bubble'.

Most cystic structures seen in the fetal abdomen are related to gastrointestinal or urinary tract and these systems should be thoroughly scanned for any sign that can help in making an accurate diagnosis. Parameters important in making the diagnosis are location in abdomen, relation to other structures, amount of amniotic fluid and fetal gender. In female fetuses one of the more common cystic structures is the ovarian cyst whereas most obstructive uropathies are seen in male fetuses. Polyhydramnios is common in bowel obstructions whereas oligohydramnios is a common feature of abnormal urinary tract development.

Ascites

The differential diagnosis of ascites and fetal hydrops is outlined in chapter 14. A sonolucent band often seen under the abdominal skin represents the musculature of the anterior abdominal wall and is termed pseudoascites (Figure 9). In the presence of true ascites fluid is seen between bowel loops and around the liver (Figure 10). True ascites is often a part of fetal hydrops and associated with polyhydramnios, thick umbilical cord and large placenta[15]. True isolated ascites is often associated with structural abnormalities such as persistent cloaca (Figure 11) or with infections.

URINARY TRACT

Urinary tract abnormalities are relatively common and account for approximately half of the structural abnormalities detected *in utero*. Urine production in the fetus begins at 10 weeks gestation and is the major source of amniotic fluid after 16 weeks. The fetal bladder is easily detected by ultrasonography and most abnormalities of the urinary tract impact on the anatomy and function of the bladder (Table 4).

The fetal kidneys are best seen in the transverse view of the fetal abdomen. They appear as round hypoechogenic structures adjacent to the fetal spine (Figure 12). The ureters can only be seen if a distal obstruction results in their abnormal dilatation and the bladder appears as a round hypoechoic

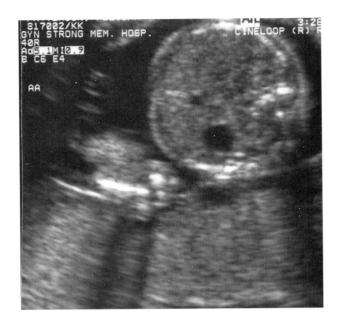

Figure 9 The ultrasonographic appearance of pseudoascites

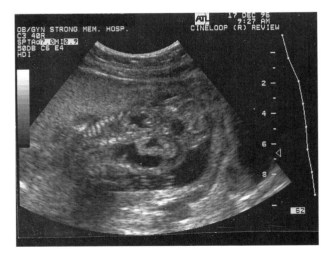

Figure 10 Ultrasonographic appearance of true fetal ascites

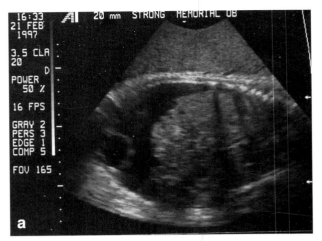

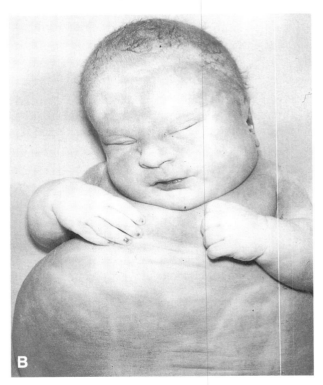

Figure 11 (a) Fetal ascites in persistent cloaca. (b) Newborn female with persistent cloaca

structure in the lower anterior fetal abdomen. Normal function is associated with filling and emptying of the bladder.

Urinary tract abnormalities can be classified as belonging to one of the following groups: renal agenesis or hypoplasia; abnormal position of kidney; cystic renal disease; renal tumors; and obstructive uropathy.

Renal agenesis or hypoplasia

Primary renal agenesis occurs in 1 in 4000 births. It also occurs in association with other congenital syndromes such as VACTERL and chromosomal anomalies. Oligohydramnios, fetal crowding, Potter facies with low-set ears, limb abnormalities and pulmonary hypoplasia are often detected after 18 weeks in fetuses with renal agenesis[16]. The differential diagnosis includes severe growth restriction and ruptured membranes. In the absence of fetal kidneys the adrenal glands may be mistaken for kidneys although the oligohydramnios seen in these cases should lead to the right diagnosis. Unilateral renal agenesis is more common and is associated with normal bladder and amniotic fluid volume[17].

Abnormal position of kidney

Pelvic ectopic kidney occurs in 1 in 1000 live births[18,19]. Fusion of the upper or lower kidney poles results in a horseshoe kidney[20]. Careful scanning

Table 4 Fetal genitourinary abnormalities, ultrasonographic appearance

Bladder dilation
   Urethral obstruction – posterior urethral valve (PUV)
   Urethral atresia
   Megacystis-microcolon-intestinal hypoperistalsis
      syndrome
   Urethral meatus agenesis
   Prune-belly syndrome
   Cloacal persistence
Non-visualization of bladder
   Renal agenesis
   Multicystic dysplastic kidneys
   Infantile polycystic kidney disease
   Adult polycystic disease
   Bilateral ureteropelvic junction obstruction
   Bladder and cloacal exstrophy

should be performed to detect an abnormal location of a kidney before the diagnosis of renal agenesis is made. Most of these abnormally located kidneys have no effect on the development of the fetus if not associated with other abnormalities.

Cystic renal disease

Numerous conditions cause a cystic appearance of the kidneys and the differential diagnosis by ultrasonography is not straightforward. The names of the different conditions are confusing and the ultrasonographic appearance often changes during pregnancy making the diagnosis even more problematic (Figure 13). Some of the cystic conditions of the kidneys are associated with chromosomal anomalies and counseling regarding outcome is important. Four major types of cystic renal diseases occur; their features are outlined in Table 5[21,22].

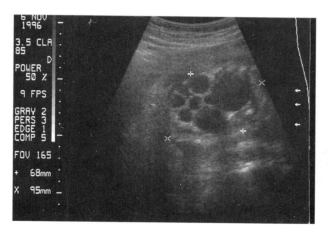

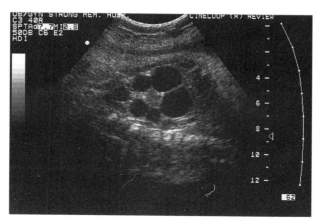

Figure 13 Two cases of multicystic-dysplastic kidney with non-communicating cysts

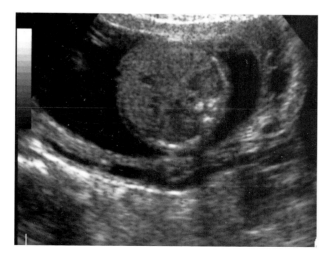

Figure 12 Normal appearance of fetal kidneys

Renal and adrenal tumors

The most common renal and adrenal tumors are adrenal cysts, mesoblastic nephroma, Wilm's tumor or nephroblastoma and adrenoblastoma. These tumors are rare and their ultrasonographic appearance is similar, consisting of a complex solid and cystic mass in the renal fossa. The specific diagnosis is made only in the neonatal period.

Obstructive uropathy

Obstructive conditions of the urinary tract are the most frequent renal anomalies detected *in utero*.

Ureteropelvic junction obstruction (UPJ)

This is the most common cause of obstructive uropathy and hydronephrosis. It is more frequently seen in males and is unilateral in 70% of cases. Pyelectasis may occur secondary to UPJ obstruction and the degree of dilatation of the renal pelvis determines outcome. Mild dilatation (< 5 mm) is generally associated with normal outcome. Moderate dilatation (5 to 9 mm) can be associated with abnormal development and warrants follow-up[23,24] (Figure 14).

Table 5 Major renal cystic diseases and their ultrasonographic appearance

---

Potter Type I – Infantile polycystic kidney disease
   Autosomal recessive transmission with a frequency of 1/50 000 births. Renal parenchyma replaced by microcystic cysts that give the kidneys an echogenic appearance. Kidneys are enlarged, bladder absent and oligohydramnios present and fetuses develop pulmonary hypoplasia

Potter Type II – Multicystic-dysplastic kidneys (Figure 13)
   1/10 000 births and unilateral in 50–75%. Multiple large non-communicating cysts with no renal parenchyma. If unilateral, normal amniotic fluid can be demonstrated, good outcome is to be expected

Potter Type III – Adult polycystic kidney disease
   Autosomal dominant disorder with variable expression. Kidneys are enlarged and appear echogenic

Potter Type IV
   Secondary to obstructive uropathy and hydronephrosis. The characteristic ultrasonographic sign is an enlarged main renal pelvis communicating with dilated calyces

Renal pelvis diameter of 10 mm or greater is an indication of hydronephrosis and is often associated with the need for surgical intervention (Figure 15). Pyelectasis has also been associated with chromosomal abnormalities and especially trisomy 21[25]. One study noted that 25% of fetuses with trisomy had pyelectasis on prenatal ultrasonography. With severe hydronephrosis the characteristic cysts communicate with the main renal pelvis, thus differentiating them from those of polycystic disease where the cysts do not communicate. In the presence of bilateral UPJ obstruction severe oligohydramnios is present and intervention may be indicated.

Ureterovesical junction obstruction (UVJ)

This is the most common cause of hydroureter (Figure 16); it occurs more frequently in male fetuses. In ureteral stenosis or ureterocele the

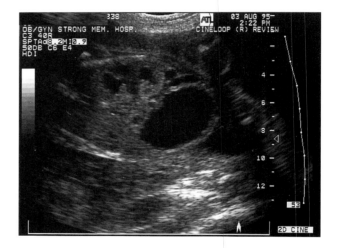

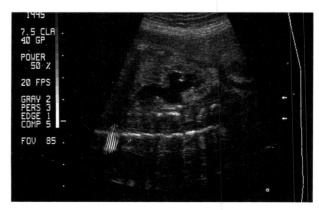

Figure 14 Two fetuses with moderate hydronephrosis

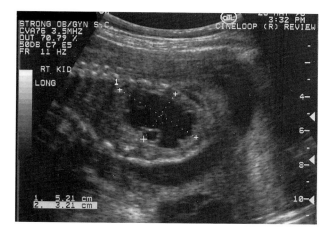

Figure 15 Ultrasonographic appearance of severe hydronephrosis

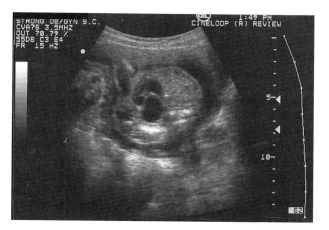

Figure 16 Hydroureter in fetus with ureterovesical junction obstruction

ureter dilates and eventually hydronephrosis may develop. Hydroureter may also develop in other bladder abnormalities such as posterior urethral valve. The ureters appear tortuous and dilated on ultrasonography and may be difficult to distinguish from the appearance of normal bowel.

Posterior urethral valve (PUV)

This is the most common cause of a dilated bladder (Figure 17). If the obstruction is complete bladder and ureters appear dilated and eventually hydronephrosis develops with oligohydramnios. These fetuses often do not survive due to pulmonary hypoplasia caused by the elevation of the diaphragm by the distended bladder. In these cases the severely distended bladder may also leak with the development of urine ascites. In partial obstruction fetal urine is produced and excreted and amniotic fluid volume may be normal or slightly decreased.

Prune-belly syndrome refers to a group of abnormalities including dilated bladder, lax abdominal wall and cryptorchidism[26]. An additional condition associated with a distended bladder is cloacal persistence which results from non-separation of cloaca into bladder, vagina and rectum. This results in a large bladder, dilatation of ureter and hydronephrosis. This condition is often associated with urine leakage and ascites (Figure 11).

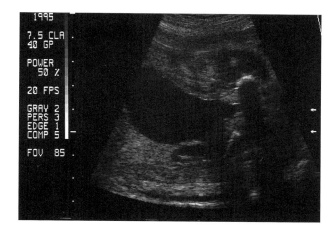

Figure 17 Fetus with posterior urethral valve and large bladder

Bladder exstrophy

This anomaly occurs in 1 in 30 000 births and more frequently in females. It is caused by an abdominal and bladder wall defect below the umbilical cord insertion. In this condition the bladder is open into the amniotic sac and urine flows directly from ureters into the amniotic cavity. As there is no accumulation of urine in the bladder it is non-visualized throughout the pregnancy (Figure 3).

References

1. Palomaki GE, Hill LE, Knight GJ, et al. Second-trimester maternal serum alpha-fetoprotein levels in pregnancies associated with gastroschisis and omphalocele. *Obstet Gynecol* 1988;71:906–9

2. Redford DHA, McNay MB, Whittle MJ. Gastroschisis and exomphalos: precise diagnosis by mid-pregnancy ultrasound. *Br J Obstet Gynaecol* 1985;92:54–9

3. Jaffe R, Schoenfeld A, Ovadia J. Sonographic findings in the prenatal diagnosis of bladder exstrophy. *Am J Obstet Gynecol* 1990;162:675–8

4. Erb R, Jaffe R, Braren V, et al. Exstrophy of the cloaca sequence. *Fetus* 1992;2:1–5

5. Meizner I, Bar-Ziv J. *In utero* prenatal ultrasonic diagnosis of a rare case of cloacal exstrophy. *J Clin Ultrasound* 1985;13:500–2

6. Benaceraff BR, Saltzman DH, Estroff JA, et al. Abnormal karyotype of fetuses with omphalocele: prediction based on omphalocele content. *Obstet Gynecol* 1990;75:317–19

7. Pretorius DH, Drose JA, Dennis MA, et al. Tracheo-esophageal fistula *in utero*: 22 cases. *J Ultrasound Med* 1987;6:509–13

8. Zimmerman HB. Prenatal demonstration of gastroschissi and duodenal obstruction by ultrasound. *J Assoc Can Radiol* 1978;29:138–41

9. Vermesh M, Mayden KL, Confino E, et al. Prenatal diagnosis of Hirschsprung's disease. *J Ultrasound Med* 1986;5:37–9

10. Weaver DD. *Catalog of Prenatally Diagnosed Conditions*, 2nd Edn. Baltimore: Johns Hopkins University Press, 1992;2–35

11. Caspi N, Elchalal U, Lancet U, et al. Prenatal diagnosis of cystic fibrosis: ultrasonographic appearance of meconium ileus in the fetus. *Prenat Diagn* 1988;8:379–82

12. Dicke JM, Crane IP. Sonographically detected hyperechoic fetal bowel: significance and implications for pregnancy management. *Obstet Gynecol* 1992:80:778–82

13. Sciosca AL, Pretorius DH, Budorick NE, et al. Second-trimester echogenic bowel and chromosomal abnormalities. *Am J Obstet Gynecol* 1992;167:889–94

14. Nyberg DA, Resta RG, Luthy DA, et al. Prenatal sonographic findings of Down's syndrome: review of 94 cases. *Obstet Gynecol* 1990;76:370–7

15. Santolaya J, Alley D, Jaffe R, et al. Antenatal classification of hydrops fetalis. *Obstet Gynecol* 1992;79:256–9

16. Romero R, Cullen M, Grannum P, et al. Antenatal diagnosis of renal anomalies with ultrasound. III. Bilateral renal agenesis. *Am J Obstet Gynecol* 1985;151:38–43

17. Jeanty P, Romero R, Kepple D, et al. Prenatal diagnoses in unilateral empty renal fossa. *J Ultrasound Med* 1990;9:651–4

18. Hill LM, Peterson CM. Antenatal diagnosis of fetal pelvic kidneys. *J Ultrasound Med* 1987;6:393–6

19. King KL, Kofinas AD, Simon NV, et al. Prenatal diagnosis of fetal pelvic kidney: a case report. *J Reprod Med* 1993;38:225–6

20. Sherer DM, Cullen JBH, Thompson HO, et al. Prenatal sonographic findings associated with a fetal horseshoe kidney. *J Ultrasound Med* 1990;9:477–9

21. Rizzo N, Gabrielli S, Pilu G, et al. Prenatal diagnosis and obstetrical management of multicystic dysplastic kidney disease. *Prenat Diagn* 1987;7:109–18

22. Pretorius DH, Lee E, Manco-Johnson ML, et al. Diagnosis of autosomal dominant kidney disease *in utero* in the young infant. *J Ultrasound Med* 1987;6:249–55

23. Corteville JE, Gray DL, Crane JP. Congenital hydronephrosis: correlation of fetal ultrasonographic findings with infant outcome. *Am J Obstet Gynecol* 1991;165:384–8

24. Ouzounian JG, Castro MA, Fresquez M, et al. Prognostic significance of antenatally detected fetal pyelectasis. *Ultrasound Obstet Gynecol* 1996;7:424–8

25. Wickstrom E, Maizels M, Sabbagha RE, et al. Isolated fetal pyelectasis: assessment of risk for postnatal uropathy and Down's syndrome. *Ultrasound Obstet Gynecol* 1996;8:236–40

26. Manivel JC, Pettinato G, Reinberg Y, et al. Prune-Belly syndrome: clinicopathologic study of 29 cases. *Pediatr Pathol* 1989;9:691–711

Fetal echocardiography

11

Susie C. Truesdell

Fetal echocardiography is an exciting field which requires knowledge of normal fetal intracardiac anatomy and physiology as well as the major forms of congenital heart disease and their fetal hemodynamics. Until recently, close attention to the fetal heart was reserved for women with a history of a previous child with severe congenital heart disease and for those fetuses with abnormal cardiac rhythms. Currently, however, most high-risk obstetrical practices evaluate the heart routinely in the four-chamber view and, if abnormal, perform a more intensive evaluation of the fetal heart prior to referral to a pediatric cardiologist for definitive diagnosis and counseling of the family.

Past obstetrical studies have documented that a normal four-chamber view will rule out approximately 80% of congenital heart disease in newborns. The unfortunate part of that statistic, however, is that the 20% not ruled out include those abnormalities which are potentially lethal to the newborn or which require immediate surgical or medical intervention to sustain the newborn infant's life. For example, the following list of defects includes the more complex defects which may be missed by a 'normal four-chamber view' at 16–18 weeks gestation: tetralogy of Fallot; truncus arteriosus; pulmonary atresia; tricuspid atresia; aortic atresia/mitral atresia/hypoplastic left heart syndrome; anomalous pulmonary venous return.

Congenital heart disease is estimated to occur in 8–15 children out of every 1000 live births; the incidence of congenital heart disease in the fetus is higher than this, but is not measurable, currently. Congenital heart disease can be so trivial as to cause no significant health effects or so severe as to be lethal to the fetus. The anomalies which can be detected prenatally involve atrioventricular (AV) valves, semilunar valves, systemic veins, pulmonary veins, systemic arteries and pulmonary arteries. The heart itself may have one, two, or three atrial chambers, and one or two ventricular chambers. The connections of atria to ventricles and ventricles to great vessels may be very abnormal. In addition, many severe defects are associated with chromosomal abnormalities or genetic syndromes.

The purpose of this chapter is to: (1) describe the standard views utilized by pediatric cardiologists and sonographers to evaluate the structure and function of a fetal heart; (2) describe the defects which may be associated with the abnormalities seen in the standard views; (3) describe the defects most often seen with chromosomal and syndromic abnormalities, maternal diseases, and maternal drug ingestion (Tables 1, 2 and 3), and to briefly describe the surgical treatment for the more common defects. In addition, this chapter has a flow chart for evaluating fetal hearts. This may be copied and kept near the ultrasound equipment for easy reference.

A thorough evaluation of the fetal heart must include a real-time study; that is, recording or at least viewing the movement of the ventricles and valves. Freeze-frame evaluation of a four-chamber view will not allow appreciation of depressed valve movement or diminished ventricular function. This information is required to fully assess the fetal heart. A full fetal echocardiographic evaluation also includes the use of color and pulsed wave Doppler.

STANDARD ECHOCARDIOGRAPHIC VIEWS

The standard echocardiographic views include:

(1) Inferior vena cava (IVC)/superior vena cava (SVC)/right atrium (RA) view;

(2) Four-chamber view;

(3) Great vessel view;

(4) Aortic arch view;

(5) Ductal arch view.

Since atria and ventricles are not always associated with one another in congenital heart disease and since the heart itself may be displaced to an unusual position, we evaluate fetal hearts by defining the morphology of each chamber. That is, there are specific criteria which help define a right atrium from a left atrium, for example. Once all the

Table 1 Syndromes most often associated with congenital heart disease[1-3]

Syndrome	Cardiac anomalies	Percentage with cardiac anomalies
T21 (Down's syndrome)	Atrioventricular canal (63%); VSD (16%); tetralogy of Fallot (8%); patent ductus arteriosus (4%); double outlet right ventricle (2%)	50%
T13	VSD; bicuspid aortic valve; bicuspid pulmonary valve; polyvalvular dysplasia	>90%
T18	VSD, bicuspid aortic valve; bicuspid pulmonary valve; coarctation of aorta; polyvalvular dysplasia	>90%
Turner's	Coarctation of aorta; aortic stenosis; aortic atresia; asplenia; D-transposition of great vessels; truncus arteriosus	
DiGeorge	Truncus arteriosus; interrupted aortic arch; tetralogy of Fallot; pulmonary atresia; double outlet right ventricle	>50%
Goldenhar	Tetralogy of Fallot; VSD	
Holt–Oram	VSD; atrial septal defect; pulmonary stenosis; aortic stenosis; TAPVR	20–30%
VACTERL	Tetralogy of Fallot; VSD; ASD; heterotaxy; truncus arteriosus; double outlet right ventricle; D-transposition of great vessels; AVCD; coarctation of aorta	
William	Supravalvular aortic stenosis; supravalvular pulmonary stenosis; pulmonary artery stenosis	>50%
Noonan	Dysplastic pulmonary valve; VSD; cardiomyopathy	>50%
Pierre Robin	Coarctation of aorta; D-transposition of great vessels; VSD; cardiomyopathy	20–30%
CHARGE	Pulmonary atresia; Ebstein's anomaly of tricuspid valve; pulmonary artery stenosis; VSD	80%

Table 2 Cardiac anomalies associated with maternal disease[4,5]

Maternal disease	Fetal heart disease
Systemic lupus erythematosus, Sjögren's complex, rheumatoid arthritis	Congenital complete heart block
Diabetes mellitus	Increased LV wall thickness; conotruncal defects; D-transposition of great vessels; LV; single ventricle; hypoplastic left heart syndrome; coarctation of aorta
Phenylketonuria	Tetralogy of Fallot; LV; coarctation of aorta; single ventricle; atrial septal defect
Rubella	Patent ductus arteriosus; pulmonary valve stenosis; branch pulmonary artery stenosis; aortic stenosis; coarctation of aorta; cardiomyopathy
Cytomegalovirus	Mitral stenosis; pulmonary stenosis; tetralogy of Fallot; myocarditis
Enterovirus (ECHO, Coxsackie, Polio)	Myocarditis, patent ductus arteriosus; VSD
Toxoplasmosis	Myocarditis with focal necrosis

Table 3 Cardiac anomalies associated with maternal drug ingestion[6,7]

Maternal drug ingestion	Fetal heart disease
Thalidomide	Tetralogy of Fallot; VSD; ASD
Hydantoin	Pulmonary stenosis; aortic stenosis; coarctation of aorta; VSD; ASD
Trimethadione	D-transposition of great vessels; tetralogy of Fallot; VSD
Lithium	Ebstein's anomaly of tricuspid valve; tricuspid atresia
Alcohol	VSD; ASD; patent ductus arteriosus; subpulmonic stenosis; subaortic stenosis
Cocaine	Ventricular ectopy; VSD with aortic valve prolapse; pulmonary artery stenosis; EKG changes (RVH, ST-T wave changes)
Retinoic acid	Conotruncal abnormalities; aortic arch abnormalities
ACE inhibitors, warfarin, anticonvulsants, poor maternal nutrition	Unknown effect on fetal hemodynamics

ASD, atrial septal defect; VSD, ventricular septal defect; TAPVR, total anomalous pulmonary venous return; AVCD, atrioventricular canal defect; ACE, angiotensin-converting enzymes

morphologic chambers are defined, the process of defining the abnormality is much easier.

The IVC/SVC/RA view (Figure 1) is obtained by orienting the transducer in the longitudinal plane, slightly to the right of center. You should be able to visualize the IVC in most of its length (certainly from below the diaphragm to the RA), the rightward atrium, and the SVC above it. If both SVC and IVC enter the rightward atrium, it is assumed to be the morphologic RA.

The four-chamber view (Figure 2) is obtained by orienting the transducer in a transverse plane just above the diaphragm. Usually this view is obtained in the plane of the fetal ribs, thus the two ribs are seen in their entirety in this view; this is not always the case, however, and does not indicate abnormalities if the full four-chamber is slightly off this plane. In this view, the following questions must be answered to confirm a normal study:

(1) Is the cardiac apex to the left?

(2) Are the right and left atrial volumes approximately equal?

(3) Are the right and left ventricular volumes approximately equal?

(4) Do the AV valves open equally widely?

(5) Is the tricuspid valve annulus (right AV valve) displaced apically beyond the mitral annulus?

(6) Is the moderator band identified in the apex of the rightward ventricle?

(7) Is there a break in the ventricular septum or the atrial septum (other than the foramen ovale)?

(8) Are the right and left ventricular free walls approximately the same thickness and are they normal for gestational age? (Figure 3)

(9) Are the mitral and tricuspid inflow velocities laminar by color Doppler and normal in velocity and configuration (Figures 4 and 5)

(10) is left ventricular contractility normal?

The great vessel view can be obtained from two different orientations. First, the great vessels may be visualized in the same transverse plane as the four-chamber, but angled toward the head. In this view you visualize the aortic valve in cross-section (Figure 6), the tricuspid valve to the right of the aortic valve, the right ventricular outflow tract wrapped anteriorly around the aortic valve, and

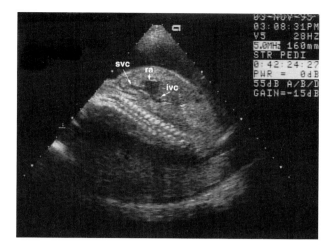

Figure 1 SVC-RA-IVC view. In the longitudinal plane, with spine posterior and head to the left of the screen, the superior vena cava (svc) is seen entering the right atrium (ra) from the upper thorax, the inferior vena cava (ivc) from the lower thorax

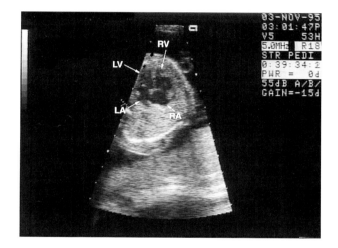

Figure 2 Four-chamber view. In the transverse plane, with spine posterior, the four-chamber view is visualized. The ventricle which is most anterior is usually the right ventricle (RV). This is confirmed by the presence of the moderator band of the RV seen just below the tip of the arrow (muscle extending across apex of RV approximately 1/4 to 1/3 distance from apex to tricuspid valve). The right atrium (RA), left ventricle (LV) and left atrium (LA) are also visualized

the pulmonary valve to the left of the aortic valve. Beyond the pulmonary valve the main pulmonary artery (PA) is seen with bifurcation into right and left pulmonary arteries. If the pulmonary valve is

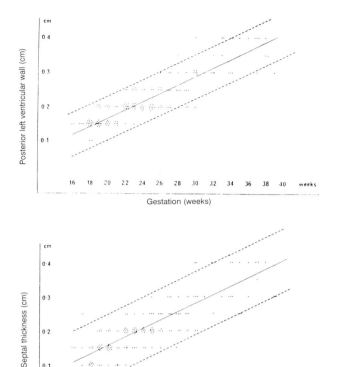

Figure 3 M-mode measurements of left ventricular posterior wall and interventricular septum by gestational age[8]

anterior to the aorta and to the fetus's left, the great vessels are normally oriented.

The second orientation for the great vessel view is the long-axial view (Figure 7), obtained by rotating the transducer toward the fetal right shoulder. In this view the left atrium (LA), left ventricle (LV), and aorta are visualized. Rotating the transducer slightly toward the head, the right ventricle (RV) and PA are visualized. If these two great vessels are seen to 'cross' each other above the valves, then the great vessels are normally oriented.

In this view, the questions to be asked are:

(1) Are there two separate great vessels?

(2) Does the anterior great vessel arise from the RV and course posteriorly, then bifurcate? Does the posterior great vessel arise from the LV and course superiorly?

(3) Do the great vessels 'cross' at the base?

(4) Are the great vessels of approximately the same size?

(5) Is color Doppler flow in each great vessel laminar and of normal velocity?

The aortic arch view is obtained from a longitudinal view (Figure 8); the best evaluations are angled either from the fetal abdomen or head. In this view, the 'candy cane' of the aorta can be easily

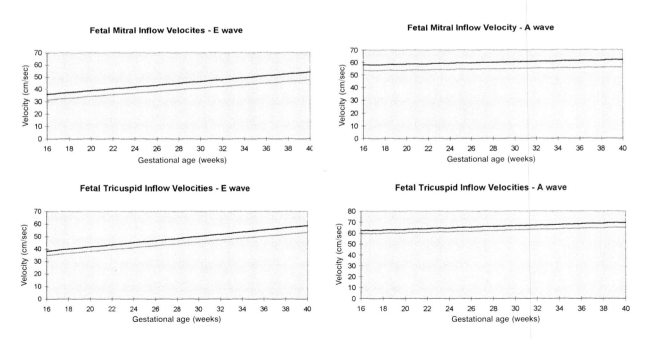

Figure 4 Mitral and tricuspid inflow velocities by gestational age (E wave is first wave seen, A wave is second)[9]

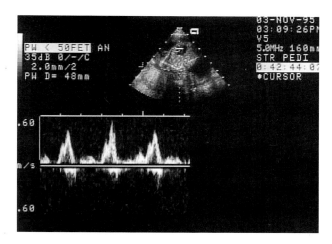

Figure 5 Normal fetal atrioventricular flow configuration. Doppler placement in ventricle just below atrioventricular valves (mitral or tricuspid) shows this configuration: E wave which is seen first is of lower velocity than the second A wave

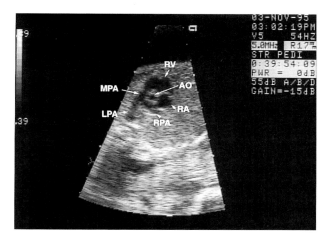

Figure 6 Short axis view. In a modified transverse plane (angled slightly counterclockwise toward left shoulder), this view of the short axis of the heart is seen. The circle in the center is the aorta (AO) and aortic valve. The right ventricle (RV) is seen anteriorly. The right ventricular outflow tract, comprised of the pulmonary valve, main pulmonary artery (MPA), and left (LPA) and right (RPA) pulmonary arteries, 'wraps' around the aorta. Posterior to the aorta, the right atrium (RA) can be visualized

visualized. Angling slightly to the left produces the usual 'hockey stick' configuration of the ductal arch view (Figure 9), comprised of left PA, ductus arteriosus, and descending aorta. For this evaluation to be normal, there must be two separate arch views, and the aortic arch must continue below the ductus arteriosus.

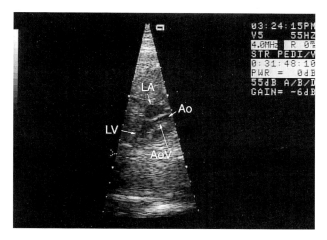

Figure 7 Long axis parasternal view of left ventricular outflow tract (LVOT). In a longitudinal plane, angled toward the right shoulder, this view of the LVOT is seen. The usual 'ballet slipper' shape of the left ventricle (LV) is seen with the aorta (Ao) being the ballet dancer's ankle and the aortic valve (AoV) closure in the center of the aorta. Compare this to the shape of the right ventricular outflow tract in Figure 6. LA, left atrium

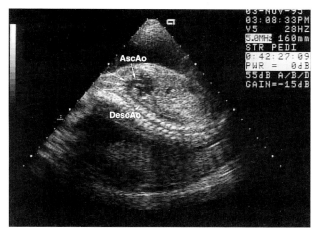

Figure 8 Aortic arch view. In a longitudinal plane, the ascending aorta (AscAo), aortic arch, and descending aorta (DescAo) are visualized. The three small arrows near the head indicate the takeoff of the three arch vessels (innominate artery, left carotid artery, left subclavian artery). Note the 'candy cane' shape of the arch; it rises superiorly, makes a tight arch, and descends

Questions to be asked are:

(1) Does the ductal arch look like a 'hockey stick'?

(2) Is there a separate aortic arch which has a 'candy cane' appearance to it?

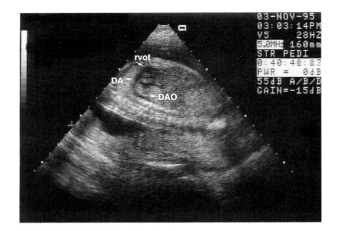

Figure 9 Ductal arch view. In a modified longitudinal plane, the ductal arch is visualized. In this view, the anterior structure is the right ventricle. From the right ventricle arises the right ventricular outflow tract (rvot), ductus arteriosus (DA), and its connection with the descending aorta (DAO). Note the 'hockey stick' shape of the arch; it courses immediately posterior and has a 'squared off' angle as it enters the descending aorta

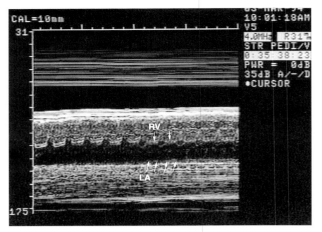

Figure 10 Arrthythmia evaluation. M-mode through the right ventricle (RV) and left atrium (LA) demonstrates contractions of the RV (top arrows) and the contractions of the LA (bottom arrows). In a normal rhythm, there should be one ventricular contraction for each atrial contraction. In this fetus, there are two atrial contractions for each ventricular contraction. This was seen over a long scanning period and represents atrial flutter with 2:1 block

Finally, if there is any question about the fetal heart rhythm, an arrhythmia evaluation should be performed. The main focus of this evaluation is to determine the rate of contraction of the atria and of the ventricles, and whether one atrial contraction is followed by one ventricular contraction. In a four-chamber view, place an M-mode cursor through one ventricle's free wall and an atrial wall (Figure 10). It may be opposite atria and ventricles or those on the same side, depending on the view you have obtained. Record an M-mode study for several minutes making sure that the atrial and ventricular contractions are visible on the recording. After this evaluation, an M-mode evaluation of the ventricular contractility should be performed to measure the thickness of the LV and its contractility. Finally, a pulsed wave Doppler study should be performed for each AV valve inflow.

Questions to be asked are:

(1) Is the heart rate normal for gestational age?

(2) Is there one atrial beat for each ventricular rate?

(3) Is the pulsed wave Doppler signal normal for each AV valve? (Figure 5). Is the rate normal for gestational age? Is there evidence of premature AV valve flow?

(4) Is the left ventricular function normal?

(5) Are there signs of fetal hydrops?

WHAT IF?

The following section is designed to help answer the question 'What if the view is not normal?' for each view of the fetal heart. Associated with each view are abnormalities which may be seen in fetal structural heart disease and suggestions as to how to refine the diagnosis.

Four-chamber view

(1) Cardiac apex not to left of the thorax:

    (i)   If the cardiac apex is to the right side of the thorax and stomach in the rightward portion of the abdomen, this is 'situs inversus' (meaning thoracic and abdominal contents are on the opposite side from usual) and may be associated with a normal heart. Close attention needs to be paid, however, to the intracardiac connections, making sure that the morphology of each ventricle is appropriate for the side of the heart and the AV valve with which it is associated.

    (ii)   If the cardiac apex is to the right of the thorax and the stomach is in the left portion of the abdomen, this is dextrocardia.

Children with dextrocardia may have a normal heart.

(iii) If the cardiac apex is to the left and the stomach to the right, this is situs ambiguous (meaning that abdominal and thoracic contents are not associated with one side or the other) and this is usually associated with complex congenital heart disease. Close attention should be paid to the intracardiac connections (as above).

(iv) If the cardiac apex is in the midline and the stomach is on the left, this is mesocardia and is usually associated with a normal heart.

(2) Right atrium is larger than left atrium:

(i) This implies there is more blood returning to the RA than to the left, or that the RA has encroached on the RV, making it larger.

(ii) This could be 'total anomalous pulmonary venous return' (TAPVR). In this defect, the pulmonary venous flow does not return to the LA (Figure 11). Sometimes the return is directly to the back of the RA; more often pulmonary veins return to a common vertical vein, then either run superiorly and enter the SVC near the SVC/RA junction or run through the diaphragm and enter the IVC via a hepatic vein. In order to rule out this anomaly, pulmonary veins should be evaluated and at least two veins seen entering the LA.

(iii) This could represent 'Ebstein's anomaly of the tricuspid valve' (Figure 12), in which the valve leaflets are 'tethered' or 'tacked down' to the RV for a portion of the length of the valve. In the four-chamber view, the atrium appears large because it has 'taken over' part of the right ventricle; likewise the right ventricle appears small for the same reason. In this view, the hinge points of the valve will appear displaced apically more than usual and there is usually at least moderate insufficiency by color Doppler (Figure 13, Color plate 21).

(3) Left atrium is larger than right atrium:

(i) This implies that there is more blood flow returning to the LA than RA.

(ii) This is most likely mitral insufficiency.

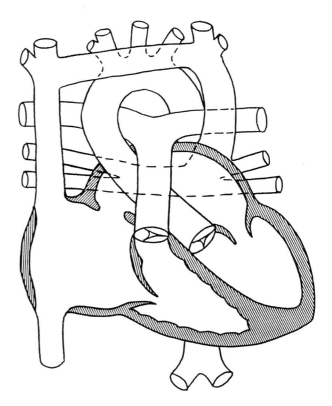

Figure 11 Total anomalous pulmonary venous return. Although there are several different sites of the anomalous pulmonary venous return, the most common is to the superior vena cava. Note blood flow is RA–RV–PA, pulmonary venous return–RA–RV–PA. There will always be an atrial septal defect in these children, so some of the blood entering the right atrium can cross the atrial septum and enter the left atrium; this represents the only source of blood flow to the left atrium and left ventricle

Mitral insufficiency may be the result of a structural abnormality of the valve or left ventricular dysfunction. If the mitral valve is not formed normally, although blood flows from LA to LV with ease, the valve leaflets are not able to close completely; thus there is a 'leak' of blood from LV to LA during systole. This is best demonstrated by color Doppler. In addition, LV function may be diminished and the LV may be dilated; this may be secondary to the degree of mitral insufficiency or may represent a primary abnormality of the ventricular myocardium (cardiomyopathy).

(iii) This may represent the acute phase of a viral myocarditis.

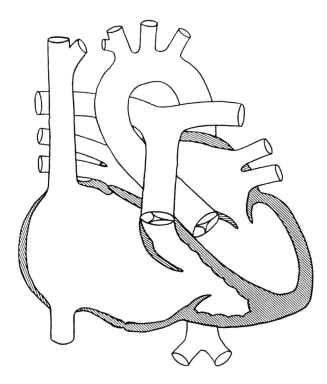

Figure 12 Ebstein's anomaly of the tricuspid valve. The hinge points of the tricuspid valve are located deep within the ventricle, thus enlarging the effective right atrial volume and diminishing the effective right ventricular volume. These valves usually function poorly and there will be tricuspid insufficiency

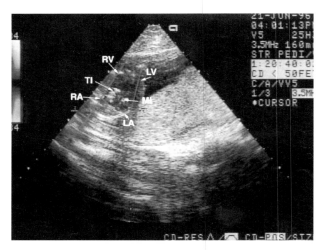

Figure 13 Ebstein's anomaly of the tricuspid valve. In the transverse plane, with the right ventricle (RV) anterior, the right atrium (RA) appears quite large. Color Doppler demonstrates a wide band of retrograde flow from RV to RA (tricuspid insufficiency, TI) which begins deep in the ventricle, suggesting that the tips of the tricuspid valve hinge at that point. In addition, there is a small amount of mitral insufficiency (MI). LA, left atrium; LV, left ventricle (see also Color plate 21)

(iv) If the left sided AV valve is displaced apically and the moderator band seen in the left sided ventricle, consider ventricular inversion. The great vessels will be abnormally oriented with the aorta anterior and to the left of the PA (L-transposition of the great vessels).

(4) Only one atrium is seen:

(i) This could represent a large break in the atrial septum, such as seen in complete AV canal defect, a large primum atrial septal defect (ASD), or a common atrium.

(5) Left ventricle is smaller than right ventricle:

(i) This happens if the volume coming into the LV is diminished or if egress from the LV is obstructed.

(ii) Aortic atresia (Figure 14) represents a failure of the aortic valve tissue to form normally, such that there is a bar of tissue where the valve would usually be. If there

is no ventricular septal defect (VSD), blood cannot leave the LV and it becomes increasingly difficult for blood to enter the LV through the mitral valve. Eventually, the mitral valve, also, will become atretic (mitral atresia). This combination represents the hypoplastic left heart syndrome. If there is a large VSD, blood can exit the LV via the VSD and thus the mitral valve. The LV may be nearly normal in size and function.

(iii) Double outlet right ventricle represents a failure of complete 'looping' of the embryonic heart. Blood flow into the atria and into their respective ventricles is normal. Both great vessels, however, come off the RV. There is always an associated VSD. Blood entering the LV must leave through the VSD, mix with blood in the RV, and leave via both the PA and the aorta. Often, the LV will appear somewhat smaller than the right, though not always. The great vessel relationships in this defect are very difficult to define on fetal echo. However, the large VSD should warrant immediate referral to a pediatric cardiologist for further definition of the anatomical defect.

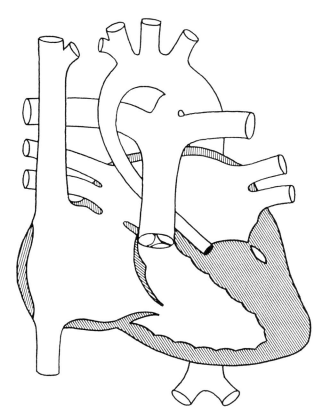

Figure 14 Aortic atresia with mitral atresia. The lack of formation of aortic valve leads to a very thin ascending aorta with no forward flow. Since there is no flow into the left ventricle through the mitral valve due to the lack of formation of that valve, and no flow out of it through the aortic valve, the left ventricle will be very small, with thick walls and poor contractility. Blood flow is RA–RV–PA, pulmonary veins–LA–RA–RV–PA, blood flow in PA can go either to the pulmonary arteries or through the ductus arteriosus to the aorta

(6) Right ventricle is smaller than left ventricle:

    (i)   Just as in aortic atresia, pulmonary atresia (Figure 15) causes diminished flow through the RV such that it fails to grow at the same rate as the LV. In this case, finding the PA will be very difficult and, if found, it will be quite small. In the presence of a VSD, there will be more growth of the RV, but it still will not be normal in size or function.

    (ii)   Tricuspid atresia, likewise, inhibits blood flow into the RV; thus the RV does not grow with the LV. With this defect, tricuspid valve motion is not seen and there is no color Doppler evidence of right ventricular inflow.

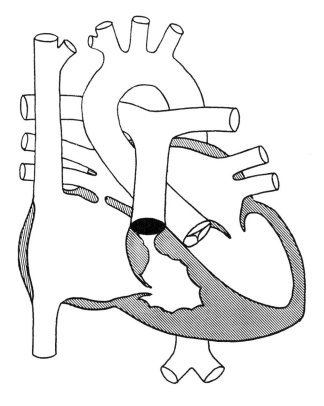

Figure 15 Pulmonary atresia, intact interventricular septum. The lack of formation of the pulmonary valve leads to a very thin pulmonary artery with no forward flow. Since there is no flow out of the right ventricle, the ventricle is small, with thick walls and poor contractility. Blood flow is RA–RV–RA–LA–LV–Ao–PDA–PA

(7) Tricuspid valve leaflets do not move freely:

    (i)   Three anomalies of the tricuspid valve may cause abnormalities of valve tissue movement. First, as discussed above, is tricuspid atresia. In this instance, valve tissue is not seen; only a bar of tissue across the tricuspid annulus is detected.

    (ii)   Tricuspid stenosis, which may be the intermediary form of tricuspid atresia, can be seen in early second trimester. The tricuspid annulus is narrow and motion of the leaflets is diminished. The tricuspid valve tissue extending into the body of the RV is shortened and moves poorly. The RV may already show signs of poor growth (chamber size smaller than the LV, globular appearance to ventricle, thick muscular walls). Color Doppler may demonstrate turbulent flow into the RV or may show laminar flow into the RV with the majority of flow leaving the RV by crossing the foramen ovale.

(iii) Ebstein's anomaly of the tricuspid valve (Figure 12), discussed earlier, involves tricuspid valve tissue which is adherent to the right ventricular walls below the tricuspid annulus. The valve tissue tends to look elongated. In addition, the RA appears large and the RV small. There is usually tricuspid insufficiency by color Doppler.

(8) The mitral valve leaflets do not move freely:

(i) If the mitral valve leaflets do not move freely and the annulus is narrow, consider mitral stenosis or mitral atresia. In these diagnoses, the left ventricular cavity will appear small. If there is a VSD associated, the aorta may be normal in size. If there is no VSD, the aortic valve will also appear abnormal and the aorta will be very narrow. This combination of mitral atresia, hypoplastic LV, and aortic atresia represents the 'hypoplastic left heart syndrome'.

(9) There is a break in the atrial septum:

(i) The most common kind of ASD is the secundum ASD. Such a break occurs in the middle of the atrial septum such that there is tissue between the defect and the mitral/tricuspid valve leaflets and there is tissue between the defect and the back wall of the atria. This defect occurs in the same position as the foramen ovale. Unless the defect is large, it is usually difficult to distinguish between the two by fetal or neonatal echocardiography.

(ii) The second most common defect is the primum ASD which is associated with the 'complete atrioventricular canal defect'. This defect is seen most often in children with Down's syndrome. This defect is in the atrial septum where the mitral and tricuspid valves hinge. It is often associated with a large defect in the ventricular septum which begins in the same area. In this defect, the mitral and tricuspid valve appear to be one large valve with a wide valve annulus.

(iii) The third type of atrial septal defect, the sinus venosus ASD, occurs in the septum near the posterior atrial wall and is a difficult area to visualize in a fetus.

(10) There is a break in the IVS:

(i) Is aorta coming off LV and PA off RV? If not, there are three diagnoses to consider. The first three appear very similar on echo: tetralogy of Fallot, double outlet right ventricle, truncus arteriosus. In all three defects there is a large VSD.

(a) In tetralogy of Fallot (Figure 16) the aorta appears to 'straddle' the ventricular septum such that it receives blood from both RV and LV. This is called an 'overriding aorta'. There will be small pulmonary arteries coming off the RV, but they are often difficult to visualize in the fetus.

(b) In truncus arteriosus (Figure 17), there is only one great vessel which looks like an aorta. Pulmonary arteries come off this great vessel.

(c) In double outlet right ventricle (Figure 18), both great vessels seem to be committed to the RV, although the aorta also receives some blood from the LV.

(ii) Is mitral motion normal? If mitral motion appears diminished or the mitral annulus diameter appears small, the diagnosis of mitral stenosis or mitral atresia (Figure 19) must be considered. Since there is a VSD associated, the aortic valve may be grossly normal and the aorta normal sized.

(iii) Is the aortic arch clear? If there is a narrowing in the aortic arch, coarctation of the aorta (Figure 20), associated with the VSD, this presents a combination of defects which may compromise cardiovascular stability in the first few days of life. In coarctation of the aorta, the 'candy cane' appearance of the aorta is still seen, but it appears to narrow just as the transverse portion meets the descending portion. Color Doppler demonstrates turbulence in this area and pulsed wave Doppler will show increased flow velocity here.

(iv) Is the PA normal in size? In pulmonary atresia with VSD (Figure 21), there may be visible but small pulmonary arteries associated with the RV, but there will be no blood flow by color Doppler from the RV to the PA.

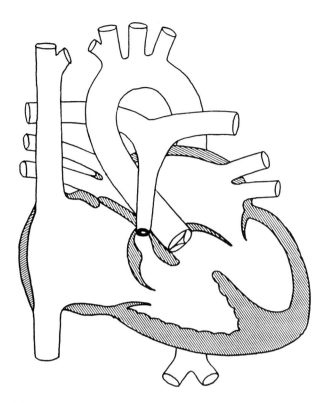

Figure 16 Tetralogy of Fallot involves a ventricular septal defect, overriding aorta, muscular narrowing of the right ventricular outflow tract below the pulmonary valve and right ventricular hypertrophy. The pulmonary arteries are usually small. Blood flow is normal, but flow out of the right ventricle is difficult because of the subpulmonary obstruction and small pulmonary arteries. Thus a variable degree of flow into the right ventricle exits via the aorta

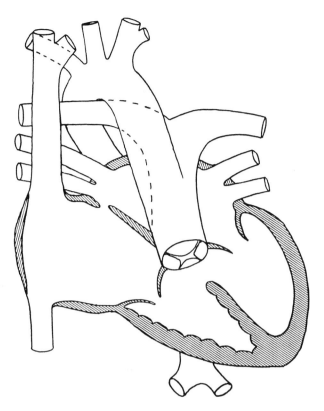

Figure 17 Truncus arteriosus. There is only one large great vessel seen which exits the heart in the center, overriding the ventricular septum above a ventricular septal defect. Pulmonary arteries will come off the aorta in one of several positions (see text), but this drawing shows the most common presentation, with pulmonary artery and branches coming off the posterior aspect of the ascending aorta

    (v) The diagnosis of an isolated ventricular septal defect can only be considered after the great vessel orientation is defined as normal and the pulmonary arteries are visualized with color Doppler evidence of normal flow from RV to PA.

(11) The left ventricular wall and ventricular septum are thick (Figure 22):

    (i) The most common cause of thickened LV walls in a fetus or newborn is that the mother of the fetus is diabetic ('infant of a diabetic mother'). Even gestational diabetes can cause a fetus to develop thickened walls. It is rarely a problem, but after delivery can sometimes present obstruction to blood flow out into the aorta.

    (ii) If the mother is not a known diabetic, then a primary or secondary cardiomyopathy should be considered. There are many different metabolic and genetic causes of cardiomyopathy. Secondary causes include viral infection and maternal drug ingestion. Of particular interest in these fetuses is whether the right and left ventricular outflows remain unobstructed. Color Doppler in each outflow tract will be turbulent if there is obstruction. Likewise, pulsed wave Doppler in the outflow tracts will show an increase in the velocity and turbulence.

(12) The right ventricle is thick:

    (i) The RV and LV should be approximately the same thickness, with the septum slightly thicker than either one.

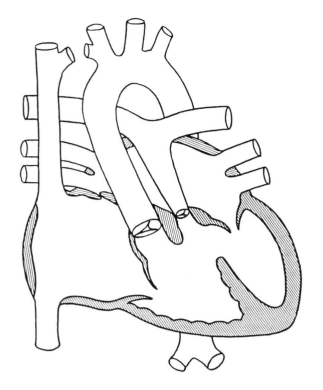

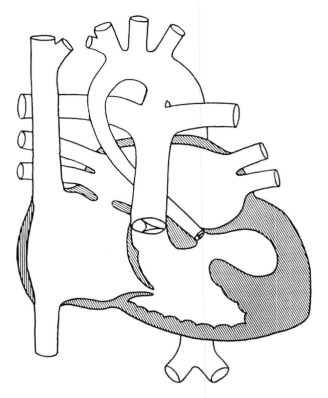

Figure 18   Doublet outlet right ventricle. There is a large ventricular septal defect and both great vessels are committed to the right ventricle. The orientation of the great vessels is variable between patients (see text), but is usually abnormal. The posterior great vessel may appear to override the ventricular septum as in tetralogy of Fallot

Figure 19   Mitral stenosis/mitral atresia. Depending on the amount of blood crossing the mitral valve, there may be a relatively normal sized left ventricle (early mitral stenosis) or a small, thick walled, poorly contractile left ventricle (mitral atresia). If there is a ventricular septal defect, the aorta may be normal in size or may be narrow. Blood flow is LA–RA–RV–PA or across VSD to Ao

(ii) Is the aortic arch clear? If there is a coarctation of the aorta (Figure 20), the RV will be thick, since the RV is the one which pumps most of the blood to the body past the obstruction.

(iii) Is there a VSD? If so, is the aorta overriding the ventricular septum? This may be tetralogy of Fallot (Figure 16); small pulmonary arteries may be seen coming off the RV.

(13) The mitral and tricuspid inflow velocities are not laminar by color Doppler or are abnormal in velocity and configuration:

(i) If flow across either valve is turbulent by color Doppler, consider valve stenosis. If mitral flow is turbulent and valve annulus appears narrow, consider mitral stenosis. If tricuspid flow is turbulent and valve annulus is narrow, consider tricuspid stenosis. If configuration of inflow is

abnormal, and if contractility is diminished, consider cardiomyopathy.

(14) The left ventricle is dilated and poorly contractile:

(i) This is called dilated cardiomyopathy. There are several etiologies including maternal/fetal infection, intrinsic myocardial disease (mitrochondrial abnormalities, carnitine deficiency) or idiopathic. Often there will be fetal hydrops including a pericardial effusion. Figure 23 demonstrates an M-mode evaluation through the right and left ventricles. While the RV appears to contract well, the LV motion is poor.

(15) There is fluid surrounding the heart (pericardial effusion):

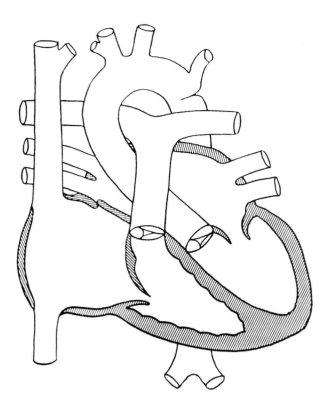

Figure 20 Coarctation of the aorta. The narrowing in the aorta is opposite to the point where the ductus arteriosus connects with the aorta. In fetal life, the obstruction may not be evident on 2D, but should be appreciated by the turbulent color Doppler flow below the obstruction

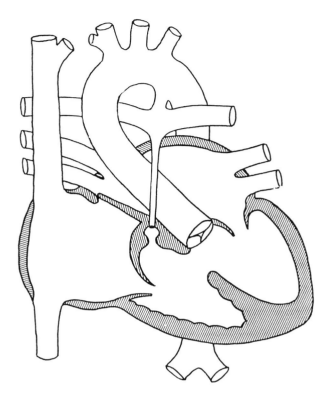

Figure 21 Pulmonary atresia with ventricular septal defect. The lack of formation of the pulmonary valve leads to a very thin pulmonary artery with no forward flow. Blood flow is RA–RV–Ao, LA–LV–Ao, pulmonary arteries are filled retrograde via the ductus arteriosus

(i) Pericardial effusion can be the result of hydrops, an intrauterine infection or long-standing congestive heart failure. The cardiac causes of fetal congestive heart failure include myocarditis and arrhythmia. For these reasons, careful attention to ventricular function and atrial/ventricular rhythm are important. See related sections below for a description of these studies.

Great vessel views

(1) Two great vessels are not seen:

(i) If one great vessel is seen with a 'candy cane' configuration and vessels coming off going toward the head, and if pulmonary arteries are not visualized, this may represent either pulmonary atresia

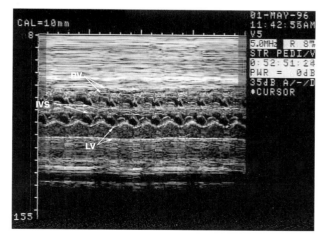

Figure 22 Thick ventricular walls. This M-mode through the anterior right ventricle (RV), ventricular septum (IVS), and posterior left ventricle (LV) shows moderate thickening of the right ventricle and ventricular septum and severe thickening of the left ventricular free wall

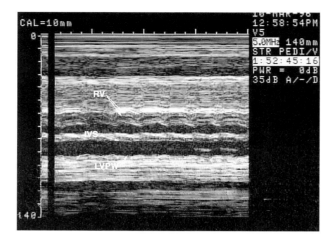

Figure 23 Dilated cardiomyopathy. This M-mode through the anterior right ventricle (RV), ventricular septum (IVS), and posterior left ventricle shows normal right ventricular contractility and minimal contractility of the ventricular septum and the left ventricular posterior wall (LVPW). In addition, the left ventricular cavity (between IVS and LVPW) is dilated

or truncus arteriosus. In pulmonary atresia (Figure 15), there is no formation of the pulmonary valve; there is only a thick bar of tissue where the valve should be. Since no blood leaves the RV to go to the pulmonary arteries, the RV is usually small and the pulmonary arteries are often difficult to identify. In truncus arteriosus (Figure 17), there is only one great vessel which is a combination of aorta and PA. It is the embryonic truncus which never septates. Thus the vessel will look somewhat like an aorta with the typical arching and vessels going toward the head, but there will also be pulmonary arteries coming off the vessel. They may come off together behind the ascending aorta, each off the side of the ascending aorta, or off the anterior portion of the descending aorta. In any case, the differentiation between pulmonary atresia and truncus arteriosus *in utero* is very difficult to determine.

(ii) If there is a dilated vessel coming off the anterior RV which immediately courses posteriorly, and if no ascending aorta is seen, this probably represents aortic atresia (Figure 14). The ductal arch will

be easily visible and the PA portion of it will be quite large. Aortic atresia is associated either with a large VSD or with mitral atresia and hypoplastic left heart syndrome.

(2) The anterior great vessel does not arch posteriorly and bifurcate:

(i) If the anterior great vessel does not course posteriorly and bifurcate, but instead courses superiorly and gives rise to vessels which go toward the head, then this anterior great vessel is the aorta. If you see another great vessel coming off the posterior ventricle, this represents D-transposition of the great vessels (DTGA) (Figure 24). DTGA is often associated with a VSD.

(3) The great vessels are not approximately the same size:

(i) If aorta is narrow and PA dilated, consider aortic atresia. If PA is narrow and aorta dilated, consider pulmonary atresia. If pulmonary arteries are not visualized and the great vessel visualized is dilated, consider also truncus arteriosus.

(4) Color Doppler in each great vessel is not laminar and normal in velocity:

(i) If color Doppler in aorta is turbulent and velocity is above normal, consider aortic stenosis. If color Doppler in PA is turbulent and velocity is above normal, consider pulmonary stenosis.

(5) The aortic arch is not visualized as a 'candy cane':

(i) If the aortic arch is not visualized, consider aortic atresia. The ductal arch will be easily visible and the PA portion of it will be quite large. Aortic atresia is associated either with a large LV or with mitral atresia and hypoplastic left heart syndrome.

(ii) If the ascending aorta is visualized with head vessels coursing cephalad, but the descending aorta is not visualized, this may represent 'interrupted aortic arch'. In this defect, the ascending and descending aorta are not connected. The ascending aorta takes all its blood flow to

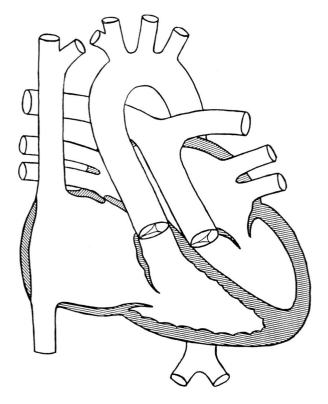

Figure 24 D-transposition of the great vessels. The aorta arises anteriorly from the right ventricle; the pulmonary artery arises posteriorly from the left ventricle. Blood flow is RA–RV–Ao–RA, LA–LV–PA–LA

the head and neck. The descending aorta is fed through the ductus arteriosus.

(6) The ductal arch is not visualized as a 'hockey stick':

(i) If a normal ductal arch is not visualized, consider pulmonary atresia or truncus arteriosus. In pulmonary atresia (Figure 15), there is no formation of the pulmonary valve; there is only a thick bar of tissue where the valve should be. Since no blood leaves the RV to go to the pulmonary arteries, the RV is usually small and the pulmonary arteries are often difficult to identify. In truncus arteriosus (Figure 17), there is only one great vessel which is a combination of aorta and PA. It is the embryonic truncus which never septates. Thus the vessel will look somewhat like an aorta with the typical arching and vessels going toward the head, but there will also be pulmonary arteries coming off the vessel. They may

come off together behind the ascending aorta, each off the side of the ascending aorta, or off the anterior portion of the descending aorta. In any case, the differentiation between pulmonary atresia and truncus arteriosus *in utero* is very difficult to determine (Figure 25).

CLINICAL SIGNIFICANCE OF DEFECTS AND SURGICAL REPAIR

Atrial septal defect

An isolated ASD is rarely associated with symptoms in childhood. Approximately 40% will spontaneously close within the first eight years of life[10]. Those which do not show evidence of closure are commonly treated with surgical or device closure, usually before school age. Because the foramen ovale is patent by definition during the first months of life, it is difficult to distinguish between a secundum ASD and a patent foramen ovale in the fetus and infant.

Surgical repair

Some ASDs are closed with only a suture, others by using a pericardial patch.

Aortic stenosis

Aortic valve stenosis is seen more predominantly in males than in females. It is part of the syndrome of left heart obstructive disease and may range in severity from a bicuspid aortic valve with no obstruction or insufficiency to critical aortic stenosis of infancy which requires immediate relief of the obstruction and which has a poor long-term prognosis. Relief of obstruction may be via surgery or balloon valvuloplasty during cardiac catheterization.

Surgical repair

Many children will have sufficient relief of aortic valve obstruction with a valvulotomy; the commissures of the native valve are incised such that function of the valve is much more normal.

Aortic atresia

Aortic atresia implies that there is no antegrade flow into the aorta from the LV. Since the aorta provides blood flow to the body, this is a lethal form of congenital heart disease.

Surgical repair

There are two surgical palliations available at this time for aortic atresia: Norwood procedure and heart transplantation. The Norwood procedure is performed primarily for infants with hypoplastic left heart syndrome and involves three stages. In the first stage, the small aorta and the dilated PA are combined to form one large great vessel. Since the coronary arteries come off the aorta, they are now part of the single great vessel. The branch pulmonary arteries are disconnected from the main PA and a shunt is created between the descending aorta and the pulmonary arteries. The second stage is a Fontan procedure, in which the SVC is transected and each end sewn into the right PA (bidirectional Glenn shunt). At the third stage, the IVC and SVC are baffled away from the RA, such that systemic venous return does not enter the RA but goes directly to the pulmonary arteries. Pulmonary venous return thus enters the LA, crosses the atrial septum to the RA, passes through the tricuspid valve into the RV and is pumped out into the new aorta. Although morbidity and mortality are relatively high, many children survive these stages and live comfortably. Others require cardiac transplantation before the second or third stage.

While cardiac transplantation is available for children, it has problems which are specific to children. Availability of infant heart donors is a significant problem. Immunosuppression in infants carries major long-term risks. Finally, the incidence of early coronary artery disease in the transplanted heart appears to be a long-term problem in all children with transplanted hearts.

Atrioventricular canal defect (AVCD)

AVCD encompasses a range of defects including the following: a cleft in the anterior mitral valve leaflet; a defect in the atrial septum; a large defect involving the atrial septum, ventricular septum, and AV valves (complete AVCD). Some children with complete AVCD will have left ventricular outflow tract obstruction and some will have unbalanced ventricular sizes. Children with the classic complete AVCD tend to have a significant degree of tricuspid and mitral insufficiency as well as shunting at the atrial and ventricular levels. In the perinatal period they are usually not symptomatic, but may develop congestive heart failure within the first few months of life. Those children with trisomy 21 are at risk of developing pulmonary hypertension and, as such, are watched closely for this. Surgical repair usually happens within the first year of life. For those children with unbalanced ventricular sizes or left ventricular outflow tract obstruction, the timing of surgery and the type of repair varies from patient to patient. Those children with an isolated ASD or cleft mitral valve may require surgery, but this is not usually performed in infancy. Because of the high association of AVCD with trisomy 21, fetuses identified with AVCD should have a more thorough evaluation for genetic abnormalities.

Surgical repair

Repair of AVCD involves placement of a patch which closes the atrial defect and one which closes the ventricular defect. The common AV valve is divided and each side is reattached to the patch at the appropriate level.

Dilated cardiomyopathy

Dilated cardiomyopathy may be acquired or familial. Those children with familial dilated cardiomyopathy usually have a poor prognosis; the cause is not understood and there is no definitive treatment. Acquired cardiomyopathy may be due to an underlying systemic disease (acquired immunodeficiency syndrome, carnitine deficiency) or to an infectious process (usually viral). Those with underlying disease also tend to do poorly. Those children with viral cardiomyopathy may recover completely, recover partially, or succumb to the illness. Although not well documented, we have evaluated fetuses with dilated, poorly contractile ventricles and evidence of mild hydrops whose mothers had antecedent viral illness-like symptoms; some of these fetuses have gone on to recover from their illness and postnatally had normal ventricular function and no evidence of hydrops. In general, however, fetuses with hydrops and congestive heart failure have a poorer prognosis.

Surgical repair

There is no 'repair' available for dilated cardiomyopathy. Some children will obtain relief of symptoms and improvement in ventricular function by myoplasty, implantation of LV assist devices, resection of the LV, or heart transplantation.

Hypertrophic cardiomyopathy

Hypertrophic cardiomyopathy can be familial or sporadic. In most cases, the degree of hypertrophy progresses with time. Some children will survive a few years, some a few decades. There is no definitive treatment.

Coarctation of the aorta

Coarctation of the aorta varies in severity from very mild to severe enough to cause diminished lower body blood flow, from a single phlange obstructing flow in the descending aorta to a complex form with tubular narrowing of the transverse arch and 'kinking' of the descending aorta. The combination of a moderate degree of obstruction and an associated moderate-sized LV is a serious and life-threatening situation for an infant. The increased afterload from the coarctation leads to a large degree of shunting across the VSD and increase in pulmonary blood flow. This causes congestive heart failure in the infant and is usually not amenable to medical management. Surgery to repair the coarctation and close the VSD in infancy is usually required. Congestive heart failure can also be seen in some infants with isolated coarctation. Surgical repair involves removing the stenotic portion of the aorta and sewing the ends together. The majority of children with coarctation of the aorta will also have a bicuspid aortic valve. Since this can progress to valvular aortic stenosis, these children will need to be followed by a pediatric cardiologist.

Surgical repair

There are two types of repair of coarctation of the aorta. In older children, the area of narrowing is simply excised and the two ends of the aorta reattached (end-to-end anastomosis). In younger children, since this area of the aorta can be quite narrow, the subclavian artery is ligated and divided. This tissue is pulled down over the area of the coarctation and sewn into a longitudinal incision in the aorta, acting as a living tissue graft (subclavian flap procedure). In addition, many institutions are effecting relief of the obstruction via balloon dilatation angioplasty in the cardiac catheterization laboratory.

D-transposition of the great vessels

DTGA without an associated moderate-sized ASD or VSD presents a medical emergency at delivery. The infant is profoundly cyanotic and will develop severe acidosis since deoxygenated blood cannot travel through the lungs where its acid/base status is restored. The use of intravenous prostaglandin E1 to maintain patency of the ductus arteriosus provides the only mixing of systemic and pulmonary blood in these infants and can stabilize them for a period of days until surgical repair is feasible. Otherwise, these children often require a Rashkind procedure (balloon atrial septostomy) in the catheterization laboratory as an emergency procedure. Surgical repair of DTGA is usually in the form of an arterial switch procedure. If there is a large VSD associated, or if there are associated anatomical abnormalities, other procedures may be warranted.

Surgical repair

Arterial switch involves transection of the aorta and PA above the valves and reanastomosis, establishing normal patterns of blood flow. Coronary arteries, which had arisen from the aorta on the right, are removed and reattached to the new aorta on the left.

Double outlet right ventricle (DORV)

DORV is associated with cyanosis in infancy because both great vessels receive blood from the right ventricle (deoxygenated). If there is associated pulmonary stenosis, the child may be stable for weeks to months. Otherwise, surgical repair is required.

Surgical repair

The Rastelli procedure is usually performed for children with DORV or pulmonary atresia and VSD; the VSD is closed in such a way that the left ventricular outflow only goes out to the aorta. A tube graft with or without a valve is attached from the body of the RV to the PA.

Ebstein's anomaly of the tricuspid valve

This defect is associated with variable degrees of tricuspid regurgitation. If the regurgitation is moderate or severe, the child may develop congestive heart failure. Treatment usually consists of medical management. If severe clinical symptoms persist, surgical palliation may be considered.

Surgical repair

Surgical repair for this defect is difficult and is reserved for those children who continue to have severe clinical debilitation despite maximal medical management. If undertaken, it may involve replacement of the tricuspid valve with a prosthetic valve.

Hypoplastic left heart syndrome (HLHS)

In its most classic form, HLHS involves mitral atresia, aortic atresia, and hypoplastic LV. As in aortic atresia (described above) this form of congenital heart disease is lethal; unoperated children with HLHS live several days to a few weeks. Surgical palliation is via a Norwood procedure or heart transplantation (see section on aortic atresia).

Infant of diabetic mother

Although the ventricular thickness associated with this entity can be severe, most children are not symptomatic. Once the child is born and circulating insulin levels normalize, the thickness resolves, usually over a period of weeks to months. Occasionally these children will experience some obstruction to left ventricular outflow as a result of the thickened septum. Under these circumstances, these children may be managed with beta blockers.

Mitral atresia

In the absence of a large VSD, this is part of the hypoplastic left heart syndrome. If there is a large VSD associated with mitral atresia, there may be a recognizable LV and a normal sized aorta. These

children will be cyanotic, but may survive unoperated for several months. Surgical repair is tailored to the combination of specific defects.

Mitral insufficiency

Severe mitral insufficiency in infancy is usually related to an intrinsic abnormality of the mitral valve and is not tolerated well. Medical management will be maximized prior to surgical intervention, since surgical repair of this defect is difficult and replacement of the valve requires life-long anticoagulation.

Pulmonary atresia

These children are cyanotic, since there is no way for blood in the RV to get to the PA. Once the diagnosis is made, intravenous prostaglandin E1 will be used to maintain patency of the ductus arteriosus until surgery can be performed. Timing of surgical repair depends on the child's clinical status and the size of the pulmonary arteries. Those children with VSD will fare better than those without since those without VSD have minimal growth of the RV cavity during fetal development and thus the RV is very small and has poor function.

Surgical repair

Surgery to repair pulmonary atresia depends on the size and configuration of the pulmonary arteries. If there are pulmonary arteries of significant size, a valved conduit or right ventricular outflow tract patch across the right ventricular outflow tract, pulmonary valvulotomy, or other reconstruction of the right ventricular outflow tract will be used to establish continuity between the RV and PA. If no discrete pulmonary arteries are seen and pulmonary blood flow is supplied by collaterals from the aorta, a unifocalization procedure will be done. In this procedure, ideally the arteries arising from the aorta which supply the lungs are combined into one central vessel which can be eventually connected to the RV.

Pulmonary stenosis

There are some infants with severe pulmonary valve stenosis who will require intervention in the

a

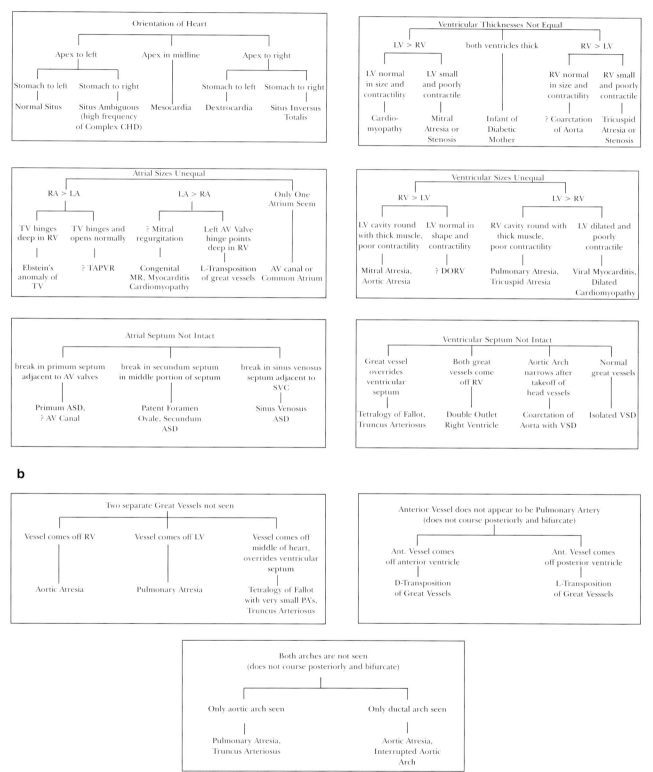

b

Figure 25   Flow charts for evaluating fetal echo views. (**a**) Abnormalities of the four-chamber view. (**b**) Abnormalities of great vessel views

neonatal period. Most, however, will have adequate pulmonary blood flow despite the obstruction.

Surgical repair

This may take the form of surgical valvulotomy or balloon valvuloplasty in the catheterization laboratory.

Tricuspid atresia

Children with tricuspid atresia will be cyanotic since there is mixing of oxygenated and deoxygenated blood in the LA. If necessary, immediate surgical palliation consists of the placement of a shunt which provides flow from a systemic artery into the pulmonary arteries.

Surgical repair

Final repair is usually via a Fontan procedure. The classic Fontan procedure separates the RA from the rest of the heart via a Goretex® baffle. The SVC and IVC blood flows into the RA. The right atrial appendage is attached to the PA and the pulmonary valve is oversewn; thus right atrial systemic venous blood flows via the right atrial appendage into the PA.

Total anomalous pulmonary venous return

These children have increased pulmonary blood flow, since all pulmonary venous return goes back to the RA. If venous return to the RA is unobstructed, these children may have congestive heart failure. If venous return to the RA is obstructed, these children will suffer pulmonary edema and require immediate surgical relief.

Surgical repair

Surgical repair is usually performed in infancy and is tailored to the anatomical insertion of the veins.

Tetralogy of Fallot

Many, though not all, of these children tend to be cyanotic. If the right ventricular outflow tract obstruction is significant and the pulmonary arteries are of reasonable size, a primary repair can be undertaken in infancy. If the pulmonary arteries are very small the placement of a shunt may be necessary to ensure reasonable pulmonary blood flow until a repair can be done.

Surgical repair

Repair involves patch closure of the VSD, relief of the subpulmonic muscle obstruction, and, if necessary, the insertion of a diamond-shaped patch across the RV outflow tract and pulmonary annulus, thus enlarging the outflow tract diameter.

Truncus arteriosus

Since all blood from both ventricles exits the heart through one great vessel, these children will be cyanotic. In addition, if there is no obstruction to pulmonary blood flow, they may suffer from early congestive heart failure.

Surgical repair

Repair is usually performed in infancy and consists of removing the pulmonary arteries from the truncus, joining them to make a single PA, then attaching the PA to the RV by insertion of a valved or non-valved conduit between RV and PA. The VSD is closed with a patch.

Ventricular septal defect

An isolated VSD, unless large, does not usually cause symptoms in infancy or childhood. A significant number of small VSDs (75–80%) will close spontaneously before adulthood. A large, isolated VSD may be associated with congestive heart failure in infancy, due to the increase in pulmonary blood flow. If medical management is unsuccessful, surgical closure would be performed, usually within the first two years of life.

Surgical repair

Most VSDs are closed with a patch of Goretex®.

FUTURE DIRECTIONS OF FETAL CARDIOLOGY

As we learn more about the effects of changes in fetal hemodynamics on fetal heart structure, interest is shifting toward defining early changes in hemodynamics. Thus, studies of ventricular function and the quantification of fetal blood flow characteristics are now being conducted. Transvaginal fetal echo is being performed at some centers as early as 8–9 weeks gestation with surprising resolution. These studies may help define a subset of fetal patients with defects caused by alterations in hemodynamics and may suggest means of effecting a realignment of hemodynamics which would alter the long-term outcome for these fetuses. As the sensitivity and specificity of the diagnosis of fetal heart disease and fetal arrhythmias improves, the issue of intervention will become more important. The growth of the fields of intrauterine fetal surgery and fetal intravascular drug therapy are expected as the definition of preclinical alterations in hemodynamics improves.

References

1. Fyler DC. Report of the New England Regional Cardiac Program. *Pediatrics* 1980;Suppl 65:375–461
2. Boughman JA, Neill CA, Ferencz C, *et al*. The genetics of congenital heart disease. In Anderson RH, Loffredo C, eds. *Perspectives in Pediatric Cardiology, Volume 4: Epidemiology of Congenital Heart Disease – The Baltimore-Washington Infant Study. 1981–1989.* Mount Kisco, NY: Future Publishing, 1993:123–68
3. Noonan JA. Chromosomal abnormalities. In Long WA, ed. *Fetal and Neonatal Cardiology.* Philadelphia: WB Saunders, 1990:578–94
4. Daniels SR. Epidemiology. In Long WA, ed. *Fetal and Neonatal Cardiology.* Philadelphia: WB Saunders, 1990:425–38
5. Rose V, Clark E. Etiology of congenital heart disease. In Freedom RM, Benson LN, Smallhorn JF, eds. *Neonatal Heart Disease.* New York: Springer-Verlag, 1992:3–17
6. Harned HS, Teratogenic agents. In Long WA, ed. *Fetal and Neonatal Cardiology.* Philadelphia: WB Saunders, 1990:595–603
7. Lipshultz SE, Frassica JJ, Orav EJ. Cardiovascular abnormalities in infants prenatally exposed to cocaine. *J Pediatr* 1991;118:44–51
8. Alan LD, Joseph MC, Boyd EGCA, *et al*. M-mode echocardiography in the developing human fetus. *Br Heart J* 1982;47:573–83
9. van der Mooren K, Barendregt LG, Vladimiroff JW. Fetal atrioventricular and outflow tract flow velocity waveforms during normal second half of pregnancy. *Am J Obstet Gynecol* 1991;165:668–74
10. Mahoney LT, Truesdell SC, Krzmarzick TR, *et al*. Atrial septal defects that present in infancy. *Am J Dis Child* 1986;140:1115–18

Skeletal disorders: *in utero* diagnostic approach

12

Israel Meizner

The term dysplasia means intrinsic growth disturbance occurring during the early stages of fetal development. Prior to the introduction of sonography in obstetrics, recognition and diagnosis of these disturbances was practically not feasible during pregnancy. Radiographs obtained from newborns suspected of having a skeletal dysplasia have opened new horizons in recognizing and diagnosing skeletal disorders. Once sonography was proven to be useful routinely during pregnancy, the accumulated experience appearing in the radiological literature was immediately adopted for the prenatal detection of skeletal abnormalities of various forms. Indeed, sonography is being applied everywhere for detection of anomalies including skeletal dysplasia starting as early as the first trimester of pregnancy.

BIRTH PREVALENCE OF SKELETAL DISORDERS

It is difficult to estimate correctly the birth prevalence of skeletal dysplasia since this is a heterogenous group of different anomalies. The data currently available concerning birth prevalence of skeletal disorders are summarized in Table 1. Thanatophoric dysplasia, achondroplasia, achondrogenesis and osteogenesis imperfecta represent the four most frequent skeletal dysplasias diagnosed prenatally. Out of almost 125 documented cases of skeletal dysplasias, around 50 are clinically apparent and recognizable at birth.

CLASSIFICATION

In 1977, a sub-committee of the European Society of Pediatric Radiology met in Paris and adopted an international nomenclature of constitutional (intrinsic) diseases of bone. This classification underwent revision in 1983 and is now the most commonly used classification of skeletal dysplasias

Table 1 Birth prevalence of specific skeletal disorders

Skeletal dysplasia	Birth prevalence
Lethal dysplasias	
Thanatophoric dysplasia	1 : 6-14 000
Achondrogenesis type I	1 : 43 000
Achondrogenesis type II	1 : 40 000
Hypophosphatasia	1 : 100 000
Camptomelic dysplasia	1 : 200 000
Diastrophic dysplasia	1 : 500 000
Osteogenesis imperfecta type II	1 : 54 000
Chondrodysplasia punctata, rhizomelic type	1 : 90 000
Others	1 : 200 000 or less
Non-lethal dysplasias	
Achondroplasia	1 : 26 000
Cleidocranial dysplasia	1 : 200 000
Asphyxiating thoracic dysplasia	1 : 100 000
Chondroectodermal dysplasia	1 : 100 000
Others	1 : 200 000 or less

(a modified version is presented in Table 2). This classification divides the skeletal disorders into five categories: (1) osteochondrodysplasia (abnormalities of cartilage or bone growth and development), (2) dysostoses (malformations of individual bones singly or in combination), (3) idiopathic osteolyses (disorders associated with multifocal resorption of bone), (4) skeletal disorders associated with chromosomal aberrations, (5) primary metabolic disorders.

Useful terms associated with skeletal disorders and their diagnosis are presented in Table 3.

Currently, diagnosis of many skeletal disorders is feasible due to improved ultrasound resolution, better sonographic skill and experience, and a more precise understanding of fetal embryology and development. With the increased utilization of ultrasound screening programs, the rising trend in detection of skeletal malformation will continue. Table 4 provides a list of well-described skeletal

Table 2   International nomenclature of constitutional diseases of bone

I.   Osteochondrodysplasias: abnormalities of cartilage and/or bone growth and development.

A.   *Defects of growth of tubular bones and/or spine**

Usually lethal before or shortly after birth
1.   Achondrogenesis type I (Parenti–Fraccaro)
2.   Achondrogenesis type II (Langer–Saldino)
3.   Hypochondrogenesis
4.   Fibrochondrogenesis
5.   Thanatophoric dysplasia
6.   Thanatophoric dysplasia with cloverleaf skull
7.   Atelosteogenesis
8.   Short-rib syndrome (with or without polydactyly)
     a.   Type I (Saldino–Noonan)
     b.   Type II (Majewsky)
     c.   Type III (Verma–Naumoff)
     d.   Type Beemer
9.   Schneckenbecken dysplasia
10.   de la Chapelle dysplasia
11.   Boomerang dysplasia
12.   Thanatophoric variants
13.   Antley Bixler dysplasia
14.   Opsisimo dysplasia

Usually non-lethal dysplasia
15.   Chondrodysplasia punctata
     a.   Rhizomelic form autosomal recessive
     b.   Dominant X-linked form
     c.   Conradi–Hunermann
     d.   X-linked recessive
     e.   Common mild form (Sheffield)
16.   Camptomelic dysplasia
17.   Kyphomelic dysplasia
18.   Achondroplasia
19.   Diastrophic dysplasia
20.   Metatropic dysplasia (several forms)
21.   Chondroectodermal dysplasia (Ellis–van Creveld)
22.   Asphyxiating thoracic dysplasia (Jeune)
23.   Spondyloepiphyseal dysplasia congenita
     a.   Autosomal dominant form
     b.   Autosomal recessive form
24.   Kniest dysplasia
25.   Dyssegmental dysplasia
     a.   Type Rolland–Desbuqois
     b.   Type Silverman–Handmaker
26.   Mesomelic dysplasia
     a.   Type Nievergelt
     b.   Type Langer
     c.   Type Robinow
     d.   Type Reinhardt
     e.   Type Werner
     f.   Osebold–Remondini dysplasia

27.   Acrosomelic dysplasia
28.   Cleidocranial dysplasia
29.   Oto-palato-digital syndrome
     a.   Type II (Andre)
30.   Pseudodiastrophic dysplasia
31.   Spondylomegaepiphyseal-metaphyseal dysplasia (SMMD)
32.   Geleophysic dysplasia
33.   Yunis–Varon
34.   Grebe dysplasia
35.   Thoraco-laryngeo-pelvic dysplasia
36.   Hypochondroplasia
37.   Dyschondrosteosis
38.   Spondylo-metaphyseal dysplasia
     a.   Type Koslowski
     b.   Other forms
39.   Oto-spondylo-megaepiphyseal dysplasia (OSMED)
40.   Acromicric dysplasia
41.   Weissenbacher – Zweymuller

B.   *Disorganized development of cartilage and fibrous components of skeleton*

C.   *Abnormalities of density of cortical diaphyseal structure and/or metaphyseal modeling*
1.   Osteogenesis imperfecta (several forms)
2.   Osteogenesis
     a.   Autosomal recessive lethal
     b.   Intermediate recessive
     c.   Autosomal dominant
     d.   Recessive with tubular acidosis
3.   Pyknodysostosis
4.   Osteodysplasty

II.   Dysotoses: malformations of individual bones, singly or in combination

A.   *Dysotoses with cranial and facial involvement*
1.   Craniosynostosis (several forms)
2.   Craniofacial dysotosis (Crouzon)
3.   Acrocephalosyndactyly
     a.   Type Apert
     b.   Type Chotzen
     c.   Type Pfeiffer
     d.   Other types
4.   Acrocephalopolysyndactyly (Greig)
5.   First and second branchial arch syndromes
     a.   Mandibulofacial dysotosis (Treacher–Collins, Franceshetti)
     b.   Acro-facial dysotosis (Nager)
     c.   Oculi-auriculo-vertebral dysotosis (Goldenhar)
     d.   Hemifacial microsomia
     e.   Others
6.   Oculi-mandibulo-facial syndrome (Hallermann–Steriff–Francois)

Table 2 *continued overleaf*

Table 2 *continued*

B.   Dysotoses with predominant axial involvement
1.   Vertebral segmentation defects (including Kliger–Feil)
2.   Cervico-oculo-acoustic syndrome (Weildervanck)
3.   Sprengel anomaly
4.   Spondylocostal dysotosis
     a.   Dominant form
     b.   Recessive forms
5.   Occulovertebral syndrome (Weyers)
6.   Cerebro-costo-mandibular syndrome

C.   Dysotoses with predominant involvement of extremities
1.   Acheiria
2.   Apodia
3.   Tetraphocomelia syndrome (Roberts)
4.   Ectrodactyly
5.   a.   Isolated
     b.   Ectrodactyly–ectodermalodysplasia cleft palate syndrome
     c.   Ectrodactyly with scalp defects
6.   Symphalangism
7.   Polydactyly (several forms)
8.   Syndactyly (several forms)
9.   Poly-syndactyly (several forms)
10. Camptodactyly

11. Rubinstein–Taybi syndrome
12. Pancytopenia–dysmelia syndrome (Fanconi)
13. Blackfan–Diamond anemia with thumb anomalies (Aase syndrome)
14. Thrombocytopenia–radial aplasia syndrome
15. Cardiomelic syndromes (Holt–Oram and others)
16. Femoral focal deficiency (with or without facial anomalies)
17. Multiple synostoses
18. Scapuloiliac dysotosis (Kosenow–Sinios)

III.   Idiopathic osteolyses

IV.   Miscellaneous disorders with osseous involvement
1.   Neurofibromatosis

V.   Chromosomal aberrations

VI.   Primary metabolic abnormalities

A.   Calcium and/or phosphorus
1.   Hypophosphatasia (several forms)

B.   Complex carbohydrates
1.   Mucopolysaccharidosis types 1–7

Modified with persmission[1]
*IA. 1–35, identifiable at birth; IA. 36–41, identifiable in later life

dysplasias identifiable at birth, many of which are diagnosable during the second trimester of pregnancy. Specific diagnostic clues, natural history and mode of inheritance are provided.

GENETICS AND SKELETAL DYSPLASIAS

Many of the skeletal abnormalities detected by ultrasound have a genetic basis. Therefore, attempts to identify the true nature of the disorder are important and may rely on a detailed family history which in many cases will provide information as to the probable mode of transmission of a particular disorder. The two main forms of inheritance associated with skeletal dysplasias are autosomal dominant and autosomal recessive. In many chromosomal disorders, one may expect to encounter skeletal abnormalities. Ten per cent of infants with trisomy 18 and a few reported cases of trisomy 13 have fetal limb reduction malformations[3]. An X chromosome deletion has been

observed in two cases of chondrodysplasia punctata, and Robert's syndrome has been associated with premature centromere division[4–6].

THE DIAGNOSIS OF SKELETAL DYSPLASIAS AND OTHER SKELETAL DEFORMITIES

An organized and comprehensive examination of the fetal skeleton is needed. A complete look at all the bones of the skeleton should be performed.

Long bones

All long bones should be measured in all extremities. If limb shortening is present, it should be established whether all segments are involved. A detailed examination of each bone is necessary to exclude the absence of hypoplasia of individual bones (e.g. radius, fibula) or malformation of individual bones (e.g. rounded tibia). Not only bone curvature should be depicted but also the degree

Table 3 Terminology and nomenclature of useful terms frequently associated with skeletal disorders

Acheiria	Complete absence of the hands
Acheiropodia	Complete absence of both hands and feet
Acromelia	Shortening of the middle and distal portion of limb
Acromesomelia	Shortening of the middle and distal segments of the limb
Adactyly	Lack of fingers or toes
Amelia	Absence of a limb
Apodia	Absence of the feet
Arthrogryposis	Contractures of the limbs
Axial	Trunk portion of the skeleton
Camptomelia	Bowed or bent limb
Cavus	Exaggeration of arch
Clinodactyly	Overlapping digits or deviation of a digit
Diaphysis	Middle segment of the shaft of a long bone
Diastrophic	Twisted
Dysostosis	A defect related to ossification or modeling
Dysplasia	Intrinsic growth abnormality
Dystrophy	Growth abnormalities moderated by external factors
Equinus	Extension of the foot
Hemimelia	Absence of extremity below the knee or elbow
Hexadactyly	Six fingers
Hypertelorism	Wide space between the orbits
Hypotelorism	Narrow gap between the orbits
Mesomelia	Shortening of middle segment of limb
Metaphysis	Extremity of the shaft of a long bone
Metatropic	Changeable
Micrognathia	Small mandible
Micromelia	Shortening of an extremity
Nanism	Dwarfism
Phocomelia	Lack of development of middle portion of limb with preservation of proximal and distal portions
Platyspondyly	Flattening of vertebrae
Polydactyly	Extra digits
Post-axial	Ulnar or fibular side
Pre-axial	Radial or tibial side
Rhizomelia	Shortening of proximal segment of limb
Sirenomelia	Fusion of legs
Symphalangism	End to end fusion of contiguous phalanges
Syndactyly	Fused adjacent digits (soft tissue or bony)
Talipes	Clubfoot
Thanatophoric	Death bearing
Vagus	Bent outward
Varus	Bent inward

of curvature should be measured. An attempt should be made to assess the degree of mineralization by examining the acoustic shadowing behind the bone and the echogenicity of the bone itself. However, there are limitations in the sonographic evaluation of bone mineralization. The reflection of ultrasound waves or the interface between the skull and amniotic fluid may lead to an overestimation of bone density. Finally, the possibility of fractures should be considered. The fractures may be extremely subtle or may lead to angulation and separation of the segments of the affected bones.

Thorax

Hypoplastic thorax occurs in many skeletal dysplasias. It is the main neonatal cause of death in the lethal forms of skeletal dysplasias secondary to severe pulmonary hypoplasia. Thoracic dimensions can be assessed by measuring the thoracic circumference at the level of the four-chamber view of the heart (Figure 1). Special note should also be given to the shape and integrity of the thorax. The clavicles are important landmarks within the thorax. Their shape is easily recognized, and they may be abnormal in several skeletal deformities. The clavicles can be easily measured[7].

Hands and feet

Hands and feet should be evaluated to exclude missing bones, polydactyly, syndactyly and postural deformities as observed in diastrophic dysplasia (hitchhiker thumb) and a few other deformities. Club feet or club hands may also be detected, and should always be looked for.

Skull

Skull shape and bone mineralization and degree of ossification should be evaluated. Orbits must be measured (the biorbital diameter) to exclude hypotelorism or hypertelorism[8]. Other findings like micrognathia, short upper lips, abnormally shaped ears, frontal bossing and cloverleaf skull deformity must be sought thoroughly. Measurements of head circumference and biparietal diameter should be performed routinely, in order to exclude cranial abnormalities such as macrocephaly (thanatotrophic dysplasia, achondroplasia).

Table 4   Specific skeletal dysplasias which are potentially diagnosable

Skeletal dysplasia
a.   Significant features for possible fetal imaging diagnosis in second trimester
b.   Inheritance
c.   Natural history

Achondrogenesis
Type I   (Parenti–Fraccoro)
a.   Short, fractured ribs; fetal hydrops; very short long bones; edema of head and neck; distended abdomen; deficient vertebral body ossification
b.   Autosomal recessive (AR)
c.   Uniformly lethal. The pregnancy may be complicated by polyhydramnios and premature labor. Diagnosis of this disorder has been made reliably with ultrasound in the second and third trimesters

Type II (Langer–Saldino)
a.   Same as achondrogenesis type I. The phenotype is somewhat less severe, with variable ossification of the vertebrae and skull. The ribs are shortened, however, with no rib fractures
b.   AR
c.   Same as achondrogenesis type I

Atelosteogenesis
a.   Absent or hypoplastic to distally tapered humerus, femoral shortening, cleft vertebrae, twisted fingers
b.   Sporadic and AR forms
c.   Usually lethal before or shortly after birth

Hypochondrogenesis
a.   Like achondrogenesis type II but milder part of achondrogenesis II/hypochondrogenesis spectrum
b.   Sporadic, probably AR
c.   Usually lethal; however, there are occasional survivors. Like achondrogenesis type II, hypochondrogenesis is thought to represent one of a heterogeneous group of disorders involving type II collagen defects
Comment: Probably not usually diagnosable in the second trimester

Fibrochondrogenesis
a.   Very short, broad long bones, ectopic ossification; short ribs, small thorax, frontal bossing. Omphalocele has been reported in one case
b.   AR
c.   Lethal before or shortly after birth

Achondroplasia
a.   Short femur, short humerus, flat vertebral bodies, large skull

b.   Autosomal dominant (AD)
c.   Homozygous condition – lethal
Comment: Probably very few cases are diagnosable in the second trimester, except for homozygous achondroplasia

Antley – Bixler dysplasia
a.   Bowed femur, radius, ulna; humeri-radial synostosis, midface hypoplasia
b.   AR
c.   Non-lethal

Asphyxiating thoracic dysplasia (Jeune, ATD)
a.   Short ribs, no polydactyly
b.   AR
c.   Variable clinical course

Boomerang dysplasia
a.   Edema, omphalocele, absent humerus and femur, small tibia, radius and ulna
b.   Sporadic
Comment: Similar to atelostenogenesis

Camptomelic dysplasia
a.   Elongated bent femur, short bent tibia, milder similar changes in upper extremities, sex reversal (XY females)
b.   AR
c.   Commonly lethal but variable

Chondrodysplasia punctata – Conradi – Hunermann type
a.   Mild asymmetric long bone shortening, ascites
b.   AD
c.   Usually non-lethal

Chondrodysplasia punctata – rhizomelic type
a.   Several femoral (and humeral) shortening, otherwise mild long bone shortening
b.   AR
c.   Usually non-lethal at birth but fatal in first year of life

Chondrodysplasia punctata – other types
a.   Similar to chondrodysplasia punctata – Conradi–Hunermann type
b.   Sporadic, X-linked dominant (XLD)
c.   X-linked recessive forms usually lethal in males
Comment: Probably not diagnosable in second trimester

Chondroectodermal dysplasia (Ellis – van Creveld)
a.   Short hands, radius and ulna; congenital heart disease (primum defect – atrium), short ribs, femoral bowing, polydactyly

Table 4 *Continued overleaf*

Table 4 *continued*

b.   AR
c.   Usually non-lethal

Cleidocranial dysplasia
a.   Absent or hypoplastic clavicles
b.   AD
c.   Mild short stature, non-lethal

De La Chapelle dysplasia
a.   Short ribs, small thorax; flat vertebrae; clubbed short humerus; short curved radius; absent ulna; short femur and tibia; absent (triangular remnant) fibula, ocular hypertelorism
b.   AR
c.   Often lethal

Diastrophic dysplasia
a.   Hitchhiker (small) thumb; short long bones; severe clubbed feet
b.   AR
c.   Usually non-lethal

Dyssegmental dysplasia
a.   Bizarre vertebral ossification (scattering big, tiny, and absent vertebral bodies); very short dumbbell long bones; encephalocele
b.   AR
c.   Rolland–Desbuquois type – often survival to 3 years; Silverman–Handmaker type – lethal
Comment: Probably not usually diagnosable in second trimester

Kyphomelic dysplasia
a.   Short bent femurs, short ribs
b.   AR
c.   Usually non-lethal

Mesomelic dysplasia
a.   Shortened radius, ulna, tibia, fibula
b.   AD, AR, sporadic
c.   Variable expression, usually non-lethal

Metatropic dysplasia
a.   Long trunk (spine), flat vertebral bodies, small thorax (short ribs), short long bones (dumbbell-shaped)
b.   AR, AD
c.   Several lethal and non-lethal forms

Osteogenesis imperfecta, especially type II
a.   Decreased skull ossification, short ribs, beaded ribs, fractures of ribs and long bones, short accordion femurs, bent short long bones, poorly ossified bones, ascites
b.   Usually AD, occasional AR or germline mosaicism
c.   Type II usually lethal

Osteopetrosis
a.   Fractures, macrocephaly (hydrocephalus), increased bone density ('increased bone echoes'), cerebral calcifications (carbonic anhydrase deficiency)
b.   AR, AD
c.   Lethal and non-lethal forms

Robinow syndrome, especially recessive form (Covesdem syndrome)
a.   Short radius, ulna, tibia, fibula, rib fusions, hydronephrosis (renal duplications)
b.   AR
c.   Usually lethal at or near birth

Thanatophoric dysplasia
a.   Large skull or cloverleaf skull, very short long bones (curved femurs), flat vertebral bodies, small hands and feet, polyhydramnios, very small thorax, hydrops
b.   Sporadic, probably spontaneous new AD mutations
c.   Lethal
Comment: The most common form of lethal skeletal dysplasia

Hypophosphatasia
a.   'Boneless' skull, prominent falx cerebri, scattered marked absence of ossification throughout skeleton (especially long bones, vertebrae, and ribs); bent short long bones; fractures; polyhydramnios
b.   AR
c.   Several congenital forms usually lethal at or near birth
Comment: Monoclonal antibodies to isoenzyme and alkaline phosphatase analysis at chorionic villus sampling

Modified with permission[2]

Spine

Careful examination of the spine is important. The relative length of the spine to the length of the limbs can be important for the diagnosis of certain skeletal abnormalities, and the mineralization of vertebral bodies and neural arches can be crucial in establishing the diagnosis of certain dysplasias (e.g. achondrogenesis type II). Evaluation of the vertebral size is important since in many cases of skeletal dysplasias platyspondyly (flat vertebrae) is a common finding. However, it should be kept in mind that this finding is not always easily detected even by experienced sonographers.

Pelvis

The shape of the pelvis and individual pelvic bones can be important in the diagnosis of certain dysplasias and dysotoses (e.g. limb-pelvic hypoplasia and scapuloiliac dysotosis).

AN ALGORITHMIC APPROACH TO THE DIAGNOSIS OF SKELETAL ABNORMALITIES

When approaching the diagnosis of skeletal dysplasia one should ask the following questions (see also Figure 2).

(1)   Is the skeleton of normal appearance? This question can be answered easily by correlating the skeletal age to the gestational age using normal charts available for pregnancy. If the answer to this question is short stature, then the next question should be:

(2)   Do we have a proportionate short stature, like in symmetrical intrauterine growth restriction (IUGR) and endocrine disorders like hypothyroidism, or is it disproportional short stature?

The third question should be:

(3)   Which parts are mainly affected by the disproportion: the limbs, the spine, the thorax or a combination of all three?

If the disproportion mainly affect the limbs, then the following questions will be considered:

(a)   Is the shortening affecting the proximal part of the limb (rhizomelic shortening), the middle

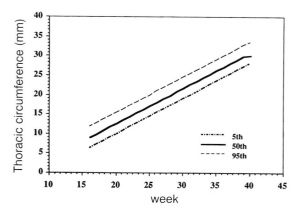

Figure 1   Growth of thoracic circumference versus gestational age

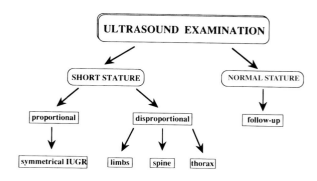

Figure 2   An algorithmic approach to the diagnosis of skeletal dysplasia. IUGR, intrauterine growth restriction

part of the limb (mesomelic shortening) or the distal part of the limb (acromelic shortening)?

(b)   Is polydactyly (preaxial or postaxial), ectrodactyly, clinodactyly, syndactyly etc. present?

(c)   Are there any fractures in the limb bones?

(d)   Are the bones curved?

(e)   Are joint deformities present?

(f)   Is there a club foot or a club hand?

(g)   Are limb dislocations present? (e.g. Larsen syndrome)

(h)   Are any metaphyseal changes present?

(i)   Is there premature appearance of ossification centers? (e.g. Ellis–Van Creveld)

(j)   Is there hypoplastic or absent bone? (e.g. radius, ulna, fibula, tibia, femur, clavicle, scapula)

Special consideration should be given to the examination of the big toe and thumb finger (e.g. hitchhiker thumb in diastrophic dysplasia, and large big toe in Rubinstein-Taybi syndrome or Proteus syndrome).

If the disproportion mainly affects the spine, the following questions must be answered.

(a) Is the spine shorter because of missing parts? (e.g. sacral agenesis)
(b) Is it shorter due to abnormal curvature? (e.g. Klippel–Feil syndrome)
(c) Is there a shortening of the vertebral bodies? (e.g. Spondyloepiphyseal dysplasia congenita)
(d) Are all parts of the spine equally ossified? (e.g. achondrogenesis types I and II)
(e) Is platyspondyly present? (e.g. thanatophoric dysplasia)
(f) Is the spinal canal of normal width?
(g) Is there any meningomyelocele (posteriorly, anteriorly or laterally)?

When the disproportion mainly affects the thorax, one should pose these questions:

(a) Is the thorax extremely small? (e.g. thanatophoric dysplasia)
(b) Is the thorax long and narrow? (e.g. Jeune syndrome)
(c) Are the ribs extremely short? (e.g. Short-rib polydactyly syndrome)
(d) Are there fractures in the ribs? (e.g. osteogenesis imperfecta type II)
(e) Is there clavicular aplasia or hypoplasia?
(f) Are the clavicles intact or partitioned? (e.g. cleido-cranial dysotosis)
(g) Is the scapula normal or abnormal?
(h) Are there gaps between the ribs? (e.g. Jarcho–Levine syndrome)

Additional clues to the detection of skeletal dysplasias can be associated anomalies. These may appear as external anomalies (ears, tail or caudal appendage which can occur in metatrophic dysplasia), facial deformities (short upper lip, facial cleft, micrognathia, short nasal bridge, hypertelorism and hypotelorism) and internal anomalies. Congenital cardiac anomaly is a common finding in several skeletal disorders (e.g. chondroectodermal dysplasia-Ellis–Van Creveld). Anomalies of the urinary tract may also be encountered (e.g. short-rib polydactyly syndrome type II). Genital abnormalities may sometimes accompany skeletal abnormalities (e.g. Robert's syndrome). The alimentary tract may also be affected, e.g. anorectal anomalies in achondrogenesis type I or esophageal atresia in VATER association. Abnormalities of the brain, although uncommon, may sometimes be encountered.

Skull anomalies should be looked at thoroughly. These may include asymmetry, acrocephaly-syndactyly syndrome, basilary invagination (e.g. achondroplasia), cloverleaf skull (e.g. thanatophoric dysplasia), craniosynostosis (e.g. acrocephalo-syndactyly), cranium bifidum, medial cleft syndrome, defective ossification (e.g. osteogenesis imperfecta type II), large or small foramen magnum, frontal bossing, macrocephaly or microcephaly.

Finally, three sonographic markers are well documented in skeletal disorders of various forms: polyhydramnios, oligohydramnios and the presence of hydrops fetalis.

Prior to the introduction of sonography, the prenatal detection of skeletal disorders *in utero* was possible only by using radiographs. This was achieved by performing either flat X-ray of the maternal abdomen (antero-posterior, lateral or both), or amniography.

The amniography was important in order to clearly delineate fetal contour. Lipidol was injected into the amniotic fluid and a radiograph was performed several hours thereafter. Using this technique, one could also inject Urografin to be swallowed by the fetus, so that the radiograph would detect the contrast material in the fetal alimentary tract, thus revealing any signs of bowel obstruction. However, this technique has been abandoned. I still believe that in selected cases of skeletal dysplasia there is still room for radiographs of the gravid uterus, provided they will contribute important clues for the diagnosis of skeletal disorders not obtainable by sonography (e.g. degree of mineralization, etc.)

The role of magnetic resonance imaging in diagnosing skeletal disorders during pregnancy is still under investigation. One should bear in mind that the most difficult problem while performing the examination in a pregnant patient is fetal movements. Also, imaging of bony structures is limited using this modality in comparison to ultrasonography or even X-ray fetography.

POSTNATAL EVALUATION

A substantial percentage of fetuses having skeletal dysplasias spontaneously abort, are stillborn or die as neonates. It is therefore of utmost importance to try and establish a correct diagnosis of the abnormality present. The postnatal work-up should provide essential information for further counseling the parents regarding their future pregnancies. Formulating the recurrence risk in future pregnancies is certainly the most important issue. The postnatal work-up should be done by an experienced team of specialists including a neonatologist and a geneticist, both experts in the field of prenatal diagnosis of skeletal disorders.

In our experience, the postnatal evaluation should include:

(1) A detailed physical examination of the neonate or abortus;
(2) Radiographs of the skeleton;
(3) Chromosomal analysis;
(4) Microscopic examination of chondro-osseous tissue;
(5) In selected cases, one may consider performing special tests including biochemical analysis, DNA studies and specific enzymatic assays. These may be achieved by establishing a tissue culture line.

In all cases of autopsy, the above tests should also be routinely performed.

SPECIFIC BONE DYSPLASIAS

Achondrogenesis type I

Synonym

Achondrogenesis type Parenti-Fraccaro.

Mode of inheritance

Autosomal recessive.

Incidence

0.23 per 10 000 births.

Definition and morphology

Very short limb dysplasia with fetal hydrops. Distended abdomen and barrel shaped thorax, short trunk and enlarged skull are the main features.

Sonographic and radiologic manifestation

Limbs: The limbs are grossly shortened with regular metaphysis. Often the degree of shortening is that of rudimentary ossicles.
Spine: The spine shows deficient ossification of vertebral bodies from complete absence to small ossified centers.
Thorax: The thorax is small compared to the protuberant abdomen, and the ribs are thin with flared anterior ends, and often with multiple fractures.
Head: The skull has variable degree of under-ossification of the vault, while the ossification of the base and facial bones is relatively normal.
Pelvis: The pelvis is small with poorly ossified iliac bones. The sacrum and pubic bones are absent.

Associated malformations

A wide spectrum of associated anomalies can be present. These may include: blue sclera, urinary tract duplication and hydronephrosis, auditory canal atresia, cleft palate, corneal clouding, ear deformities, aplastic testes and anal atresia[9-13].

Other findings

Polyhydramnios, fetal hydrops and redundancy of subcutaneous tissue are common.

Achondrogenesis type II

Synonym

Achondrogenesis type Langer-Saldino.

Mode of inheritance

Autosomal recessive pattern.

Incidence

1:40 000 births.

Definition and morphology

Very short-limb dysplasia with fetal hydrops. The soft tissue edema is mainly marked around the skull. Distended abdomen and barrel shaped thorax, short trunk and enlarged skull are the main features. Cleft palate is also sometimes encountered.

Sonographic and radiologic manifestations

Limbs: The limbs are markedly shortened. There is lack of ossification of the talus and calcaneous, the long bones are shortened and broad, and the metaphyses are concave.
Spine: The spine is shortened and there is lack of mineralization of all or many vertebral bodies.
Thorax: The thorax is markedly narrowed with shortened ribs. The clavicles, however, are well developed and often of the bucket-handled type. The abdomen is very protuberant.
Head: The head, which is well developed and appears enlarged, is normally ossified.
Pelvis: The pelvis is small. The iliac wings are small with concave inferior and medial margins.

Associated malformations

Cleft palate.

Other findings

These may include fetal hydrops and poly-hydramnios. Redundancy of subcutaneous tissue is evident.

Achondroplasia

Mode of inheritance

Autosomal dominant. Sporadic mutation occurs more frequently.

Incidence

1:26 000 live births. The most common non-lethal skeletal dysplasia.

Definition and morphology

Short limb, short trunk dysplasia with relatively large head with prominent forehead and saddle nose. Kyphosis of the thoracolumbar region and prominent buttock are present.

Sonographic and radiologic manifestations

Limbs: Rhizomelic type shortening of the limbs. The long bones are short and broad and slightly bowed. The tubular bones of hands and feet are short and broad. The fingers of the hands are of equal length and are separated in a trident fashion.
Thorax: The thorax has decreased dimensions.
Head: Large skull with relatively small base. Small posterior fossa is apparent. The forehead is prominent anteriorly, and the nasal bridge is depressed – the so called 'saddle nose' (Figure 3).
Spine: There is narrowing of the spinal canal both in the anterior–posterior and transverse diameters. This gives the vertebral body a concave posterior border. The interpediculate distance is narrowed progressively from above downward in the lumbar region. There is posterior tilting of the sacrum causing prominence of the buttocks.
Pelvis: The lilac wings are squared and the sciatic notches are narrowed. The acetabular roofs are irregular and horizontal. The iliac bones thus appear as a tombstone.

Associated malformations

Hydrocephalus malformations: hydrocephalus has been reported in some cases[14,15].

Arthrogryposis multiplex congenita (AMC)

Synonym

Congenital contractures.

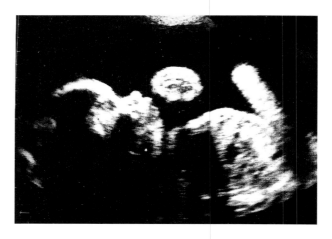

Figure 3   Achondroplasia. Sonogram of the fetal head showing marked prominence of the forehead. The skull base is shortened. Note the depressed nasal bridge

Mode of inheritance

Variable, depending on the condition leading to AMC.

Incidence

Depends on the condition.

Definition and morphology

AMC is a descriptive term, not a specific disease, that refers to a heterogeneous group of conditions characterized by multiple congenital joint contractures. Some of the conditions may belong to specific syndromes.

Sonographic and radiologic manifestations

Arthrogryposis multiplex congenita manifests by (1) immobility of involved joints, (2) joint contractures and (3) polyhydramnios. Other manifestations can occur depending on conditions leading to AMC. It is to be remembered that whole body movements of the fetus can still be perceived by the mother and observed during ultrasound assessment[16,17].

Comment

The Pena–Shokeir syndrome belongs to the AMC group. Besides the other features of AMC, this syndrome is characterized by loss of breathing movements, polyhydramnios and micrognathia. In this syndrome central nervous system anomalies may occur.

Asphyxiating thoracic dysplasia

Synonym

Jeune syndrome, thoracopelvic-phalangeal dystrophy.

Mode of inheritance

Autosomal recessive pattern.

Incidence

1 : 100 000–1 : 130 000 live births.

Definition and morphology

A skeletal disorder characterized by small, long, and narrow thorax, causing severe pulmonary hypoplasia. The pelvis is small and the phalanges of the hands are shortened[18–20].

Sonographic and radiologic manifestations

Limbs: The limbs are either normal or mildly shortened, and polydactyly may be present. Premature ossification of femoral heads can appear. The phalanges of the hands are shortened.
Spine: The spine is normal.
Thorax: The thorax is elongated and narrow. The ribs are horizontally directed with bulbus and irregular rib ends. The clavicles have a handlebar shape.
Head: The skull is normal.
Pelvis: The pelvis is small with short flared iliac bones and trident acetabular roofs.

Associated malformations

The main accompanying anomalies include progressive nephropathy, hepatic fibrosis and polycystic liver disease. Other visceral and metabolic abnormalities have been described which are probably undetectable *in utero*. Cleft lip and palate and polydactyly have been reported in some cases.

Chondroectodermal dysplasia

Synonym

Ellis–van Creveld syndrome.

Mode of inheritance

Autosomal recessive pattern.

Incidence

1 : 100 000 births. High incidence in closed societies like among Amish and the Arabs of the Gaza strip.

Definition and morphology

Disproportional short-limb dysplasia with polydactyly and ectodermal dysplasia involving nails, teeth and hair. Congenital heart disease is present in 50–60% of the cases, usually in the form of ASD.

Sonographic and radiologic manifestations

Limbs: The tubular bones are short and mildly bowed. Shortening of the hands and feet is more marked than of the bones of arm and leg, and these are shorter than the humerus and femur. In other words, there is acromesomelic shortening or the so-called 'centrifugal shortening'. Polydactyly of the hands is almost always present, and is post-axial. Polydactyly of the feet is present in only one-quarter of the cases. Premature ossification of the proximal femur is noticed in many cases. Marked shortening of the fibula may appear[21,22].
Spine: The spine is normal.
Thorax: The chest is long and narrow with shortened ribs.
Head: The skull is normal.
Pelvis: The pelvis is small with flared iliac wings and trident acetabular roofs.

Associated malformations

Various congenital heart defects have been reported, however, ASD is the most frequent malformation detected. Other anomalies may include: cerebral heterotopia, cleft palate, situs inversus, nephro-calcinosis, gallstones, Dandy–Walker malformation and cryptorchidism.

Diastrophic dysplasia

Synonym

Diastrophic dwarfism.

Mode of inheritance

Autosomal recessive pattern.

Incidence

0.2 per 100 000 live births.

Definition and morphology

The term 'diastrophic' implies 'twisted' and describes the twisted habitus appearing in this syndrome. Micromelic dysplasia with clubfeet, hand deformities in the form of 'hitchhiker'

thumb, and contractures of other joints are characteristic. Deformed ears and cleft or high arched palate are also present.

Sonographic and radiologic manifestations

Limbs: Micromelia with short, broad and clubbed tubular bones is present. The metacarpals and metatarsals and phalanges are short, irregular in length, with ovoid first metacarpal and proximal located thumb ('hitchhiker thumb'). Joint deformities in the form of contractures and dislocations are present, especially severe talipes equinovarus.
Spine: Scoliosis, kyphosis, platyspondyly and hypoplasia of vertebrae especially in the cervical spine can be present.
Thorax: Unremarkable.
Pelvis: Hypoplastic acetabulum is present.

Associated malformations

These may include facial anomalies (micrognathia, cleft palate), inguinal hernia and cryptor-chidism[23–25].

Dyssegmental dysplasia

Synonym

Lethal anisospondylic camptomicromelic dwarfism, dyssegmental dwarfism.

Mode of inheritance

Autosomal recessive pattern.

Incidence

Uncommon.

Definition and morphology

This is a lethal short-limbed dysplasia, characterized by micromelia, marked disorganization of the vertebral bodies and, infrequently, an occipital encephalocele.

Sonographic and radiologic manifestations

Limbs: Severe shortening of the long bones is present. The bones are also broad with flared ends, and bowed.

Spine: Anisospondyly is present, including severe segmentation defects, and absent, oversized or clefted vertebral bodies of the entire spine.
Thorax: The chest is narrowed with very short and flared ribs.
Head: Occipital defect with or without encephalocele may appear in 50% of cases.
Pelvis: Small round iliac bones with very dense ossification may be present.

Associated malformations

Micrognathia, ear anomalies, flat face and orbital hypoplasia may be present. Also, congenital heart disease, urinary tract anomalies and Dandy–Walker malformation have been reported[26–28].

Hemivertebra

Definition and morphology

Malformation of the spine usually occurring separately or as part of a syndrome or a dysplasia. In this anomaly, only half the vertebral body develops, thus causing scoliosis and often kyphoscoliosis[29,30].

Sonographic and radiologic manifestations

Spine: Absence of half of the vertebral body is associated with scoliosis at the site of the defect (Figures 4–6).

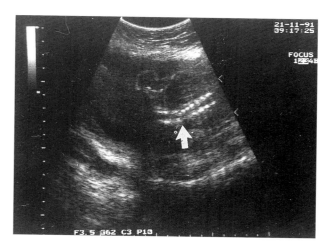

Figure 5   Hemivertebra. Coronal sonogram showing marked distortion of spine (arrow)

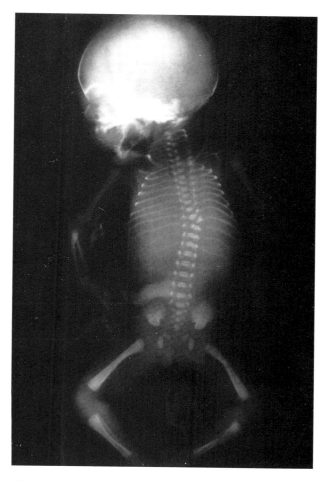

Figure 6   Hemivertebra. Radiograph of the abortus. Note the hemivertebra. Only 11 ribs are present on the right side, while there are 12 on the left

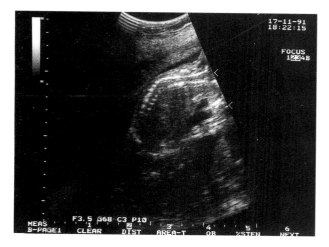

Figure 4   Hemivertebra. Longitudinal sonogram showing abnormal curvature of the spine

Associated malformations

These may include anomalies of the ribs, spinal cord and lower limbs. Other anomalies may appear in the gastrointestinal tract, central nervous system and genitourinary system.

Kyphomelic dysplasia

Synonym

Pseudocampomelia.

Mode of inheritance

Autosomal recessive pattern.

Incidence

Rare.

Definition and morphology

Severe rhizomelic limb shortening with bowed extremities, especially lower. Narrow chest, facial hemangiomatoma and whistling face appearance are present[31].

Sonographic and radiologic manifestations

Limbs: The femurs are markedly shortened and kyphotic with a lateral convex curve. The other long bones are also shortened and bowed but to a lesser degree. All tubular bones are slightly bowed with flared irregular metaphyses. Joint stiffness is present[29].
Spine: Mild platyspondyly, otherwise unremarkable.
Thorax: Narrow thorax is present, and the ribs are short with flared ends.
Head: Unremarkable.
Pelvis: Unremarkable.

Associated malformations

These include facial hemangiomata.

Osteogenesis imperfecta

Mode of inheritance

Depending on the type, see below.

Incidence

4 : 100 000 births. The most common second trimester ultrasound diagnosis of short bent limbs.

Definition and morphology

Osteogenesis imperfecta comprises a heterogeneous group of disorders of defective collagen, characterized by multiple fractures of brittle bone (Table 5)[32–39].

Osteogenesis imperfecta type I

Mode of inheritance

Autosomal recessive.
   Up until now, prenatal sonographic detection was attempted but rarely successful, due to the fact that the manifestations of this condition are only blue sclera and occasional isolated fractures (in 5% of the cases). The fractures are mainly postnatal without any obvious dysplasia at birth. Deafness has been noted in one-third of the patients.

Osteogenesis imperfecta type II

Type II osteogenesis imperfecta has been further subdivided into types IIa, IIb and IIc, according to mode of inheritance and appearance of the bone. Type IIa is mainly autosomal dominant with many new mutations. In only 5% of the cases, the mode of inheritance is autosomal recessive. The long

Table 5   Prenatal sonographic appearance of different types of osteogenesis imperfecta

Type	Bone echogenicity	Fractures	Limb length	Skull ossification
I	Normal	Isolated	Normal	Normal
II	Normal to decreased	Multiple (accordion like)	Moderate to severe shortening	Poor
III	Slightly decreased	Multiple	Moderate femoral shortening	Decreased
IV	Normal	Isolated	Normal	Normal

bones are broad and 'accordion like', and the ribs are beaded. Type IIb is inherited via an autosomal recessive pattern, with the long bones being broad and crumpled. Type IIc is characterized by an autosomal recessive mode of inheritance, and the long bones are thin with multiple fractures.

Sonographic and radiologic manifestations

Limbs: In most of the cases of type II, the fractured bones are broad, bent and short, with an 'accordion' or 'telescope like' appearance.
Spine: The spine is fractured and undermineralized.
Thorax: The ribs are broad with multiple fractures, giving them a beaded appearance.
Head: The head mark demineralization of the skull bones results in softening of the skull and permits compression when pressure is applied by the ultrasound transducer. This permits an abnormally clear view of the brain anatomy.
Pelvis: The pelvis is unremarkable except for flattened acetabulae and iliac wings (Figures 7–10).

Osteogenesis imperfecta type III

A rare autosomal recessive disorder. Type III is similar to type II except for moderate shortening of the long bones and less fractures of the long bones.

Osteogenesis imperfecta type IV

This type is inherited by autosomal dominant pattern and is similar to type I.

Associated malformation

Polyhydramnios is common. Cleft palate may be present.

Short-rib polydactyly syndrome (SRPS)

SRPS represents a group of lethal dysplasias having in common short limbs, polydactyly (postaxial) and

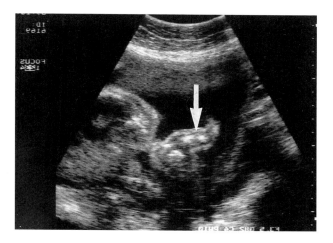

Figure 8   Osteogenesis imperfecta type II. A fractured humerus is evident (arrow)

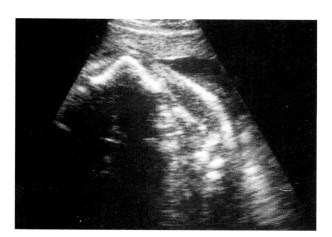

Figure 7   Osteogenesis imperfecta type II. Ultrasound scan of a lower limb; the femur is markedly bowed due to a fracture

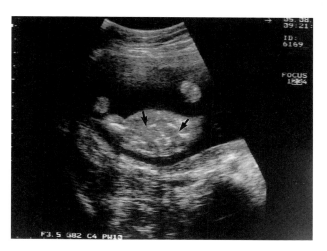

Figure 9   Osteogenesis imperfecta type II. Ultrasound scan of the fetal thoracic inlet demonstrating fractured clavicles (arrows)

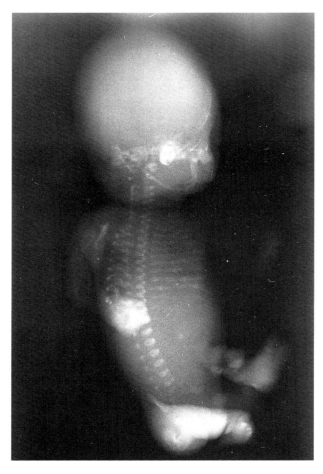

Figure 10 Osteogenesis imperfecta type II. Postmortem radiograph of an abortus at 21 weeks of gestation. Note the beaded appearance of the ribs

narrowed thorax internal organ abnormalities. They are subdivided into three groups: type I (Saldino–Noonan), type II (Majewski) and type III (Verma–Naumoff). Recently, a fourth group of SRPS, type Beemer has been added. Table 6 summarizes the differences between SRPS, types one to three, and also shows features of other skeletal dysplasias associated with a narrow thorax.

Short-rib polydactyly syndrome type I

Synonym

SRPS Saldino–Noonan.

Mode of inheritance

Autosomal recessive.

Incidence

Uncommon.

Definition and morphology

This is a short-rib type of dysplasia with severely shortened limbs. There are 'flipper-like' extremities. Postaxial polydactyly with occasional preaxial co-existing polydactyly is present. The chest is extremely short and narrow. Ambiguous genitalia and imperforated anus may be present[40,41].

Table 6 Ultrasonic approach to the diagnosis of short-rib polydactyly syndrome (SRPS), chondro-ectodermal dysplasia (CED) and asphyxiating thoracic dysplasia (ATD)

	SRPS I (Saldino–Noonan)	SRPS II (Majewski)	SRPS III (Naumoff)	CED	ATD
Short limbs	++	+	++	(+)	(+)
Narrow thorax	++	++	++	++	+
Polydactyly	++	++	++	++	+
Cleft lip and palate	–	++	–	–	–
CVS abnormalities	+	+	+	+	–
Polycystic kidneys	+	+	–	–	+
Genital anomalies	++	+	++	–	–
Metaphyseal dysplasia					
a. Pointed metaphyses	++	–	–	–	–
b. Widened metaphyses with marginal spurs	–	–	++	–	–
Disproportional short tibia	–	++	–	–	–

++, present; +, inconsistently present; –, absent; (+), present to a mild degree; CVS, cardiovascular system

Sonographic and radiologic manifestations

Limbs: The limbs are very short and 'flipper-like'. The long bones are pointed with metaphyseal spurs, the fibula is absent, and there is deficiency in ossification of metacarpals, metatarsals and phalanges. Postaxial polydactyly with occasional co-existing preaxial polydactyly is present. Premature ossification of the proximal epiphyseal centers of the humerus and femur may occur.

Spine: The vertebral bodies are square and hypoplastic with coronal clefts.

Thorax: The thorax is shortened and narrowed. The ribs are severely shortened and horizontally oriented, and the scapulae are small in contrast to almost normal appearing clavicles.

Head: The head is dolichocephalic with poor mineralization of the frontal bones. Mandibular hypoplasia is present.

Pelvis: The pelvis is small, with small iliac bones, and the acetabular roofs are flattened.

Associated malformations

Renal, genital, cardiac and alimentary system anomalies have all been reported with SRPS type I.

Other findings

Polyhydramnios is present in most reported cases (Figures 11–13).

Short-rib polydactyly syndrome type II

Synonym

SRPS Majewski type.

Mode of inheritance

Autosomal recessive.

Incidence

Rare.

Definition and morphology

The description and appearance are similar to SRPS type I except for:

(a)   In type Majewski the limbs are less shorter than in type I.

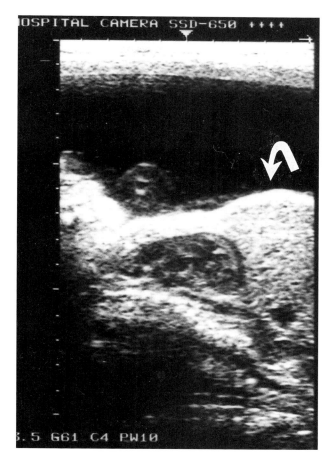

Figure 11   Short-rib polydactyly syndrome type I. Ultrasound scan of the fetal chest and abdomen. The abdomen is protruberant (curved arrow)

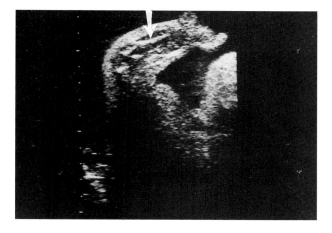

Figure 12   Short-rib polydactyly syndrome type I. Ultrasound scan of an upper limb. Note the pointed metaphysis of the ulna (arrow)

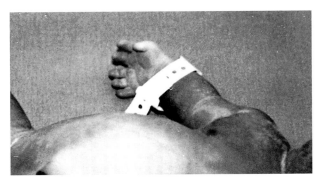

Figure 13   Short-rib polydactyly syndrome type I. Picture of a newborn after delivery showing postaxial polydactyly

(b)   Shortened lower leg is present (mesomelic dysplasia) due to short tibia.
(c)   Cleft lip and palate are present[42,43].

Sonographic and radiologic manifestations

Limbs: Mesomelia of the lower limb with marked shortening of tubular bones, in particular, extreme shortening of the tibia which often has an ovoid configuration, are the main features. The metaphyseal ends of long tubular bones are rounded. Premature ossification of proximal epiphyses of femur and humerus may appear. Postaxial and preaxial polydactyly can be present with distal phalangeal hypoplasia and symphalangism.
Spine: The spine usually is normal.
Thorax: The thorax is extremely short and narrowed, and the ribs are very short and horizontal. The scapulae and clavicles are normal.

Associated malformations

These may include cardiovascular malformations, renal anomalies (polycystic kidney), genital anomalies, pancreatic fibrosis, gastrointestinal tract anomalies, brain anomalies (arrhinencephaly), and hypoplastic epiglottis and larynx.

Other findings

Polyhydramnios is frequent.

Short-rib polydactyly syndrome type III

Synonym

SRPS type Verma–Naumoff.

Mode of inheritance

Autosomal recessive.

Incidence

Uncommon.

Definition and morphology

SRPS type III is similar to types I and II.

Sonographic and radiologic manifestations

Limbs: The limbs are very shortened. The metaphyseal ends of the long bones are widened with marginal spurs. Postaxial and preaxial polydactyly is present. Progressive distal shortening of all tubular bones (hands and feet) is a pathognomic feature[44,45].
Spine: The vertebral spine exhibits hypoplastic thin vertebrae with irregular margins of vertebral bodies. Coronal clefts of the vertebral bodies can be present.
Thorax: The thoracic cage is extremely short and narrowed with short ribs.
Head: The head is dolichocephalic with short cranial base and flattened occiput. The nasal bridge is depressed.
Pelvis: The pelvis is shortened cranio-caudally with horizontal trident acetabulae.

Associated malformations

Urogenital, alimentary tract and cardiovascular anomalies may be present.

Other findings

Both polyhydramnios and hydrops fetalis may be present (Figures 14–16).

Thanatophoric dysplasia

Synonym

Thanatophoric dwarfism.

Mode of inheritance

Sporadic.

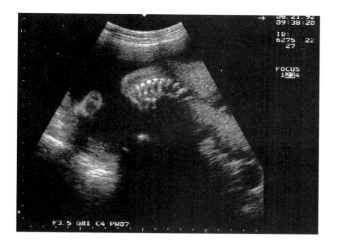

Figure 14 Short-rib polydactyly syndrome type III. Longitudinal scan of the thorax showing shortened limbs

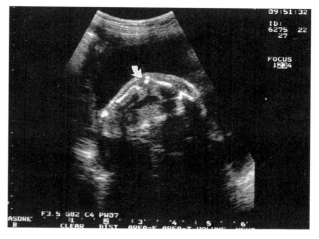

Figure 16 Short-rib polydactyly syndrome type III. Ultrasound picture of an upper limb. Note the widened metaphyses (arrow)

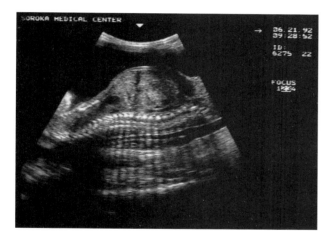

Figure 15 Short-rib polydactyly syndrome type III. Longitudinal scan of the fetus showing severely shortened thorax and protruberant abdomen

Incidence

Between 0.69–1.7 : 10 000 births. The most common form of lethal neonatal skeletal dysplasia.

Definition and morphology

Thanatophoric dysplasia is derived from the Greek 'thanatophoros' which means 'bearing death'. It is a form of short limb dysplasia. The limbs are markedly shortened, while the trunk is almost of normal length. The thorax is narrowed and the abdomen is protuberant, and often markedly protuberant. The skull is of normal size and often with mild frontal bossing. Rarely, the skull is of a cloverleaf appearance. The cloverleaf appearance is secondary to premature closure of the coronal and lambdoid sutures, resulting in prominence of the forehead and the temporal areas[46–50].

Sonographic and radiologic manifestations

Limbs: Marked shortening and bowing of long bones. The curved femur has been described as having the appearance of a 'telephone receiver'. The tubular bones of hands and feet are extremely shortened and broadened. The tubular bones, long and short, show widened irregular metaphyses.

Spine: Although the spine is of normal length, the vertebral bodies show severe platyspondyly with apparent wide disk spaces. In the frontal projection the vertebral bodies reveal a characteristic 'H' or inverted 'U'. The spinal canal is short as there is shortening of both the distance between the pedicles and that in the anteroposterior diameter.

Thorax: The thorax is narrowed but elongated compared to the abdomen, which is protuberant. The shortening of the thorax is secondary to very short ribs. There is wide cupped costo-chondral junction with posterior rib scalloping. The scapulae are small and deformed.

Head: In many cases of thanatophoric dysplasia frontal bossing of head and nasal depression are apparent. The skull is otherwise of normal dimensions. Rarely, cloverleaf appearance exists with closure of the coronal and the lambdoid sutures and widening of the anterior fontanelle. In such cases, hydrocephalus may be present.

Pelvis: The pelvis is small and there are small iliac bones with horizontal acetabular roofs and small sacroiliac notches. There are medial and lateral spikes at the lower part of the iliac bones.

Associated malformations

Hydrocephalus is often present in cases of associated cloverleaf skull. Other malformations which are sometimes present include horseshoe kidney, hydronephrosis, cardiac defects, agenesis of corpus callosum and radioulnar synostosis (Figures 17–20).

Other findings

Polyhydramnios is present in almost 50% of cases. Redundant subcutaneous soft tissue is a common finding.

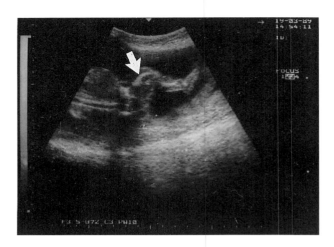

Figure 18   Thanatophoric dysplasia. Scan of the fetal femur (arrow) showing the typical 'telephone receiver' appearance of the femur

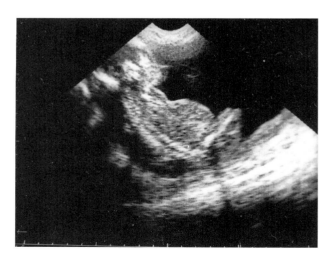

Figure 17   Thanatophoric dysplasia. Longitudinal scan of the fetus showing short thorax and protruberant abdomen

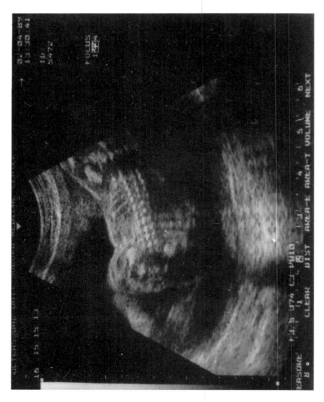

Figure 19   Thanatophoric dysplasia. Anteroposterior sonogram of the chest, abdomen and pelvis. The vertebral bodies are flat and have an 'H' like configuration

Special note

(1) Thanatophoric variants have been reported but are extremely rare.

(2) In cases where cloverleaf skull deformity is present, the long bones are sometimes not bowed.

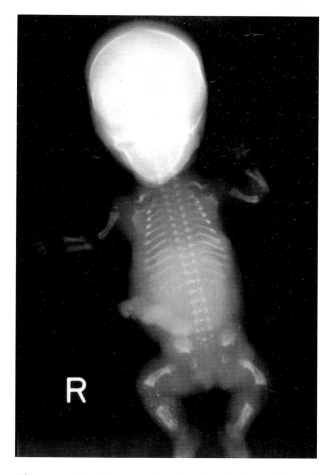

Figure 20 Thanatophoric dysplasia. Frontal radiograph after termination of pregnancy. Marked shortening of the limbs compared with normal size of the spine is apparent. Note the 'telephone receiver' appearance of the femur

References

1. International Nomenclature of Constitutional Diseases of Bone, revision May 1983. *Ann Radiol* 1983;26:457

2. Lachman RS, Rappaport V. Fetal imaging in the skeletal dysplasias. *Clin Perinatol* 1990;17:703–22

3. Rabinovitz JG, Mosseley JE, Mitty HA, *et al.* Trisomy 18, esophageal atresia, anomalies of the radius and congenital hypoplastic thrombocytopenia. *Radiology* 1967;89:488

4. Warkany J, Passarge E, Smith LB. Congenital malformations in autosomal trisomy syndromes. *Am J Dis Child* 1966;112:502

5. Curry CJR, Magenis RE, Brown M. Inherited chondrodysplasia punctata due to deletion of the terminal short arm of an X chromosome. *N Engl J Med* 1984;311:1010

6. Tomkins D, Hunter A, Roberts M. Cytogenetic findings in Roberts-SC phocomelia syndrome(s). *Am J Med Genet* 1979;4:17

7. Yarkoni S, Schmidt W, Jeanty P. Clavicular measurement: a new biometric parameter for fetal evaluation. *J Ultrasound Med* 1985;4:467

8. Jeanty P, Cantraine F, Consaret E, *et al.* The binocular distance: a new way to estimate fetal age. *J Ultrasound Med* 1984;3:741

9. Bencerraf B, Osathanondth R, Rieber FR. Achondrogenesis type I: ultrasound diagnosis *in utero. J Clin Ultrasound* 1984;12:357

10. Smith WL, Breitweiser TD, Dinno N. *In utero* diagnosis of achondrogenesis type I. *Clin Genet* 1981;19:51

11. Graham D, Tracy J, Winn K. Early second trimester sonographic diagnosis of achondrogenesis. *J Clin Ultrasound* 1983;11:336–41

12. Andersen PE. Achondrogenesis type II in twins. *Br J Radiol* 1981;54:61

13. Cohen H, Liu CT, Yang SS. Achondrogenesis: a review with special consideration of achondrogenesis type II (Langer-Saldino). *Am J Med Genet* 1981;10:379

14. Filly RA, Golbus MS, Carey JC. Short-limbed dwarfism: ultrasonographic diagnosis by measurement of fetal femoral length. *Radiology* 1981; 138:653

15. Kurtz AB, Filly RA, Wapner RJ. *In utero* analysis of heterozygous achondroplasia: variable time of onset as detected by femur length measurements. *J Ultrasound Med* 1986;5:137

16. Goldberg JD, Chervenack FA, Lipman RA. Antenatal sonographic diagnosis of arthrogryposis multiplex congenita. *Prenat Diag* 1986;6:45

17. Hagman G, Willemsw J. Arthrogryposis multiplex congenita. Review with comment. *Neuroped* 1983;14:6

18. Schnizel A, Savoldelli G, Briner J. Prenatal sonographic diagnosis of Jeune syndrome. *Radiology* 1985;154:777

19. Skiptunas SM, Weinwe S. Early prenatal diagnosis of asphyxiating thoracic dysplasia (Jeune syndrome): value of fetal thoracic measurement. *J Ultrasound Med* 1987;6:41

20. Elejalde BR, de Elajalde MM, Pausch D. Prenatal diagnosis of Jeune syndrome. *Am J Med* 1985;433:21

21. Bui TH, Marsk L, Eklof O. Prenatal diagnosis of chondroectodermal dysplasia with fetoscopy. *Prenat Diagn* 1984;4:155

22. Mahoney MJ, Hobbins JC. Prenatal diagnosis of chondroectodermal dysplasia (Ellis-Van Creveld syndrome) with fetoscopy and ultrasound. *N Engl J Med* 1977;297:258

23. Kaitila I, Ammala P, Karjalainin D. Early prenatal detection of diastrophic dysplasia. *Prenat Diagn* 1983;3:237

24. Mantagos S, Weiss RR, Mahoney M. Prenatal diagnosis of diastrophic dwarfism. *Am J Obstet Gynecol* 1981;139:111

25. Gollop RR, Eigier A. Prenatal ultrasound diagnosis of diastrophic dysplasia at 16 weeks. *Am J Med Genet* 1987;27:321

26. Kim HJ, Costales F, Bouzouki M. Prenatal diagnosis of dyssegmental dwarfism. *Prenat Diagn* 1986;6:143

27. Handmaker SD, Campbell IA, Robinson LD. Dyssegmental dwarfism: a new syndrome of lethal dwarfism. *Birth Defects* 1977;13:79

28. Andersen PE Jr, Hauge M, Bang J. Dyssegmental dysplasia in siblings: prenatal ultrasonic diagnosis. *Skeletal Radiol* 1988;17:29

29. Abrams SL, Filly RA. Congenital vertebral malformations: prenatal diagnosis using ultrasonography. *Radiology* 1988;155:762

30. Benacerraf BR, Greene MF, Brass VA. Prenatal sonographic diagnosis of congenital hemivertebra. *J Ultrasound Med* 1986;5:257

31. Macklean RN, Prater WK, Lozzio CB. Brief clinical report: skeletal dysplasia with short, angulated femoral (kyphomelic dysplasia). *Am J Med Genet* 1983;14:373

32. Silence DO, Senn A, Danks DM. Genetic heterogeneity in osteogenesis imperfecta. *Am J Med Genet* 1979;16:101

33. Chervenack FA, Romero R, Berkovitz RL. Antenatal sonographic findings of osteogenesis imperfecta. *Am J Obstet Gynecol* 1983;143:228

34. Kuller J, Bellantoni J, Dorst J. Obstetric management of fetus with nonlethal osteogenesis imperfecta. *Obstet Gynecol* 1988;74:477

35. Dinno ND, Yacoub UA, Kadlec JF. Midtrimester diagnosis of osteogenesis imperfecta, type II. *Birth Defects* 1982;18:125

36. Stephens JD, Filly RA, Callen PW. Prenatal diagnosis of osteogenesis imperfecta type II by real-time ultrasound. *Hum Genet* 1983;64:191

37. Elejalde BR, de Elejalde MM. Prenatal diagnosis of perinatally lethal osteogenesis imperfecta. *Am J Med Genet* 1983;14:353

38. Meizner I, Levy A, Yosef S, *et al*. Prenatal ultrasonic diagnosis of type II osteogenesis imperfecta in the second trimester. *Isr J Obstet Gynecol* 1991;2:26

39. Robinson LP, Worthen NJ, Lacham RS. Prenatal diagnosis of osteogenesis imperfecta type III. *Prenat Diagn* 1987;7:7

40. Meizner I, Bar-Ziv J. Prenatal ultrasonic diagnosis of short rib polydactyly syndrome type I. A case report. *J Reprod Med* 1989;34:668

41. Johnson VP, Peterson LP, Holzworth DR. Midtrimester prenatal diagnosis of short-limb dwarfism (Saldino–Noonan Syndrome). *Birth Defects* 1982; 18:133

42. Cooper CP, Hall CM. Lethal short-rib polydactyly syndrome of the Majewski type: a report of three cases. *Radiology* 1982;144:513

43. Thomson GSM, Reynolds CP, Cruickshank J. Antenatal detection of recurrence of Majewski dwarf (short-rib polydactyly syndrome type II Majewski). *Clin Radiol* 1982;33:509

44. Meizner I, Bar-Ziv J. Prenatal ultrasonic diagnosis of short-rib polydactyly syndrome (SRPS) type III: a case report and a proposed approach to the diagnosis of SRPS and related conditions. *J Clin Ultrasound* 1985;13:284

45. Naumoff P, Young LW, Mazar J. Short-rib polydactyly syndrome type III. *Radiology* 1977;122:443

46. Meizner I, Levy A, Carmi R, *et al*. Early prenatal ultrasonic diagnosis of thanatophoric dwarfism. *Isr J Med Sci* 1990;26:287

47. Camera G, Dodero D, de Pascale S. Prenatal diagnosis of thanatophoric dysplasia at 24 weeks. *Am J Med Genet* 1984;18:39

48. Chervenak P, Blackmore KJ, Issacson G. Antenatal sonographic findings of thanatophoric dysplasia with cloverleaf skull. *Am J Obstet Gynecol* 1983; 146:894

49. Fink IJ, Filly RA, Callen PW. Sonographic diagnosis of thanatophoric dwarfism *in utero. J Ultrasound Med* 1982;1:337

50. Elejalde BR, de Elejalde MM. Thanatophoric dysplasia: fetal manifestations and prenatal diagnosis. *Am J Med Genet* 1985;22:669

The fetal spine

13

The-Hung Bui, Richard Jaffe, Henry Lindholm and Mark I. Evans

INTRODUCTION

Neural tube defects (NTDs) and other spinal anomalies are common congenital malformations in humans. Hence examination of the fetal spine is an integral and important part of any sonographic fetal evaluation[1,2], whether ultrasound is performed as a screening test for malformations in a low-risk population[3], or used as a diagnostic test in high-risk pregnancies defined by either family history, maternal conditions (e.g. maternal diabetes mellitus or epilepsy)[4-6], potentially teratogenic exposure (e.g. anti-epileptic drugs, warfarin)[6-7], or as a result of biochemical screening tests such as maternal serum α-fetoprotein (MSAFP) for open NTDs or, more recently, maternal serum screening test for Down's syndrome in the second trimester since MSAFP is included as one of the biochemical markers[8].

This chapter deals with evaluation and anomalies of the fetal spine including spinal dysraphism, spinal deformities, dysostoses with predominantly axial involvement, syndromes in which spinal defects are a major feature among the constellation of findings, and sacrococcygeal teratoma. The spondylodysplasias are discussed in the chapter on skeletal dysplasias (chapter 12). The recent introduction of three-dimensional (3D) ultrasound into clinical use carries promise for improved assessment of the fetal spine, in particular when the anatomy is complex. Early experience with this new modality is accumulating. A short summary of important embryonic events related to the formation of the spine and associated structures that will allow a better comprehension of spinal defects is also given.

NORMAL EMBRYONIC DEVELOPMENT OF THE SPINE

The normal development of human embryos is by convention categorized into 23 stages[9]. This classification is based on specific external features and on somite development during the early stages, and on crown–rump length (CRL) during the later stages.

At the end of the 4th and beginning of the 5th gestational week (Carnegie stages 6–7) the primitive streak forms along the caudal midline of the bilaminar germ disc and establishes the fundamental craniocaudal axis and bilateral symmetry of the developing embryo. The definitive endoderm and intra-embryonic mesoderm form by a process of cell ingress and invagination called gastrulation, thus converting the bilaminar germ disc into the trilaminar embryo (Carnegie stage 7). The ectodermal central part of the embryonic disc is induced to thicken and differentiate into the neural plate by the underlying paraxial mesoderm around 18–19 days postconception (Carnegie stage 8). By the end of the 5th week of gestation, neurulation and somite formation are initiated with appearance of the neural plate which will form the neural groove along the long axis of the embryo. The underlying paraxial mesoderm on each side of the neural groove undergoes segmentation known as somites (Carnegie stage 9). This process occurs in craniocaudal succession and progresses until the end of the 6th week of pregnancy. The somites will later differentiate into most of the axial skeleton including part of the occipital bone of the skull, the segmental bones, cartilages and ligaments of the vertebral column; the voluntary muscles of the neck, body wall, and limbs; and to part of the dermis and subcutaneous tissue of the neck and trunk.

During the 6th week of gestation (Carnegie stages 10 to 12), the neural folds arch over and gradually meet in the dorsal midline through a process of folding called neurulation[10]. The neural folds fuse in the midline to form the neural tube, first in the region of the embryo's future neck, and extend from there simultaneously toward the cephalic and caudal ends of the embryo. At the end of stage 10, the neural tube is closed opposite the somites, but is still widely open at the cranial and caudal neuropores. The human neural tube appears to close segmentally requiring the orchestration of a number of developmental genes with specific genetic and environmental susceptibilities and modifiers[11,12], but little is known about these factors in humans. Both neuropores close during stage 12, when the rostral end starts to enlarge to form the forebrain, midbrain and hindbrain. The remainder of the neural tube will become the spinal cord. The caudal neuropore corresponds to the future lumbar region. The sacral and coccygeal regions of the neural tube arise subsequently by another process, called canalization or secondary neurulation. Cells are added to the caudal end of the neural tube from the undifferentiated caudal cell mass forming a solid neural cord. A lumen along the central axis of the neural cord is gradually formed by cavitation. It then joins with the neural canal previously formed by neurulation. This process is completed by 8 weeks' gestational age.

It is generally accepted that NTDs occur because the neural tube somehow fails to close. Neurulation defects occur within Carnegie stages 8 to 12, corresponding to 17th to 30th days postconception; craniorachischisis (inionschisis) within 17 to 23 days postconception (Carnegie stages 8 to 10), anencephaly within 23 to 26 days postconception (Carnegie stage 11) and myelomeningocele (spina bifida) within 26 to 30 days postconception (Carnegie stage 12). Defects that occur during neurulation result in open defects, whereas defects arising after neurulation are closed NTDs, i.e. the defect is covered by skin.

Ossification of the fetal spine

The axial skeleton, including the base of the skull, is formed through cartilage models and endochondral ossification which can be observed by ultrasound at the earliest at 8 weeks' gestation[13] (Figure 1). The first spinal structures that can be visualized are the three ossification centers in individual vertebrae: a ventral center for the vertebral body and two paired dorsal centers that will become the central masses and the posterior arch. There is some variability with regard to ossification times[13–17] (Table 1). As the vertebrae acquire ossification centers, they become increasingly accessible to ultrasound examination. Whereas the ossification centers of the vertebral bodies are first observed in the lower thoracal and upper lumbar vertebrae with spreading in both rostral and caudal directions (Table 1), the dorsal ossification centers appear in a cephalic to caudal direction beginning in the cervical spine and progressing to the sacrum[15]. Dorsal ossification in lower lumbar

vertebrae is not seen before 19 weeks of gestation, and the arch of the upper sacral region is not consistently seen until 22–25 weeks[16,17]. With each new generation of ultrasound machines and probes, it is expected that the times of ossification detection of the spine will become earlier.

The notochord within the vertebral body will degenerate and persist as the nucleus pulposus in the invertebral disc. Skeletal maturation in females is more advanced than in males, and this is most evident at term. However, opinions on this issue differ regarding the early stages of development[18,19]. Multiple pregnancy and fetal growth restriction are often associated with slower skeletal

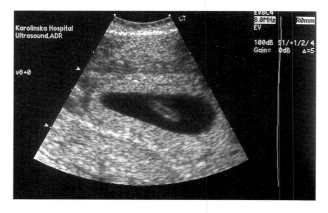

Figure 1 Fetal spine in the 8th week gestation. Two parallel rows of separate centers of ossification are noted. This is the earliest stage that these should be expected to be visualized

Table 1 Approximate detection times by sonography of bone elements in the fetal spine and adjacent osseous structures

Bone structures	Gestational age (weeks)
Vertebral bodies	8–20
lower thoracic, upper lumbar	8–12
lower cervical	12–14
midcervical	14–16
upper cervical	16–20
Clavicle	6–8
Scapula	8–12
Sternum	21–33
Ribs	8–10
Os ilium	7–8
Os pubis	20–23

development, whereas maternal diabetes and anencephaly are usually associated with accelerated maturation[18,19].

ULTRASONOGRAPHIC EXAMINATION OF THE FETAL SPINE AND SPINAL CORD

During the second and third trimesters, the fetal spine and spinal cord can be systematically scanned[20]. However, given the ontogeny of the fetal spine, ultrasonographic evaluation is not generally meaningful before 15 weeks. By 16 to 17 weeks of pregnancy, the fetal spine is clearly seen and can be evaluated. Examination of the fetal spine consists of a systematic imaging and evaluation of the ossification centers within the fetal vertebrae. The coronal (frontal) (Figure 2), sagittal/parasagittal (Figure 3) and transverse (axial) (Figure 4) scanning planes are used to assess the fetal spine from the cervical to the coccygeal regions. In the longitudinal planes, the spine has the appearance of a 'railroad track' or 'string of beads' with gradual widening toward the fetal neck and gradual tapering in the sacrococcygeal region (Figure 5). Demonstration of the cord and dura mater is feasible when an exact midsagittal scan is achieved; on an oblique scan these structures are obscured by acoustic shadows. If the spine is arched, care should be taken to adjust the position of the transducer to the particular area of the back that is being examined. In the transverse plane, the three ossification centers in each vertebra should be visualized, and the paramedially located ossification centers of the neural arches should be parallel or converging. At the level of the thoracic spine, an exact transverse scan is evidenced by the three vertebral ossification centers and by the paired ossification centers of the ribs (Figure 6). For detailed examination, a series of transverse scans are performed, proceeding slowly in a cranio-caudal direction, to allow visualization of the ossification centers at each level.

During real-time examination in the second trimester, the most popular view of the fetal spine for parents-to-be is either one of two oblique longitudinal planes because nearly all the fetal spine can be captured in one frame. However, this scanning plane is the least sensitive to demonstrate small spina bifida since only the ossification centers of the vertebral bodies and the ones at the base of the transverse processes on one side can be visu-

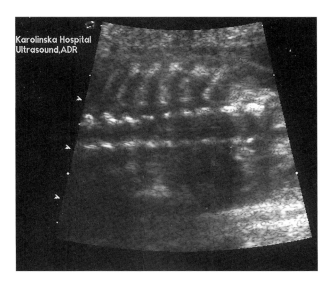

Figure 2 In this coronal view of the spine of a fetus at 19 weeks gestation we see the splaying of the dorsal ossification centers. This, however, is the result of dorsal convergence of these centers appearing at different times in development. This finding is a potential pitfall and should not be mistaken for a dysraphy

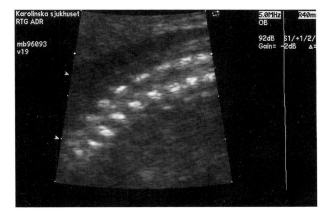

Figure 3 The convergence of the dorsal ossification centers has progressed enough in this 19-week fetus to produce an even echo as seen in the sagittal view

alized concomitantly. Axial (transverse) views are generally superior to longitudinal views (sagittal, parasagittal, and coronal) for demonstrating small spinal defects since all three ossification centers can be imaged in the same plane. However, anomalies such as scoliosis, hemivertebrae, disorganized or hypomineralised vertebrae are optimally demonstrated with sagittal and coronal views because many vertebrae can be imaged in the same plane.

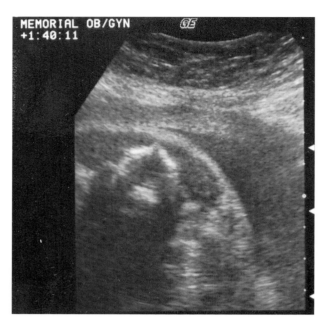

Figure 4   Transverse view of a normal spine of a second-trimester fetus

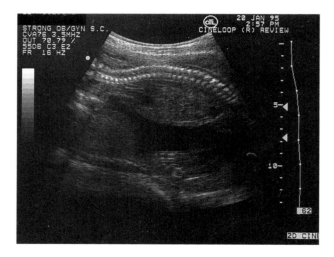

Figure 5   Normal appearance of the spine in the longitudinal view

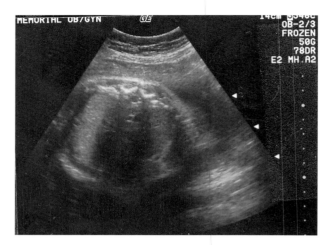

Figure 6   Transverse view of the fetal spine at the level of the thorax

Pitfalls when scanning the fetal spine

Apparent splaying at the thoracic level may be created by inadvertent imaging through a part of the fetal ribs in the parasagittal plane[23]. The dorsal ossification centers of the lower lumbar spine and sacral region during the mid-trimester may appear parallel to one another rather than converging to the midline on axial views[24]. This may lead to an erroneous diagnosis of spinal defect if the sonographer is unaware that posterior ossification centers at these levels develop late in the second trimester[16,17]. Furthermore, 'pseudodysraphic defects' may also be produced by oblique angulation of the probe in the axial scanning plane giving an impression of splaying of the dorsal ossification centers[25] (Figure 7).

Fetal position may affect the ability to examine the posterior neural arch. This examination cannot be carried out when the fetus is supine. When oligohydramnios is present detailed fetal survey is much more difficult. Transabdominal amnio-infusion may be needed to allow visualization of fetal structures as discussed in the chapter on ultrasound guided invasive procedures (chapter 17).

SPINA BIFIDA

NTDs are commonly occurring congenital malformations in humans. Their prevalence decreases from 2.5% of embryos at the end of the 6th gestational week to 0.6% or less at term[26]. The three main types of NTDs include anencephaly, encephalocele and spina bifida. The two most

When the fetus is in breech presentation, transperineal or transvaginal ultrasound can alternatively be used to evaluate the distal fetal spine since the transabdominal imaging technique may give suboptimal views[21,22].

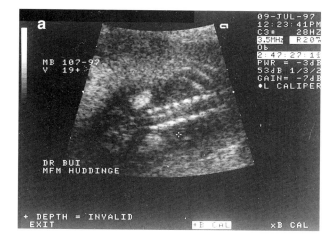

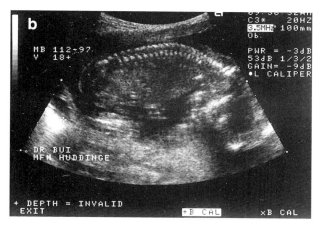

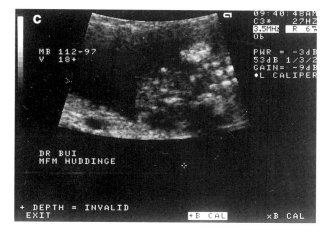

Figure 7 (a) Coronal view of unossified posterior lower sacral and coccygeal vertebrae mimicking 'pseudosacral agenesis'. (b) Parasagittal and (c) oblique views of same fetus

common are anencephaly and spina bifida with similar overall frequencies of about 1 in 1000 births[27]. The incidence of NTDs varies with ethnicity and geography, with the highest incidences seen in Northern Ireland, Scotland and Wales, whereas one of the lowest rates is observed in Japan[8]. In the USA, NTDs are superseded only by congenital heart defects[27].

NTDs are generally considered one entity. However, only about 70% of presently observed NTDs are folic acid sensitive and may be prevented by periconceptional maternal folic acid consumption[28,29]. Successful programs using this form of primary prevention still need to be established[30]. It is now clear that not all NTDs in humans can be prevented by folic acid. Moreover, about 10% of NTDs are due to a number of monogenic diseases, chromosomal defects and teratogenic agents[31–33]. Most cases, however, are thought to be multifactorial in origin, being the result of polygenic and environmental factors.

Since the majority of infants with NTDs are born to families with no history of these defects, MS-AFP screening programs at 16–18 weeks of gestation for open NTDs are currently offered in low-risk populations in many parts of the world[8]. Presently, well-organized population screening programs detect all fetuses with anencephaly and 70–80% of those with spina bifida[34]. Sonography plays an essential role in the management of those pregnancies with an increased MS-AFP level and suspected NTDs[35,36]. Amniocentesis is generally recommended when no obvious defects can be imaged although the MS-AFP is elevated for gestational age, or in pregnancies at known high risk for NTDs. However, it has been argued that ultrasound in experienced centers may be used as a diagnostic test in both situations[37–41]. Anencephaly can be diagnosed by ultrasound alone. Both amniotic fluid biochemistry and ultrasound have a false-positive rate of about 2 per 1000 when carried out in high-risk pregnancies[34]. The results are likely to be better if the two methods are performed in parallel.

The terminology used to describe different types of NTDs is not standardized[42]. Anencephaly, encephalocele and other NTDs involving craniocerebral structures are discussed in chapter 8.

Spinal dysraphism refers to a failure of part of the neural tube to close. This will disrupt not only the differentiation of the central nerve system but also the induction of the vertebral arches along the spine resulting in a number of developmental anomalies. When the vertebral arches fail to fuse along the dorsal midline to enclose the vertebral canal, the resulting open vertebral canal is called spina bifida. The contents of the vertebral canal may bulge into a membranous sac or cele that is continuous with the surrounding skin. In meningocele, only the meninges are incorporated into the overlying skin, whereas in myelomeningocele both meninges and spinal cord tissue are incorporated into the skin. Spina bifida is commonly found in the lower lumbar and upper sacral region, suggesting that failure of caudal neuropore closure or secondary neurulation may be involved in the pathogenesis of these malformations. The most severe NTD is craniorachischisis totalis, a failure of the entire neural tube to fuse resulting in spontaneous abortion. If the neurulation defect involves the occipital and upper spinal region the lesion is called inionschisis (craniorachischisis).

Occult spinal dysraphism

Spina bifida occulta or occult spinal dysraphism are terms that may be sources of confusion. Occult spinal dysraphism is a condition in which the conus has an abnormal attachment to neighboring structures and may be elongated, with one or more of a variety of anomalies of the spinal cord, vertebrae and skin. These include spinal lipoma, lipomeningocele, diastematomyelia, dorsal dermal sinuses and the split notochord syndrome[43]. They all have in common the lack of association with hydrocephalus. Postnatally, cutaneous or subcutaneous anomalies such as an angioma, a lipoma, a pigmented nevus, a tuft of hair or skin dimple indicate the site of the vertebral lesion. Occult spinal dysraphism is part of the NTD spectrum and has the same genetic implications[44].

Sometimes, the term spina bifida occulta is used to describe incomplete ossification of the posterior vertebral laminae, most often at L5 or S1, in a healthy individual. This lesion has no clinical or genetic consequences. This is a normal variant in children younger than 2 years and occurs in about 20% of adults.

Associated malformations

Hydrocephalus, scoliosis, dilated urinary tract, or club foot are generally considered secondary consequences of the primary NTD. Other non-randomly associated malformations include cleft palate, diaphragmatic hernia, heart defects, omphalocele, renal hypoplasia, and imperforated anus (reviewed by Medeira et al.[45]). Overall, about 20% of cases with NTDs have other major malformations, although they are less frequent in surviving children, among whom they are found in 6–10%[46–48]. The term schisis association has been coined to a non-random tendency for malformations such as omphalocele, orofacial clefts, tracheoesophageal fistulae, diaphragmatic defects to be found with each other and with NTDs in the absence of a chromosomal disorder[49].

Ultrasonographic findings

The NTDs involving the cranial region such as anencephaly and encephalocele together with the important sonographic cranial signs of spinal anomalies are discussed in chapter 7. Recognition of associated sonographic abnormalities in the fetal skull and cerebellum has enhanced the prenatal detection of open spina bifida[50], and may allow accurate diagnosis of low NTDs already in the early second trimester[51]. Frontal bone scalloping (lemon sign) and abnormal curvature of the cerebellum (banana sign), often associated with obliteration of the cisterna magna, are two of the most common cranial findings in the fetus with open spina bifida[52–55] (Figure 8). These signs, however, differ in sensitivity and specificity depending upon the gestational age and which particular sign is found. It is therefore appropriate to discuss further here, in some more detail, these issues. The lemon sign is strongly associated with open spina bifida and is seen in 98% of fetuses of less than 24 weeks' gestational age with myelomeningocele. After 24 weeks, it is much less consistent being found in only 13–25% of fetuses with NTDs[56,57]. However, this sign alone is not specific for spina bifida as it has been reported both in normal fetuses and in those with other structural abnormalities[58,59]. Although the banana sign is less frequently observed in the second-trimester fetus with a NTD than the lemon sign, its specificity and positive predictive value is higher[56]. Thus, these findings alone or in combination should alert the sonographer and prompt a detailed examination of the fetal spine. Other important craniocerebral signs of the presence of spina bifida are small biparietal diameter, Arnold–Chiari type II malformation and secondary cerebral ventricular enlargement (hydrocephalus)[57]. However, the diagnosis of myelomeningocele and spina bifida should always be based on direct imaging of the spinal anomaly and not on secondary signs.

Although spina bifida involving three or more segments may be easily visualized on longitudinal scans, smaller defects can only be detected through meticulous examination of each vertebra in the transverse plane. Diagnosis is based on imaging the outward splaying of the posterior ossification centers which are further apart than corresponding ossification centers above or below the defect in coronal views (Figure 9). The cleft in soft tissue is often recognized and is, sometimes, more easily seen than the bony defect itself. When the sac is intact in myelomeningocele, it bulges into the amniotic cavity and is easily recognized as a cystic extension from the posterior aspect of the spine moving and 'shimmering' with fetal movements (Figures 10 and 11). When the fetal spine pushes on the placenta or myometrial wall, the sac of a myelomeningocele, even when present and intact, may be difficult to demonstrate. Light pressure on both sides of the uterus may allow amniotic fluid to flow between the fetal spine and the surrounding structures for better visualization. In the third trimester, posterior vertebral elements including the laminae and spinous processes are normally seen by ultrasound. Hence, absence of these structures support a diagnosis of spina bifida.

Diastematomyelia

In diastematomyelia the spinal cord is divided sagitally by a fibrocartilagenous or bony structure. Most cases are sporadic and the malformation is either isolated or seen in association with vertebral defects such as spina bifida, kyphoscoliosis, hemivertebra or butterfly vertebra[60]. However, affected sisters were reported by Kapsalakis[61], and Gardner[62] described a family in which three sisters had diastematomyelia and other dysraphic malformations in various combinations.

Prenatal diagnosis of diastematomyelia by ultrasound can be made in the second trimester (18–20 weeks of gestation) by the finding of an extra posterior echogenic focus between the fetal spinal laminae and splaying of the posterior elements in the axial plane (reviewed by Sepulveda et al.[63]). Prognosis is good when the malformation is isolated, but is guarded when associated with

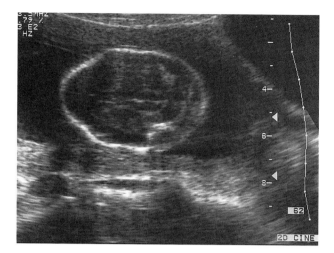

Figure 8 Lemon and banana signs of fetus with spina bifida

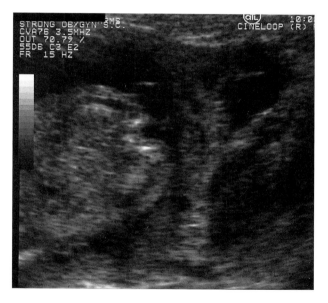

Figure 9 Wide splaying of vertebral ossification centers in fetus with spina bifida

more severe NTDs[60,63,64]. A fourth echogenic area in the lumbosacral midline may also be caused by a lipomyelomeningocele, a rare teratomatous tumor of the spinal cord[65].

DYSOSTOSES WITH PREDOMINANTLY AXIAL INVOLVEMENT

The dysostoses include conditions in which there are malformations or absence of an individual bone or group of bones. They differ from the

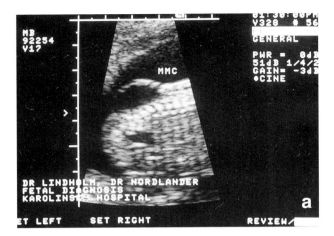

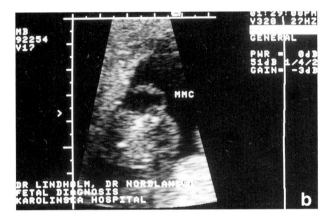

Figure 10   (**a**) Sagittal and (**b**) transverse views of a lumbo-sacral myelomeningocele (MMC) in a 17-week fetus. When only meninges are incorporated it is termed meningocele

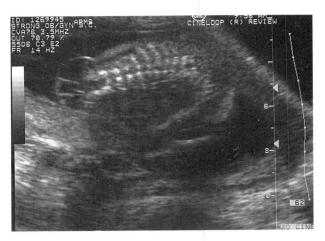

Figure 11   Oblique view of spina bifida with splaying of vertebrae and myelomeningocele

osteochondrodysplasias, which are characterized by a generalized abnormality in bone or cartilage. Frequently, there are additional congenital anomalies. Our knowledge of the pathogenesis of dysostoses is limited, and this is reflected in the difficulty in classifying them. Indeed, no classification was given in the revised International Nomenclature of Constitutional Diseases of Bones[66]. Thus, a major challenge for the sonographer resides in demonstrating whether the spinal anomaly is an isolated defect, or part of a malformation sequence or association, a developmental field defect, a complex, or a syndrome (i.e. chromosomal, autosomal dominant, autosomal recessive, X-linked). Many times, the prenatal diagnosis will be only descriptive. Clinically, dysostoses may be subdivided into three broad categories based on the most affected part of the skeleton: those with primarily craniofacial bone defects, those with predominantly axial involvement, and those affecting only the extremities. In this chapter, discussion of the dysostoses with predominant axial involvement which have been relatively well described and which are potentially amenable to prenatal diagnosis by ultrasound are only included.

Klippel–Feil anomaly

Abnormal vertebral segmentation is most commonly seen in the cervical region although any part of the vertebral column can be involved. The Klippel–Feil anomaly or sequence refers to segmentation anomalies of the cervical vertebrae, whether the entire cervical spine or only two segments are affected. It is the most common form of axial dysostosis. Subclassification into three morphological types has been defined by Gunderson et al.[67]: type I shows massive synostosis of many cervical and upper thoracic vertebrae into bony blocks; type II is characterized by fusion at only one or two interspaces although hemivertebrae, occipito-atlantal fusion and other anomalies might be associated; and type III which includes both cervical and lower thoracic or lumbar fusions. The existence of a fourth type associated with sacral agenesis has been suggested[68]. There are clearly several entities in the general category of Klippel–Feil anomaly. One or more may be autosomal recessive or autosomal dominant, and some may have no simple genetic basis. C2–C3 fusion (a subcategory of type II) is the most common form of congenital fused cervical vertebrae and is probably an autosomal dominant condition with variable expression, whereas C5–C6 fusion may be recessive[67,69–71].

Hemivertebrae, defective posterior elements leading to spina bifida occulta, anterior clefting of the vertebral body, missing vertebrae have all been reported together with the Klippel–Feil anomaly[72]. Other associated anomalies include congenital heart defects, cleft palate, renal hypoplasia or bilateral agenesis, and limb anomalies[67] which, therefore, should be looked for when there is evidence of a Klippel-Feil anomaly in the fetus. The mechanism that leads to the malformations seen in the Klippel-Feil anomaly appears to be a failure of the normal segmentation and fusion processes of the mesodermal somites, which occur between 5–9 weeks gestation.

Wildervanck syndrome

The Wildervanck or cervical-oculo-acoustic syndrome consists of congenital perceptive deafness, Klippel–Feil anomaly, and abducens palsy with retraction of the bulb of one or both eyes (Duane syndrome)[73–75]. It is limited, or almost completely limited, to females, raising the question of sex-linked dominance with lethality in the hemizygous male[76]. This syndrome may be responsible for at least 1% of deafness among females[77]. Multifactorial inheritance was favored by Kongismark and Gorlin[78], whereas Wildervanck[79] concluded that polygenic inheritance with limitation to females is most likely, after an extensive review of the syndrome.

Fetal scoliosis

Abnormal curvature of the fetal spine such as fetal scoliosis, lordosis and kyphosis may result from a multitude of causes. The deformity can be a component of a syndrome, some of the skeletal dysplasias (e.g. diastrophic dysplasia), a chromosome abnormality, or arise as a result of mechanical forces (e.g. abdominal wall defects) (Figure 12). It can be diagnosed by ultrasound when angulation of the spine persists on coronal and parasagittal scans[80]. Often the deformity is due to vertebral anomalies as a result of abnormal segmentation or failure of formation of part of a vertebra such as block vertebrae, hemivertebrae, butterfly vertebrae and absent vertebral body[81–83]. NTDs are most commonly observed with scoliosis of varying severity[80]. Examples of conditions associated with fetal scoliosis include the dysostoses with predominant axial involvement[83], the limb–body wall complex and other abdominal wall defects[84,85] (Figure 12), the amniotic band sequence[86], the VATER association[87,88], or the MURCS association[89], among other rare disorders. Thus, a search for associated anomalies is warranted when fetal scoliosis is found.

VATER and MURCS associations

The VATER and MURCS association also includes vertebral anomalies. Thus, consideration should be given to examination of the fetus with Klippel–Feil anomaly or with multiple segmentation defects for signs of these associations.

The VATER association is an acronym for **V**ertebral anomalies, **A**nal anomalies, **T**racheal, **E**sophageal, and **R**adial ray defects. This combination of associated defects was pointed out by Quan and Smith[87]. Nearly all cases have been sporadic with no recognized teratogen or chromosomal abnormality[88]. A few familial instances have been reviewed[90]. Iafolla et al.[91] described three patients with hydrocephalus secondary to aqueductal stenosis in addition to the multisystemic features of the VATER association. The VATER association was later expanded to the VACTERL association[92]. VACTERL is an acronym for **V**ertebral anomalies (similar to those of spondylocostal dysplasia), **A**nal atresia, **C**ardiac malformations, **T**racheoesophageal fistula, **Re**nal anomalies (urethral atresia with hydronephrosis), and **L**imb anomalies (hexadactyly, humeral hypoplasia, radial aplasia, and proximally placed thumb). The vertebral malformations are

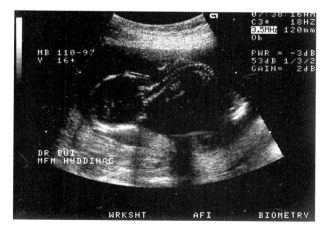

Figure 12 Scoliosis in fetus with limb–body wall complex and normal karyotype

often located in the caudal region. Recently, a mitochondrial mutation has been found in a patient with the VACTERL association[93].

MURCS is an acronym for the leading features, namely, **Mu**llerian duct aplasia, **R**enal aplasia, dysgenesis or ectopia, and **C**ervicothoracic **S**omite dysplasia[89,94]. Lin *et al.*[95] described the combination of MURCS association and occipital encephalocele in a stillborn girl of 41 weeks' gestation. The malformations in this disorder are compatible with a defect in the organization of the paraxial mesoderm that gives rise to occipital, cervical, and thoracic somites and adjoining intermediate mesoderm or a developmental field defect. These structures contribute to the occipital bone, cervical spine, upper limbs, and urogenital system. Differential diagnosis includes Goldenhar (oculo-auriculo-vertebral) syndrome[96] and VATER/VACTERL association.

Sprengel deformity

Sprengel deformity or sequence is characterized by a congenital upward displacement of the scapula. It can be unilateral or bilateral, isolated, or part of a more complex malformation constellation. Although most cases have been sporadic, familial occurrence of Sprengel deformity has been reported with an autosomal dominant pattern of inheritance[97,98]. It is presumably the result of failed descent of the scapula from the neck to the thorax during the second month of gestation.

The scapula is generally hypoplastic and with an abnormal shape. In up to 50% of cases, there is accumulation of connective tissue or even bony fusion between the scapula and ribs or vertebrae. Frequently, there are also skeletal anomalies such as scoliosis, hemivertebrae, fused vertebrae, spina bifida occulta, cervical or missing ribs, fused ribs, anomalies of the clavicles, and hypoplasia of the shoulder girdle muscles. Thus, the osseous anomalies may be detected by ultrasound. The diagnosis may be suspected if the fetus in addition cannot move one or both shoulders and there is a positive family history.

Bouwes Bavinck and Weaver[99] suggested that Klippel–Feil anomaly, Sprengel anomaly and some other conditions are each the result of interruption of the early embryonic blood supply in the subclavian arteries, the vertebral arteries and/or their branches. The term subclavian artery supply disruption sequence (SASDS) was coined for this group of birth defects.

Multiple vertebral segmentation defects and Jarcho–Levin syndrome

Jarcho and Levin[100] are credited with first describing a syndrome characterized by extensive vertebral segmentation defects, in a black brother and sister in Baltimore, but they mistakenly believed it to be the same condition as the one described by Klippel and Feil in 1912. Numerous patients with multiple spinal segmentation defects have since been reported under a variety of names including Jarcho–Levin syndrome, spondylocostal or spondylothoracic dysostosis (or dysplasia), and costovertebral dysplasia (reviewed by Mortier *et al.*[101]). Both autosomal recessive and autosomal dominant forms have been postulated. There is still considerable semantic and nosological confusion concerning syndromes characterized by extensive vertebral segmentation anomalies. Based on radiographic and clinical findings at least three distinct entities have been recognized: a lethal autosomal recessive form associated with a symmetric 'crab-like' radiologic appearance of the thoracic skeleton called Jarcho–Levin syndrome[102,103]; an autosomal recessive form, spondylothoracic dysostosis, with striking intrafamilial variability and considerable clinical and radiographic overlap with spondylocostal dysostosis[104]; and a benign autosomal dominant condition, spondylocostal dysostosis, with a normal life span and lack of associated anomalies[101,105]. Sporadic cases of vertebral segmentation defects probably represent a heterogeneous group and are difficult to classify as to genetic versus non-genetic forms. Associated anomalies are more common in this group than in the familial types and may involve both mesodermally and ectodermally derived structures. In the severe forms, early death in infancy occurs secondary to respiratory distress at birth or recurrent respiratory tract infections.

Cervical spine involvement results in a short neck, and postnatally also in a low posterior hairline. The trunk is short due to vertebral segmentation defects such as fusion or absence of vertebrae, hemivertebrae and butterfly vertebrae resulting in kyphosis or scoliosis. The ribs can vary in number and shape, and are often fused at the costovertebral junctions. Pectus deformities are due to multiple ribs anomalies. Prenatal diagnosis may be difficult[106,107], as illustrated by the case presented by Poor *et al.*[108] where repeated ultrasound examinations in a known at-risk pregnancy failed to demonstrate the characteristic findings of the Jarcho–Levin syndrome. However, prenatal diagnosis by ultrasound in the second trimester has since been reported both in families with known increased risk but also in those without prior specific risk[109–111] (Bui and Lindholm, unpublished cases) (Figure 13).

Cerebro-costo-mandibular syndrome

Rib gaps due to uncalcified fibrous or cartilaginous tissue in the posterior part of the ribs, Pierre Robin anomaly (micrognathia, cleft palate, glossoptosis) and vertebral dysplasia are characteristics of this syndrome[112]. Other malformations have also been reported. Both autosomal dominant with variable expressivity and autosomal recessive inheritance have been reported[113]. Prenatal diagnosis is based on rib gaps and family history. In sporadic cases there may be difficulties in reaching a specific diagnosis as rib gaps are also seen in other syndromes including Jarcho–Levin syndrome, Goldenhar syndrome and the oculovertebral syndrome.

Caudal regression syndrome

The caudal regression syndrome is the generic name for a continuum of congenital malformations ranging from agenesis of the lumbosacral spine to the most severe cases of sirenomelia (mermaid syndrome) (Figure 14) with lower extremities fusion and major visceral anomalies[114]. Maternal diabetes, genetic predisposition, and vascular hypoperfusion have been implied as possible etiologic factors[4,114,115]. The development of this syndrome is believed to result from a disruption of the maturation of the caudal portion of the spinal cord prior to 4 weeks gestation[116]. The degree of associated anomalies usually parallels the severity of the primary defect. The anomalies that have been associated with this syndrome are anomalies of the central nervous system, musculoskeletal system, genitourinary system and heart. Early prenatal diagnosis by ultrasonography is important and typically shows the absence of vertebrae in the caudal region of the fetal spine (Figure 15). In lumbosacral agenesis the umbilical cord generally contains three vessels. This is in

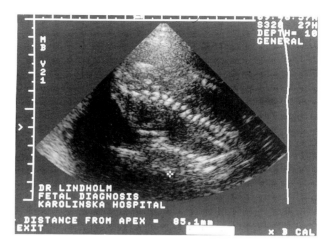

Figure 13 Multiple vertebral fusion defects in a fetus at 20 weeks gestational age with Jarcho–Levin syndrome

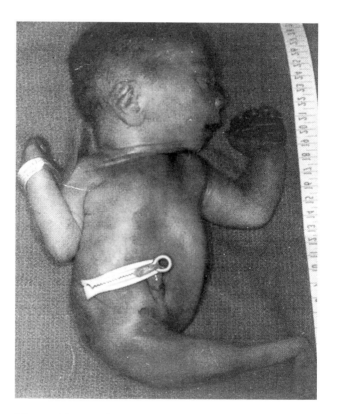

Figure 14 Newborn with sirenomelia syndrome

contrast to the two-vessel umbilical cord found typically in cases of sirenomelia, suggesting that sirenomelia is a separate entity, distinct from caudal regression syndrome[117] (Figure 16). Amnio-infusion and magnetic resonance imaging (MRI) may allow a better evaluation of the fetal anatomy in cases with severe oligohydramnios. The syndrome in general appears to have a low recurrence risk, although it is higher in diabetic women.

Sacral defect with anterior meningocele is a form of caudal dysgenesis. It is present at birth and becomes symptomatic later in life, usually because of obstructive labor in females, chronic constipation, rectal fistula and abscess, or meningitis. The inheritance is autosomal dominant. Demonstration by ultrasound of abrupt termination of the fetal lumbar spine together with smaller lower extremities would suggest the diagnosis of sacral agenesis.

SACROCOCCYGEAL TERATOMA

Sacrococcygeal teratoma, although rare, is the most common congenital tumor with a reported incidence of 1 in 35 000 to 40 000[118]. The tumor has a male to female ratio of 1:4 and is assumed to be derived from the multipotent cells of Hensen's node located anterior to the coccyx. Sacrococcygeal teratomas are usually benign. They are composed of a wide diversity of tissues not inherent to the sacrum and contain all three germ cell layers. Neuroglias are the most common histologic finding in these teratomas.

With the increase in utilization of prenatal ultrasonography the tumor is increasingly diagnosed *in utero*. On ultrasonography these tumors most often appear as heterogeneous complex masses external to the lower fetal pole[119]. In some cases they are mostly cystic and some are completely presacral with no external element. Sacrococcygeal teratomas have been classified according to their location following a system developed by Altman[120] and the American Academy of Pediatrics Surgical Section:

Type I: predominantly external tumor with minimal presacral involvement;
Type II: predominantly external tumor with significant intrapelvic component;
Type III: partially exterior tumor with predominantly intrapelvic and abdominal extensions;
Type IV: presacral and entirely interior with no external presentation.

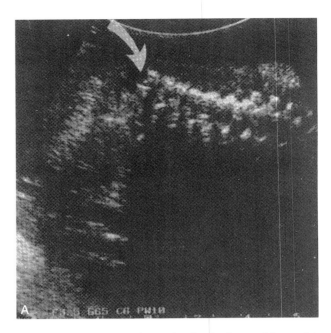

Figure 15   Absence of sacral spine in fetus with caudal regression syndrome

Presentation and differential diagnosis

The majority of sacrococcygeal teratomas are diagnosed on routine ultrasound examination. Depending on location of the mass the differential diagnosis differs[121] (Figure 17). In the presence of external masses the differential diagnosis includes myelomeningoceles, extrarenal Wilms' tumors, hamartomas, neuroblastomas and other soft tissue masses. With an internal, presacral location the differential diagnosis includes fetal ovarian cyst, rectal, bowel or bladder duplication, neuroblastoma, meconium pseudocyst and hydronephrosis. MSAFP can be elevated in these tumors but with experienced ultrasonographic examination they should be distinguished from NTDs.

Management and outcome

Most sacrococcygeal teratomas are external and benign. Prognosis is variable and although location is an important prognostic factor there are other issues involved. If the diagnosis is made early in pregnancy and any poor prognostic factors such as hydrops, placentomegaly or other anomalies are

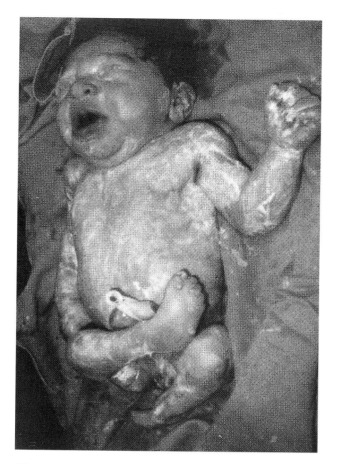

Figure 16 Classical 'buddha' posture of newborn with caudal regression syndrome

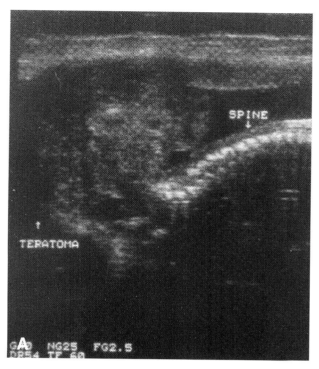

Figure 17 Ultrasonographic appearance of sacro-coccygeal teratoma of lower spine

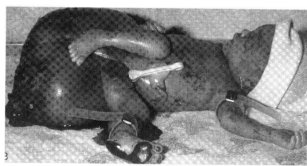

Figure 18 Newborn with large sacrococcygeal teratoma

demonstrated, pregnancy termination should be offered. In general the more solid tissue within the tumor, the higher the incidence of malignancy. Malignancy may also increase in type IV as diagnosis is often delayed in the absence of any external component[122]. In the absence of hydrops the fetus should be followed with serial ultrasound with the attempt to reach fetal lung maturity before delivery. As with any external fetal mass the mode of delivery is sometimes controversial. It is widely believed that in the case of sacrococcygeal teratomas, delivery should be by Cesarean section to avoid trauma and bleeding of the tumor. Immediate surgical intervention with complete excision of the mass is indicated as soon as the diagnosis is made postnatally (Figure 18).

NEW DIRECTIONS

With recent advances in technological development we are now faced with a new generation of ultrasound equipment: three-dimensional ultrasonography (chapter 20). This technology has the potential to greatly enhance our understanding of morphogenesis and improve the diagnosis of fetal

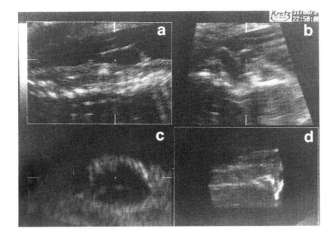

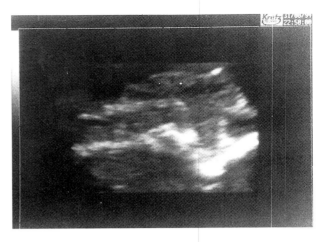

Figure 19 A 25.3-week fetus with a thoracic neural tube defect and meningomyelocele. (**a**) Sagittal view of the spine and meningomyelocele projecting up into the amniotic fluid. (**b**) Transverse view through the meningomyelocele and spinal defect. (**c**) Coronal view posterior to the spine through the meningomyelocele. (**d**) Three-dimensional reconstruction

Figure 20 The enlarged three-dimensional reconstruction of the fetus in Figure 19. The image illustrates the upper thoracic spine to the middle of the meningo-myelocele in a sagittal view

structural anomalies, in particular when the anatomy is complex. Multiplanar imaging of the fetal spine appears to be a useful technique. The entire length of the spinal column can be visualized in one frame and the exact level of any anomaly can be more easily determined[123] (Figures 19 and 20).

Ultrafast magnetic resonance imaging (MRI) is another new technology that, with its enhanced visualization of soft tissue and faster imaging, eliminates the effects of fetal movements on image reconstruction and thus the exact extent of a spinal abnormality and its content may be better delineated[124].

References

1. American Institute for Ultrasound in Medicine. Guidelines for performance of the antepartum obstetrical ultrasound examination. *J Ultrasound Med* 1991;10:577–8

2. American College of Obstetricians and Gynecologists. *Ultrasound in Pregnancy*. Washington, DC: ACOG Technical Bulletin Number 187, 1993

3. Seeds JW. The routine or screening obstetrical ultrasound examination. *Clin Obstet Gynecol* 1996;39:814–30

4. Goto MP, Goldman AS. Diabetic embryopathy. *Curr Opin Pediatr* 1994;6:486–91

5. Garner P. Type I diabetes mellitus and pregnancy. *Lancet* 1995;346:157–61

6. Samrén EB, Lindhout D. Major malformations associated with maternal use of antiepileptic drugs. In: Tomson T, Gram L, Sillanpää M, Johannessen SI, eds. *Epilepsy and Pregnancy*. Petersfield, UK, Bristol, PA, USA: Wrightson Biomedical Publishing Ltd, 1997:43–61

7. Howe AM, Webster WS. The warfarin embryopathy: a rat model showing maxillonasal hypoplasia and other skeletal disturbances. *Teratology* 1992;46:370–90

8. Ross HL, Elias S. Maternal serum screening for fetal genetic disorders. *Obstet Gynecol Clin N Am* 1997;34:33–47

9. O'Rahilly R, Muller F. *Human Embryology and Teratology*. New York: Wiley-Liss Inc., 1992

10. O'Rahilly R, Muller F. Neurulation in the normal human embryo. *Ciba Foundation Symposium* 1994;181:70–82

11. Van Allen MI, Kalousek DK, Chernoff GF, *et al.* Evidence of multi-site closure of the neural tube in humans. *Am J Med Genet* 1993;47:723–43

12. Seller MJ. Sex, neural tube defects, and multisite closure of the human neural tube. *Am J Med Genet* 1995;58:332–6

13. Bareggi R, Grill V, Zweyer M, *et al.* A quantitative study on the spatial and temporal ossification patterns of vertebral centra and neural arches and their relationship to the fetal age. *Anat Anzeiger* 1994;176:311–7

14. Bagnall KM, Harris PF, Jones PR. A radiographic study of the human fetal spine. II. The sequence of development of ossification centres in the vertebral column. *J Anat* 1977;124:791–802

15. Cochlin DL. Ultrasound of the fetal spine. *Clin Radiol* 1982;33:641–50

16. Filly RA, Simpson GF, Linkowski G. Fetal spine morphology and maturation during the second trimester. Sonographic evaluation. *J Ultrasound Med* 1987;6:631–6

17. Budorick NE, Pretorius DH, Grafe MR, *et al.* Ossification of the fetal spine. *Radiology* 1991;181:561–5

18. Pryse-Davies J, Smitham JH, Napier KA. Factors influencing development of secondary ossification centers in the fetus and newborn. A postmortem radiological study. *Arch Dis Child* 1974;49:425–31

19. Russell JGB. Radiological assessment of age, retardation and death. In Barson AJ, ed. *Laboratory Investigation of Fetal Disease*. Chicago: Yearbook Medical Publishers, 1981

20. Budorick NE, Pretorius DH, Nelson TR. Sonography of the fetal spine: technique, imaging findings, and clinical implications. *Am J Roentgenol* 1995;164:421–8

21. Weber TM, Hertzberg BS, Bowie JD. Use of endovaginal ultrasound to optimize visualization of the distal fetal spine in breech presentations. *J Ultrasound Med* 1990;9:519–24

22. Weber TM, Hertzberg BS, Bowie JD. Transperineal US: alternative technique to improve visualization of the presenting fetal part. *Radiology* 1991;179:747–50

23. Russ PD, Pretorius DH, Manco-Johnson ML, *et al.* The fetal spine. *Neuroradiology* 1986;28:398–407

24. Gray DL, Crane JP, Rudloff MA. Prenatal diagnosis of neural tube defects: origin of midtrimester vertebral ossification centers as determined by sonographic water-bath studies. *J Ultrasound Med* 1988;7:421–7

25. Dennis MA, Drose JA, Pretorius DH, *et al.* Normal fetal sacrum simulating spina bifida: 'pseudo-dysraphism'. *Radiology* 1985;155:751–4

26. Shiota K. Development and intrauterine fate of normal and abnormal human conceptuses. *Congenital Anom* 1991;31:67–80

27. Main DM, Mennuti MT. Neural tube defects: issues in prenatal diagnosis and counseling. *Obstet Gynecol* 1986;67:1–16

28. MRC Vitamin Study Research Group. Prevention of neural tube defects: results of the MRC vitamin study. *Lancet* 1991;338:132–7

29. Czeizel AE, Dudas I. Prevention of the first occurrence of neural-tube defects by periconceptional vitamin supplementation. *N Engl J Med* 1992;327:1832–5

30. Czeizel AE. Prevention of congenital abnormalities by periconceptional multivitamin supplementation. *Br Med J* 1993;306:1645–8

31. Holmes LB, Driscoll SG, Atkins L. Etiologic heterogeneity of neural tube defects. *N Engl J Med* 1976;294:365–9

32. Jones KL. *Smith's Recognizable Patterns of Human Malformation*, 4th ed. Philadelphia: WB Saunders, 1988:32–3

33. Hall JG. Give the embryo a chance. *Nature Med* 1997;24–5

34. Cuckle HS. Screening for neural tube defects. *Ciba Foundation Symposium* 1994;181:253–66

35. Watson WJ, Chescheir NC, Katz VL, *et al.* The role of ultrasound in evaluation of patients with elevated maternal serum alpha-fetoprotein: a review. *Obstet Gynecol* 1991;78:123–8

36. Platt LD, Feuchtbaum L, Filly RA, *et al.* The California maternal serum alpha-fetoprotein screening program: the role of ultrasonography in the detection of spina bifida. *Am J Obstet Gynecol* 1992;166:1328–9

37. Richards DS, Seeds JW, Katz VL, *et al.* Elevated maternal serum alpha-fetoprotein with normal ultrasound: is amniocentesis always appropriate? A review of 26 069 screened patients. *Obstet Gynecol* 1988;71:203–7

38. Nadel AS, Green JK, Holmes LB, *et al.* Absence of need for amniocentesis in patients with elevated levels of maternal serum alpha-fetoprotein and normal ultrasonographic examinations. *N Engl J Med* 1990;323:557–61

39. Anonymous. Sensitivity of ultrasound in detecting spina bifida. *N Engl J Med* 1991;324:769–72

40. Katz VL, Seeds JW, Albright SG, *et al.* Role of ultrasound and informed consent in the evaluation of elevated maternal serum alpha-fetoprotein. *Am J Perinatol* 1991;8:73–6

41. Morrow RJ, McNay MB, Whittle MJ. Ultrasound detection of neural tube defects in patients with elevated maternal serum alpha-fetoprotein. *Obstet Gynecol* 1991;78:1055–7

42. Dolk H, Seller MJ. Neural tube defects: a survey of lesion descriptions made by different European pathologists. *J Med Genet* 1993;30:942–6

43. Aicardi J. *Diseases of the Nervous System in Childhood*. London: McKeith Press, 1992

44. Carter CO, Evans KA, Till K. Spinal dysraphism: genetic relation to neural tube malformations. *J Med Genet* 1976;13:343–50

45. Medeira A, Dennis N, Donnai D. Anencephaly with spinal dysraphism, cleft lip and palate, and limb reduction defects. *Clin Dysmorph* 1994;3:270–5

46. Bamforth SJ, Baird PA. Spina bifida and hydrocephalus: a population study over a 35 year period. *Am J Hum Genet* 1989;44:225–32

47. Dolk H, De Wals P, Gillerot Y, *et al*. Heterogeneity of neural tube defects in Europe: the significance of other anomalies in relation to geographic differences in prevalence. *Teratology* 1991;44:547–59

48. Simpson JL, Mills J, Rhoads GG, *et al*. Genetic heterogeneity in neural tube defects. *Ann Genet* 1991;34:279–86

49. Czeizel AE. Schisis-association. *Am J Hum Genet* 1981;10:25–35

50. Nicolaides KH, Campbell S, Gabbe SG, *et al*. Ultrasound screening for spina bifida: cranial and cerebellar signs. *Lancet* 1986;2:72–4

51. Blumenfeld Z, Siegler E, Bronshtein M. The early diagnosis of neural tube defects. *Prenat Diagn* 1993;13:863–71

52. Campbell J, Gilbert WM, Nicolaides KH, *et al*. Ultrasound screening for spina bifida: cranial and cerebellar signs in a high-risk population. *Obstet Gynecol* 1987;70:247–50

53. Gabbe SG, Mintz MC, Mennuti MT, *et al*. Detection of open spina bifida by the lemon sign: pathologic correlation. *J Clin Ultrasound* 1988;16:399–402

54. Nyberg DA, Mack LA, Hirsch J, *et al*. Abnormalities of fetal cranial contour in sonographic detection of spina bifida: evaluation of the 'lemon' sign. *Radiology* 1988;167:387–92

55. Benacerraf BR, Stryker J, Frigoletto FD Jr. Abnormal US appearance of the cerebellum (banana sign): indirect sign of spina bifida. *Radiology* 1989;171:151–3

56. Van den Hof MC, Nicolaides KH, Campbell J, *et al*. Evaluation of the lemon and banana signs in one hundred thirty fetuses with open spina bifida. *Am J Obstet Gynecol* 1990;162:322–7

57. Thiagarajah S, Henke J, Hogge WA, *et al*. Early diagnosis of spina bifida: the value of cranial ultrasound markers. *Obstet Gynecol* 1990;76:54–7

58. Ball RH, Filly RA, Goldstein RB, *et al*. The lemon sign: not a specific indicator of meningomyelocele. *J Ultrasound Med* 1993;12:131–4

59. Johnson DD, Nager CW, Budorick NE. False-positive diagnosis of spina bifida in a fetus with triploidy. *Obstet Gynecol* 1997;89:809–11

60. Pang D, Hoffman HJ, Rekate HL. Split cord malformation. Part 2: clinical syndrome. *Neurosurgery* 1992;31:481–500

61. Kapsalakis Z. Diastematomyelia in two sisters. *J Neurosurg* 1964;21:66–7

62. Gardner WJ. The dysraphic states from syringomyelia to anencephaly. Amsterdam: Excerpta Medica, 1973:89–94

63. Sepulveda W, Kyle PM, Hassan J, *et al*. Prenatal diagnosis of diastematomyelia: case reports and review of the literature. *Prenat Diagn* 1997;17:161–5

64. Anderson NG. Diastematomyelia: diagnosis by prenatal sonography. *Am J Roentgenol* 1994;163:911–4

65. Seeds JW, Powers SK. Early prenatal diagnosis of familial lipomeningocele. *Obstet Gynecol* 1988;72:469–71

66. Spranger J. International classification of osteochondrodysplasias. The International Group on Constitutional Diseases of Bone. *Eur J Pediatr* 1992;151:407–15

67. Gunderson CH, Greenspan RH, Glaser GH, *et al*. The Klippel–Feil syndrome: genetic and clinical reevaluation of cervical fusion. *Medicine* 1967;46:491–512

68. Raas-Rothschild A, Goodman RM, Grunbaum M, *et al*. Klippel–Feil anomaly with sacral agenesis: an additional subtype, type IV. *J Craniofac Genet Dev Biol* 1988;8:297–301

69. Juberg RC, Gershanik JJ. Cervical vertebral fusion (Klippel–Feil) syndrome with consanguineous parents. *J Med Genet* 1976;13:246–9

70. da-Silva EO. Autosomal recessive Klippel–Feil syndrome. *J Med Genet* 1982;19:130–4

71. Clarke RA, Singh S, McKenzie H, *et al*. Familial Klippel–Feil syndrome and paracentric inversion (8)(q22.2q22.3). *Am J Hum Genet* 1995;57:1364–70

72. Goldberg MJ. *The Dysmorphic Child: an Orthopedic Perspective*. New York: Raven Press, 1987

73. Wildervanck LS. Een Cervico-oculo-acusticus-syndroom. *Nederl T Geneesk* 1960;104:2600–5

74. Everberg G, Ratjen E, Sorensen H. Wildervanck's syndrome: Klippel–Feil's syndrome associated with deafness and retraction of the eyeball. *Br J Radiol* 1963;36:562–7

75. Fraser WI, MacGillivray RC. Cervico-oculo-acoustic dysplasia ('the syndrome of Wildervanck'). *J Ment Defic Res* 1968;12:322–9

76. Wettke-Schafter R, Kantner G. X-linked dominant inherited diseases with lethality in hemizygous males. *Hum Genet* 1983;64:1–23

77. Cremers CWRJ, Hoogland GA, Kuypers W. Hearing loss in the cervico-oculo-acoustic (Wildervanck) syndrome. *Arch Otolaryng* 1984;110:54–7

78. Konigsmark BW, Gorlin RJ. *Genetic and Metabolic Deafness*. Philadelphia: WB Saunders, 1976:189

79. Wildervanck LS. The cervico-oculo-acusticus syndrome. In: Vinken PJ, Bruyn GW, Myranthopoulos NC, eds. *Handbook of Clinical Neurology*. Amsterdam: North Holland, 1978;32:123–30

80. Harrison LA, Pretorius DH, Budorick NE. Abnormal spinal curvature in the fetus. *J Ultrasound Med* 1992;11:473–9

81. Benacerraf BR, Greene MF, Barss VA. Prenatal sonographic diagnosis of congenital hemivertebrae. *J Ultrasound Med* 1986;5:257–9

82. Zelop CM, Pretorius DH, Benacerraf BR. Fetal hemivertebrae: associated anomalies, significance, and outcome. *Obstet Gynecol* 1993;81:412–6

83. Mortier GR, Lachman RS, Bocian M, et al. Multiple vertebral segmentation defects: analysis of 26 new patients and review of the literature. *Am J Med Genet* 1996;61:310–9

84. Van Allen MI, Curry C, Gallagher L. Limb body wall complex: I. Pathogenesis. *Am J Med Genet* 1987;28:529–48

85. Van Allen MI, Curry C, Walden CE, et al. Limb body wall complex: II. Limb and spine defects. *Am J Med Genet* 1987;28:549–65

86. Bamforth JS. Amniotic band sequence: Streeter's hypothesis reexamined. *Am J Med Genet* 1992;44:280–7

87. Quan L, Smith DW. The VATER association: vertebral defects, anal atresia, tracheoesophageal fistula with esophageal atresia, radial dysplasia. *Birth Defects Orig Art Ser* 1972;8:75–8

88. Weaver DD, Mapstone CL, Yu P. The VATER association: analysis of 46 patients. *Am J Dis Child* 1986;140:225–9

89. Braun-Quentin C, Billes C, Böwing B, et al. MURCS association: case report and review. *J Med Genet* 1996;33:618–20

90. Auchterlonie IA, White MP. Recurrence of the VATER association within a sibship. *Clin Genet* 1982;21:122–4

91. Iafolla AK, McConkie-Rosell A, Chen YT. VATER and hydrocephalus: distinct syndrome? *Am J Med Genet* 1991;38:46–51

92. Khoury MJ, Cordero JF, Greenberg F, et al. A population study of the VACTERL association: evidence for its etiologic heterogeneity. *Pediatrics* 1983;71:815–20

93. Damian MS, Seibel P, Schachenmayr W, et al. VACTERL with the mitochondrial NP 3243 point mutation. *Am J Med Genet* 1996;62:398–403

94. Duncan PA, Shapiro LR, Stangel JJ, et al. The MURCS association: mullerian duct aplasia, renal aplasia, and cervicothoracic somite dysplasia. *J Pediatr* 1979;95:399–402

95. Lin HJ, Cornford ME, Hu B, et al. Occipital encephalocele and MURCS association: case report and review of central nervous system anomalies in MURCS patients. *Am J Med Genet* 1995;61:59–62

96. Rodriguez JI, Palacios J, Lapunzina P. Severe axial anomalies in the oculo-auriculo-vertebral (Goldenhar) complex. *Am J Med Genet* 1993;47:69–74

97. Wilson MG, Miksity VG, Shinno NW. Dominant inheritance of Sprengel's deformity. *J Pediatr* 1971;79:818–21

98. Hodgson SV, Chiu DC. Dominant transmission of Sprengel's shoulder and cleft palate. *J Med Genet* 1981;18:263–5

99. Bouwes Bavinck JN, Weaver DD. Subclavian artery supply disruption sequence: hypothesis of a vascular etiology for Poland, Klippel–Feil, and Moebius anomalies. *Am J Med Genet* 1986;23:903–18

100. Jarcho S, Levin PM. Hereditary malformation of the vertebral bodies. *Bull Johns Hopkins Hosp* 1938;62:216–26

101. Mortier GR, Lachman RS, Bocian M, et al. Multiple vertebral segmentation defects: analysis of 26 new patients and review of the literature. *Am J Med Genet* 1996;61:310–19

102. Karnes PS, Day D, Berry SA, et al. Jarcho–Levin syndrome: four new cases and classification of subtypes. *Am J Med Genet* 1991;40:264–70

103. Aurora P, Wallis CE, Winter RM. The Jarcho–Levin syndrome (spondylocostal dysplasia) and complex congenital heart disease: a case report. *Clin Dysmorph* 1996;5:165–9

104. Turnpenny PD, Thwaites RJ, Boulos FN. Evidence for variable gene expression in a large inbred kindred with autosomal recessive spondylocostal dysostosis. *J Med Genet* 1991;28:27–33

105. Lorenz P, Rupprecht E. Spondylocostal dysostosis: dominant type. *Am J Med Genet* 1990;35:219–21

106. Apuzzio JJ, Diamond N, Ganesh V, et al. Difficulties in the prenatal diagnosis of Jarcho–Levin syndrome. *Am J Obstet Gynecol* 1987;156:916–8

107. Marks F, Hernanzz-Schulman M, Horii S, et al. Spondylothoracic dysplasia. Clinical and sonographic diagnosis. *J Ultrasound Med* 1989;8:1–5

108. Poor MA, Alberti O, Griscom NT, et al. Nonskeletal malformations in one of three siblings with Jarcho-Levin syndrome of vertebral anomalies. *J Pediatr* 1983;103:270–2

109. Tolmie JL, Whittle MJ, McNay MB, et al. Second trimester prenatal diagnosis of the Jarcho–Levin syndrome. *Prenat Diagn* 1987;7:129–34

110. Romero R, Ghidini A, Eswarara MS, et al. Prenatal findings in a case of spondylocostal dysplasia type I (Jarcho–Levin syndrome). *Obstet Gynecol* 1988;71:988–91

111. Lenoir S, Rolland M, Sarramon MF, et al. Diagnostic prénatal échographique due syndrome de Jarco–Levin. *J Génét Hum* 1989;37:425–30

112. Tachibana K, Yamamoto Y, Osaki E, et al. Cerebro-costo-mandibular syndrome: a case report and review of the literature. *Hum Genet* 1980;54:283–6

113. Merlob P, Schonfeld A, Grunebaum A, et al. Autosomal dominant cerebro-costo-mandibular syndrome: ultrasonographic and clinical findings. *Am J Med Genet* 1987;26:195–202

114. Adra A, Cordero D, Mejides A, et al. Caudal regression syndrome: etiopathogenesis, prenatal diagnosis, and perinatal management. *Obstet Gynecol Surv* 1994;49:508–16

115. Källen B, Castilla EE, Lancaster PA, *et al*. The cyclops and the mermaid: an epidemiological study of two types of rare malformation. *J Med Genet* 1992;29:30–5

116. Jaffe R, Zeituni M, Fejgin M. Caudal regression syndrome. *Fetus* 1991;4:1–4

117. Twickler D, Budorick N, Pretorius D, *et al*. Caudal regression versus sirenomelia: sonographic clues. *J Ultrasound Med* 1993;12:323–30

118. Gross RE, Clatworthy HW, Meeker IA. Sacrococcygeal teratoma in infants and children. *Surg Gynecol Obstet* 1951;92:341–5

119. Holzgreve W, Miny P, Anderson R. Experience with 8 cases of prenatally diagnosed sacrococcygeal teratomas. *Fetal Therapy* 1987;2:88–94

120. Altman RP, Randolph JG, Lilly JR. Sacrococcygeal teratoma: American Academy of Pediatrics Surgical Section Survey-1973. *J Pediatr Surg* 1973;9:389–98

121. Shipp TD, Shamberger RC, Benacerraf BR. Prenatal diagnosis of a Grade IV sacrococcygeal teratoma. *J Ultrasound Med* 1996;15:175–7

122. Winderl LM, Silverman RK. Prenatal identification of a complete cystic internal sacrococcygeal teratoma (Type IV). *Ultrasound Obstet Gynecol* 1997;9:425–8

123. Mueller GM, Weiner CP, Yankowitz J. Three-dimensional ultrasound in the evaluation of fetal head and spine anomalies. *Obstet Gynecol* 1996;88:372–8

124. Colleti PM. Computer assisted imaging of the fetus with magnetic resonance imaging. *Comput Med Imag Graphics* 1996;20:491–6

Hydrops fetalis

14

Shyla Vengalil, William J. Meyer and Joaquin Santolaya-Forgas

Fetal hydrops represents a condition characterized by pathologic accumulation of fluid within fetal extravascular spaces. This fluid accumulation represents the clinical manifestation of an underlying disorder of fetal water balance[1]. The clinical presentation of fetal hydrops is variable both in onset and severity depending on the gestational age and etiology. The prognosis in most cases is poor. However, there are some cases of hydrops fetalis which may resolve spontaneously or can be successfully treated *in utero*.

Fetal hydrops has been generally classified as immune or non-immune (Figure 1). Immune hydrops results from maternal alloimmunization to fetal antigens[2]. The basic pathologic mechanism of immune hydrops is progressive fetal anemia leading to congestive heart failure and death. Non-immune hydrops occurs when there is no evidence of maternal alloimmunization. The incidence of non-immune hydrops has been estimated from 1 : 1500 to 1 : 3700 births[3]. Potential causes of non-immune fetal hydrops include genetic diseases, congenital infections, and anatomic abnormalities of the fetus, placenta or umbilical cord (Figure 1).

Ultrasonography is the method by which fetal hydrops is diagnosed. Once recognized, it is important to determine the etiology and to evaluate fetal hemodynamic and, sometimes, metabolic status. Advances in animal research, ultrasound technology, and invasive fetal testing have helped in understanding the pathophysiology of hydrops fetalis in relation to the precise etiology. This in turn has become important in counseling the patients with regards to the prognosis and recurrence risk. Knowledge of the primary etiology will allow the physician to determine if an aggressive clinical strategy is indicated or, in cases with dismal fetal prognosis, to avoid potential maternal morbidity such as that related to cesarean delivery for fetal distress. Immune and genetically mediated cases of hydrops may recur while other causes rarely do.

There are several recent texts on the topic of hydrops fetalis, with particular emphasis on the clinical aspects. No attempt will be made here to duplicate all aspects of those sources and the clinical detail they provide, and the interested reader is referred to those sources for further information[1,2]. In this chapter, we will concentrate on the ultrasonographic techniques used to diagnose and evaluate a fetus with hydrops.

ULTRASONOGRAPHIC DIAGNOSIS OF HYDROPS FETALIS

The ultrasonographic diagnosis of hydrops is not difficult. The hallmark feature of fetal hydrops is the finding of fluid in fetal extravascular tissue. This occurs either in fetal subcutaneous tissue or in more than two serous body cavities. Isolated fluid collections such as ascites, pleural or pericardial effusions may represent a pre-hydropic state or may be related to a specific fetal condition that may not progress to hydrops fetalis.

Skin edema is an ominous finding in patients with hydrops[4] regardless of the etiology. A fetus is hydropic when the skin thickness exceeds 5 mm. Skin edema is usually measured in a transverse view of the fetal abdomen or head (Figure 2).

Fetal ascites may be detected by identifying sonolucent areas surrounding bowel loops or outlining the intra-abdominal umbilical vein[5–7]. The fluid provides very clear definition of intra-abdominal structures which are not appreciated in the normal fetus (Figures 3 and 4). True ascites must be differentiated from pseudoascites which gives the appearance of sonolucent fluid within the fetal abdomen[8,9]. The latter is always seen at the periphery of the abdomen or retroperitoneal space and does not outline intra-abdominal structures such as the bowel or umbilical vein. As the amount of ascitic fluid increases the diagnosis is straightforward: the abdomen will progressively enlarge, the bowel loops will be outlined, the umbilical vein and falciform ligament will straighten out and the liver will appear suspended from these structures. In severe cases, the small bowel will freely float in fluid and the omental sacs become visible.

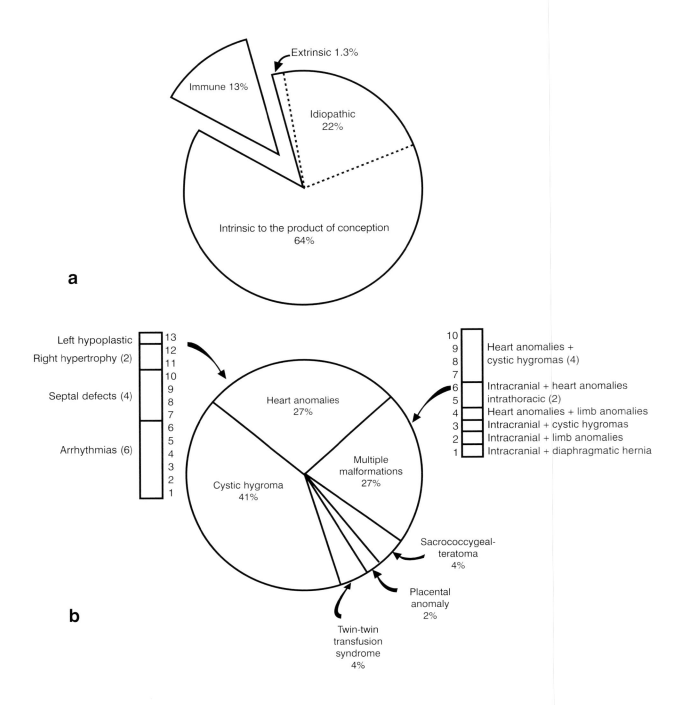

Figure 1 Distribution of immune and non-immune cases of fetal hydrops in which the etiology could be diagnosed by ultrasound. Intrinsic: origin in the product of conception; extrinsic: origin outside the product of conception; idiopathic: no etiologic factor found. (**a**) Ultrasonographic classification of fetal hydrops (n = 76). (**b**) Ultrasonographic findings in fetal hydrops due to causes intrinsic to the product of conception

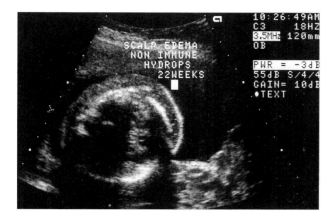

Figure 2 Fetal skin edema can be noted at the level of the head

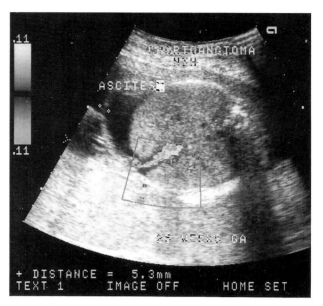

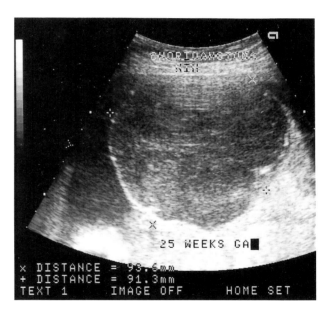

Figure 3 The intrahepatic portion of the umbilical vein can easily be visualized in a fetus with hydrops due to a placental chorioangioma (lower panel)

Pleural effusions are diagnosed by visualizing sonolucent spaces between the inner chest wall and the fetal lung[10]. They are most commonly found at the base of the lung. The diagnosis is best made using a cross sectional or sagittal view of the fetal thorax (Figure 5). Fluid on both sides of the diaphragm will make the diagnosis easier.

Pericardial effusions are diagnosed by imaging the fetal thorax sagittally and transversely[11]. Small amounts of fluid surrounding the heart can be normal after 20 weeks gestation. Sonolucent spaces within the pericardium may also be observed during fetal systole on two dimensional real-time imaging and should not be confused with true pericardial effusions. Both two dimensional and M-mode images can be used to document effusions. A pathologic pericardial effusion has been defined as a sonolucent ring of pericardial fluid exceeding 2 mm in diameter[12] (Figure 6).

There are other findings that may be seen in association with hydrops fetalis. Hepatospleno-megaly is most commonly seen in immune hydrops but can also occur in some cases of non-immune hydrops. Hepatomegaly is diagnosed by measuring the sagittal length of the right lobe of the liver and comparing with established nomograms[13]. This can be a technically difficult measurement to obtain and some disagreement exists regarding the value of liver size measurements in predicting the severity of fetal anemia in the immune type of hydrops. Nicolaides et al.[14] found no correlation between liver size and fetal anemia, while Vintzileos et al.[15] showed that increases of 5 mm per week in liver length correlated well with severe anemia and the need for transfusion within 2 weeks of the examination. The usefulness of this measurement in the assessment of the hydropic fetus remains questionable[14-16].

Skin edema, placental edema and polyhydramnios are frequently associated. Polyhydramnios has been suggested to occur prior to frank hydrops in cases of alloimmunization. Amniotic fluid volume can be assessed by both qualitative and quantitative

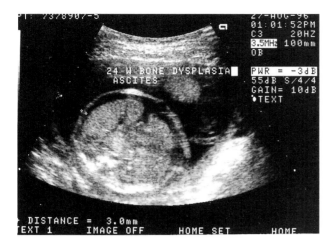

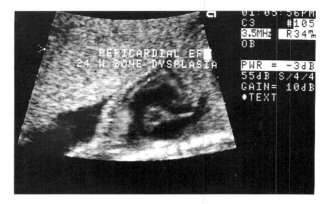

Figure 6 Pericardial effusion was noted in a hydropic fetus due to a severe bone dysplasia with thoracic hypoplasia

Figure 4 The fetal liver and bowel are well delineated in this hydropic fetus

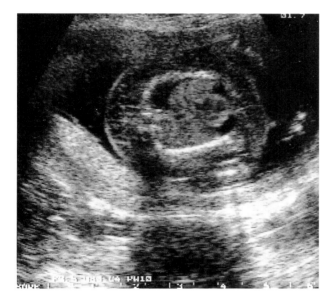

Figure 5 Skin edema and bilateral hydro-thorax can be noted in this hydropic fetus due to cystic hygromas (not shown) and Turner syndrome (45,X)

means. The four quadrant amniotic fluid index (AFI) is the most commonly used method after 20 weeks gestational age[17]. This method involves dividing the uterus into four quadrants and measuring the maximal vertical pocket of fluid in each quadrant. Polyhydramnios is diagnosed when the AFI exceeds 20 cm or is greater than the 95th centile for that gestational age[18]. Subjectively polyhydramnios is diagnosed when the fetal abdomen fails to touch both the anterior and posterior wall

of the uterus in the third trimester. The authors prefer to use the AFI when following patients with polyhydramnios. Placental edema may also occur causing an increase in its thickness. A placental thickness greater than 4 cm is considered abnormal[19]. However, placental thickness varies with the location, gestational age and amniotic fluid volume and hence limits the sensitivity of this parameter in predicting hydrops. Sonographically, edema of the placenta gives it a ground glass appearance with disappearance of the chorionic plate, loss of cotyledon formation and buckling of the fetal surface[20]. It should be remembered that all of these associated findings are symptoms of a primary problem occurring within the fetus itself who is having problems maintaining water homeostasis.

HEMODYNAMIC ASSESSMENT OF THE HYDROPIC FETUS

Hutchinson classified the etiologies of hydrops based on the physiologic mechanisms[21]. Alterations in hydrostatic pressure, colloid osmotic pressure, cardiac output, venous and lymphatic drainage and membrane permeability all contribute to the clinical manifestation of hydrops. Fetal edema and hydrops may reflect or lead to chronic congestive heart failure.

Doppler velocimetry has become useful in assessing fetal hemodynamic function and prognosis[22,23]. Fetal bradycardia and tachyarrhythmias can be diagnosed with conventional Doppler echocardiography. Hydrops can occur as a result

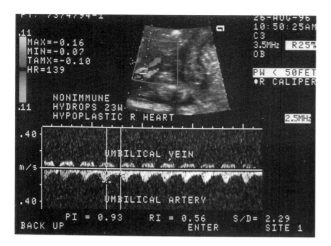

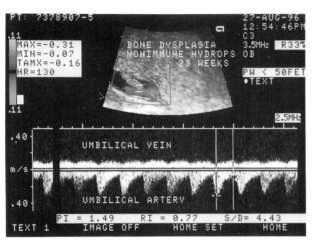

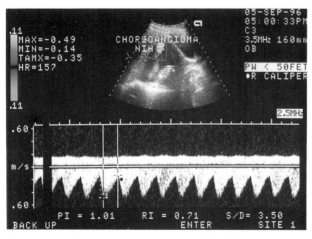

Figure 7 All three panels show umbilical blood velocity waveforms in three very similar fetuses of the same gestational age. Upper panel demonstrates severe umbilical venous pulsation in a fetus with hypoplastic right heart, mid-panel demonstrates less severe umbilical venous pulsation in a fetus with bone dysplasia and a restrictive thoracic pattern, and lower panel shows normal vein waveforms in a fetus with a placental chorioangioma (see Color plate 22)

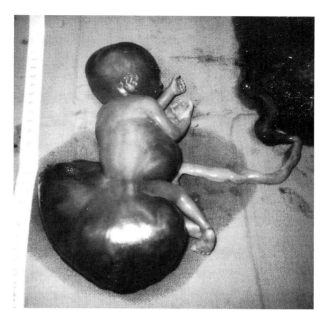

Figure 8 Fetal tumors such as sacrococcygeal teratomas can cause non-immune fetal hydrops

of altered ventricular filling time, ejection fraction or reduced or absent atrial contractions which can be assessed with real-time, B- or M-mode imaging. These techniques allow for documentation of heart rate, fractional shortening index and valvular excursion during systole. Arterial blood impedance, a measure of cardiac afterload, may be assessed by measuring different pulsatility indices in the umbilical and fetal arterial vascular beds[24]. In addition, Doppler velocimetry can assess the status of the fetal venous system, which is useful in evaluating the degree of congestive heart failure (Figure 7, Color plate 22). This involves assessment of the character of the blood velocity waveforms in the inferior vena cava (IVC), umbilical vein and ductus venosus[25–28]. Clinically, assessment includes calculation of the peak velocity, minimum velocity and the time-averaged maximum velocity during a cardiac cycle. In the normal fetus there is continuous forward flow within the venous system during diastole. Umbilical venous velocities are monophasic during fetal apnea with average flow rates of approximately 120 ml/kg/min in the second and third trimesters. Assessment of the IVC is normally performed in a sagittal plane where the IVC is seen entering the right atrium[26]. A triphasic waveform is obtained reflecting systolic flow, diastolic ventricular filling, and a small retrograde wave secondary to atrial contraction.

The ratio of flow velocity during systole and diastole is constant throughout gestation at 3.5 to 3.7. The ratio of reverse flow with atrial contraction relative to forward flow during systole and early diastole should be less than 10%. Velocities within the ductus venosus range between 65 and 75 cm/s and are highest during ventricular systole and lower during diastole[28,29]. There is normally a continuous forward flow, even during atrial contraction when the lowest velocities occur (30–40 cm/s).

Reversal of flow within the venous system is typical of fetal congestive heart failure. With progressive congestive heart failure, central venous pressure is elevated which then reduces the venous velocities. In contrast, increased resistance to flow within the liver causes portal hypertension and subsequently increased velocities within the ductus venosus. In a study of 24 cases of non-immune hydrops, Tulzer *et al.*[30] found that perinatal death was associated with a high percentage of retrograde flow in the IVC, decreased IVC E/V ratio and the presence of umbilical venous pulsations. Gudmundsson *et al.*[31] and other investigators have also confirmed that the presence of umbilical venous pulsations carries a grave prognosis for the fetus and may also help define the etiology of hydrops. Those hydropic fetuses with umbilical vein pulsations are felt to have functional cardiac abnormalities while those without umbilical venous pulsations have other causes of hydrops such as placental chorioangiomas (Figure 8).

MANAGEMENT OF IMMUNE FETAL HYDROPS

Immune fetal hydrops implies a maternal antibody response to a foreign fetal antigen. Hydrops occurs when this fetal antigen is expressed on the red blood cell membrane and the maternal antibody (IgG) attached to the fetal blood cell membrane leads to hemolysis and anemia.

The frequency of potential incompatible materno-fetal antigens in humans varies depending on ethnicity. However, approximately 97% of all cases of immune fetal hydrops are caused by maternal alloimmunization against the Rh(D) antigen present in the fetal red blood cells[32]. Despite the use of anti-D immunoprophylaxis in Rh (D) negative women and the dramatic advances made in the field of fetal medicine alloimmunizations

due to incompatible blood group systems remains a clinical problem[33]. Causes of immune hydrops include alloimmunization to other fetal blood group antigens such as C, c, E, e, K, k, Fya, M, and Jka[34]. Rare cases of immune hydrops have been described due to ABO incompatibility[35].

The pathophysiology of immune fetal hydrops is related to progressive fetal anemia leading to tissue hypoxia, acidosis, hepatic and cardiac failure. The fetus responds to anemia by increasing hematopoiesis and by adjusting hemodynamically to facilitate oxygen delivery to tissues[36]. Since the main erythropoietic tissues vary through pregnancy, the increase in hematopoiesis may lead to secondary effects reflecting the abnormal function of the organ that has been superactivated as erythropoietic tissue. Gestational age at which anemia occurs and acuteness of the process are, therefore, important parameters to consider when analyzing fetal adaptive mechanisms to anemia. These two factors also explain the different sequences in which the ultrasonographic hydropic signs may occur in anemic fetuses.

Failure of fetal adaptive mechanisms to anemia results in hypoxemia, acidemia, hypoproteinemia and increased capillary permeability with extravasation of fluids into different body cavities. In anemic fetuses it is not uncommon to find hepatomegaly, impaired hepatocyte function and decreased fetal serum concentration of albumin and total proteins[37,38]. The metabolic dysfunction of the fetal hepatocyte is thought to be related both to hypoxia and to the progressive compression of the hepatocyte and hepatic sinusoids by the hyperplastic erythropoietic tissue. Fetal hypoproteinemia may also result from increased protein transfer to the interstitium through damaged endothelial vascular cells secondary to hypoxemia. Very anemic fetuses develop acidemia[39]. Severe hypoxemia and acidemia may result in myocardial insufficiency and cardiac failure[40]. Hypervolemia and subsequent increased hydrostatic pressure in cases of high output cardiac failure should also contribute to the extravasation of fluids[41,42].

Alloimmunization is diagnosed when the indirect Coombs test is positive. Classically, serial titers were obtained and if they reached the critical level of 1 : 16 after 25 weeks gestation, an amniocentesis was recommended to determine the concentration of bilirubin in the amniotic fluid (delta O.D. 450). Today, at any gestational age, fetal Rh (D), C, c, E, e, and Kell status can be determined by analysis of fetal cells obtained after a chorionic villous sampling or amniocentesis using the polymerase chain reaction (PCR) technique[43]. If the alloimmunization is against an antigen for which molecular diagnostic techniques are not yet available, serial ultrasounds and amniotic fluid delta O.D. 450 determinations remain the way to determine the need for performing fetal blood sampling to determine fetal blood group and hemoglobin concentration. The fetus is unlikely to become hydropic until the fetal hemoglobin is less than 5 g/l.

Ultrasound-guided intravascular fetal transfusion is the treatment of choice for anemic fetuses and has been successfully performed after 17 weeks of gestational age. The techniques for fetal transfusions have been well described. The overall survival rate in fetuses undergoing intravascular transfusion for Rh alloimmunization has been reported to be around 96%[44] and 85% for hydropic fetuses.

MANAGEMENT OF NON-IMMUNE FETAL HYDROPS

The term non-immune hydrops fetalis (NIH) describes all those hydropic fetuses in whom no evidence of maternal–fetal blood group incompatibility exists. Currently, it is the largest group of recognized cases of hydrops and the list of reported etiologies is extensive. Cardiac abnormalities, chromosomal aneuploidies in association with congenital anomalies and recognizable syndromes represent the largest subgroups of NIH. Less common causes included twin to twin transfusion syndrome, pulmonary–gastro intestinal–genitourinary abnormalities, neoplastic conditions and congenital infections[45–49] (Figure 8).

Most NIH series report that in 40–50% of cases of hydrops there is an identifiable etiology. However, according to Holzgreve and colleagues[50,51], a careful evaluation can identify as many as 84% of the cases. Although the etiology of NIH may be recognized in many cases, the exact pathophysiological mechanism is not always understood.

NIH is usually detected after referral to a fetal medicine unit due to causes such as uterus fundus height/dates discrepancy or decreased fetal movements. Occasionally it is detected on a routine ultrasonographic evaluation requested for morphologic fetal assessment or determination of fetal growth: in one series, 63% of all cases of NIH were discovered on routine ultrasonography and 30% were referred for suspected polyhydramnios[52]. While polyhydramnios is frequently associated with fetal hydrops there are cases in which oligohydramnios occurs.

Once the immune type of hydrops is ruled out, a systematic approach investigating all the potential causes of NIH is necessary. A detailed medical and genetic history should be obtained including history of prior pregnancy losses, congenital anomalies, consanguinity, ethnicity and racial background. Also important is a history of recent maternal infections or exposure to chemicals or drugs.

A detailed survey of fetal anatomy is essential to establish the etiology of non-immune hydrops. Since fetal cardiac anomalies are the most common cause of NIH, a fetal echocardiogram should be performed. Fetal tachyarrhythmia, most commonly supraventricular tachycardia, leading to hydrops fetalis may be intermittent and can be missed by a single ultrasound scan. If suspected, prolonged tococardiography to rule out intermittent tachyarrhythmia is necessary. If arrhythmia or myocarditis is suspected, a viral etiology should be considered. Fetal bradycardia is often detected in mothers who have clinical evidence of collagen disorders or the presence of anti-Ro antibodies[53]. Complete fetal heart block occurs in approximately 15% of patients who have anti-Ro antibodies and the risk increases to 33% if the mother has already had a child with congenital heart block[54].

Maternal blood studies should include a complete blood count with differential and indices, glucose levels, Kleihauer-Betke smear for fetal hemoglobin identification, acute phase titers for toxoplasmosis, cytomegalovirus, parvovirus B19, serological test for syphilis, hemoglobin electrophoresis and glucose-6 phosphate dehydrogenase enzyme levels.

Ultrasound-guided invasive diagnostic procedures such as amniocentesis, chorionic villus sampling and fetal blood sampling are used for accurate determination of the etiology. Fetal blood sampling has the advantage of allowing karyotypic analysis as well as evaluation of the hematological, biochemical and metabolic status. Serological testing and PCR studies can also be performed on fetal blood. The sensitivity of cytomegalovirus IgM antibody detection in fetal blood is 69%[55]. On the other hand amniotic fluid cultures and/or PCR studies have a sensitivity of 81–100% and a specificity close to 100% in diagnosing presence of cytomegalovirus after 22 weeks[56–59]. It is important to counsel the patients about the role of fetal blood sampling and its attendant risks since in NIH the procedure may be associated with a fetal loss rate of up to 25%[60].

The perinatal mortality of NIH in most published series ranges between 50 and 98%[52,61]. In cases of hydrops detected prior to fetal viability, pregnancy termination may be offered as the prognosis is poor regardless of the etiology. In many cases no effective intrauterine therapy exists. In patients who continue the pregnancy, careful follow-up is indicated to determine whether early intervention in terms of delivery is in the best interests of the fetus.

MATERNAL COMPLICATIONS DUE TO FETAL HYDROPS

In rare cases, maternal complications related to non-immune fetal hydrops can occur. These include pre-eclampsia, anemia, retained placenta and postpartum hemorrhage. A very interesting complication is the Ballentyne syndrome[62], mirror syndrome, pseudotoxemia[63], or triple edema[64]. It is a 'pre-eclampsia like' disease in which the mother exhibits typical symptoms of pre-eclampsia characterized by excessive fluid accumulation and often hypertension. This syndrome can be associated with low hematocrit, as opposed to the hemoconcentration usually seen in pre-eclampsia. The etiology of this maternal hydrops syndrome is unknown although it may be associated with a large placental mass[65]. The authors have seen this in patients with maternal parvovirus B19 infection, fetal sacrococcygeal teratoma and alloimmunization. In cases of parvovirus infection, the condition may be managed conservatively and may resolve with good prognosis for the fetus and mother[66,67].

POSTPARTUM EVALUATION OF THE HYDROPIC FETUS

Following delivery of hydropic fetuses, neonatal evaluation and if necessary autopsy may identify the etiology not previously suspected. If the parents do not wish an autopsy, permission for skin biopsy and needle biopsy of the liver should be attempted and taken as soon as possible. The skin biopsy can be used to establish a fibroblast culture for biochemical and DNA analysis of inherited disorders. Liver tissue should be frozen immediately in liquid nitrogen and stored at $-70°F$[68]. Liver tissue is valuable for iron quantification and for other enzyme assays.

Other helpful investigations include skeletal radiographs and clinical photographs. The placenta should be sent fresh to the histopathology laboratory and not placed in formalin. All these tests may not be indicated in every case of hydrops. Clinical judgment is of utmost value in getting appropriate specimens and studies. However, identification of inborn errors of metabolism or aneuploidy may alter the risk of recurrence and will help the parents make appropriate decisions regarding future pregnancies.

CONCLUSIONS

Hydrops fetalis is diagnosed using ultrasonographic studies. A detailed prenatal and postnatal diagnostic evaluation of the hydropic fetus will very likely elicit an etiology. Hydrops due to maternal alloimmunization may have an excellent outcome. Most cases of non-immune hydrops can not be effectively treated *in utero*. However, effective parental counseling when confronted with NIH requires understanding of the etiology and potential outcome in these cases.

References

1. Santolaya J, Warsof SL. Hydrops and associated anomalies. In Brock DJ, Rodeck CH, Ferguson-Smith MA, eds. *Prenatal Diagnosis and Screening.* Edinburgh: Churchill Livingstone, 1993;329–47
2. Rodeck CH, Santolaya J, Nicolini U. Management of the fetus with immune hydrops. In Harrison MR, Golbus S, Filly RA, eds. *The Unborn Patient. Prenatal Diagnosis and Treatment;* 2nd edn. Philadelphia: WB Saunders, 1990;215–27
3. Im SS, Rizos N, Joutsi P, *et al.* Nomimmunologic hydrops fetalis. *Am J Obstet Gynecol* 1984;148: 566–9

4. Warsof SL, Nicolaides KH, Rodeck C. Immune and non-immune hydrops. *Clin Obstet Gynecol* 1986;29: 533–42

5. Cederqvist LL, Williams LR, Symchych PS, *et al.* Prenatal diagnosis of fetal ascites by ultrasound. *Am J Obstet Gynecol* 1977;128:229–30

6. Hadlock FP, Deter RL, Garcia-Platt J, *et al.* Fetal ascites not associated with Rh incompatibility: recognition and management with sonography. *Am J Roentgenol* 1980;134:1225–30

7. Benacerraf B, Frigoleto FD. Sonographic sign for the detection of early fetal ascites in the management of severe isoimmune disease without intra-uterine transfusion. *Am J Obstet Gynecol* 1985;152: 1039–41

8. Hashimoto B, Filly MA, Callen PW. Fetal pseudo-ascites, further anatomic observations. *J Ultrasound Med* 1986;5:151–2

9. Rosenthal SJ, Filly RA, Callen PW. Fetal pseudo-ascites. *Radiology* 1979;131:195–7

10. Mahony BS, Filly RA, Callen PW. Severe non-immune hydrops fetalis: sonographic evaluation. *Radiology* 1984;151:757–67

11. Jeanty P, Romero R, Hobbins JG. Fetal pericardial fluid: a normal finding of the second half of gestation. *Am J Obstet Gynecol* 1984;149:529–32

12. Shenker L, Reed K, Anderson CF. Fetal pericardial effusion. *Am J Obstet Gynecol* 1989;160:1505–7

13. Roberts AB, Mitchell JM, Pahison NS. Fetal liver length in normal and isoimmunized pregnancies. *Am J Obstet Gynecol* 1989;161:42–6

14. Nicolaides KH, Fontanarosa M, Gabbe SG, *et al.* Failure of ultrasonographic parameters to predict the severity of fetal anemia in Rhesus isoimmunization. *Am J Obstet Gynecol* 1988;158:920–6

15. Vintzileos AM, Campbell WA, Storlazzi E, *et al.* Fetal liver ultrasound measurements in isoimmunized pregnancies. *Obstet Gynecol* 1986;68:162–7

16. Chitkara U, Wilkins I, Lynch L, *et al.* The role of sonography in assessing severity of fetal anemia in Rh and Kell isoimmunized pregnancies. *Obstet Gynecol* 1988;71:393–8

17. Phelan JP, Ahn MO, Smith CV, *et al.* Amniotic fluid index measurements during pregnancy. *J Reprod Med* 1987;32:601–4

18. Phelan JP, Smith CU, Broussard P, *et al.* Amniotic fluid volume assessment with the four-quadrant technique at 36–42 weeks gestation. *J Reprod Med* 1988;32:540–2

19. Hoddick WK, Mahony BS, Callen PW, *et al.* Placental thickness. *J Ultrasound Med* 1988;4: 479–82

20. Harman CR, Manning FA, Bowman JM, *et al.* Severe Rh disease: poor outcome is not inevitable. *Am J Obstet Gynecol* 1983;45:823–29

21. Hutchinson AA. Pathology of hydrops fetalis. In Long WA, ed. *Fetal and Neonatal Cardiology.* Philadelphia: WB Saunders, 1990:197–210

22. Silverman NH. Fetal heart failure. In Copel JA, Reed KL, eds. *Doppler Ultrasound in Obstetrics and Gynecology.* New York: Raven Press, 1995:231–52

23. Reed KL. The fetal venous system. In Copel JA, Reed KL, eds. *Doppler Ultrasound in Obstetrics and Gynecology.* New York: Raven Press, 1995:291–5

24. Gill RW, Warren PS. Doppler measurement of umbilical blood flow. In Sanders RC, James AE, eds. *The Principles and Practice of Ultrasonography in Obstetrics and Gynecology.* 3rd edn. Norwalk, CT: Appleton-Century-Crofts, 1985:85–97

25. Huisman TWA, Stewart PA, Wladimiroff JW. Flow velocity waveforms in the fetal vena cava during the second half of normal pregnancy. *Ultrasound Med Biol* 1991;17:679–82

26. Reed KL, Appleton CP, Anderson CF, *et al.* Doppler studies of vena cava flows in human fetuses. *Circulation* 1996;81:498–505

27. Huisman TWA, Stewart PA, Wladimiroff JW. Ductus venosus blood flow velocity waveforms in the human fetus: a Doppler study. *Ultrasound Med Biol* 1992;18:33–7

28. Kiserud T, Eik-Nes SH, Blaas HK, *et al.* Ultra-sonographic velocimetry of the fetal ductus venosus. *Lancet* 1991;338:1412–14

29. Kiserud T, Eik-Nes SH, Hellevik LR, *et al.* Ductus venosus: a longitudinal Doppler velocimetric study of the human fetus. *J Mat–Fet Invest* 1992;2:5–11

30. Tulzer G, Gudmundsson S, Huhta JC, *et al.* The value of Doppler in evaluation and prognosis of fetuses with non-immunologic hydrops fetalis. *Gynakologische Rundschau* 1991;31(Suppl. 2):152–3

31. Gudmundsson S, Huhta JC, Wood DC, *et al.* Venous Doppler ultrasonography in the fetus with non-immune hydrops. *Am J Obstet Gynecol* 1991;164:33–7

32. Arias F (ed). *Erythroblastosis Fetalis*, 2nd edn. *Practical Guide to High Risk Pregnancy and Delivery.* St. Louis: Mosby-Year Book, 1993:114–30

33. Bowman JM. Controversies in Rh prophylaxis. *Am J Obstet Gynecol* 1985;151:289–94

34. Santolaya J, Meyer W, Gauthier W, *et al.* Trans-placental passage of erythropoietin (EPO-ALFA): a case control study. *Am J Obstet Gynecol* 1997;176:583

35. Sherer DM, Abramowicz JS, Ryan RM, *et al.* Severe fetal hydrops resulting from ABO incompatibility. *Obstet Gynecol* 1991;78:897–9

36. Nicolaides KH, Rodeck CH, Millar DS, *et al.* Fetal haematology in rhesus isoimmunization. *Br Med J* 1985;290:661–3

37. Nicolaides KH, Warenski JC, Rodeck CH. The relationship of fetal plasma protein concentration and hemoglobin levels to the development of hydrops in rhesus isoimmunisation. *Am J Obstet Gynecol* 1985;152:341–4

38. Grannum PA, Copel JA, Moya FR, *et al.* The reversal of hydrops fetalis by intravascular intrauterine transfusion in severe isoimmune fetal anemia. *Am J Obstet Gynecol* 1988;158:914–19

39. Soothill PW, Nicolaides KH, Rodeck CH. Effect of anaemia on fetal acid-base status. *Br J Obstet Gynaecol* 1987;94:880–3

40. Phibbs RH, Johnson P, Tooley WH. Cardio-respiratory status of erythroblastic newborn infants. II. Blood volume, hematocrit and serum albumin concentration in relation to hydrops fetalis. *Pediatrics* 1974;53:13–23

41. Diamond LK, Blackfan KD, Baty JM. Erythroblastosis fetalis and its association with universal edema of the fetus, icterus gravis neonatorum and anemia of the newborn. *Pediatrics* 1932;1:269–309

42. Mollison PL, Veall N, Cutbush M. Red cell volume and plasma volume in newborn infants. *Arch Dis Child* 1950;25:242–53

43. Graves GR, Baskett TF. Nonimmune hydrops fetalis: antenatal diagnosis and management. *Am J Obstet Gynecol* 1984;148:563–9

44. Weiner CP, Williamson RA, Wenstrom KD, *et al.* Management of fetal hemolytic disease by cordocentesis. *Am J Obstet Gynecol* 1991;105:1302–7

45. Hutchinson AA, Drew JH, Yu YY, *et al.* Non-immunologic hydrops fetalis: a review of 61 cases. *Obstet Gynecol* 1982;59:347–52

46. Hansmann M, Genbruch U, Bald R. New therapeutic aspects in nonimmune hydrops fetalis on four hundred and two prenatally diagnosed cases. *Fet Ther* 1989;4:29–37

47. Machin GA. Hydrops revisited: literature review of 1414 cases published in the 1980s. *Am J Med Genet* 1989;34:366–90

48. Turkel SB. Conditions associated with nonimmune hydrops fetalis. *Clin Perinatol* 1982;9:613

49. Santolaya J, Alley D, Jaffe R, *et al.* Antenatal classification of hydrops fetalis. *Obstet Gynecol* 1992;79:256–9

50. Holzgreve W, Curry CJR, Golbus MS, *et al.* Investigation of nonimmune hydrops fetalis. *Am J Obstet Gynecol* 1984;150:805–12

51. Holzgreve W, Holzgreve B, Curry JR. Non-immune hydrops fetalis: diagnosis and management. *Semin Perinatol* 1985;9:52–67

52. Watson I, Campbell S. Antenatal evaluation and management in nonimmune hydrops fetalis. *Obstet Gynecol* 1986;67:589–93

53. Scott JS, Esscher E. Congenital heart block and maternal systemic lupus erythematosus. *Br Med J* 1979;1:1235–8

54. Olaf KS, Gee H. Fetal heart block associated with maternal anti-Ro (SS-A) antibody-current management: a review. *Br J Obstet Gynaecol* 1991;98:751–5

55. Bonner C, Liesnard C, Content J. Prenatal diagnosis of 52 pregnancies at risk for congenital cytomegalovirus infection. *Obstet Gynecol* 1993;82:481–6

56. Weiner CP, Grose C. Prenatal diagnosis of congenital cytomegalovirus infection by virus isolation from amniotic fluid. *Am J Obstet Gynecol* 1990;163:1253–5

57. Hohlfeld P, Vial Y, Maillard-Brignon C, *et al.* Cytomegalovirus fetal infection: prenatal diagnosis. *Obstet Gynecol* 1991;78:615–8

58. Lynch L, Daffos F, Emanuel D, *et al.* Prenatal diagnosis of fetal cytomegalovirus infection. *Am J Obstet Gynecol* 1991;165:714–8

59. Lamy ME, Mulongo KN, Gadisseux JF, *et al.* Prenatal diagnosis of fetal cytomegalovirus infection. *Am J Obstet Gynecol* 1992;166:91–4

60. Maxwell DJ, Johnson P, Hurley P, *et al.* Fetal blood sampling and pregnancy loss in relation to indication. *Br J Obstet Gynaecol* 1991;98:892–7

61. Castillo RA, Devoe LD, Hadi HA, *et al.* Nonimmune hydrops fetalis: clinical experience and factors related to a poor outcome. *Am J Obstet Gynecol* 1986;155:812–16

62. Kaiser IH. Ballantyne and triple edema. *Am J Obstet Gynecol* 1917;110:115–20

63. Hirsch MR, Mark MS. Pseudotoxemia and erythroblastosis. Report of a case. *Obstet Gynecol* 1964;24:47–48

64. Rigsby WC, Vorys N, Copeland WE, *et al.* Antenatal diagnosis of the Rh and erythroblastotic fetus. *Obstet Gynecol* 1961;18:579–90

65. Selm MV, Kanhai HHH, Gravenhorst JB. Maternal hydrops syndrome: a review. *Gynecol Surv* 1991;46:785–8

66. Sheikh AU, Ernest JM, O'Shea M. Long-term outcome in fetal hydrops from parvovirus B19 infection. *Am J Obstet Gynecol* 1992;167:337–41

67. Smoleniec JS, Pillai M. Management of fetal hydrops associated with parvovirus B19 infection. *Br J Obstet Gynaecol* 1994;101:1079–81

68. Stephenson T, Zucollo J, Mohajer M. Diagnosis and management of non-immune hydrops in the newborn. *Arch Dis Child* 1994;70:F151–4

Multiple gestation

15

Steven L. Warsof, David E. Patton and Richard Jaffe

Although the news of twins frequently brings unexpected joys to the parents, in fact the prudent obstetrician should greet this news with respect and concern. Among the problems that should immediately come to mind are the increased risks for prematurity, congenital anomalies, abnormal presentation, intrauterine growth delay, discordant fetal growth, and exacerbation of underlying maternal medical problems. Prior to diagnostic ultrasonography the obstetrician frequently had minimal advance warning to deal with these issues. Today the role of diagnostic obstetrical ultrasonography is paramount for the diagnosis and management of these critical issues related to multiple gestation, and allows monitoring and optimization in critical situations.

DIAGNOSIS

As recently as the 1970s it was commonly recognized that 50% of twins were undiagnosed prior to the onset of labor and one-third of twins remained undiagnosed until after the first twin was delivered. In fact is was not uncommon for second twins to be delivered in the recovery room. Prenatal ultrasonography has changed this picture completely. In countries where obstetrical scans are used in all pregnancies 99–100% of twins are diagnosed at the time of scan[1]. When routine scanning programs in the first or second trimester are in place then the diagnosis is readily made, allowing for early recognition of twins with subsequent serial scans to follow fetal development and problems. The earlier diagnosis is made the more likely that obstetrical intervention may have a positive impact.

In the USA, where the debate persists between routine scanning versus indicated scanning, the recent RADIUS[2,3] study sheds important light on the impact of routine scanning. Although every patient in this study was under close clinical scrutiny for any size, dates, or other clinical discrepancy, the study confirms that in the indicated scanning group the diagnosis of multiple gestation was late in 37% and missed in 13%. In the routine scanning group the diagnosis of twins was made in 99% by 26 weeks (missed in one non-compliant patient who missed her ultrasound appointments). Early diagnosis has numerous self-evident advantages for the expectant couple, and may also allow earlier clinical therapeutic intervention. These authors take issue with the RADIUS study conclusions and stand firmly in support of routine ultrasonography for every expectant patient.

FREQUENCY

The incidence of multiple gestation varies from population to population. On closer scrutiny, however, it appears that the incidence of monozygotic (identical) twins is stable among populations, but that dizygotic (fraternal) gestations do vary considerably. In the USA, the incidence of twins is approximately 1.5% of all live births[1], with approximately one-third being monozygotic (MZ) and two-thirds being dizygotic (DZ). Internationally the incidence of DZ twins ranges from a low of 1.3/1000 in Japan to a high of 49/1000 among the Nigerians. Exactly which genetic or environmental factors play a role in the incidence of multifetal gestation remain uncertain. Having noted all of this, statistics describing the natural occurrence rates for multiple gestations are rapidly being relegated to the 'historical interest only' category by the emergence of assisted reproduction technologies (ART). The last 20 years have witnessed a virtual epidemic of multifetal pregnancy due to ovulation induction and various *in vitro* fertilization techniques. While the majority of twins today still result from spontaneous conception, the majority of triplets (>83%) and higher order gestations result from ART[5–7].

This low frequency, however, belies the significant contribution of twins to neonatal morbidity and mortality. It is estimated that the incidence of congenital malformations (per fetus) is essentially doubled in twins[8,9]. The majority of these malformations are structural and related to monozygocity[10]. In addition, while twins account for only 1.5% of live births, they account for approximately 11% of neonatal deaths[3,11].

SEPARATION ANXIETY

Many of the complications in twin pregnancy can be related to the degree of 'separateness' of the embryos and their supporting structures. The most straightforward and usually less complicated circumstance is the set of dizygotic (fraternal) twins. In this case two separate sperm fertilize two separate ova, resulting in two completely separate pregnancies that just happen to occupy the same uterus at the same time. While complications may still occur, the fetuses are entities distinct from each other, and their fates are much less intertwined than those of their monzygotic counterparts. Monozygotic twins result from fertilization of a single ovum by a single sperm, followed by early cleavage (which is often incomplete to a greater or lesser degree) into two identical embryos. The phenomenon of incomplete cleavage will be dealt with below in discussions regarding chorionicity, twin transfusion syndrome (TTS), and conjoined twins.

CHORIONICITY

Twin gestations may be characterized as being dichorionic diamniotic (di di), monochorionic diamniotic (mo di), or monochorionic mono-amniotic (mo mo). Dizygotic twins are always di di. Depending on the time span from fertilization to cleavage, monozygotic twins can be di di, mo di, or mo mo, with earlier separations being more complete. Table 1 lists the various membrane configurations, the interval from fertilization to separation, and the associated mortality rates.

The 'separateness' alluded to above refers to the degree which monozygotic twins separate at cleavage. Most identical twins have some degree of cleavage failure, resulting in some connection between the twins. This connection ranges from insignificant benign anastomoses of like vessels across the placenta (arterial–arterial or venous–venous), to pathologic anastomoses of unlike vessels (anterial–venous) which can result in various degrees of twin transfusion sequence, to

Table 1   Identical twins[12]

	Days of separation	Incidence	PNMR*
Di di	0–3	30	9
Mo di	4–8	68	25
Mo mo	8–13	2	50+
Conjoined twins	>13	0.002	N/A

Di di, dichorionic diamniotic; Mo di, monochorionic diamniotic; Mo mo, monochorionic monoamniotic; *PNMR, perinatal mortality rate as x/1000 live births; N/A, not available

conjoined twins and its attendant hazards. Given the significance of chorionicity, it is important for the sonographer to attempt to distinguish chorionicity any time twins are studied.

A number of criteria can be used to predict chorionicity. Fetuses of opposite sex will always be di di. The presence of separate placentas or a thick dividing membrane also indicates di di (Figures 1 and 2). A single placental mass, same sex, and a thin wispy membrane indicate mo di. Although Kurtz and colleagues[13] were able to correctly ascertain chorionicity in 96% of di di twins and 88% of mo di twins using the above criteria, they identified the so-called 'Lambda' or T-zone sign (Figure 3) in only 6 of 85 di di twins, and noted this sign in two mo di sets, bringing the value of this sign into question. It appears that the reliability of these ultrasound findings to determine chorionicity are greatly affected by gestational age. The best time to identify thickened membranes and the 'Lambda' sign appears to be the first trimester (Figure 1). Recent reports have demonstrated a membrane thickness of > 2 mm in the first trimester to be a frequent indicator of di di twins (Figures 1 and 4). While absence of a membrane generally indicates mo mo, several recent works[14,15] have demonstrated that inability to visualize a dividing membrane is inadequate to complete the diagnosis of monochorionic monoamniotic twins. To support the diagnosis of monoamniotic twins, in addition to being unable to visualize the membrane, there should be only a single placental mass, the fetuses should be of the same sex, and both fetuses should be able to move freely within the entire amniotic cavity[16]. Intertwining of the two umbilical cords may also be seen. Recently it has been demonstrated that with high-frequency ultrasonography the number of layers in the membrane and chorionicity can be predicted in most twin pregnancies[17].

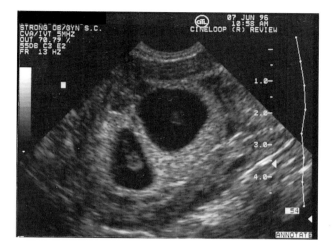

Figure 1   Thick membrane separating two early gestational sacs in dichorionic diamniotic gestation

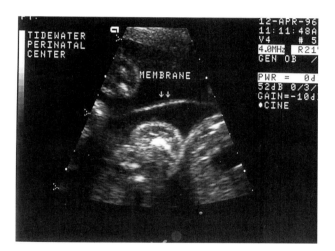

Figure 2   Thick membrane of a 17-week dichorionic diamniotic twin gestation

ESTABLISHMENT OF GESTATIONAL AGE

Perhaps the single most important role that ultrasound plays in modern obstetrics is the determination or confirmation of gestational age. Nearly all obstetrical decisions are dependent on gestational age.

While ART can often provide the time of conception accurate down to the minute, the misleading clinical clues of first trimester bleeding, accelerated uterine growth, and the high incidence of premature labor continue to keep sonographic establishment of gestational age a critical factor in management of multiple gestation. There has been some debate regarding ultrasonographic determination of gestational age, and whether separate 'twin

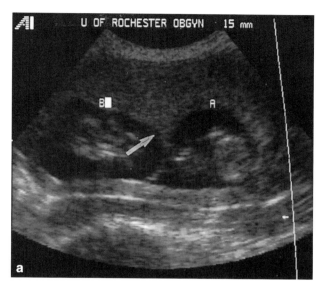

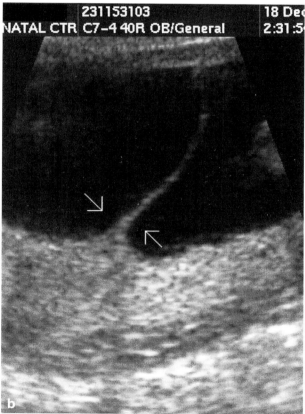

Figure 3   The Lambda, or twin peak, sign of (**a**) first trimester (arrow) and (**b**) second trimester (arrows) dichorionic diamniotic pregnancy

babies' growth charts should be used. If one accepts the premise that ultrasonographic dating of pregnancy is most accurate when performed at

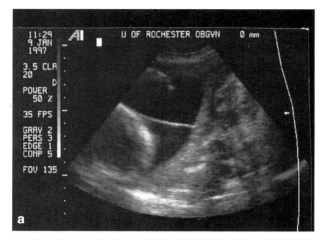

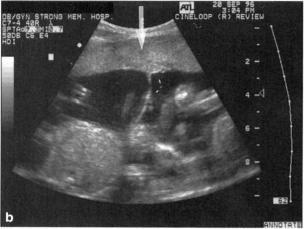

Figure 4 (a,b) Two monochorionic diamniotic pregnancies demonstrating single placental mass (arrow) and thin separating membranes

multiples. Furthermore, since genetic and uteroplacental factors influence fetal growth significantly after 20 weeks, fetal biometrics should rarely if ever be used to establish gestational age in any pregnancy, let alone multiples, after 20 weeks. Since separate tables or methods are unnecessary for multiples, the reader is referred to chapter 4 in this text for detailed discussions regarding ultrasonographic establishment of fetal gestational age.

PRESENTATION

Although the incidence of various twin presentations at birth have long been recognized, it is important to recognize that earlier in gestation the frequency of abnormal presentation is much greater leading to higher cesarean section rates in premature multiple births. Vertex leading twins rise from 59 to 81% from 15 to 30 weeks. Vertex second twins range from 49–60% in the same gestational age period. Decisions regarding mode of delivery of twins are strongly based on presentation, and will be addressed in the section below on intrapartum management. Table 2 depicts the statistics on presentation at various gestational ages.

FETAL GROWTH

It has been well established that fetal growth disturbances are much more common in multiple than singleton gestations[4]. It is also clear that intrauterine growth restriction (IUGR) is a major contributor to twin perinatal morbidity and mortality rates[21,22]. While it is true that 'twin tables' for fetal growth exist, it is the opinion of these authors that utilization of these tables only serves to decrease sensitivity in detecting IUGR, and may allow important diagnoses or opportunities for therapeutic intervention to be missed. Again, these tables are mentioned only to be dismissed. It is our recommendation that standard growth tables, presented elsewhere in this text, be employed, and

less than 20 weeks' gestation, then data comparing biometrics on singletons versus members of multiples should clarify the issue. Recent literature establishes that there is little difference in the biometrics[18,19] and birthweight[20] between singletons and members of multiples until the late third trimester. Accordingly, there appears to be no need nor rationale for separate dating tables for

Table 2   Number of scans and non-vertex fetal presentations on ultrasonography[21]

Gestational age (weeks)	Scans (n)	Non-vertex 1st twin (%)	Non-vertex 2nd twin when 1st vertex (%)	Total with at least 1 non-vertex (%)
15–20	124	41.0	50.8	90.3
21–25	62	27.5	46.7	74.2
26–30	145	22.0	51.0	73.0
31–34	144	25.0	39.5	64.5
35–38	47	19.0	40.4	59.5
26–38	336	22.9	44.6	67.5

that fetuses who are in less than the 10th percentile or who demonstrate abnormal head/abdominal circumference ratios be considered to be at risk due to IUGR, just as their singleton counterparts would be.

Inasmuch as (nearly) every twin or multiple is at its most basic also a singleton, every member of a multiple gestation is subject to the same influences on growth as are singleton gestations. Uteroplacental insufficiency is probably the primary cause of IUGR in multiple gestations[12]. This conclusion is not only intuitive, but is also supported by studies showing premature advancement of placental grade in twins[23]. IUGR may also be caused by isolated viral infection[24], aneuploidy, structural malformation, or the twin transfusion syndrome. Therefore, before the conclusion 'Of course they're small...they're twins!' is drawn, all of these possible causes for IUGR must be entertained and excluded.

DISCORDANT TWIN GROWTH

Discordant twin growth occurs in up to 29% of twin pairs[20] and has long been a vexing issue. The occurrence of growth discordance in many series is dependent upon the proportion of monozygotic versus dizygotic twins in those same series. Differences of opinion persist today regarding the definition and significance of discordant twin growth. In the not too distant past discordance was felt to be a universally ominous finding indeed. Today, when taken in context with information regarding zygosity, chorionicity, and biophysical evaluation of fetal well-being, the finding of discordance may be regarded as ranging in significance from clinically insignificant to critically important. For instance, in a set of dizygotic opposite sex twins who are both normally grown, discordance may merely be a manifestation of healthy differences in genetic predisposition. However, the same discordance in a monochorionic diamniotic same sex pair of twins in the setting of one twin with IUGR and oligohydramnios may forecast lethal consequences for one or both of the fetuses.

The causes of discordant twin growth are many. Obviously, any factor that can influence singleton growth *in utero* may be operative in twins as well. Accordingly, factors such as genetic predisposition, aneuploidy, structural malformations, metabolic disturbances, intrauterine infection, and uteroplacental insufficiency may all play a role in discordant twin growth. In addition, syndromes unique to twins which will be dealt with later, such as twin transfusion syndrome or acardia/acephalus, need to be considered.

While a universally accepted definition of discordance remains elusive, some headway is being made. One of the earliest and most persistently cited criteria utilized a 5 mm difference in the biparietal diameter measurements[25] (Figure 5). This method, however, lacks sensitivity for actually predicting birthweight discordance[26], and should probably be abandoned. Similarly, use of any individual biometric parameter should probably be abandoned in favor of methods utilizing fetal weight calculations[27–30]. Blickstein[31] published responses from 61 authors of internationally distributed twins literature, and suggested a two-tiered schema. Using the larger twin as the 100% value, he suggested that a fetal weight discordance of 15–25% be classified as 'mild', and a discordance of >25% be classified as 'severe discordance'. These authors support this classification, but caution that the clinician must take other factors such as the absolute fetal weight, chorionicity, presence or absence of IUGR, and the fetal biophysical evaluation into consideration before making clinical decisions based on the diagnosis of discordance. Discordant twins, when both are within normal growth ranges, is much less ominous than similarly discordant twins when one or both twins is growth delayed.

AMNIOTIC FLUID VOLUME

As with amniotic fluid volume (AFV) assessments for singletons, until recently AFV assessments for multiple gestations have been made on a subjective 'adequate or inadequate' scale. Recently, the introduction of the amniotic fluid index (AFI) has allowed the standardization of reporting methods for amniotic fluid volumes. These methods have been shown to be reliable, reproducible, and clinically useful[32,33]. Information is currently available which allows reliable quantification and communication of amniotic fluid volume in twin gestations. In studies limited to 'normal' twin gestations, Porter and colleagues[34] and Magann[35] have contributed greatly to the understanding of amniotic fluid volume in twin pregnancy. Utilizing a direct, reliable dye-dilution technique, Magann showed that mean amniotic fluid volume for the third trimester is approximately 877 ml. This is not significantly different from the amniotic fluid

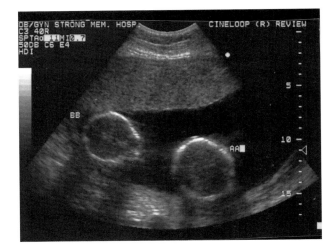

Figure 5 Significant difference in head diameter as a sign of discordant growth

Table 3 Amniotic fluid index (cm) by percentile distribution for estimated gestational age (EGA) in uncomplicated twin pregnancy[34]

EGA (weeks)	5th Percentile	50th Percentile	95th Percentile
28	1.0	16.3	24.0
30	9.8	16.1	23.8
34	9.3	15.6	23.3
38	8.9	15.2	22.9
40	8.7	15.0	22.7

Table 4 Amniotic fluid index (cm) by percentile distribution for estimated gestational age (EGA) in uncomplicated singleton pregnancy[37]

EGA (weeks)	5th Percentile	50th Percentile	95th Percentile
28	9.4	14.6	22.8
30	9.0	14.5	23.4
34	8.1	14.2	24.8
38	7.3	13.2	23.9
40	7.1	12.3	24.0

volume reported for third trimester singletons[36]. Utilizing a standardized technique for determining AFI, Porter and colleagues were able to construct normative data tables for AFI in normal twin gestations. As the participants in this study were excluded for cases of IUGR, anomaly, twin transfusion syndrome, and multiple other criteria, they were able to measure the AFI without regard to the separating membrane. Their data reveal the (surprising) conclusion that total AFI for the twin gestation is remarkably similar to that of singletons[37]. Of interest, fluid indices at the 5th and 50th percentile for twins was slightly higher than that for singletons of the same gestational age, whereas the 95th percentile values for twins were slightly lower. These statistics are presented in Tables 3 and 4; the message appears to be that amniotic fluid volume differs little between normal twin and normal singleton gestations.

PRENATAL DIAGNOSIS IN MULTIPLE GESTATION

Two major considerations predominate regarding prenatal diagnosis in twins. The first is the ability to identify any anomaly relevant to any singleton pregnancy; the second refers to the ability to recognize anomalies unique to twins. As the scope of this text is limited, this discussion will be limited to ultrasonographically related diagnoses and diagnostic procedures. Genetic amniocentesis has long been available to singleton gestations. Numerous studies have recently addressed the relative safety of genetic amniocentesis in twins, and the only conclusion that can be reached is that genetic amniocentesis in twins is no more hazardous than it is in singletons[38,39]. The most common approach to twin amniocentesis involves two separate procedures, with the instillation of indigo carmine into the first sac sampled (after the genetic specimen has been taken). This assures the operator that upon withdrawing colorless fluid on the second puncture that in fact both sacs have been sampled, rather than inadvertently sampling the same sac twice. At times the instillation may be unnecessary with close ultrasound guidance. Some authors advocate a single needle technique wherein one sac is sampled, and the needle is advanced through the intervening membrane for the second sample. This technique raises the issues of some mixing of specimens and possible rupture of the intervening membranes. In fact, one author (DP) is aware of a case of diamniotic twins rendered mono-amniotic by an errant amniocentesis procedure. Accordingly, this technique should be used only under research settings. In addition, recent studies of chorionic villus sampling (CVS) would indicate that the risks of the first trimester CVS do not differ from those of second trimester amniocentesis for twin gestations[40].

DOPPLER

Numerous studies exist regarding the use of Doppler velocimetry in normal and abnormal twin gestations[41]. Suffice it to say that the application of Doppler technology in twins is essentially the same as in singletons, and the reader is referred to the appropriate chapters elsewhere in this text for further discussions regarding Doppler. Needless to say absent, reverse, or discordant flow between a set of twins may be critically important, and this type of analysis should be available in any multifetal pregnancy, especially when growth discordance is present.

MULTIFETAL PREGNANCY REDUCTION

A parallel outgrowth of rising rates of higher order multifetal gestations has been the development of sonographically guided multifetal pregnancy reduction techniques. This procedure is typically performed between 10–14 weeks of gestation in order to enhance the likelihood of normal pregnancy outcome. It can be done to 'selectively terminate' an abnormal member of a multiple gestation (selective termination), or simply to reduce in a 'non-targeted' way the number of fetuses to a lower number in order to enhance the survival and decrease severe morbidity associated with prematurity in high order multiple gestations (multifetal pregnancy reduction). Reduction procedures are usually performed in the out-patient setting, utilizing ultrasound guidance and local anesthesia. Both transabdominal and transvaginal approaches have been used. In cases of anomalous fetus(es) the choice of which fetus to reduce is obvious. When the goal is simply to reduce the number of fetuses present, the choice is more controversial. One school of thought argues for the preservation of the presenting fetus in order to preserve the viability of the presenting membranes, while another argues simply for reduction based on ease and accessibility. Neither approach has been shown to be definitively superior. Specifically, the procedure involves injecting 2–10 millequivalents of potassium chloride (2Meq/ml) into the fetal thorax, resulting in instantaneous asystole. Reduced fetuses resorb to a lesser or greater degree, and are either not evident at delivery, or may present as a 'fetus papyraceous'. Although early efforts had as much as a 10% loss of the entire pregnancy, more recent experience indicates the loss rate will probably settle at approximately 3–5% in experienced hands.

This improvement in outcome has led to discussions as to when reduction is appropriate. Originally it was used only in quadruplets or greater, where the risk of severe prematurity was greatest. By continuing the ethical principles of autonomy and beneficence recently triplets and even twins have been considered appropriate candidates for reduction. Further discussion and clarification of the ethical issues surrounding fetal reduction is expected to continue in the literature for some time to come[42].

The possibility of higher order multifetal pregnancy should be discussed in any ART procedure. Fortunately, although utilization of ART is continuing to increase, the incidence of high order multifetal pregnancies can be reduced by limiting the number of embryos replaced, and by cryopreservation rather than replacement of extra embryos.

ANOMALIES UNIQUE TO TWINS

Twin transfusion syndrome (TTS)

As noted above, a significant portion of the morbidity and mortality related to twins is due to the failure of complete cleavage during the monozygotic twinning process. Pathologic studies have demonstrated that in fact the majority of MZ placentas share vasculature to some degree[43,44]. Fortunately, most of these anastomoses are of like vessels and are hemodynamically insignificant. On occasion, however, a hemodynamically significant arteriovenous anastomosis occurs, and results in a life-threatening complication called twin transfusion syndrome. TTS is characterized by one twin who serves as the 'donor' with the other as the 'recipient'. The donor is on the arterial side of the transplacental anastomosis and essentially pumps its blood, calories, and virtually its life into the recipient. This is thought to cause hypovolemia, oliguria, oligohydramnios, and growth failure. The donor fetus ultimately becomes so oligohydramniotic that it may become a 'shrink-wrapped stuck twin' (Figure 6). The shrink-wrapped stuck twin phenomenon occurs when the amniotic fluid for the donor twin is completely non-existent, such that the amniotic membrane essentially envelopes the donor and becomes an adherent shroud around it. In fact, the amnion can adhere so closely that it not only binds the fetus to the uterine wall (hence the term 'stuck twin') but it also becomes very difficult to identify.

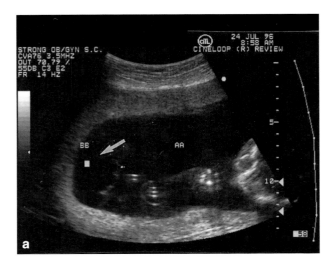

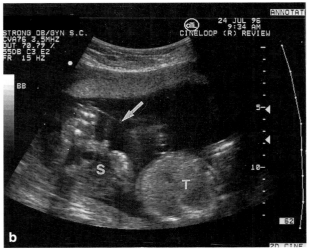

Figure 6   Twin pregnancy with twin to twin transfusion syndrome (**a**) One sac demonstrating oligohydramnios (arrow). (**b**) Thin membrane (arrow) separating 'stuck twin' (S) from other twin (T)

It is not uncommon for the inexperienced ultrasonographer to mislabel a stuck twin as a set of monoamniotic twins due to failure to identify the amnion around the stuck donor twin, or to miss the diagnosis of stuck twin altogether. This is a significant error as clinical management of TTS versus monoamniotic twins is very different, as is the outcome. It is often helpful to observe the fetal limbs for the characteristic shrouded effect of the amnion surrounding the limb. Meanwhile, as the donor twin is literally pumping its life away, the recipient twin has its own worries. This twin generally becomes volume overloaded, plethoric, hydramniotic, and often hydropic due to high

output cardiac failure (Figure 7). This syndrome is extremely difficult to manage, and is frequently lethal to both twins. While the future holds the promise of fetoscopic laser ablation of the offending vessels[45], the only readily available successful therapy involves aggressive repeated 'decompression' amniocenteses of the hydramniotic twin[46,47]. This decompression or therapeutic amniocentesis may involve removal of 3–5 liters of amniotic fluid in serial treatments performed as frequently as once or more per week. Outcome with this management can reverse an otherwise frequently lethal process. Recently removal, puncture, or destruction of the intervening membrane in order to equalize pressures between the two sacs has been attempted, but this remains highly experimental. Precise, accurate diagnosis of twins discordant for size and/or amniotic fluid volume is critical because the etiologies and treatments are so diverse, as are the outcomes. Minimum diagnostic criteria must include the findings of: a single placental mass, same sex fetuses, a fetal size and/or amniotic fluid discordance, a separating amnion must be identified, and other anomalies must be excluded.

Monoamniotic twins

This occurs in approximately 1 in 500 twin sets. It is thought to be the result of later embryonic cleavage (Table 1), and carries with it a mortality rate of approximately 50%. Mortality is related predominantly to cord entanglement. Stuck twin or TTS is frequently misdiagnosed as monoamniotic twins. Before the diagnosis of monoamniotic twins can be made, one must demonstrate a single (or fused) placental mass, same sex fetuses, both of whom have 'free range' within the entire amniotic cavity, and a dividing amniotic membrane must be unequivocally absent. Delivery in monoamniotic twins is fraught with hazards associated with cord entanglement or prolapse. As antenatal fetal surveillance by any means cannot predict catastrophic cord accident, most authors advocate delivery by cesarean section between 32 and 34 weeks to avoid late fetal death due to cord accident.

Polyhydramnios–oligohydramnios sequence (Poly–oli sequence)

In the past the finding of polyhydramnios (or more commonly normal amniotic fluid) in one twin and

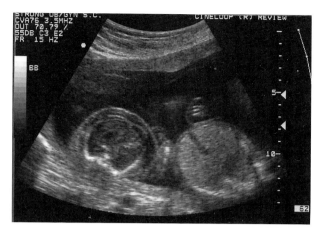

Figure 7 Twin to twin transfusion with severely hydropic twin on the left

oligohydramnios in the other was considered diagnostic of TTS (above). It is now known that there are multiple causes for these findings. Any time there is excessive fluid in one sac and decreased or normal fluid in the other, individual fetal disorders must be considered before labeling the condition TTS[24] as the true pathology may in fact be with the other fetus. Isolated hydramnios may result from aneuploidy, neural tube defects, gastrointestinal anomalies or other complications, and oligohydramnios may result from aneuploidy, uteroplacental insufficiency, genitourinary disorders, premature rupture of membranes or other complications. All of these individual possibilities must be ruled out when discordant fetal size or amniotic fluid volumes are noted.

Acardia–acephalus

There are numerous synonyms for this syndrome which can be considered as the ultimate expression of the twin transfusion syndrome[48]. It is characterized by the finding of one (initially) normal twin and an acardiac twin (the term acardiac monster should be avoided, especially when talking with parents). The normal twin essentially provides cardiac output for both fetuses. Diagnostic criteria include documenting a twin pregnancy (usually monochorionic diamniotic), a single placental mass, one essentially normal (though often growth restricted) fetus

(Figure 8a), and one fetus with demonstrable movement and arterial pulsations (Doppler), but complete absence of a heart. The acardiac fetus usually has multiple other defects, commonly including acephalus (Figure 8b). Surprisingly, the outcome is often more favorable than one might expect, and vigilance may provide up to a 50% survival of the normal twin. This should be remembered prior to embarking on invasive treatments such as hysterotomy and removal of the acardiac twin.

Vanishing twins

The recent use of ultrasonography in early pregnancy has shed considerable light on the twinning phenomenon. It has been estimated that up to 4% of conceptions are twin conceptions[49], yet only 1.5% of deliveries are twin deliveries. One must conclude, then, that the majority of multiple conceptions fail, and one or more of the conceptuses simply disappears.

This phenomenon is known as the 'vanishing twin'. The diagnosis is characterized by the finding of two gestational sacs in the uterus. One sac contains a normal embryo, while the other may contain an embryo but more often is empty and in various states of collapse. There may be associated vaginal bleeding. This phenomenon does not seem to have an adverse effect on the pregnancy[50]. This situation needs to be differentiated from a single fetal demise in the late second or third trimester in a twin pregnancy. In this case, consideration for immediate delivery of the surviving twin, especially if monozygotic, should be given, as there have been many cases of poor outcome in the surviving twin in this setting. Damage noted in the surviving twin has included encephalomalacia and splanchnic organ infarcts. While the theoretical details are beyond the scope of this chapter, the possible etiologies for such damage may relate to embolization of histamines, other tissue factors and necrotic products, and 'watershed' hemodynamics.

Conjoined twins

A detailed discussion of conjoined twins is beyond the scope of this chapter, so the subject will be touched on only briefly. First, please note the terminology. 'Conjoined' is the appropriate description. The archaic term 'Siamese twins' is not only nondescriptive but is also offensive and should be

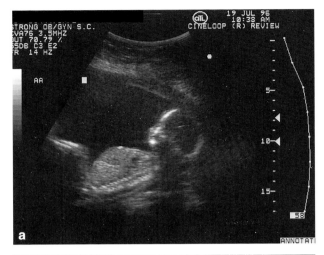

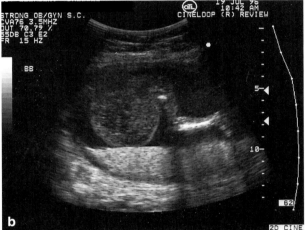

Figure 8   (**a**) Normal twin and acardiac twin (**b**) with acephalus

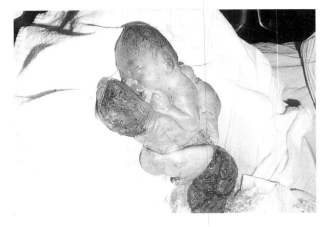

Figure 9   Conjoined twins attached at chest and abdomen

INTRAPARTUM MANAGEMENT

Delivery of twin gestations generates considerable controversy. Delivery of monoamniotic twins has already been addressed. Primary cesarean section appears most appropriate. In other settings extreme caution and clinical judgment must be employed. When the leading twin is non-vertex almost all authorities today advocate cesarean section if the fetuses have reached viability. When both twins are vertex most would recommend trial of vaginal birth. However, if there is considerable prematurity, discordancy (especially if the lead twin is smaller), or other confounding problems are present, then abdominal delivery should be considered. When there is a vertex/non-vertex situation there are three possibilities: cesarean section for the benefit of the following twin; vaginal delivery of the lead twin with breech vaginal delivery of the second twin; or vaginal delivery of the lead twin with external cephalic version of the second fetus to a vertex presentation to allow subsequent vaginal delivery. In any trial of labor in multiple gestations close intrapartum surveillance with continual electronic fetal heart rate monitoring is needed. In addition, intrapartum ultrasound for guidance and verification of presentation is required. Anesthesia, pediatric and nursing assistance must be available both to assist with vaginal delivery, or to proceed expediently with cesarean section should events go awry. Higher order gestations should always be delivered by cesarean section if the fetuses have reached viability.

abandoned. Conjoined twins are perhaps the ultimate expression of monozygotic cleavage failure. They are usually the result of cleavage occurring 13 days or more after fertilization and occur in approximately 1 in 1500 twin gestations, or 1 in 100 000 pregnancies[12] (Figure 9). The diagnosis of conjoined twins can be difficult in late gestation due to fetal crowding and other factors. Earlier in gestation the diagnosis is suggested by: the absence of dividing amnion, single or fused placenta, constant relationship of fetal parts, and the inability to document tissue planes between homologous fetal parts. While notable exceptions have occurred, conjoined twins rarely survive *ex utero* when there is major sharing of critical organ systems.

CONCLUSION

Ultrasonography plays a critical role in the diagnosis, treatment, and management of multiple pregnancy. If we anticipate being able to reduce the morbidity and mortality associated with this condition, then diagnostic obstetrical ultrasound will need to play an important role.

References

1. Persson PH, Kullander S. Long-term experience of general ultrasound screening in pregnancy. *Am J Obstet Gynecol* 1983;146:942–7

2. LeFevre ML, Bain RP, Ewigman BG, *et al*. A randomized trial of prenatal ultrasonography screening: impact on maternal management and outcome. *Am J Obstet Gynecol* 1993;169:483–9

3. Ewigman BG, Crane JP, Frigoletto FD, *et al*. Effect of prenatal ultrasound screening on perinatal outcome. *N Engl J Med* 1993;329:821–7

4. ACOG Technical Bulletin: *Multiple Gestation*. August 1989;131

5. Collins MS, Bleyl JA. Seventy-one quadruplet pregnancies: management and outcome. *Am J Obstet Gynecol* 1990;162:1384–92

6. Elliott JP, Radin TG. Quadruplet pregnancy: contemporary management and outcome. *Obstet Gynecol* 1992;80:421–4

7. Weissman A, Yoffe N, Jakobi P, *et al*. Management of triplet pregnancies in the 1980s: are we doing better? *Am J Perinatol* 1991;8:333–7

8. Gall S, Wenstrom K. Incidence, morbidity and mortality, and diagnosis of twin gestations. *Clin Perinatol* 1988;15:1–12

9. Hay S, Wehrung DA. Congenital malformations in twins. *Am J Hum Genet* 1970;22:662–78

10. Schinzel AA, Smith DW, Miller JR. Monozygotic twinning and structural defects. *J Pediatr* 1979;95:921–30

11. Powers WF, Kiely JL. The risk confronting twins: a national perspective. *Am J Obstet Gynecol* 1979;170:456–61

12. Gall SA. *Multiple Pregnancy and Delivery*. St. Louis MO: Mosby, 1996

13. Kurtz AB, Wapner RJ, Mata J, *et al*. Twins pregnancies: accuracy of first trimester abdominal ultrasound in predicting chorionicity and amnionicity. *Radiology* 1992;185:759–62

14. Barss VA, Benacerraf BR, Frigoletto FD. Ultrasonographic determination of chorion type in twin gestation. *Obstet Gynecol* 1985;66:779–83

15. Blane CE, DiPietro MA, Johnson MZ, *et al*. Sonographic detection of monoamniotic twins. *J Clin Ultrasound* 1987;15:394–6

16. Rodis JF, Vintzileos AM, Campbell WA, *et al*. Antenatal diagnosis and management of monoamniotic twins. *Am J Obstet Gynecol* 1987;157:1255–7

17. Vayssiere CF, Heim N, Camus EP, *et al*. Determination of chorionicity in twin gestations in high-frequency abdominal ultrasonography: counting the layers of the dividing membrane. *Am J Obstet Gynecol* 1996;175:1529–33

18. Reece EA, Yarkoni S, Abdalla M, *et al*. A prospective longitudinal study of growth in twin gestations compared with growth in singleton pregnancies. I. The fetal head. *J Ultrasound Med* 1991;10:439–43

19. Reece EA, Yarkoni S, Abdalla M, *et al*. A prospective longitudinal study of growth in twin gestations compared with growth in singleton pregnancies. II. The fetal limbs. *J Ultrasound Med* 1991;10:445–50

20. Luke B. The changing pattern of multiple births in the United States: maternal and infant characteristics, 1993 and 1990. *Obstet Gynecol* 1994;84:101–6

21. Santolaya J, Sampson M, Abramowicz J, *et al*. Twin pregnancy: ultrasonographically observed changes in fetal presentation. *J Reprod Med* 1992;37:328–30

22. Luke B, Minogue J, Witter FR. The role of fetal growth restriction and gestational age on length of hospital stay in twin infants. *Obstet Gynecol* 1993;81:949–53

23. Ohel G, Granat M, Zeevi D, *et al*. Advanced ultrasonic placental maturation in twin pregnancies. *Am J Obstet Gynecol* 1987;156:76–8

24. Weiner CP. Challenge of twin-twin transfusion syndrome. *Contemporary Ob-Gyn* 1992;37:83–104

25. Crane JP, Tomich PG, Kopta M. Ultrasonic growth patterns in normal and discordant twins. *Obstet Gynecol* 1980;55:678–83

26. Erkkola R, Ala-Mello S, Piiroinen O, *et al*. Growth discordancy in twin pregnancies: a risk factor not detected by measurement of the biparietal diameter. *Obstet Gynecol* 1985;66:203–6

27. Barnea ER, Romero R, Scott D, *et al*. The value of biparietal diameter and abdominal perimeter in the diagnosis of growth retardation in twin gestations. *Am J Perinatol* 1985;2:221–2

28. Brown CEL, Guzick DS, Leveno KJ, *et al*. Prediction of discordant twins using ultrasound measurement of biparietal diameter and abdominal perimeter. *Obstet Gynecol* 1987;70:677–81

29. Chamberlain P, Murphy M, Comerford FR. How accurate is antenatal sonographic identification of discordant birthweight in twin? *Eur J Obstet Gynecol Reprod Biol* 1991;40:91–6

30. Storlazzie E, Vintzileos AM, Campbell WA, et al. Ultrasonic diagnosis of discordant fetal growth in twin gestations. Obstet Gynecol 1987;69:363–7

31. Blickstein I. The definition, diagnosis, and management of growth-discordant twins: an international census survey. Acta Genet Med Bemellol (Roma) 1991; 40:345–51

32. Phelan JP, Smith CV, Broussard P, et al. Amniotic fluid volume assessment with the 4 quadrant technique at 36–42 weeks gestation. J Reprod Med 1987; 32:540–2

33. Dildy GA, Liva N, Moise KJ, et al. Amniotic fluid volume assessment: comparison of ultrasound estimation versus direct measurement with a dye dilution technique in human pregnancy. Am J Obstet Gynecol 1992;167:986–94

34. Porter TF, Dildy GA, Blanchard JR, et al. Normal values for amniotic fluid index during uncomplicated twin pregnancy. Obstet Gynecol 1996;87: 699–702

35. Magann EF, Whitworth NS, Bass JD, et al. Amniotic fluid volume of third trimester diamniotic twin pregnancies. Obstet Gynecol 1995;85:957–60

36. Brace RA, Wolf EJ. Normal amniotic fluid changes throughout pregnancy. Am J Obstet Gynecol 1989; 161:382–8

37. Moore TR, Cayle JE. The amniotic fluid index in normal human pregnancy. Am J Obstet Gynecol 1990;162:1168–73

38. Elias S, Gerbie AB, Simpson JL. Genetic amniocentesis in twin gestation. Am J Obstet Gynecol 1980; 138:169–74

39. Anderson RL, Goldberg JD, Golbus MS. Prenatal diagnosis in multiple gestation: 20 years experience with amniocentesis. Prenatal Diagn 1991;11:263–70

40. Wapner RJ, Johnson A, Davis G, et al. Prenatal diagnosis in twin gestation: a comparison between second trimester amniocentesis and first trimester chorion villus sampling. Obstet Gynecol 1993;82: 49–56

41. Giles WB. Doppler assessment in multiple pregnancy. Semin Perinatol 1987;11:369–74

42. Evans MI, Dommergues M, Johnson MP, et al. Multifetal pregnancy reduction and selective termination. Curr Opin Obstet Gynecol 1995;7:126–9

43. Benirschke H. Twin placenta in perinatal mortality. NY State J Med 1961;61:1499–508

44. Robertson EG, Neer KJ. Placental injection studies in twin gestation. Am J Obstet Gynecol 1983;147: 170–4

45. De Lia JE, Cruikshank DP, Keye WR. Fetoscopic neodymium: yag laser occlusion of placental vessels in severe twin-twin transfusion syndrome. Obstet Gynecol 1990;75:1046–53

46. Elliott JP. Amniocentesis for twin-twin transfusion syndrome. Contemporary Ob-Gyn 1992;37:30–47

47. Pinette MG, Pan Y, Pinette SG, et al. Treatment of twin-twin transfusion syndrome. Obstet Gynecol 1993; 82:841–6

48. Van Allen MI, Smith DW, Shepard TH. Twin reversed arterial perfusion (TRAP) sequence: a study of 14 twin pregnancies with acardius. Semin Perinatol 1983;7:285–93

49. Landy HJ, Weiner S, Corson SL, et al. The 'vanishing twin'. Ultrasonographic assessment of fetal disappearance in the first trimester. Am J Obstet Gynecol 1986;155:14–19

50. Spellacy WN. Antepartum complications in twin pregnancies. Clin Perinatol 1988;15:79–86

Antenatal fetal assessment technologies

16

J. Christopher Glantz

Perinatal mortality is the sum of all fetal deaths ≥ 20 weeks gestation plus neonatal deaths through the first 28 days of life. The perinatal mortality rate (PMR) is the number of perinatal deaths per 1000 births. Between 1950 and 1970, the PMR in the USA fell from 39 to 29[1]. The most common causes of death during this time were: placental and umbilical cord complications (47%), intra-amniotic infection (17%), premature rupture of the membranes and congenital anomalies (≈ 10% each), with 20% unknown[2]. In an effort to reduce PMR due to uteroplacental factors, methods for antepartum fetal surveillance were devised to detect early signs of intrauterine hypoxia and to identify fetuses at risk for hypoxic damage. The goal of antepartum fetal surveillance is to enable delivery before such damage occurs. Concurrently, neonatologists developed and refined expertise in caring for preterm and compromised newborns.

Antepartum fetal heart rate monitoring became available in the 1970s. Through the use of antepartum fetal heart rate monitoring along with improvements in antenatal management and neonatal care, PMR in the USA declined from 29 to 17.5 by the end of the decade. Further refinements in antepartum heart rate testing interpretation and more frequent use of ultrasound for fetal assessment occurred in the 1980s so that PMR fell to 13.7. As fetal monitoring and neonatal care progressed, mortality associated with birth asphyxia and prematurity decreased, leaving fetal anomalies as the greatest single contributor to infant mortality[3].

In a 1989 study of fetal death certificates in Massachusetts, ≈ 60% of fetal deaths were equally divided between antepartum asphyxia and maternal complications, 12% from fetal anomalies, 4% from infection, and the remaining quarter from unknown causes[4]. Of these fetal deaths, 86% were antepartum and 14% were intrapartum. The majority of intrapartum fetal deaths were due to either congenital anomalies or infections, and only 12% were due to asphyxia. Stubblefield and Berek[5] reported that in term fetal deaths, 81% were antepartum and 19% intrapartum. Although this was similar to the 1989 study, the causes of death were distributed differently. For antepartum deaths, three-quarters were from perinatal hypoxia, ≈ 10% apiece from anomalies and fetal growth restriction, and 3% from infection. Of intrapartum deaths, ≈ 40% were due to hypoxia, ≈ 30% to anomalies, and ≈ 15% to infection. The majority of term, antepartum fetal deaths from asphyxia occurred in the setting of chronic hypoxia (e.g. placental infarction) rather than acute events (abruption or cord accidents), and the authors suggested that antepartum fetal assessment may lower the perinatal mortality rate.

Before 1980, perinatal mortality was divided relatively equally between fetal and neonatal deaths, with slightly more neonatal than fetal deaths contributing to total perinatal mortality. Due to recent advances in neonatal technology, the neonatal death rate is now less than the fetal death rate[6]. In 50% or more of perinatal deaths, avoidable factors can be identified (albeit some in cases in which fetal demise was inevitable for other reasons)[7]. Most of these factors are obstetrical rather than neonatal[8]. Not all avoidable factors are medical, however. Delke and colleagues[9] reported that social and maternal factors were present in 39% of perinatal deaths in New York City.

This chapter will discuss the use of fetal heart rate and ultrasonographic monitoring to assess fetal status. The primary purpose of these techniques is to detect signs of fetal compromise early enough to intervene in an effort to decrease perinatal morbidity and mortality. Although mortality is an objective measure by which to evaluate effectiveness of surveillance techniques, death is an extreme measure and fails to account for significant morbidity. Surveillance techniques should improve on both outcomes to be most useful to clinicians.

FETAL HEART RATE MONITORING

The first known description of fetal heart sounds was in the 17th century, but auscultation of fetal heart sounds was not thought to be of potential clinical benefit until the 1800s[10]. Fetal heart rates <100 or >180 beats per minute were thought to be associated with unfavorable perinatal outcomes. The fetoscope, a specialized stethoscope held against the maternal abdomen by pressure from the listener's forehead, was developed in the early 1900s to hear fetal heart sounds.

The fetal heart rate (FHR) was first monitored electronically in 1906, but such technology was used primarily to confirm fetal viability. In the 1950s and 1960s, fetal electrocardiograph recording did not prove useful in predicting fetal compromise, but did lead to the development of external FHR monitoring. Different FHR deceleration patterns were described in association with pathological perinatal conditions. In 1959, Hon[11] described variable and late decelerations in humans following umbilical cord compression and uteroplacental insufficiency, respectively. In 1963, Caldeyro-Barcia and colleagues reported on the prognostic value of these deceleration patterns, and in 1967 Hammacher described the importance of FHR variability. Prototype electronic fetal monitors were very bulky and expensive, but in 1968 the first commercial monitors were marketed using microphones to detect fetal heart sounds. Fetal heart rate monitoring standards and terminology were developed in the 1970s, and Doppler recording of fetal cardiac activity replaced phonocardiography.

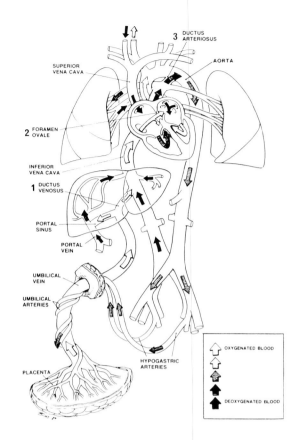

Figure 1 Fetal circulation. Reproduced with permission[1]

FETAL CARDIOVASCULAR PHYSIOLOGY

The fetus must have oxygen to live, and depends on transplacental exchange of carbon dioxide and oxygen to and from maternal blood. Blood flows from the fetal hypogastric arteries into the umbilical arteries and through the umbilical cord into the placenta (Figure 1). Maternal uterine arteries carry oxygenated blood through the myometrium to the intervillus spaces within the placenta. The oxygenated blood bathes the placental villi, which contain fetal capillaries filled with relatively deoxygenated fetal blood. Oxygen diffuses from the maternal blood across the villus trophoblast into the fetal capillaries, while carbon dioxide diffuses from fetal blood across the trophoblast into maternal blood. Partial pressure gradients between the maternal and fetal blood drive oxygen and carbon dioxide diffusion.

Oxygenated blood returns to the fetus via the umbilical vein, passing into the fetal liver and inferior vena cava. Oxygenated blood carried by the inferior vena cava into the right atrium of the fetal heart is preferentially shunted across the foramen ovale into the left atrium, where it is pumped into the left ventricle and out into the aortic arch to perfuse the head and arms. Less-well-oxygenated blood entering the right atrium from the superior vena cava mixes slightly with oxygenated blood from the inferior vena cava. It is pumped into the right ventricle and out the pulmonary artery, where most of it flows through the ductus arteriosus into the descending aorta (thus the less-oxygenated blood is in the hypogastric arteries).

Limitation of placental blood flow

Anything that interferes with the flow of maternal blood into the placenta potentially interferes with fetal oxygenation. Supine maternal position places the weight of the uterus on the inferior vena cava, compressing it against the spine, slowing flow and decreasing venous return to the heart. With less venous return, there is less blood for the heart to pump, so cardiac output and blood pressure fall. Compression of the aorta also limits flow below the compression point. Lower cardiac output and impaired aortic flow result in less delivery of oxygenated maternal blood to the placenta, less oxygen exchange, and eventually fetal hypoxia[12]. Turning the woman to a lateral position alleviates these effects.

Uterine contractions constrict spiral arteries as they traverse the myometrium, lessening flow of maternal blood into the placenta and decreasing maternal–fetal oxygen exchange. In normal pregnancy, baseline fetal oxygenation is high enough so that the drop in fetal oxygen tension during contractions does not exceed fetal reserve. However, for cases in which fetal oxygenation is borderline – just barely adequate – this decline in oxygen exchange during a contraction may result in transient fetal hypoxemia. Because it takes 30–60 seconds for fetal oxygen tension to drift downwards during a contraction, and additional seconds to recover following relaxation of the myometrium and restoration of blood flow, the period of hypoxemia is delayed until after the peak of the contraction. Fetal chemoreceptors respond to this transient hypoxemia by reflexively decreasing the fetal heart rate through vagal parasympathetic outflow[13]. The resulting late deceleration is so-named because it occurs after the peak of a contraction (Figure 2). It represents a response to acute hypoxemia in a fetus with compromised baseline oxygenation.

Conditions that decrease placental surface area limit the amount of placenta available to participate in gas exchange. Examples of such conditions include placental abruption, infarction, and hypoplasia. Maternal vascular disease, as in hypertension, diabetes, and collagen-vascular disease, may limit the flow of maternal blood into the placenta. Umbilical cord compression obstructs flow of blood to and from the placenta, even though the placenta itself may be functioning normally.

Control of fetal heart rate

The FHR is controlled by the combined effects of the sympathetic and parasympathetic nervous systems. The normal FHR is between 110–160

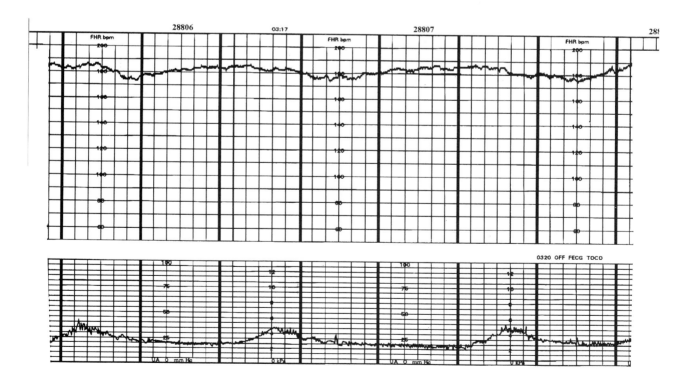

Figure 2 Late decelerations. The fetal heart rate tracing on the upper panel demonstrates repetitive decelerations occurring after uterine contractions recorded in the lower panel

beats per minute. Sympathetic nerve endings release norepinephrine, which causes the FHR to increase. Systemic epinephrine from the adrenal medulla has the same effect. The parasympathetic vagus nerve releases acetylcholine, which slows the heart rate. At any given moment, the two components of the autonomic nervous system interact. The result is constant modulation of the heart rate, with continual instantaneous rate changes from one beat to another, called 'beat-to-beat variability'. Mild stimulation of the sympathetic nervous system produces short, low-grade heart rate accelerations ($\approx$ 5 beats), while mild stimulation of the parasympathetic nervous system produces brief, modest decelerations. These slower responses yield 'long-term variability' (Figure 3)[14].

Beginning in the second trimester, fetal movements are associated with FHR accelerations. This is a normal sympathetic response and is called 'reactivity'. The earlier in gestation, the less frequent the accelerations tend to be, and the lower their magnitude[15]. Fetal behavioral states affect the FHR pattern. A fetus who is awake or in REM sleep normally manifests a reactive pattern with good variability, whereas a fetus in quiet sleep may be minimally reactive and have decreased variability. Variability and FHR reactivity undergo periodic fluctuations according to sleep cycles, with episodes of reactivity lasting 20–40 minutes interspersed with less-reactive episodes usually lasting $\leq$ 80 minutes[16].

Inherent in the concept of autonomic control of FHR is that the brain must have adequate oxygen in order for the autonomic nervous system to function normally. A hypoxic central nervous system cannot function properly and the heart may not receive normal signals from autonomic nerves. One manifestation of hypoxia is loss of normal FHR patterns. The baseline FHR may lose variability and appear flat, without discernible accelerations. This 'non-reactive' pattern with decreased variability is highly suggestive of fetal hypoxia, although the same effect may be seen in association with certain drugs (sedatives, magnesium sulfate, anticholinergics, or adrenergic antagonists), some congenital anomalies (e.g. anencephaly), or with central nervous system injury. The key tenet of antepartum fetal monitoring is that normal FHR patterns require normal central nervous system function, which requires normal fetal oxygenation. The non-stress test (NST) and contraction stress test (CST) were developed using FHR patterns to indirectly measure fetal oxygenation.

NON-STRESS TESTING

Fetal heart rate accelerations accompanying fetal movements are associated with normal fetal oxygenation. Using an external fetal monitor, FHR patterns can be recorded for 20 minutes during which time the woman marks the tracing whenever fetal movements occur. This is the concept of the NST to evaluate fetal well-being, popularized in the 1970s.

Interpretation of non-stress testing

Many different criteria have been proposed to define a reactive NST, including 1–5 accelerations of 10–15 beats over a period of 15–40 minutes[17]. It is uncertain whether any one of the various definitions of reactivity has significantly better or worse predictive properties than any other. Specific criteria are somewhat arbitrary; probably the most important issue is differentiating 'accelerations' from small changes in FHR constituting long-term variability[18]. To end the confusion of multiple proposed criteria, a standardized definition of reactivity was adopted that includes two or more accelerations within 20 minutes, of 15 seconds' duration from beginning to end, peaking at least 15 beats above baseline[19]. Normal baseline heart rate, variability, and the absence of non-reassuring decelerations are also requirements for a reassuring NST (Figure 4). Although performance of the

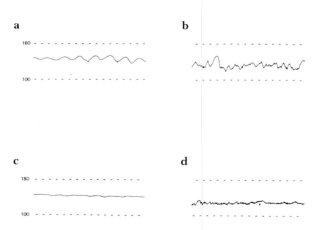

Figure 3   Variability. (**a**) Long-term variability present, short-term variability absent; (**b**) Long- and short-term variability present; (**c**) Long- and short-term variability absent; (**d**) Short-term variability present, long-term variability absent. Reproduced with permission[14]

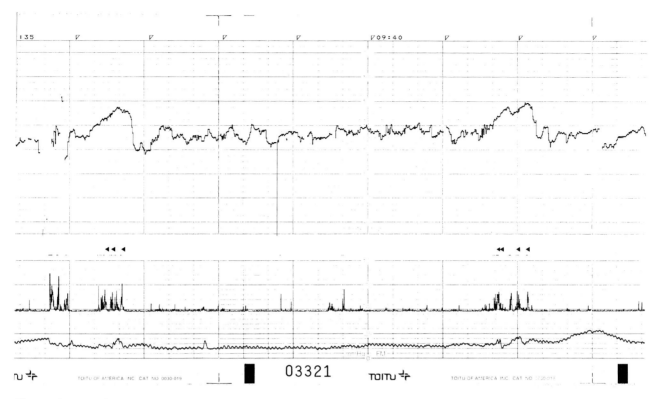

Figure 4   Reactive non-stress test. Several accelerations meeting the 15-beats for 15-seconds criteria are present, with normal baseline rate, normal variability, and no decelerations

test includes notation of fetal movements, nearly all accelerations are associated with movements[20], and tend to be counted even in the absence of maternal perception of fetal motion.

If the NST is not reactive after 20 minutes, the fetus may be asleep and the test duration extended. In a study using reactivity criteria of 5 accelerations per 20-minute interval, 75% of NSTs were reactive within 20 minutes, and 95% within 40 minutes[16]. Another approach to the non-reactive NST is fetal vibroacoustic stimulation (VAS), which stimulates the fetus by application of an artificial larynx to the maternal abdomen for 3 seconds in an effort to rouse the fetus from sleep. Accelerations in response to VAS correlate with normal fetal pH (which correlates with normal fetal oxygenation)[21], and reactivity following VAS has the same significance as 'spontaneous' reactivity[22,23]. The benefits of uterine manipulation, maternal ambulation, or glucose administration in an effort to convert a non-reactive NST into a reactive test are controversial[23].

Predictive value of non-stress testing

The efficacy of fetal testing depends on the definition of outcome. A positive test can be based on fetal death (a definite criterion), fetal distress (a vague criterion), operative delivery (multifactorial), etc. Fetal death is much easier to ascertain than fetal distress. 'Fetal distress' is meant to connote possible fetal hypoxia or asphyxia, but is imprecise and correlates poorly with these adverse outcomes. A test that predicts 'fetal distress' may or may not be relevant to the outcomes of fetal asphyxia or death. The choice of outcome will influence the sensitivity and specificity of the test.

Whatever the chosen outcome, the ideal test should have high sensitivity and specificity. Since it is difficult to have both in the same test, a balance between the two yields the most useful test. Because fetal demise is a catastrophic outcome that is potentially preventable, the sensitivity of a test of fetal well-being should be as high as possible to prevent as many such occurrences as possible. To do this, the criteria for defining an abnormal NST should be set overly inclusive to minimize false negatives, although this means the positive predictive value will be low. As a consequence of this, many false-positive tests will occur, necessitating follow-up testing and engendering anxiety in those patients.

Unfortunately, because of the occurrences of unpredictable events (placental abruption, for example), the sensitivity of NSTs is only ≈ 50% for perinatal mortality, although the specificity is high[24]. The patient with a positive test needs further testing, but the patient with a negative test can be reassured that fetal death is very unlikely to occur within a specified time period (usually one week).

The false-positive rate of non-stress testing is approximately 75%[18]. A false-positive NST refers to a non-reactive NST that is followed by a good perinatal outcome. Five to 15% of NSTs will initially be non-reactive[25,26], but most non-reactive NSTs will become reactive with further testing and not lead to adverse perinatal outcome. Prolonging the duration or using VAS during a NST that does not meet criteria for reactivity will decrease the false-positive rate. Persistently non-reactive NSTs are associated with uncorrected perinatal mortality rates of about 30–60/1000 and a three-fold increase in fetal distress[25,26]. Correcting for fetal anomalies, cord accidents, and placental abruption decreases the mortality rate by half.

Non-stress testing is considered a first line antenatal test because of its ease, time-efficiency, high negative predictive value, and relatively low cost. A reactive NST correlates well with normal central nervous system function at the time the test is performed but does not exclude past fetal hypoxemia or necessarily reflect fetal chronic state[18]. Despite these concerns, the risk of adverse perinatal outcome following a reactive NST is low. In eight studies (each including ≥ 500 patients) reviewed by Manning[18] and corrected for fetal anomalies, perinatal mortality after a reactive NST was 2–9 per 1000 (false-negative rate). Although this is higher than with CSTs or biophysical profiles (BPPs), when BPPs were prospectively compared with NSTs as a primary method of surveillance, the BPP's predictive value for adverse perinatal outcome was not statistically different from the NST[27,28]. None of these tests predict cataclysmic events (such as placental abruption) which can cause demise of an otherwise-healthy fetus.

Despite efforts to standardize NST criteria, there is a significant subjective element in its interpretation[29]. Because of the high false-positive rate associated with non-reactivity, delivery decisions are rarely made on the basis of a non-reactivity alone. The NST is best at predicting which fetus will be safe *in utero* for another 4–7 days: a normal test result is a good predictor of fetal well-being, but an abnormal result is not as good at predicting abnormal outcome. The NST serves as a screening test to determine which fetuses warrant additional testing modalities, such as a CST or BPP.

Indications for non-stress testing

Because non-stress testing is intended to detect signs of fetal hypoxia, it is used to assess fetal well-being in conditions potentially compromising fetal oxygenation. There are many conditions in which fetal hypoxia could conceivably occur, and so the list of possible indications for non-stress testing is indeed lengthy (Table 1). Although non-stress testing has been validated for some of these indications (intrauterine growth restriction, diabetes, postdates), other 'indications' are based on theoretical rationales and have not been tested for effectiveness in improving perinatal outcome (e.g. substance abuse, multiple gestation).

When a NST is reactive, the risk of fetal death over the following week is generally very low, so the test is repeated at weekly intervals. Fetal deaths within a week of a reactive NST may be more common in some conditions such as fetal growth

Table 1   Indications for non-stress testing

Maternal	*Fetal*
Diabetes	Growth restriction
Hypertension (chronic or	Multiple gestation
pre-eclampsia)	Hydrops (immune or
Collagen–vascular disease	non-immune)
Severe anemia or	Post-term
hemoglobinopathy	Decreased movement
Cardio-pulmonary disease	Oligohydramnios
Renal disease	
Hyperthyroidism	
Isoimmunization	
Substance abuse	
Previous stillborn	
Vaginal bleeding	
Premature rupture of	
membranes	

restriction, diabetes, or severe pre-eclampsia. Because fetal condition may deteriorate quickly in patients with these diagnoses, testing at least every 3–4 days is reasonable in such circumstances[19,30].

Non-stress testing usually begins at 32–34 weeks, but may be instituted before 30 weeks for some conditions (fetal growth restriction, severe diabetes, pre-eclampsia). Interpretation of NSTs in preterm fetuses is complicated because they are less likely to manifest reactive fetal heart rate patterns by traditional criteria. Total number of accelerations per hour, proportion of accelerations reaching 15 beats above baseline and lasting 15 seconds, and reactivity (based on the '15 beats for 15 seconds' criteria) all decrease with lower gestational age[31,32]. Using the 15×15 criteria, the frequencies of reactive NSTs at various gestational ages are shown in Table 2[31]. Gestational age dependency does not invalidate the test at early gestational ages, but using standard criteria, the clinician must accept that the false-positive rate of a non-reactive NST will be proportionally higher the earlier the gestational age, and ancillary testing will often be required.

In healthy fetuses below 30 weeks gestational age, the frequency of 10-beat accelerations is similar to the proportion of 15-beat accelerations in healthy fetuses $\geq$ 30 weeks gestation[15]. With this in mind, some authors have proposed modifying the criteria for reactivity in preterm gestations to require 10-beat rather than 15-beat accelerations. Although theoretically sound, the validity of this has not been clinically verified in preterm gestations[33]. Whichever criteria are used to define reactivity, non-reactive NSTs in the very premature fetus may be due to prematurity but must be considered non-reassuring until proven otherwise. At the same time, because of the significant false-positive rate and the risk of morbidity and mortality associated with preterm delivery, intervention for non-reassuring monitoring at <30 weeks gestation should be undertaken with great caution[34].

CONTRACTION STRESS TESTING

The CST was designed to evaluate uteroplacental function. Normally, there is enough oxygen exchange across the placenta so that the fetus has reserve, enabling it to tolerate transient episodes of decreased placental perfusion (such as those occurring during a contraction, when the

Table 2 Non-stress test reactivity by gestational age[31]

Gestational age	Reactive by 15 × 15-beat criteria
20–24 weeks	27%
24–28 weeks	55%
28–32 weeks	82%
32–36 weeks	95%
36–40 weeks	99%

myometrium compresses the uterine vessels conveying blood to the placenta). If uteroplacental function is diminished (uteroplacental insufficiency; UPI), then fetal oxygenation may be barely adequate when the uterus is relaxed, but become inadequate during the stress of a contraction. When uteroplacental blood flow fails to provide adequate oxygen exchange to meet fetal needs during a contraction, the fetus becomes hypoxemic and responds with a late FHR deceleration. Whereas a non-reactive NST is suspicious for fetal hypoxia compromising central nervous system function, an abnormal CST is evidence that uteroplacental function is impaired and fetal oxygen reserve is tenuous. As such, the CST may test for earlier signs of fetal compromise than does the NST[35]. The CST has an advantage of being independent of gestational age because the neurologic responses mediating late decelerations are functional by the middle of the second trimester.

Performance of the CST

Fetal heart and contraction monitors are applied to the woman in lateral tilt position. Contractions are then induced by one of several methods, the only requirement being that palpable contractions occur with a frequency of 3 in 10 minutes. There is no requirement for absolute intensity of contractions.

The most common way of inducing contractions is by using oxytocin, in which case the test is called an oxytocin challenge test (OCT). An intravenous catheter is inserted and oxytocin infused at 0.5 mU min^{-1}. The infusion rate is doubled every 15–20 minutes until the desired contraction frequency is achieved, depending on the FHR response. The fetal heart tracing is observed, noting the presence or absence of late decelerations. Stimulation of the maternal nipples for several minutes, followed by a 5 minute rest (repeating the cycle as needed) will produce contractions in the majority of women and is an acceptable method. Occasionally, contractions will occur spontaneously, and if there are three within 10 minutes, then a 'spontaneous' CST has been performed.

Interpretation of the CST

Interpretation of the CST is outlined in Table 3[10].

If repetitive late decelerations are present even when the contraction frequency is less than 3 in 10 minutes, the CST is considered positive and should be discontinued.

Predictive value of the CST

Whenever a CST is performed, an NST-equivalent is simultaneously performed. Because of this, every CST includes an NST interpretation. Each NST can be reactive or non-reactive and each CST positive or negative, so there are four possible combinations of results.

(1) Reactive–negative: This is the most common result, with no indication of UPI or fetal hypoxia. The corrected fetal death rate within one week of a reactive–negative CST is approximately 0.4/1000 (1/1000 if uncorrected for fetal anomalies)[36]. The test is usually repeated weekly, if indicated.

(2) Reactive–positive: This is consistent with mild–moderate UPI, but without frank fetal hypoxia at the time the test was performed. Corrected perinatal mortality is 8/1000 (51/1000 uncorrected)[25]. Fetal distress during labor occurs in 28–62% of pregnancies in which the CST is reactive–positive[25,37,38]. At term, a patient with a reactive–positive CST should be delivered because of the chance that UPI will progressively worsen and result in frank fetal hypoxia. In a preterm gestation in the absence of fetal pulmonary maturity, testing should be repeated daily until maturity is reached or fetal status deteriorates.

(3) Non-reactive–negative: A true non-reactive–negative CST should be rare, and is associated with prematurity, fetal sleep cycles, and maternal medication use. Physiologically, it would be unusual for the fetus to be hypoxic (evidenced by non-reactivity) if uteroplacental function is normal (evidenced by a negative CST). In some instances, subtle late decelerations may have been missed and

Table 3   Interpretation of the contraction stress test

Negative	No late decelerations on a tracing of adequate technical quality
Positive	Repetitive late decelerations occurring after >50% of contractions, in the absence of hyperstimulation or supine hypotension
Suspicious	Late decelerations after <50% of contractions
Hyperstimulation	Decelerations after prolonged (>90 seconds) contractions or those occurring more frequently than every two minutes
Unsatisfactory	Technically inadequate tracing, either unable to document contractions or interpret fetal heart rate pattern

the test interpreted as non-reactive–negative when it should have been non-reactive–positive. Corrected perinatal mortality after a non-reactive–negative CST is 0–17/1000[39,40]. Perinatal morbidity is doubled compared with reactive–negative CSTs, and fetal distress during labor occurs in 50% of patients with non-reactive–negative CSTs[41,42]. Follow-up after a non-reactive–negative CST is controversial, with recommendations ranging from weekly to daily fetal assessment.

(4) Non-reactive–positive: This result is consistent with UPI and fetal hypoxia, and is associated with a corrected perinatal mortality rate of 176/1000 (211/1000 uncorrected)[25]. Non-reassuring intrapartum FHR patterns occur in 78–100% of patients with non-reactive–positive CSTs[25,37,38], and 33–100% require cesarean section[37,42–44]. Delivery is indicated after a non-reactive–positive CST occurring after 30–32 weeks gestational age. In gestations <30–32 weeks, further evaluation of the fetus should be considered first, because of the chance that the non-reactive NST may be due to prematurity rather than hypoxia.

Cesarean is the most common route of delivery after a non-reactive–positive CST, because these fetuses rarely tolerate labor[37,42–44]. However, induction may be attempted if the cervix is favorable and internal FHR monitoring and scalp pH determinations are readily available.

Suspicious CSTs should be repeated within 24 hours. The false-positive rate of a suspicious CST is high, and intervention based on a suspicious result alone is often unwarranted. Although the incidence of intrapartum fetal distress following a suspicious CST is twice as high as after a negative CST, perinatal mortality is unchanged[25].

The CST has been criticized for having a high false-positive rate, generally reported to be about 30%[38,45,46] but occasionally as high as 75%[47]. A false-positive CST refers to a positive CST in a fetus who tolerates labor without perinatal morbidity. It is apparent that full interpretation of the CST includes concurrent interpretation of the NST. A reactive NST lowers the perinatal morbidity and mortality associated with a positive CST, whereas a non-reactive NST increases morbidity and mortality. To minimize the false-positive CST rate, it is important that supine hypotension or other reversible causes of UPI be corrected before performing a CST.

The indications for a CST are the same as for an NST, except that a CST is rarely repeated more than once a week. Unlike the NST, there are several contraindications to the CST. Preterm labor, cervical incompetence, placenta previa, abruption, or previous classical uterine incision are contraindications, and a CST should be used with caution in patients with premature rupture of the membranes or multiple gestation.

Overall, the CST is a better predictor of fetal outcome than the NST. Freeman et al.[36] reported that, when used as a primary means of surveillance, the corrected perinatal mortality using CSTs was 0.4/1000 compared with 3.2/1000 for NSTs. However, because the CST is cumbersome, invasive, and time-consuming, the NST is better suited as a screening test, with the CST usually reserved for further evaluation of non-reactive NSTs rather than as a primary method of fetal surveillance.

ULTRASONOGRAPHIC ASSESSMENT

Whereas fetal heart rate monitoring allows indirect assessment of placental function and fetal oxygen status, ultrasonography has expanded the scope of fetal assessment to include visualization of fetal anatomy, behavioral states, amniotic fluid volume, and umbilical cord blood flow. Integration of several of these parameters into the biophysical profile improves the predictive value for fetal well-being and for fetal compromise.

Amniotic fluid volume assessment

Until approximately 18–20 weeks gestation, amniotic fluid consists primarily of transudate across the membranes and fetal skin[48]. In the second half of pregnancy, fetal urine is the main component. Amniotic fluid volume changes with gestational age, ranging from ≈ 30 ml at 10 weeks, to ≈ 190 ml at 16 weeks, peaking at ≈ 900 ml at the middle of the third trimester and then declining toward term[49]. Fetal swallowing removes amniotic fluid, through absorption of swallowed fluid into the fetal circulation where it can equilibrate over the placenta into the maternal bloodstream. Precise mechanisms regulating amniotic fluid volume (AFV) and composition are poorly understood, but involve a balance between fetal urine output, swallowing, pulmonary fluid efflux, maternal hydration, and membrane status[50].

Dye dilution is the 'gold standard' for measuring AFV. A given amount of a certain concentration of a dye is injected into the amniotic fluid, allowed to equilibrate, and an aliquot of fluid removed. The amniotic fluid dilutes the dye, and the new dye concentration can be measured. By knowing the initial amount and concentration of the dye, the total volume of fluid into which the dye has been diluted can be calculated, equaling the AFV. Although precise, this method is invasive and impractical for clinical use.

Methods of sonographically assessing amniotic fluid volume

Ultrasonographic assessment of AFV is non-invasive and can substitute for dye dilution. Several methods using ultrasound have been proposed, none of which are as precise as dye dilution, but all of which are easily performed. The first such method was to estimate total intrauterine volume to correlate with AFV[51]. Because of technical problems and the difficulty of accounting for fetal and placental volume, this method did not prove accurate. A simple method is to subjectively assess the AFV as either normal, decreased (oligohydramnios), or increased (polyhydramnios). Such assessments are dependent on the experience of the observer, although fairly reproducible if the observers are experienced[52]. The 'deepest single pocket' method measures the deepest pocket of amniotic fluid (at least 1 cm wide). A deepest pocket measuring ≥ 8 cm has been defined as polyhydramnios, and ≤ 2 cm as oligohydramnios[53,54]. More recently, the 'amniotic fluid index' (AFI) has gained popularity. To perform an AFI, the deepest pocket of amniotic fluid in each of 4 quadrants of the uterus are measured while holding the transducer perpendicular to the floor and longitudinal to the patient's spine. Umbilical cord should not be included in the measurement. The four measurements are added to yield the AFI[55]. Confidence intervals for each gestational age (based on AFI assessment of nearly 800 pregnancies) allow the clinician to determine whether or not the AFI is within the normal percentile range[56]. A normal AFI or deepest single pocket correlates well with normal AFV as measured by dye dilution, but may underestimate or overestimate AFV in cases of oligohydramnios or polyhydramnios, respectively[57–59].

Abnormal amniotic fluid volume

Polyhydramnios is associated with fetal anomalies (especially gastrointestinal and neural tube defects, in which there is obstructed swallowing or excessive fluid passage across exposed tissues), hydrops (as a result of cardiac decompensation due to either immunologic or non-immune mechanisms), aneuploidy, multiple gestation, maternal diabetes, or fetal macrosomia. Because of these associations, polyhydramnios is associated with a three to sevenfold increase in perinatal mortality (two to fourfold if corrected for fetal anomalies)[54,60]. If polyhydramnios is idiopathic and mild, 40% to 73% will resolve without sequelae. Persistent polyhydramnios (even mild) is frequently associated with adverse perinatal outcome[61,62]. In as many as 90% of pregnancies complicated by severe polyhydramnios, there is an identifiable cause for the excess amniotic fluid[63].

Oligohydramnios is associated with fetal growth restriction, anomalies (especially urinary tract obstruction, preventing passage of urine), aneuploidy, placental insufficiency, postdates, ruptured membranes, and certain medications (prostaglandin synthetase inhibitors and angiotensin converting enzyme inhibitors). Fetal hypoxia results in redistribution of fetal blood away from the kidneys, decreasing plasma filtration and urine output. Prolonged oligohydramnios may cause pulmonary hypoplasia and limb deformities. Perinatal mortality is related to the degree of oligohydramnios. In a large study using the single deepest pocket technique, corrected perinatal mortality increased 19-fold when the largest pocket measured between 1 and 2 cm, and 55-fold for a largest pocket <1 cm when compared with patients with normal AFV[53]. In that study, perinatal morbidity also correlated with the degree of oligohydramnios. Other studies have reported a threefold increase in operative deliveries when the AFI is 2 cm[64], and a twofold increase in umbilical artery acidosis at delivery when the AFI is ≤ 5 cm (positive predictive value 31%)[65]. Oligohydramnios during the second trimester is associated with very poor outcome. Under these circumstances, perinatal mortality has been reported to range from 64% to 100%, with normal outcome in less than 20%[66,67].

BIOPHYSICAL PROFILE SCORING

Ultrasonographic fetal weight estimation and evaluation of fetal anatomy popularized the use of obstetrical ultrasound in the 1970s. In the 1980s, investigators realized that ultrasound had potential beyond the ability to evaluate just fetal anatomy and weight: it could be used to observe the intrauterine environment and dynamic fetal responses therein. As with FHR monitoring, normal fetal responses require normal fetal central nervous system function, which requires adequate fetal oxygenation. BPP scoring was developed, enabling quantitative evaluation of the fetus.

Central nervous system maturation and neuromuscular function

The fetal central nervous system gradually matures throughout gestation. Manifestation of this maturation takes the form of neuromuscular activity, such as muscular tone, movements, and breathing motions, all of which are under central nervous system control. Tone and movement have been recognized as early as 6–7 weeks gestation, and breathing movements as early as 12–14 weeks. FHR accelerations with movements (reactivity) develop at 16–18 weeks[68]. Normal manifestations of these activities require adequate fetal oxygenation to ensure proper central nervous system function. There is evidence that the various subcortical centers in the brain that control these activities have differential sensitivities to oxygen, with the earliest developed being the least sensitive to hypoxia. Reactivity followed by breathing are most sensitive to decreased oxygen concentrations, with movement and tone least sensitive. With progressive hypoxia, reactivity tends to be lost first, then breathing motions, and finally movement and tone[69,70].

These parameters can be evaluated sonographically. The presence or absence of each parameter alone can be influenced not only by gestational age and absolute hypoxia, but also by fetal sleep cycles, maternal medications, fetal structural anomalies, and duration of hypoxia. Although each parameter does correlate individually with the presence or absence of acute fetal hypoxia and acidosis, they are much better predictors of fetal state when evaluated in aggregate. Not only does the aggregate score allow for graded risk prediction, but it minimizes the effect of random fluctuations of each parameter[71].

An isolated, acute, mild-to-moderate hypoxic episode may resolve. Although fetal movement, tone, breathing, and reactivity may be transiently depressed during the episode, unless significant cerebral injury is sustained these parameters will subsequently return to normal. Unless testing is done during such a hypoxic episode, its occurrence cannot be retrospectively verified by these parameters.

Fetal responses to hypoxia can be classified as either acute or chronic. In the case of sudden umbilical cord compression, flow of oxygenated blood into the fetus precipitously slows or stops. Fetal pO_2 decreases and pCO_2 increases. If compression persists, the increased pCO_2 lowers the fetal blood pH through conversion of CO_2 to carbonic acid. The immediate fetal response to hypoxia is redistribution of blood flow to the brain, heart, and adrenal glands, away from the kidneys, gut, and extremities[72]. If normal oxygenation is restored, pO_2 rises, pCO_2 declines, the pH rises back to normal, and the cardiovascular changes reverse.

With prolonged or current hypoxia, whether due to repetitive umbilical cord compression, uteroplacental insufficiency, or placental abruption, fetal cardiovascular redistribution persists. Fetal urinary output declines because of vasopressin release and decreased renal perfusion. Because fetal urine is the primary component of amniotic fluid, lower urine output results in lower AFV. In addition, prolonged hypoxia causes a shift from aerobic to anaerobic metabolism. In the absence of adequate oxygen, glucose is metabolized to lactic acid, an inefficient process leading to metabolic acidosis. In extreme cases, asphyxia and organ damage ensue.

AFV assessment provides a means of evaluating chronic hypoxic states. When the largest single pocket of amniotic fluid is ≤ 2 cm, perinatal morbidity increases[53]. When combined with assessment of the acutely-affected parameters above, the presence and contribution of both acute and chronic hypoxia can be evaluated. The BPP comprises these five parameters.

Performance and scoring of the biophysical profile

The BPP consists of a 30-minute period of sonographic observation of the fetus. This period can be extended, if necessary. The patient should be in a semi-recumbent position (not supine). During this time, fetal body movements, tone, breathing motion, and AFV are evaluated. The patient also undergoes a NST before or after the ultrasound examination. According to the criteria listed in Table 4[68] either 2 or 0 points are given for the presence or absence of each parameter, respectively. The maximum score is 10, if all five parameters are present. The lowest score is 0, if none of the parameters are present.

The BPP score correlates with the probability of perinatal morbidity and mortality. Scores of 10 or

Table 4 Biophysical profile scoring

Biophysical variable	Normal (2 points)	Abnormal (0 points)
Breathing movements	≥ 1 episode of ≥ 30 seconds	Absent or episodes <30 seconds
Body movements	≥ 2 discrete body/limb movements*	<2 body/limb movements*
Fetal tone	≥ 1 active extension and return to flexion of limb or trunk	Absent, or partial return to flexion, or movement in full extension only
FHR reactivity	≥ 2 FHR accelerations of ≥ 15 bpm (peak of ≥ 15 seconds' duration in 20 minutes)	<2 FHR accelerations ≥ 15 bpm (peak) of ≥ 15 seconds' duration in 20 minutes
Amniotic fluid volume	≥ 1 pocket of fluid of ≥ 2 cm vertical depth	No pocket of fluid of ≥ 2 cm vertical depth

*Earlier criteria use 3 movements rather than 2. FHR, fetal heart rate. Modified with permission[68]

8 are normal, while a score of 6 is equivocal. A score of 4 is non-reassuring and indicates probable fetal hypoxia. Scores of 2 or 0 are ominous, consistent with a very high likelihood of fetal asphyxia. The lower the BPP score, the lower the mean umbilical cord pH and the higher perinatal morbidity and mortality[69,73] (Figures 5, 6 and 7).

For perinatal mortality, the sensitivity of the BPP is 75%, with 33% false positives. For perinatal morbidity, the sensitivity of the BPP is 69%, with 39% false positives[74].

Non-equivalence of score combinations

Although each parameter is evaluated using the same scale (0 or 2 points), they are not all of exactly the same predictive value. Using logistic regression analysis, NST non-reactivity has the highest

correlation with perinatal mortality, and decreased AFV with morbidity[74]. Different combinations of normal and abnormal parameters may equal a certain score, but depending on the composition of that score, predictive value may vary. Gradations of predictive value for different normal and abnormal parameter combinations have been reported, but the clinical utility of these gradations is limited.

BPP interpretation, management, and modifications

Manning[68] proposed management plans that depend on the score composition and persistence, and gestational age. Any score must be interpreted in light of available clinical information about the patient, rather than in a vacuum. A normal preterm

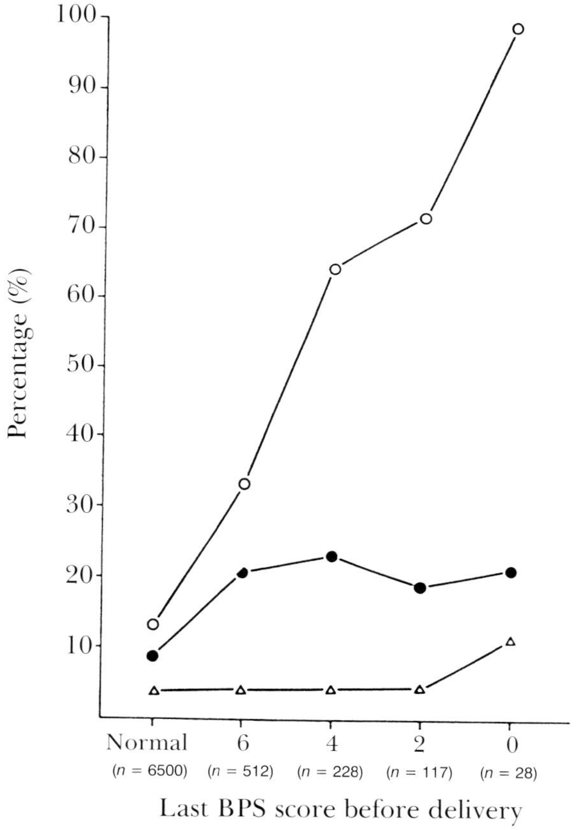

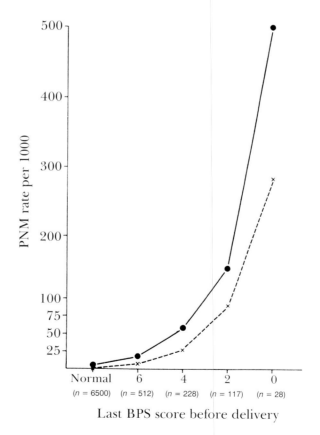

Figure 5 Perinatal morbidity by most recent biophysical profile score. Morbidity is 100% with a biophysical profile score of 0. BPS, biophysical profile score. Perinatal morbidity (any), empty circles; meconium, shaded circles; major anomaly, triangles. With permission[73]

Figure 6 Perinatal mortality by most recent biophysical profile score. The increase in perinatal mortality rises exponentially with decreasing biophysical profile score. BPS, biophysical profile score; PNM, perinatal mortality. Gross PNM rate, solid line; corrected PNM rate, broken line. With permission[73]

fetus may score lower on a BPP than a term fetus due to lower frequencies of breathing movements and NST reactivity, both of which are gestational age dependent and are less sensitive indicators of hypoxia in premature fetuses[31,75,76]. Testing intervals depend on gestational age, obstetrical complications, and the most recent BPP score, ranging from hours to 7 days (Table 5).

Several BPP modifications have been proposed. Placental grading is included in some scoring systems[77], but does not appear to improve predictive value. If a score of 8/8 is achieved on ultrasonographic evaluation before performance of an NST, proceeding to an NST is optional because, in the absence of oligohydramnios, an 8–10/10 score is normal and so the additional 0 or 2 points from the NST will not influence management. However, if a sonographic score is less than 8/8, non-stress testing must be performed[78].

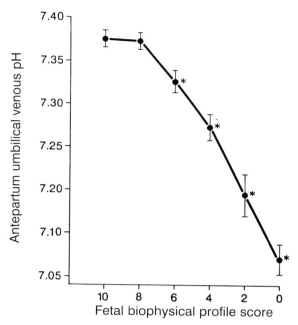

Figure 7 Antepartum umbilical artery pH by most recent biophysical profile score. Umbilical artery pH falls as the biophysical profile score decreases. *$p < 0.05$ vs. next higher value. With permission[69]

Table 5 Interpretation and management of biophysical profile score (BPS)

BPS/result	Interpretation	Risk of asphyxia (umbilical venous) metabolic acidosis <7.25) (%)	Risk of fetal death (per 1000/week)	Recommended management
10/10 8/10 (N-AFV) 8/8 (NST not done)	Nonasphyxiated	0	0.565	No indication for intervention for fetal indications
8/10 Oligo	Chronic compensated asphyxia	5–10 (estimate)	20–30	If mature (≥ 37 weeks), deliver. Serial testing (twice weekly) in the immature fetus
6/10 N-AFV	Acute asphyxia possible	10	50	If mature (≥ 37 weeks), deliver. Repeat test in 24 hours in immature fetus. Repeat test; if ≤ 6/10, deliver
6/10 Oligo	Chronic asphyxia with possible acute asphyxia	> 10 (?)	> 50	Factor in gestational age; if ≥ 32 weeks, deliver. If ≤ 32 weeks, test daily
4/10 N-AFV	Acute asphyxia likely	36	115	Factor in gestational age; if ≥ 32 weeks, deliver. If ≤ 32 weeks, test daily.
4/10 Oligo	Chronic asphyxia, acute asphyxia likely	>36	>115	If ≥ 26 weeks, deliver
2/10 N-AFV	Acute asphyxia nearly certain	73	220	If ≥ 26 weeks, deliver
2/10 Oligo	Chronic asphyxia with superimposed acute asphyxia	>73	>220	If ≥ 26 weeks, deliver
0/10	Gross severe asphyxia	100	550	If ≥ 26 weeks, deliver

Oligo, oligohydramnios (maximal fluid pocket ≤ 2 cm in vertical axis)
Reproduced with permission[68]

Several investigators have reported that performance of only an AFV assessment and an NST (the 'modified BPP') has similar predictive value to a CST, and can be done in less time than a complete BPP[79,80]. The presence of normal AFV and a reactive NST should rule out both chronic and acute hypoxia, respectively. It is unlikely that two of the remaining three parameters will be abnormal if AFV and NST are normal, making it unlikely that a total score of less than 8 will be obtained.

Indications for biophysical profile testing

The BPP is used frequently as a follow-up test after a non-reactive NST. Compared with a CST, the BPP is less invasive, easier to perform, takes less time, and has no contraindications. Although both the BPP and CST have graded prognostic value, they evaluate different physiologic variables. The CST evaluates uteroplacental function whereas the BPP evaluates fetal state as a function of oxygenation. With rare exceptions, the CST is not influenced by gestational age, fetal anomalies, or fetal sleep cycles, all of which can influence the BPP. The BPP's gradations give more information, but not all of it necessarily relates to fetal oxygen status. The BPP is better than the CST at predicting fetal morbidity, but may be difficult to interpret in pregnancies complicated by prematurity[75], fetal anomalies (central nervous system, musculo-skeletal, or restrictive cutaneous), maternal drug use (sedatives or magnesium sulfate)[81,82], or during fetal sleep cycles. These factors should be considered when choosing which test to use following a non-reactive NST.

The BPP has been evaluated as a primary means of fetal surveillance. Although it has a lower false-negative rate than the NST, it takes longer and is more expensive. Several randomized trials have failed to demonstrate superiority of the BPP over the NST as a primary means of surveillance, and so the BPP is not recommended as the initial mode of testing for the majority of patients in whom antepartum fetal assessment is indicated[27,28].

UMBILICAL ARTERY DOPPLER VELOCIMETRY

To receive oxygen, fetal blood must flow through the placenta. It is possible to measure umbilical artery flow through the use of Doppler ultrasound.

The principle is based on the Doppler shift: waves of a given frequency that are reflected by a moving surface or interface will undergo a shift in frequency that is proportional to the rate of movement of the surface. If the surface is moving towards the transducer, the frequency of the returning wave will shift upward to a higher frequency. If the surface is moving away from the transducer, the returning wave's frequency will shift downward. To use Doppler to calculate the velocity of flow of the blood cells through a vessel, the diameter of the vessel, the angle of insonation, the tissue densities through which the sound waves must pass, and the frequencies of the transmitted and received ultrasound waves must all be determined. Unfortunately, there is a certain error inherent in each measurement, so that when added together the range of error for a given calculated value is so wide that the derived rate of flow cannot be considered accurate.

Despite the intrinsic error in the absolute flow calculation, the ratio of systolic/diastolic flow can be accurately calculated (the S/D ratio). Since the vessel diameter varies only slightly during the cardiac cycle, the tissue density and angle of insonation do not change, and the transmitted ultrasound frequency remains the same, the error terms in the numerator and denominator of the ratio cancel, leaving the Doppler frequency shift as the only variable. This can be precisely measured. This ratio is proportional to the resistance to flow downstream from the measurement point. If there were no friction (resistance to flow), then the heart would only have to beat once, and blood would flow through the vessels indefinitely. Flow during systole would equal flow during diastole, and S/D would equal 1.0. Conversely, if there is high resistance to flow, blood will surge forward during systole, but nearly stop during diastole when the heart is relaxed and there is no active driving force propelling the blood forward through the high-resistance vessels. In that case, the S/D will be a very high number (approaching infinity in the case of no diastolic flow), because of the low value of the denominator. At first glance, a high S/D might be thought favorable and indicative of increased systolic flow. However, it must be remembered that, in the case of elevated S/D, both systolic and diastolic flow are actually decreased, but diastolic (denominator) more so than systolic (numerator). In the worst cases, the increased resistance is so great that the vessels reflect back the column of blood during diastole, reversing flow.

The pulsatility index $PI = \frac{(S-D)}{S}$ and resistance index $RI = \frac{(S-D)}{mean}$ can also be derived from relative systolic and diastolic flow. The mathematical properties of the PI and RI are different from the S/D, but their clinical utility is similar.

The S/D in evaluating placental resistance

Using the umbilical artery S/D (or related measurements such as the PI or RI), intraplacental resistance to flow can be assessed. The transducer should be held so that the focal point is on the umbilical artery just as it enters the placenta, otherwise resistance due to umbilical cord length will be incorporated into the S/D, artifactually elevating the ratio. Resistance to flow is inversely proportional to the total cross-sectional diameter through which a fluid flows: the greater the diameter, the lower the resistance. As the placenta grows during pregnancy, there are more and more villi, arterioles, and capillaries, so there is progressively greater cross-sectional area. Therefore, intraplacental resistance normally decreases as pregnancy progresses, and so does the umbilical artery S/D. Normal curves and confidence intervals have been derived by measuring the S/D at many gestational ages. An S/D above the 95th percentile is considered abnormal, consistent with increased resistance to flow. Conditions limiting placental vascularity, such as infarction or hypoplasia, decrease the cross-sectional area and increase the resistance to flow. The placental small-arteriole count is lower in pregnancies with high S/Ds compared with pregnancies with normal S/Ds[83] (Figures 8, 9 and 10).

Umbilical artery Doppler velocimetry in clinical practice

Umbilical artery Doppler velocimetry has been used for antenatal fetal monitoring, but uncertainty persists about its value. Several authors have reported associations of abnormal umbilical artery Doppler S/Ds with adverse perinatal outcomes in aggregate, but the positive predictive values for individual outcomes by themselves (low Apgar, acidosis, NICU admission, mortality, etc.) are variable and tend to be low (from 8% to 74%)[84–86]. In one report, umbilical artery Doppler surpassed fetal heart rate monitoring[85], but several other investigators have reported the opposite to be true[87,88]. Screening obstetrical populations with

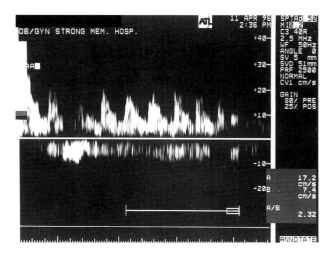

Figure 8 Umbilical artery Doppler – normal. The ratio of the systolic peak to the diastolic nadir (S/D) is low, indicating normal placental resistance to flow. Non-pulsatile flow in the umbilical vein is recorded as a continuous band beneath the pulsatile arterial flow

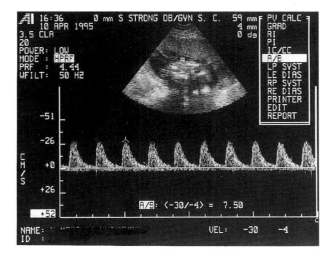

Figure 9 Umbilical artery Doppler – high. The ratio of the systolic peak to the diastolic nadir (S/D) is high, indicating increased placental resistance to flow

umbilical artery Doppler is not effective in reducing perinatal morbidity and mortality in most studies[89–94], although a recent meta-analysis concluded that perinatal mortality is lower in patients undergoing Doppler screening[95]. In some studies, statistical power may have been too low to prove significant differences, and differences in study design make direct comparisons problematic.

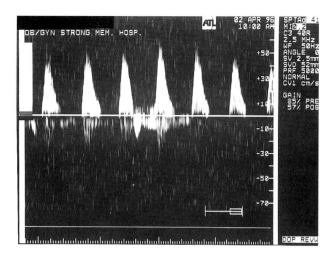

Figure 10 Umbilical artery Doppler – absent diastolic flow. Placental resistance is so high that flow stops during diastole. This is associated with poor perinatal outcome

Umbilical artery Doppler may possibly be helpful in some high-risk patients. A recent review of eight studies noted sensitivities of between 49% and 78% for detection of growth restricted fetuses, with positive predictive values of between 24% and 81% (not very different from the results using standard ultrasound size measurements alone)[96]. Several investigators have reported decreased perinatal morbidity associated with Doppler screening of patients at high risk for fetal growth restriction[97,98]. At this time, it is unclear whether there are advantages to using umbilical artery flow velocimetry in pregnancies complicated by diabetes or hypertension.

An important exception is the patient with absent or reversed diastolic flow. Reversed diastolic flow is associated with 50–90% perinatal mortality, and significant morbidity[99,100]. In this case, a patient at or near term should be delivered. However, even reversed diastolic flow can sometimes improve if reversible causes of placental insufficiency are effectively treated. For the preterm patient with absent diastolic flow, continuing the pregnancy with aggressive daily monitoring has been shown to be effective in prolonging pregnancy and achieving acceptable outcomes[101].

In summary, umbilical artery Doppler velocimetry may be useful in certain patients at risk for placental dysfunction, but for most patients does not clearly add benefits beyond those achievable with standard monitoring modalities such as non-stress testing and BPP scoring. Umbilical artery Doppler velocimetry is most often used to confirm what is already suspected, rather than as an integral part of initial fetal assessment. Management decisions are more often made based on NST, CST, or BPP results than on Doppler.

CONCLUSION

Although the NST, CST, and BPP all differ methodologically, they have a common ultimate goal of indirectly evaluating fetal oxygen status as an indicator of fetal well-being. Each test has its strengths and weaknesses. The NST is quickest, least expensive, and non-invasive, but has a high false-positive rate and is the least sensitive for the outcome of fetal death. The CST is invasive, time-consuming, and has certain contraindications, but has a very low false-negative rate and provides accurate assessment of uteroplacental insufficiency. BPP scoring based on assessment of multiple parameters is expensive and time-consuming, but provides graded perinatal morbidity and mortality risk assessment, with a very low false-negative rate. For all three tests, a normal test result is very reassuring, although an abnormal result is less predictive for significant fetal compromise. The use of these tests in high-risk pregnancies has the potential to detect compromised fetuses at a time when intervention can be life-saving.

References

1. Cunningham FG, MacDonald PC, Gant NF, *et al.* *Williams Obstetrics*, 20th edn. Norwalk, CT: Appleton & Lange, 1997
2. Naeye RL. Causes of perinatal mortality in the United States. Collaborative perinatal project. *J Am Med Assoc* 1987;238:228–9
3. Center for Disease Control. Contribution of birth defects to infant mortality – United States, 1986. *Morb Mortal Wkly Rep* 1989;38:633–5
4. Lammer EJ, Brown LE, Anderka MT, *et al.* Classification and analysis of fetal deaths in Massachusetts. *J Am Med Assoc* 1989;261:1757–62

5. Stubblefield PG, Berek JS. Perinatal mortality in term and post-term births. *Obstet Gynecol* 1980;56:676–82

6. Public Health Service. *Vital Statistics of the United States*, Vol II. *Mortality*, 1986. Hyattsville: U.S. Department of Health and Human Services

7. Mersey Region Working Party on Perinatal Mortality. Confidential inquiry into perinatal deaths in the Mersey region. *Lancet* 1982;1:491–4

8. Kirkup B, Welch G. 'Normal but dead': perinatal mortality in non-malformed babies of birthweight 2.5 kg and over in the Northern Region in 1983. *Br J Obstet Gynaecol* 1990;97:381–92

9. Delke I, Hyatt R, Feinkind L, *et al*. Avoidable causes of perinatal death at or after term pregnancy in an inner-city hospital: medical versus social. *Am J Obstet Gynecol* 1988;159:562–6

10. Freeman RK, Garite TJ, Nageotte MP. *Fetal Heart Rate Monitoring*, 2nd edn. Baltimore: Williams & Wilkins, 1991

11. Hon EH. Observations on 'pathologic' fetal bradycardia. *Am J Obstet Gynecol* 1959;77:1084–99

12. Huch A, Huch R, Schneider H, *et al*. Continuous transcutaneous monitoring of fetal oxygen tension during labour. *Br J Obstet Gynaecol* 1977;84:1–39

13. Parer JT, Krueger TR, Harris JL. Fetal oxygen consumption and mechanisms of heart rate response during artificially produced late decelerations of fetal heart rate in sheep. *Am J Obstet Gynecol* 1980;136:478–82

14. Yeh SY, Forsythe A, Hon EH. Quantification of fetal heart beat to beat interval differences. *Obstet Gynecol* 1973;41:355–63

15. Gagnon R, Campbell K, Hunse C, *et al*. Patterns of human fetal heart rate accelerations from 26 weeks to term. *Am J Obstet Gynecol* 1987;57:743–8

16. Brown R, Patrick J. The nonstress test: how long is enough? *Am J Obstet Gynecol* 1981;141:646–51

17. Devoe LD. The non-stress test. In Eden RD, Boehm FH, eds. *Assessment and Care of the Fetus: Physiological, Clinical and Medicolegal Principles*. Norwalk: Appleton & Lange, 1990:265

18. Manning FA (ed.) The fetal heart rate: antepartum and intrapartum regulation and clinical significance. In *Fetal Medicine: Principles and Practice*. Norwalk: Appleton & Lange, 1995:13–111

19. American College of Obstetricians and Gynecologists. Antepartum fetal surveillance. *ACOG Technical Bulletin* 1994;188

20. Timor-Tritsch IE, Dierker LJ, Hertz RH, *et al*. Fetal movements associated with fetal heart rate accelerations and decelerations. *Am J Obstet Gynecol* 1978;131:276–80

21. Smith CV, Nguyen HN, Phelan JP, *et al*. Intrapartum assessment of fetal well being: a comparison of fetal acoustic stimulation with acid base determinations. *Am J Obstet Gynecol* 1986;155:726–8

22. Gagnon R. Acoustic stimulation: effect on heart rate and other biophysical variables. *Clin Perinatol* 1989;16:643–60

23. Smith CV. Vibroacoustic stimulation. *Clin Obstet Gynecol* 1995;38:68–77

24. Ware DJ, Devoe LD. The nonstress test: reassessment of the 'gold standard'. *Clin Perinatol* 1994;21:779–96

25. Freeman RK, Anderson G, Dorchester W. A prospective multi-institutional study of antepartum fetal heart rate monitoring: I. Risk of perinatal mortality and morbidity according to antepartum fetal heart rate test results. *Am J Obstet Gynecol* 1982;143:771–7

26. Phelan JP. The nonstress test: a review of 3000 tests. *Am J Obstet Gynecol* 1981;139:7–10

27. Manning FA, Lange IR, Morrison I, *et al*. Fetal biophysical profile score and the nonstress test: a comparative trial. *Obstet Gynecol* 1984;64:326–31

28. Platt LD, Walla CA, Paul RH, *et al*. A prospective trial of the fetal biophysical profile versus the nonstress test in the management of high-risk pregnancies. *Am J Obstet Gynecol* 1985;153:624–33

29. Borgatta L, Shrout PE, Divon MY. Reliability and reproducibility of nonstress test readings. *Am J Obstet Gynecol* 1988;159:554–8

30. Barrett JM, Salyer SL, Boehm FH. The nonstress test: an evaluation of 1000 patients. *Am J Obstet Gynecol* 1981;141:153–7

31. Druzin ML, Fox A, Kogut E, *et al*. The relationship of the nonstress test to gestational age. *Am J Obstet Gynecol* 1985;153:386–9

32. Natale R, Nasello C, Turliuk R. The relationship between movements and accelerations in fetal heart rate at twenty-four to thirty-two weeks' gestation. *Am J Obstet Gynecol* 1984;148:591–5

33. Castillo RA, DeVoe LD, Arthur M, *et al*. The preterm nonstress test: effects of gestational age and length of study. *Am J Obstet Gynecol* 1989;160:172–5

34. Rouse DJ, Owen J, Goldenberg RL, *et al*. Determinants of the optimal time in gestation to initiate antenatal fetal testing: a decision-analytic approach. *Am J Obstet Gynecol* 1995;173:1357–63

35. Murata Y, Martin CB, Ikenoue T, *et al*. Fetal heart rate accelerations and late decelerations during the course of intrauterine death in chronically catheterized rhesus monkeys. *Am J Obstet Gynecol* 1982;144:218–23

36. Freeman RK, Anderson G, Dorchester W. A prospective multi-institutional study of antepartum fetal heart monitoring: II. Contraction stress test versus nonstress test for primary surveillance. *Am J Obstet Gynecol* 1982;143:778–80

37. Huddleston JF, Sutliff G, Carney FE, *et al*. Oxytocin challenge test for antepartum fetal assessment. *Am J Obstet Gynecol* 1979;135:609–14

38. Braly P, Freeman RK. The significance of fetal heart rate reactivity with a positive oxytocin challenge test. *Obstet Gynecol* 1977;50:689–93

39. Druzin ML, Gratacos J, Paul RH. Antepartum fetal heart rate testing: VI. Predictive reliability of

'normal' tests in the prevention of antepartum death. *Am J Obstet Gynecol* 1980;137:746–7

40. Grundy H, Freeman RK, Lederman S, *et al.* Nonreactive contraction stress test: clinical significance. *Obstet Gynecol* 1984;64:337–42

41. Lin CC, Moawad AH, River P, *et al.* An OCT-reactivity classification to predict fetal outcome. *Obstet Gynecol* 1980;56:17–23

42. Keegan KA, Paul RH. Antepartum fetal heart rate testing: IV. The nonstress test as a primary approach. *Am J Obstet Gynecol* 1980;136:75–80

43. Slomka C, Phelan JP. Pregnancy outcome in the patient with a nonreactive nonstress test and a positive contraction stress test. *Am J Obstet Gynecol* 1981;139:11–15

44. Bissonnette JM, Johnson K, Toomey C. The role of a trial of labor with a positive contraction stress test. *Am J Obstet Gynecol* 1979;135:292–6

45. Barrada MI, Edwards LE, Hakanson EY. Antepartum fetal testing: I. The oxytocin challenge test. *Am J Obstet Gynecol* 1979;134:532–7

46. Freeman RK, Goebelsman U, Nochimson D. An evaluation of the significance of a positive oxytocin challenge test. *Obstet Gynecol* 1976;47:8–13

47. Gauthier RJ, Evertson LR, Paul RH. Antepartum fetal heart rate testing: II. Intrapartum fetal heart rate observation and newborn outcome following a positive contraction stress test. *Am J Obstet Gynecol* 1979;133:34–9

48. Hill LM. Abnormalities of amniotic fluid. In Nyberg DA, Mahony BS, Pretorius DH, eds. *Diagnostic Ultrasound of Fetal Anomalies: Text and Atlas.* Chicago: Year Book Medical Publishers, 1990:38–66

49. Brace RA, Wolf ERJ. Normal amniotic fluid volume changes throughout pregnancy. *Am J Obstet Gynecol* 1989;161:382–8

50. Brace RA. Amniotic fluid dynamics. In Creasy RK, Resnik R, eds. *Maternal–Fetal Medicine: Principles and Practice.* Philadelphia: WB Saunders, 1994:106–14

51. Gohari P, Berkowitz RL, Hobbins JC. Prediction of intrauterine growth retardation by determination of total intrauterine volume. *Am J Obstet Gynecol* 1979;127:255–60

52. Halperin ME, Fong KW, Zalev AH, *et al.* Reliability of amniotic fluid volume estimation from ultrasonograms: intraobserver and interobserver variation before and after the establishment of criteria. *Am J Obstet Gynecol* 1985;153:264–7

53. Chamberlain PF, Manning FA, Morrison I, *et al.* Ultrasound evaluation of amniotic fluid volume: I. The relationship of decreased amniotic fluid volumes to perinatal outcome. *Am J Obstet Gynecol* 1984;150:245–9

54. Chamberlain PF, Manning FA, Morrison I, *et al.* Ultrasound evaluation of amniotic fluid volume: II. The relationship of increased amniotic fluid volume to perinatal outcome. *Am J Obstet Gynecol* 1984;150:250–4

55. Phelan JP, Ahn MO, Smith CV, *et al.* Amniotic fluid index measurements during pregnancy. *J Reprod Med* 1987;32:601–4

56. Moore TR, Cayle JE. The amniotic fluid index in normal human pregnancy. *Am J Obstet Gynecol* 1990;162:1168–73

57. Magann EF, Nolan TE, Hess W, *et al.* Measurement of amniotic fluid volume: accuracy of ultrasonography techniques. *Am J Obstet Gynecol* 1992;167:1533–7

58. Croom CS, Banias BB, Ramos-Santos E, *et al.* Do semiquantitative amniotic fluid indexes reflect actual volume? *Am J Obstet Gynecol* 1992;167:995–9

59. Dildy GA, Lira N, Moise KJ, *et al.* Amniotic fluid volume assessment: comparison of ultrasonographic estimates versus direct measurements with a dye-dilution technique in human pregnancy. *Am J Obstet Gynecol* 1992;167:986–94

60. Varma TR, Bateman S, Patel RH, *et al.* The relationship of increased amniotic fluid volume to perinatal outcome. *Int J Obstet Gynecol* 1988;27:327–33

61. Glantz JC, Abramowicz JA, Sherer DM. Significance of idiopathic midtrimester polyhydramnios. *Am J Perinatol* 1994;11:305–8

62. Sivit CJ, Hill MC, Larsen JW, *et al.* Second-trimester polyhydramnios: evaluation with US. *Radiology* 1987;165:467–9

63. Hill LM, Breckle R, Thomas ML, *et al.* Polyhydramnios: ultrasonically detected prevalence and neonatal outcome. *Obstet Gynecol* 1987;69:21–5

64. Grubb DK, Paul RH. Amniotic fluid index and prolonged antepartum fetal heart rate decelerations. *Obstet Gynecol* 1992;79:558–60

65. Chauhan SP, Rutherford SE, Sharp TW, *et al.* Intrapartum amniotic fluid index and neonatal acidosis. *J Reprod Med* 1992;37:868–70

66. Mercer LJ, Brown LG. Fetal outcome with oligohydramnios in the second trimester. *Obstet Gynecol* 1986;67:840–2

67. Barss VA, Benacerraf BR, Frigoletto FD. Second trimester oligohydramnios, a predictor of poor fetal outcome. *Obstet Gynecol* 1984;64:608–10

68. Manning FA (ed.) Fetal biophysical profile scoring: theoretical considerations and clinical application. In *Fetal Medicine: Principles and Practice.* Norwalk: Appleton & Lange, 1995:221–305

69. Manning FA, Snijders R, Harman CR, *et al.* Fetal biophysical profile score: VI. Correlation with antepartum umbilical venous fetal pH. *Am J Obstet Gynecol* 1993;169:755–63

70. Vintzileos AM, Flemming AD, Scorza WE, *et al.* Relationship between fetal biophysical activities and umbilical cord blood gas values. *Am J Obstet Gynecol* 1991;165:707–13

71. Manning FA, Platt LD, Sipos L. Antepartum fetal evaluation: development of a fetal biophysical profile. *Am J Obstet Gynecol* 1980;136:787–95

72. Peters LLH, Sheldon RE, Jones MD, *et al*. Blood flow to fetal organs as a function of arterial oxygen content. *Am J Obstet Gynecol* 1979;135:637–46

73. Manning FA, Harman CR, Morrison I, *et al*. Fetal assessment based on fetal biophysical profile scoring: IV. An analysis of perinatal morbidity and mortality. *Am J Obstet Gynecol* 1990;162:703–9

74. Manning FA, Morrison I, Harman CR, *et al*. The abnormal fetal biophysical profile score: V. Predictive accuracy according to score composition. *Am J Obstet Gynecol* 1990;162:918–27

75. Baskett TF. Gestational age and fetal biophysical assessment. *Am J Obstet Gynecol* 1988;158:332–4

76. Fox HE, Inglis J, Steinbrecher M. Fetal breathing movements in uncomplicated pregnancies: I. Relationship to gestational age. *Am J Obstet Gynecol* 1979;134:544–6

77. Vintzileos AM, Campbell WA, Ingardia CJ, *et al*. The fetal biophysical profile and its predictive value. *Obstet Gynecol* 1983;62:271–8

78. Manning FA, Morrison I, Harman CR, *et al*. Fetal biophysical profile scoring: selective use of the nonstress test. *Am J Obstet Gynecol* 1987;156:709–12

79. Nageotte MP, Towers CV, Asrat T, *et al*. The value of a negative antepartum test: contraction stress test and modified biophysical profile. *Obstet Gynecol* 1994;84:231–4

80. Nageotte MJ, Towers CV, Asrat T, *et al*. Perinatal outcome with the modified biophysical profile. *Am J Obstet Gynecol* 1994;170:1672–6

81. Peaceman AM, Meyer BA, Thorp JA, *et al*. The effect of magnesium sulfate tocolysis on the fetal biophysical profile. *Am J Obstet Gynecol* 1989;161:771–4

82. Carlan SJ, O'Brien WF. The effect of magnesium sulfate on the biophysical profile of normal term fetuses. *Obstet Gynecol* 1991;77:681–4

83. Giles WB, Trudinger BJ, Baird PJ. Fetal umbilical artery flow velocity waveforms and placental resistance: pathological correlation. *Br J Obstet Gynaecol* 1985;92:31–8

84. Maulik D, Yarlagadda P, Youngblood JP, *et al*. The diagnostic efficacy of the umbilical artery systolic/diastolic ratio as a screening tool: a prospective blinded study. *Am J Obstet Gynecol* 1990;162:1518–25

85. Trudinger BJ, Cook CM, Jones L, *et al*. A comparison of fetal heart rate monitoring and umbilical artery waveforms in the recognition of fetal compromise. *Br J Obstet Gynaecol* 1986;93:171–5

86. Brar HS, Medearis AL, DeVore GR, *et al*. A comparative study of fetal umbilical velocimetry with continuous- and pulsed-wave Doppler ultrasonography in high-risk pregnancies: relationship to outcome. *Am J Obstet Gynecol* 1989;160:375–8

87. DeVoe LD, Gardner P, Dear C, *et al*. The diagnostic values of concurrent nonstress testing, amniotic fluid measurement, and Doppler velocimetry in screening a general high-risk population. *Am J Obstet Gynecol* 1990;163:1040–8

88. Sarno AP, Ahn MO, Brar HS, *et al*. Intrapartum Doppler velocimetry, amniotic fluid volume, and fetal heart rate as predictors of subsequent fetal distress. *Am J Obstet Gynecol* 1989;161:1508–14

89. Whittle MJ, Hanretty KP, Primrose MH, *et al*. Screening for the uncompromised fetus: a randomized trial of umbilical artery velocimetry in unselected patients. *Am J Obstet Gynecol* 1994;170:555–9

90. Beattie RB, Dornan JC. Antenatal screening for intrauterine growth retardation with umbilical artery Doppler ultrasonography. *Br Med J* 1989;298:631–5

91. Bruinse HW, Sijmons EA, Reuwer PJHM. Clinical value of screening for fetal growth retardation by Doppler ultrasound. *J Ultrasound Med* 1989;8:207–9

92. Davies JA, Gallivan S, Spencer JAD. Randomized controlled trial of Doppler ultrasound screening of placental perfusion during pregnancy. *Lancet* 1992;340:1299–303

93. Newnham JP, O'Dea MRA, Reid KP, *et al*. Doppler flow velocity waveform analysis in high risk pregnancies: a randomized controlled trial. *Br J Obstet Gynaecol* 1991;98:957–63

94. Sijmons EA, Reuwer PJHM, Van Beek E, *et al*. The validity of screening for small-for-gestational-age and low-birth-weight-for-length infants by Doppler ultrasound. *Br J Obstet Gynaecol* 1989;96:557–61

95. Neilson JP. Doppler ultrasound in high risk pregnancies. Review 03889. In Enkin MW, Keirse MJNC, Renfrew MJ, Neilson JP, eds. *Pregnancy and Childbirth Module, Cochrane Database of Systematic Reviews*. Oxford: Update Software, 1994: Cochrane Updates on Disk, Issue 1

96. Maulik D. 1994: Doppler ultrasound velocimetry for fetal surveillance. *Clin Obstet Gynecol* 1995;38:91–111

97. Almstrom H, Axelsson O, Cnattingius S, *et al*. Comparison of umbilical-artery velocimetry and cardiotocography for surveillance of small-for-gestational-age fetuses. *Lancet* 1992;340:936–40

98. Tyrrell SN, Lilford RJ, MacDonald HN, *et al*. Randomized comparison of routine vs highly selective use of Doppler ultrasound and biophysical scoring to investigate high risk pregnancies. *Am J Obstet Gynecol* 1990;97:909–16

99. Woo JSK, Liang ST, Lo RLS. Significance of an absent or reversed end diastolic flow in Doppler umbilical artery waveforms. *J Ultrasound Med* 1987;6:291–7

100. Brar HS, Platt LD. Reverse end-diastolic flow on umbilical artery velocimetry in high-risk pregnancies: an ominous finding with adverse pregnancy outcome. *Am J Obstet Gynecol* 1988;159:559–61

101. Divon MY, Girz BA, Lieblich R, *et al*. Clinical management of the fetus with markedly diminished umbilical artery end-diastolic flow. *Am J Obstet Gynecol* 1989;161:1523–7

Current perspectives and new developments in ultrasound guided invasive procedures for prenatal diagnosis and therapy

17

The-Hung Bui, Jan A. Deprest, Eric Jauniaux and R. Douglas Wilson

Prenatal diagnosis has become an important option that has altered the outlook for many families at risk of having affected children. However, it should be viewed in the context of the entire situation for the couple, i.e. the risk of carrying a fetus affected by a genetic disorder or with severe structural defects amenable to prenatal diagnosis, the other measures such as carrier detection or screening tests which may define that risk more precisely, the potential for treatment of the disorder in question, the safety and accuracy of the diagnostic procedures offered and, of decisive importance, the attitude and wishes of the parents concerned. The risks associated with invasive testing, the inherent limitations of prenatal diagnosis and the consequences of abnormal results require detailed, diligent and non-directive explanation to the patient or couple. Whenever possible such information should be given in a genetic counseling session before a pregnancy occurs.

The remarkable advances in medical genetics in the past few years, coupled with the availability of increasingly sophisticated ultrasonographic modalities, and the rapid evolution of invasive techniques have both expanded and enhanced our ability to prenatally diagnose genetic diseases and structural abnormalities. Hence, increasing numbers of women are and will be presented with the option of invasive prenatal diagnosis[1]. Current techniques include amniocentesis, chorionic villus sampling, fetal blood sampling, fetal tissue biopsy and fetal urine sampling, whereas embryoscopy, fetoscopy, coelocentesis and cervical flushing should still be regarded as investigational methods (Table 1).

Once effective prenatal diagnostic procedures become established, the same evolutionary steps in medical concepts for postnatal life can be expected for the fetus with a correctable congenital defect or disorder[2]. The ability to achieve early diagnosis is a significant step towards the potential for fetal therapy. It allows time for counseling and to determine whether therapy is feasible or indeed appropriate. Ultrasound guided invasive fetal therapy includes minimally invasive therapeutic procedures, manipulation of amniotic fluid, direct drug provision to the fetal blood circulation, transfusion of blood products, drainage and shunting procedures, and innovative experimental therapy such as *in utero* transplantation of hematopoietic stem cells or endoscopic fetal surgery[2–7].

This chapter focuses on issues regarding the current techniques, optimal time of performance, appropriateness for a given indication, as well as safety and accuracy of ultrasound guided invasive fetal diagnosis. Important progress is also being made with various ultrasound directed surgical interventions aimed at correcting problems *in utero*, and an outline of these procedures is also briefly given.

Table 1 Techniques for prenatal diagnosis

Invasive	Amniocentesis
	Chorionic villus sampling
	Fetal blood sampling
	Fetal skin biopsy
	Fetal liver biopsy
	Fetal muscle biopsy
	Fetal urine sampling
	Embryoscopy, fetoscopy
	Coelocentesis
	Transcervical flushing
Non-invasive	Ultrasonography
	Other imaging techniques (X-ray, CT, MRI)
	Fetal cells in maternal blood

INDICATIONS, TIMING AND TECHNIQUES OF INVASIVE PRENATAL DIAGNOSIS

Effective prenatal diagnosis of genetic disorders depends on the skills of a multidisciplinary team with a wide range of clinical and laboratory expertise. In view of rapid advances in this field, contact should be made with a medical genetics unit or other specialized laboratories to inquire into current availability of prenatal diagnosis if there are any doubts about a potentially diagnosable disorder.

A detailed account of the many genetic, multifactorial and acquired disorders amenable to prenatal diagnosis by laboratory investigations is outside the scope of this chapter and can be found elsewhere[8-10]. The indications for invasive prenatal diagnostic procedures fall generally into four broad categories: cytogenetic, biochemical, molecular, and more seldom, infectious diseases (Table 2). The most common indication for invasive first- and second-trimester prenatal diagnosis is chromosome analysis for advanced maternal age (Tables 2 and 3). Table 4 shows estimates of the risks of Down's syndrome at varying gestational ages corresponding with timing for chorionic villus sampling, amniocentesis and term live births in women of advanced maternal age[11-13].

Estimates of spontaneous loss rates in fetuses with various chromosomal defects[14] are summarized in Table 5, although loss rates for fetuses with Down's syndrome differ somewhat in other studies[15-16]. This information is useful for genetic counseling when considering maternal and pregnancy risks prior to invasive prenatal diagnosis. Many pregnancies with a chromosome abnormality will be lost spontaneously but this may also occur after a procedure and therefore be considered procedure-related.

Both mid-trimester amniocentesis and first-trimester chorionic villus sampling (CVS) are now well established techniques for obtaining genetic information about the fetus (Table 2)[17,18]. Other less commonly used methods include fetal blood sampling, fetal urine sampling and fetal tissue biopsy to gain access to specialized tissues for rapid karyotyping and biochemical or histological analysis (Tables 1 and 2). The timing of invasive prenatal diagnosis has been reported as early as 6 weeks' gestation for chorionic villus sampling, 7 weeks' gestation for amniocentesis and 8–10 weeks' gestation for coelocentesis/embryoscopy[19-21]. However, earliest is not always the best.

Table 2 Categories of tests carried out on chorionic villi, amniocytes, amniotic fluid and fetal blood

Tests	Chorionic villus sampling	Amnio-centesis	Fetal blood sampling
Fetal sexing	+	+	+
Fetal karyotyping	+	+	+
Amniotic fluid biochemistry	–	+	–
Fetal enzyme assay*	+	+	(+)
Fetal DNA analysis*	+	+	(+)
Fetal hematologic analysis	–	–	+

*Chorionic villi are usually preferred to amniotic fluid cells

Table 3 The genetic indications for first-trimester and late chorionic villus sampling

A. Increased risk for chromosomal abnormalities
  1. Maternal age >35 years at estimated date of delivery
  2. Family history
      Previous stillbirth or livebirth with chromosomal abnormality
      Parent with potentially transmissible chromosome rearrangement
      Genetic disorders with identifiable chromosome abnormality, e.g. chromosomal breakage syndromes
      X-linked disorders – fetal sexing
  3. Abnormal ultrasound scan
      Chromosomal abnormalities are frequently found in association with such abnormalities as cystic hygroma, omphalocele, duodenal stenosis, intrauterine growth retardation, etc.

B. Biochemical or molecular disorders (such as cystic fibrosis, fragile-X, myotonic dystrophy, Tay-Sachs disease, hemoglobinopathies, etc.)
  1. Previous affected offspring with detectable disorder
  2. Both parents identified by screening to be carriers of detectable autosomal recessive disorder
  3. Positive family history of X-linked disorder with at-risk mother

Table 4 Maternal age at conception and fetal chromosome risks at different gestational ages

Maternal age (years)		Risk of chromosomal abnormality		
At conception	At delivery	In liveborn (>37 weeks)	At amniocentesis (16–18 weeks)	At CVS (9–12 weeks)
27	28	1/430	–	–
28	29	420	–	–
29	30	390	–	–
30	31	390	–	–
31	32	320	–	–
32	33	285	–	–
33	34	240	–	–
34	35	180	–	–
35	36	150	1/141	1/189
36	37	125	111	94
37	38	100	88	61
38	39	80	70	58
39	40	80	56	37
40	41	55	44	39
41	42	43	35	23
42	43	34	29	14
43	44	27	22	11
44	45	20	17	7
45	46	–	14	–
46	47	–	11	–
47	48	–	9	–

CVS, chorionic villus sampling

Table 5 Estimated spontaneous loss rates in fetuses with various chromosome defects[13]

Chromosome defect	Estimated spontaneous loss rate (%)	
	10 weeks–birth	16 weeks–birth
Trisomy 13 (Patau's syndrome)	83	71
Trisomy 18 (Edwards' syndrome)	86	74
Trisomy 21 (Down's syndrome)	47	31
45,X (Turner's syndrome)	76	52
47,XXY (Klinefelter's syndrome)	5	3
47,XXX	5	3
47,XYY	5	3
Triploidy	>99	>99

Amniocentesis

Amniocentesis was first used in the 1880s for reduction of polyhydramnios. In the 1930s, both placental localization and termination of pregnancy were achieved by intra-amniotic injection of X-ray contrast medium and hypertonic saline, respectively[17]. In the 1950s, amniocentesis for prenatal evaluation of hemolytic disease was introduced[22]. Fetal sexing of X-chromatin (Barr's body) was reported in 1956, chromosome analysis of amniotic fluid cells in 1966, and the first antenatal detection of trisomy 21 and a metabolic disorder in 1968[17,23–25].

Mid-trimester genetic amniocentesis has been available since 1970 and continues to be the most common form of invasive prenatal diagnosis[1,26]. The technique is efficacious for the majority of women requiring invasive prenatal diagnosis, who are at an increased risk for meiotic non-disjunctional chromosome events such as trisomy 21 (Down's syndrome) associated with advanced reproductive age. The genetic indications for amniocentesis are the same as for CVS (Tables 3 and 4) except that α-fetoprotein (AFP) determination for screening of neural tube defects can additionally be done with amniocentesis. Besides karyotyping, cultured amniocytes and amniotic fluid can be used for molecular and biochemical analyses of a wide range of genetic disorders[8]. However, chorionic villi are, today, preferred over cultured amniocytes for DNA and most biochemical investigations for genetic disorders because analyses can be performed on fresh specimen obviating the need and delay of cell culturing. Amniotic fluid and its cellular content can be analyzed biochemically and molecular studies using DNA-amplification based methods (polymerase chain reaction; PCR) can be performed without further cell culture, e.g. molecular genotyping of the common Rhesus alleles or fetal platelet antigens[8,27–31]. In many countries, routine measurement of AFP concentration in amniotic fluid is carried out in all mid-trimester genetic amnioncenteses as a highly sensitive screening test for neural tube defects. Amniocentesis is also performed during both the second and third trimesters of pregnancy for other forms of fetal evaluation such as infections and well-being[9,10].

Despite the significant advantages offered by mid-trimester amniocentesis, there are major limitations inherent in the procedure. It is usually performed between 16–18 weeks when karyotyping of cultured amniocytes can be carried out consistently within 10–14 days with a turn-around time of up to 3 weeks. When cytogenetic or other results are abnormal and termination of pregnancy is chosen by the patient, there is a higher likelihood of medical and psychological morbidity for the mother than when it is done in the first trimester[32]. Thus, a major disadvantage of mid-trimester genetic amniocentesis is that cytogenetic results are usually available only after 18 weeks' gestation.

Technique of amniocentesis

The technique is well established and mid-trimester amniocentesis is performed as an outpatient procedure. It does not require, in most cases, local anesthetics or antibiotic prophylaxis. The abdomen is prepared with an alcohol or iodine solution. Ultrasound guidance is used either continuously or, rarely so today, to initially identify an appropriate pocket of amniotic fluid followed by blind puncture. A free-hand or needle guided technique can be used to insert transabdominally a 20–22 gauge spinal needle with stylet into the amniotic cavity. Whenever possible a transplacental puncture is avoided to minimize feto-maternal hemorrhage and potential maternal cell contamination[33–35]. A small amount (10–20 ml) of amniotic fluid is removed to yield a sufficient number of viable cells to minimize the risk of

laboratory failure. The first few millilitres are discarded to decrease the risk of potential maternal cell contamination. Rh-prophylaxis is given as indicated.

A twin gestation presents unique problems in both genetic counseling and prenatal diagnosis. Amniocentesis in twin pregnancy is usually done by separate needle insertions in each gestational sac[36,37], but single needle insertion for diamniotic gestational sacs has been reported[38,39]. A technique which permits visualization of both needles simultaneously, providing proof of proper needle placements in each cavity has been described, thus rendering unnecessary the need for injection of a dye substance into the amniotic sac[40].

Early amniocentesis

Concern about safety and diagnostic accuracy of first-trimester CVS led to the introduction of early amniocentesis in the late 1980s[41,42]. This was made possible by the widespread and large experience with second-trimester amniocentesis, improved cell culture techniques, and the availability of high-resolution ultrasound machines. Early amniocentesis refers to procedures performed at 9–14 weeks' gestation. However, it has been suggested that an 'early amniocentesis' is at 12.0 –13.9 weeks and a 'very early amniocentesis' or first-trimester amniocentesis is before 12.0 weeks[43]. For convenience here, early amniocentesis will make reference to both procedures if not otherwise specified.

First-trimester amniocentesis has the additional advantage over CVS that the processing of samples in the laboratory is less labor intensive. Hence, early amniocentesis is presently being investigated as an alternative for first-trimester prenatal diagnosis as amniotic fluid cells continue to be the preferred tissue by cytogeneticists and are more cost-effective than CVS tissue[44,45]. AFP screening for neural tube defects is standard care in many countries when amniocentesis is performed after 14 weeks' gestation. Normal ranges for early amniocentesis are being developed but whether detection rate is comparable to that at standard amniocentesis has not been established[46–49]. Karyotyping of amniocytes from early amniocentesis may take on average a few more days but the turnaround time of up to 3 weeks is similar to that after the conventional mid-trimester procedure.

Technique of early amniocentesis

Although technically very similar to mid-trimester amniocentesis, early amniocentesis is more difficult than the traditional mid-trimester procedure due to the relatively smaller target area and the separation of amnion and chorion with possible amnion 'tenting' at the time of amniocentesis. For these reasons, continuous ultrasound guidance is required for amniocentesis prior to 14 weeks' gestation. A modified amniocentesis technique can reduce the failure rate in cases of tenting of the membranes. Failure to aspirate amniotic fluid may persist after advancement and rotation of the needle. In such cases, the membranes may be pierced by using a stylet that is no longer than the length of the needle. With the needle in the middle of a suitable amniotic fluid pocket, the stylet of the needle is replaced with a longer stylet. Under real-time ultrasonographic guidance, the tip of the stylet is then rapidly advanced 5–10 mm beyond the tip of the needle[50]. The amnio-chorionic separation is usually obliterated by 14 –15 weeks of gestation. The amount of amniotic fluid aspirated, about 5–10 ml, is also less than that at mid-trimester. Transplacental needle passage in amniocentesis performed before 14.9 weeks' gestation does not appear to increase the risk of pregnancy loss[51]. Early twin amniocentesis has been reported but experience is still very limited[42,52].

Other techniques for first-trimester amniocentesis have been described including amniotic fluid cell filtration[48,53–55], per-urethral transvesical[56] and transvaginal[57] amniocentesis, but their use is uncommon.

Chorionic villus sampling

Chorionic villus sampling was first reported in the late 1960s, but was soon abandoned due to a high frequency of complications and insufficient reliability to become a routine clinical method[58–61]. Although blind CVS was performed for fetal sex determination with a relatively high rate of success in the mid-1970s[62], it was not until the mid-1980s that ultrasound guided CVS was reported, allowing successful chromosome, biochemical and DNA analysis[63–68].

The main indications for CVS are still chromosome, biochemical and DNA analyses (Table 3). CVS is generally preferred over amniocentesis for the two latter categories of investigations (Table 2). While transcervical or transabdominal CVS is usually done between 10–12 weeks' gestation, later CVS by the transabdominal route has been shown to be an alternative approach to amniocentesis or cordocentesis for genetic analyses[69]. Table 6 summarizes recent reports of late CVS[70–73].

The turnaround time after CVS is 7–14 days for karyotyping owing to differences in cell culture, although direct villi processing or overnight culture may give a karyotype within hours or one day after CVS, admittedly of lower chromosome banding quality. Thus, the major advantage of CVS is that results are obtained at an earlier gestational age than with amniocentesis, allowing the option of earlier termination in the event of an abnormal result.

Techniques of CVS

Chorionic villus sampling technique uses continuous abdominal ultrasound guidance with either a transcervical or transabdominal sampling approach (Figures 1 and 2). A transvaginal CVS technique has also been described[74]. The transcervical technique uses a flexible plastic or metal catheter which can be shaped for easier ultrasound guided insertion through the cervix and into the placental

Table 6   Late chorionic villus sampling: summary of recent studies

Investigators	Number of women	Gestation weeks	Result success	Abortion	Loss rate
Dalpra *et al.* (1993)[70]	131	13–35	–	11	–
Smidt-Jensen *et al.* (1993)[71]	210 (142 normal scan, 58 abnormal scan)	13–38	209	19/58	0.7%
Cameron *et al.* (1994)[72]	551	18.2 (mean)	549	14	0.4%
Ko *et al.* (1995)[73]	124 (single gene 89, abnormal scan 35)	18.2 (mean)	124	29/89 9/35	1.8%

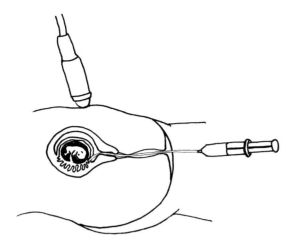

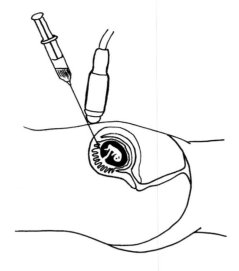

Figure 1   Transcervical chorionic villus sampling with flexible catheter

Figure 2   Transabdominal chorionic villus sampling

tissue. The transabdominal approach utilizes a free-hand technique inserting a 19 or 20 gauge spinal needle under ultrasound guidance, but needle guides attached to the ultrasound probe can also be used. Rigid straight or curved biopsy forceps have also been employed by both routes[19,75,76]. Transabdominal double needle CVS techniques have been described with a larger outer sheath (17–18 gauge) and a smaller aspirating needle (19–20 gauge)[77]. Negative pressure is applied to a 20–30 ml syringe attached to the end of the catheter or needle in order to aspirate the placental tissue into the syringe. The biopsy forceps obtain a specimen mechanically from opening and closing the jaws of the forceps. The goal of all these techniques is to retrieve at least 5 mg of chorionic villus tissue (wet weight) depending on the indication for prenatal diagnosis (cytogenetic, molecular or biochemical). For the transabdominal approach, skin preparation by iodine or alcohol solution is used. For the transcervical approach, a vaginal speculum is inserted and the cervix and vaginal walls are cleaned with either an antiseptic or just normal saline solution prior to the insertion of the catheter or biopsy forceps. The use of antibiotic prophylaxis without any maternal risk factors is controversial[78]. It has essentially been used for transcervical procedures. Rh-prophylaxis is given as indicated.

Initially CVS was only done transcervically. Presently, transcervical CVS is often chosen for posterior placental locations and the transabdominal approach for fundal and anterior placental locations. If only the transcervical approach is utilized for CVS, manipulation of the uterus by cervical tenaculum or speculum may be necessary sometimes for fundal or anterior placental positions[79]. The ability to use both transabdominal and transcervical techniques may improve procedure safety and provides increased patient choice[80–82]. The CVS techniques can be used for both singleton and twin pregnancies[37].

Fetal blood sampling

Access to fetal blood was first obtained in the early 1970s by hysterotomy during the second trimester[83]. Blind multiple needle aspirations of intraplacental blood, placentacentesis, was thereafter introduced, but the samples were frequently contaminated with maternal blood[84]. It was soon replaced by fetoscopy, which granted direct visualization of the mid-trimester fetus, placental surface vessels and umbilical cord, adding precision to sampling pure fetal blood[85,86]. In the early 1980s, as better ultrasonographic imaging became available, less traumatic access to pure fetal blood was obtained by simple needle placement to first the umbilical vein (cordocentesis)[87] and, soon thereafter, to both the hepatic vein (intrahepatic vein sampling) and, less satisfactorily, the fetal heart (cardiocentesis)[84,88].

Cordocentesis, also called percutaneous umbilical blood sampling (PUBS) or funipuncture, has now gained wide acceptance in perinatal centers due to its relative technical simplicity, reliability and safety in obtaining pure fetal blood (Figure 3). It can be performed from about 18 weeks of gestation until term to assist in the detection or elucidation of genetic fetal anomalies and acquired disorders including chromosome defects, congenital infections, hematological disorders, and evaluation of fetal metabolic state and acid–base balance[89]. However, the indications for diagnostic fetal blood sampling are changing[90] due to the rapid development of extremely sensitive molecular methods for the diagnosis of single gene disorders and congenital infections using chorionic villus tissue or amniotic fluid[91–93]. The major indications for diagnostic fetal blood sampling today include rapid karyotyping allowing results within 48–72 hours[94–96], evaluation of hematologic status for red blood cell isoimmunization and fetal hydrops[97], assessment of fetal metabolic and acid–base status[98,99], thyroid function[100], and fetal platelet count[101]. Acid–base and blood gas status in fetuses is not affected by the site of sampling. Thus, values obtained at the intrahepatic vein may be interpreted using reference ranges derived from sampling at the placental cord insertion[102].

Once a sample of blood has been aspirated it is essential to verify that it is uncontaminated and of fetal origin[89]. An advantage of fetal intrahepatic vein sampling is the certainty of the origin of the blood sample and non-contamination with amniotic fluid without further investigation.

Techniques of fetal blood sampling

Fetal blood sampling is performed as an out-patient procedure, local anesthetics and sedation rarely being needed. The use of antibiotic prophylaxis and β-mimetics is of unproved value. The abdomen is prepared with an alcohol or iodine solution. Just prior to the procedure, the preferred site of sampling is identified. This may be facilitated by use of colour Doppler. High-resolution ultrasound guidance is then used continuously as a 20–22 gauge spinal needle is advanced percutaneously toward the target fetal vessel or the fetal heart. A single operator free-hand technique holding the transducer with one hand and directing the needle with the other has the advantage of permitting adjustment of the needle pathway when the target

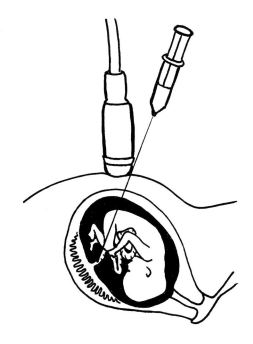

Figure 3 Cordocentesis at placental cord insertion

is moving. This is often the case when aiming at the intrahepatic vein, a free loop of the cord or, rarely, the fetal heart. An assistant can aspirate the blood once the needle is in the blood circulation. A two-operator technique requires perfect co-ordination between the ultrasonographer and the operator. A needle guide fixed to the transducer can also be used[103], although it allows less flexibility if the fetus moves or should a contraction occur with the needle in the myometrium.

The placental cord insertion is generally targeted with puncture about 1–2 cm from its root because it is its most fixed portion (Figure 4). When the placenta is anterior, the cord insertion can be reached through the placenta without entering the amniotic cavity. When the placenta is posterior, cordocentesis is transamniotic aiming either at the placental cord insertion or a free-loop which, in both cases, may be more difficult to accomplish due to possible interposition of fetal parts or when polyhydramnios is present (Figures 3 and 4).

An alternative site is the fetal intrahepatic vein when difficulties are expected or puncture of the umbilical cord fails. The needle is introduced into the fetal abdominal wall either anteriorly near the midline or from the left or right hypochondrium. It is then advanced through the liver parenchyma into the umbilical vein near the center of the fetal body, or the left portal vein, leaving the needle unheld at this stage to move with fetal movements. This is to minimize the risk of dislodgement.

The volume of fetal blood retrieved is generally 1–5 ml depending on gestational age, indication for the procedure and thus the laboratory tests to be performed. Needles used for samples taken for fetal platelet count should be siliconized as they have been reported free of platelet clumping and clots[104]. Rh-prophylaxis is given as indicated.

Diagnostic use of cordocentesis in both twins in twin pregnancies has been reported[105].

Fetal tissue biopsy

Fetal tissue biopsies were first performed by fetoscopy in the early 1980s for prenatal diagnosis of hereditary skin disease[106–108]. *In utero* sampling of fetal skin[109,110], liver[111], and muscle[112] may be required when prenatal diagnosis cannot be effected through analysis of chorionic villi or amniotic fluid cells[113]. For skin biopsy, samples should be retrieved from multiple predilection sites to allow for variable expression of certain diseases during the second trimester. When the whole skin is abnormal as in Herlitz junctional epidermolysis bullosa, convenient sites include the fetal buttock and thigh, whereas in oculocutaneous albinism, a scalp biopsy is preferable. However, many of these conditions will be detected by DNA analysis in the near future, and the need for these procedures will decrease dramatically[114]. Confirmation of fetal chromosome mosaicism by fetal skin biopsy and fibroblast culture has been described when fetal blood could not confirm the suspicion of mosaicism for trisomy 12 found at amniocentesis[115].

Technique of fetal tissue sampling

The abdomen is prepared with an alcohol or iodine solution. Fetal tissue sampling is now most frequently done by inserting transabdominally a biopsy needle or fine biopsy forceps (Figure 5) through a thin cannula under continuous ultrasonographic guidance[113]. Samples are obtained during the second trimester, usually at 15–22 weeks' gestation depending on the indication and target tissue. The procedure is done in the outpatient department under local anesthesia. Fetal immobilization by pharmacological means may be needed. Rh-prophylaxis is given as indicated.

Fetal urine sampling

The evaluation of fetal renal function is the subject of intensive research because fetuses with lower urinary tract obstruction may benefit from prenatal shunting or other experimental surgical interventions[116,117]. Once chromosome and other structural defects are excluded, the main determinant of outcome is the degree of remnant renal function. Oligohydramnios, although a poor prognostic sign, relates more to the degree of obstruction than to the severity of renal dysfunction. The ultrasonographic appearance of fetal kidneys has a limited value in the prenatal diagnosis of renal dysplasia. Fetal blood indices, even in the most severe cases of renal dysplasia, are normal due to the clearance activity through the placenta[84]. Serial percutaneous sampling of urine from the fetal

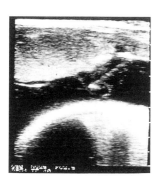
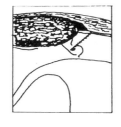
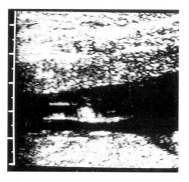
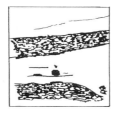

Figure 4 Ultrasound images of cordocentesis (above) at placental cord insertion, intra-abdominal cystic structure seen in the fetus in the left quadrant; insertion of needle tip in free loop of the cord (below)

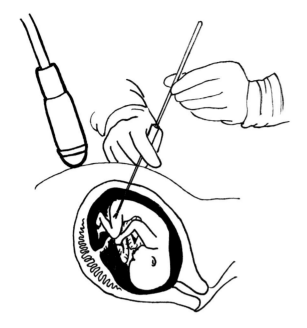

Figure 5 Transabdominal percutaneous fetal skin biopsy

fetal diagnosis ultimately led to the disappearance of diagnostic fetoscopy by the mid-1980s.

Ironically, embryoscopy or fetoscopy (depending on gestational age) have been recently reintroduced due to the shortcomings of ultrasound to diagnose fetal anomalies in the early stages of gestation. In that way, a few malformations and syndromes have been diagnosed in the first trimester[124–128]. Fetal blood sampling with this technology has also been performed in the first trimester, establishing the feasibility to access the human embryonic circulation[129]. Presently, the greatest benefit of embryoscopy – and occasionally of diagnostic needle-fetoscopy – is to confirm a diagnosis equivocally suggested by ultrasound examination[130,131]. Thus, future applications for embryoscopy include first-trimester prenatal diagnosis and, possibly, therapeutic interventions such as gene or cell therapy at a time when the embryo is immunologically tolerant[132]. In the second trimester, thin-gauge fetoscopy is emerging as a tool for fetal surgical procedures[3,4]. Fetal cystoscopy *in utero* has also been described[117].

bladder (fetal vesicocentesis) or selectively from each renal pelvis is today utilized in the assessment of renal function[118,119].

Technique of fetal urine sampling

The technique is similar to that of amniocentesis and requires continuous ultrasound guidance. Serial sampling is recommended to monitor functional reserve by biochemical evaluation of fresh urine including concentrations of sodium, chloride, calcium, beta2-microglobulin, and osmolarity. Rh-prophylaxis is given as indicated.

Embryoscopy and fetoscopy

Endoscopic fetal visualization was first reported in the 1950s[120]. In the 1970s, fetoscopy permitted fetal blood sampling in the second trimester[83,85,86]. The technique then evolved in combination with ultrasound to direct the fetoscope toward the fetal part to be investigated because of the limited field of direct vision: applications included direct visualization of parts of fetal anatomy, skin biopsy and intrauterine vascular transfusion[106,121–123]. However, the evolution of ultrasound and the introduction of new less invasive techniques for

Techniques of embryoscopy and fetoscopy

Initially, a rigid fiber-optic endoscope was passed under ultrasound guidance transcervically into the extracoelomic cavity to identify developmental milestones from 6–8 weeks' gestation[133]. Subsequently, a transabdominal approach was used and is now preferred, both in the first and second trimester of pregnancy, as semirigid fiber-endoscopes of 0.5–0.7 mm in diameter that fit through 20–18 gauge needles and solid or semi-flexible micro-endoscopes of diminutive diameters (0.7–2.0 mm) became available[131,132,134]. The procedure is performed in an out-patient setting in local or under anesthesia. Skin preparation by iodine or alcohol solution is used. The cannula containing a sharp trocar is inserted under continuous sonographic guidance into the exocoelomic cavity when performed in the first trimester, and into the amniotic cavity in the second trimester. The endoscope is connected to a xenon light source and a lightweight CCD videocamera with zooming capability. Simultaneous dual vision of both the ultrasound and the fetoscopic images is necessary throughout the procedure for better orientation, to avoid fetal trauma, and to direct the fetoscope to the fetal part to be investigated. Rh-prophylaxis is given as indicated.

Coelocentesis: a new invasive technique?

In 1991, two independent teams of investigators reported the first data on the biochemistry of the coelomic fluid[135,136]. Both teams showed that coelomic fluid could be successfully aspirated by transvaginal puncture between 6 and 12 weeks of gestation and that the coelomic fluid had different biochemical characteristics from those of early amniotic fluid and maternal serum. Normal ranges of AFP concentrations in early fetal fluid were established and the importance of identifying the site of amniocentesis in the first trimester was emphasized by Wathen and colleagues[137]. Since 1991, the purpose of Juniaux and colleagues has been twofold: firstly, within the context of risk of limb defects associated with early CVS, to develop a less traumatic technique to obtain pure fetal cells and secondly, to explore the biology of materno-embryonic exchanges at a gestational age when fetal blood can not easily be obtained[129].

Embryologic background and early studies

The extraembryonic coelom develops during the fourth postmenstrual week. It surrounds the blastocyst which is composed of two cavities separated by the bilaminar embryonic disk, i.e. the amniotic cavity and the primary yolk sac. At the end of the fourth week of gestation, the developing exocoelomic cavity splits the extraembryonic mesoderm into two layers: the somatic mesoderm, lining the trophoblast, and the splanchnic meso-derm, covering the secondary yolk sac and the embryo[135]. The exocoelomic cavity can be visualized by ultrasound from 5 to 12 weeks' gestation and coelomic fluid is aspirated with a success rate close to 100% in pregnancies between 6 and 10 weeks[135]. The amniotic cavity can only be clearly identified from the beginning of the seventh week of gestation and amniotic fluid can be obtained in all cases from 8 weeks.

Exocoelomic fluid is yellow coloured and more viscous than amniotic fluid, which is always clear. This is probably mainly due to a highly significant difference in total protein levels between the two compartments[135,138,139]. Between 6 and 12 weeks of gestation, the mean level of total protein is 18 times lower in the coelomic fluid than in maternal serum and 54 times higher in the coelomic cavity than in the amniotic cavity[140]. The results of bio-chemical analysis suggest that the thin membrane separating these two compartments, which later becomes the amniotic epithelium, is not permeable to molecules with a high molecular weight (Table 7). Sampling the exocoelomic cavity is of relevance to study and quantify drug transfer from maternal to fetal compartments in early pregnancy at a time when most damage from drugs occurs[141,142].

Coelocentesis is in theory the ideal alternative for early amniocentesis and CVS because the risk of directly injuring the growing embryo or damaging its placenta is almost non-existent. Furthermore, the procedure is easy to learn, induces only minimal discomfort to the mother and is associated with a very low rate of contamination of the sample by maternal cells[143]. Although there are still no data about the relative long-term risks of coelocentesis, the rate of fetal loss should be similar or lower than that associated with early CVS. The high failure rate of cell growth from coelomic samples limits at the moment the applications of coelocentesis to DNA analysis[144].

Technique of coelocentesis

Coelomic as well as amniotic fluid can be retrieved by transvaginal or transabdominal puncture aspira-tion performed under continuous ultrasound guidance. When the two compartments are clearly visualized, coelomic fluid is first aspirated using a 20-gauge needle (Figure 6). Subsequently, a second 20-gauge needle is reintroduced through the guide and the needle advanced into the amniotic cavity to aspirate amniotic fluid. The volume of fluid obtained from the exocoelomic cavity varies between 2 and 8 ml at 6 and 10 weeks, respectively, whereas amniotic fluid volume samples increase exponentially from 3 to 30 ml between 7 and 12 weeks.

Table 7   Comparison of coelomic versus amniotic fluid protein composition in the first trimester

Protein	Coelomic fluid	Amniotic fluid
Total protein, g/l	3.5 ± 0.7	0.2 ± 0.2
AFP, kIU/l	21 816 ± 12 667	27 096 ± 11 822
Albumin, g/l	1.7 ± 0.5	ND
Pre-albumin, g/l	0.04 ± 0.02	ND
IgG, mg/dl	32 ± 21	ND
hCG, mIU/ml	165 607 ± 78 543	1752 ± 1421
Transferrin, g/l	0.22 ± 0.05	ND

AFP, α-fetoprotein; hCG, human chorionic gonado-tropin; ND, Not detectable

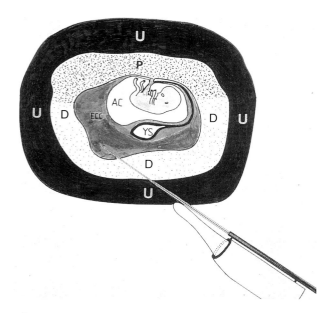

Figure 6 Diagrammatic representation of exocoelomic cavity (ECC) puncture under transvaginal ultrasound guidance (coelocentesis). The needle guide attached to the shaft of the probe is introduced inside the uterine wall. Exocoelomic fluid is first aspirated through a 20G needle and subsequently another 20G needle is introduced inside the amniotic cavity for amniocentesis. U, myometrium; D, decidua; P, placenta; YS, yolk sac. Modified with permission[139]

Transcervical flushing: a new minimally invasive technique?

The feasibility of obtaining exfoliated placental cells in the cervical mucus using cotton swabs was explored in the early 1970s but results were contradictory[145–147]. Placental cells retrieved by flushing mucus from the cervical canal or lower uterine cavity regained increased interest in the early 1990s with the availability of molecular and fluorescence *in situ* hybridization methods and the possibility to isolate fetal cells from maternal cell contaminants by flow cytometry and magnetic beads sorting[148–150]. After enrichment, these cells could possibly be used for prenatal diagnosis[150–153].

SAFETY AND ACCURACY OF INVASIVE PRENATAL DIAGNOSIS

Mid-trimester amniocentesis

Every known invasive prenatal procedure carries the risk of procedure-related fetal loss. Amnio-

centesis performed at 15 to 18 weeks' gestation has been the gold standard approach for prenatal cytogenetic diagnosis with a high accuracy (99.4%–99.8%) and an estimated procedure-related loss rate of 0.5–1%[154–156]. A small number of fetal demises has been attributed to direct needle injury or iatrogenic infection[17,157–159]. However, the mechanism behind most abortions remains unknown. The risk of serious maternal injury as a direct result of amniocentesis is negligible, but amniotic fluid leak or vaginal blood spotting may be experienced by 2–3% of patients[154,155]. Increased experience with the procedure may help reduce these complications[160].

Congenital malformations following amniocentesis have been suspected but not proven. Review of four large epidemiological studies showed two studies with an unexplained excess of neonatal respiratory disease following mid-trimester amniocentesis[154,155,161,162]. In a monkey model, amniocentesis led to suboptimal lung growth and development[163]. Babies subjected to amniocentesis during their mother's pregnancy had a significantly lower dynamic component and tended to have a higher resistance compared with controls when tested for lung function[164]. Taken together, these reports provide evidence that mid-trimester amniocentesis may have an adverse effect on lung growth and development. Similar studies have not been completed following early amniocentesis. However, no long-term effects were found in children and adolescents 7–18 years following amniocentesis except for an increased rate of ABO-immunization[165].

Maternal cell contamination is regularly observed in amniotic fluid samples from pregnancies with an anterior placenta, whereas it is rare when the placenta is posterior. The origin of maternal cells is therefore thought to be a result of placental bleeding during amniocentesis[35]. This may contribute to wrong fetal sex assignment and pseudomosaicism[166]. Although this contamination does not affect to any large extent the overall accuracy of cytogenetic analysis of cultured amniocytes, there may be implications for prenatal molecular diagnosis using uncultured amniotic fluid samples[31].

CVS versus mid-trimester amniocentesis

Studies trying to differentiate the risk between early and later invasive prenatal procedures compare total fetal loss rate (spontaneous loss, procedure-related loss, termination of pregnancy due to diagnosis) from a predetermined gestational age rather than post-procedural loss because the background fetal loss is higher in earlier gestation. Just comparing post-procedural fetal loss rates would be confounding otherwise.

Chorionic villus sampling was the initial first-trimester prenatal diagnosis technique receiving extensive evaluation. A Canadian multicenter randomized collaborative CVS trial[167,168] showed a non-significant 0.6% increase in total pregnancy losses in the CVS group compared to the amniocentesis group for an increased pregnancy loss no greater than 2.7% at the upper confidence interval. The American National Institute of Health CVS trial[169] was not randomized and found a non-significant 0.8% increased loss rate in the CVS group compared to the amniocentesis group. In these two studies CVS was done transcervically. The MRC-European multicenter randomized CVS trial[170] showed a significant 4.6% less successful pregnancy outcome in the CVS group compared with the amniocentesis group. In this study CVS was done by several different methods. However, the 95% confidence interval for that study and the Canadian study overlap, suggesting that this difference may be non-significant[156]. A possible explanation is that loss rate may be higher in less experienced centers[82,171]. Many centers in the MRC-European study contributed very few patients which may reflect less experience in CVS. As with all surgical procedures, the experience of the operator is a major determinant of risk.

Transabdominal versus transcervical CVS

Comparison of transabdominal and transcervical CVS has shown both procedures to be equally safe and accurate (diagnostic accuracy of 97.5–99.6%) in their prediction[168,172–174]. Some studies have indicated a decreased procedural risk for fetal loss with transabdominal CVS[78,79,82]. In a randomized study transcervical CVS had a relative fetal loss risk of 1.7 compared with either transabdominal CVS or amniocentesis, whereas no difference was found between transabdominal CVS and mid-trimester amniocentesis[77,175]. Another difference between the two techniques is that the transcervical technique results in a greater risk of post-procedural spotting and minimal bleeding while the transabdominal technique increases uterine discomfort with cramps.

Intrauterine infection has not been identified as a significant risk factor in a large number of patients having transcervical procedures. Maternal evaluation for infection indicates a low rate of bacteremia following CVS but antibiotic prophylaxis is recommended for women with abnormal cardiac valves[78].

Evaluation of the safety and accuracy of CVS has subsequently shifted focus: questions concerning the clinical significance of confined placental mosaicism, maternal cell contamination, and possible associations between CVS and vascular disruptive limb abnormalities if CVS was performed at gestational ages prior to 9 weeks have been raised.

Confined placental mosaicism and CVS

Confined placental or chorionic mosaicism is defined as a discrepancy between the chromosomes in the chorionic and fetal tissues, and is a complicating factor in 1–2% of patients undergoing CVS[176–178]. The cytotrophoblast cells that cover the chorionic villus are generally responsible for this confined chorionic mosaicism. These cells are rapidly dividing and may have chromosomal or molecular errors that are not representative of the fetal status. Long-term culturing is required which grows fibroblasts from the mesenchymal core of the chorionic villus. This has been shown to be more reliable in the prediction of the fetal karyotype. Confined chorionic mosaicism can only be confirmed when a normal karyotype from the amniocytes is found after an additional amniocentesis[179]. Cordocentesis may be necessary in certain specific chromosomal situations to clarify the discrepancy.

Thus, CVS mosaicism usually represents an abnormal cell line confined to the placenta and often involves chromosomal trisomy[176–178]. Such confined placental mosaicism may occur when there is complete dichotomy between a trisomic karyotype in the placenta and a normal diploid fetus or when both diploid and trisomic components are present within the placenta. Gestations with pure or significant trisomy in placental lineages associated with a diploid fetal karyotype probably result from a trisomic zygote that has lost one copy of the trisomic chromosome in the embryonic progenitor cell during cleavage (trisomic rescue)[177]. Uniparental disomy would be expected to occur in one-third of such cases. Uniparental disomy (both copies of one chromosome pair inherited from the same parent instead of the usual one chromosome from each parent) in the fetus may be associated with confined placental mosaicism for certain chromosomes[180]. Trisomy of chromosomes 7, 9, 15 and 16 are the most common among gestations with these dichotomic confined placental mosaicisms. Pregnancies with trisomy 16 confined to the placenta show intrauterine growth restriction, low birthweight or fetal death, and are correlated with high levels of trisomic cells in the term placenta. For these reasons, careful follow-up with medical and ultrasound examination for fetal growth is necessary when confined placental mosaicism is identified.

Contamination by maternal decidual tissue is possible but this potential problem can be minimized with very careful attention to cleaning and stripping off the chorionic villi of any maternal decidua cells under the dissecting microscope prior to tissue culturing[181]. Long-term tissue culturing increases the contamination risk if villi are not appropriately cleaned. This has not posed a significant problem with most cytogenetic laboratories with long-term experience in CVS but may be a problem in smaller centers with reduced patient loads[174].

Vascular disruptive anomalies have been reported in pregnancies exposed to CVS at 55–66 days gestation or earlier[182–185]. The increased risk of congenital malformations following CVS prior to 10 weeks' gestation is supported by other published data[42] (Table 8). The risk of congenital vascular disruptive anomalies secondary to CVS after 10 weeks' gestation is controversial and continues to be debated[186,188,190,191]. To evaluate the risk for limb or other defects an international registry of CVS was established by the World Health Organization (WHO) committee on chorionic villus sampling in 1992. The consensus of data based on 138 000 infants born after CVS does not support any increased risk or specific pattern of limb defects if CVS is performed after the 9th week of gestation[171]. However, utilization of CVS has been affected by this controversy[192].

CVS is technically more demanding for both obstetricians and cytogeneticists. Mid-trimester amniocentesis is somewhat safer than CVS and benefits of earlier diagnosis by CVS must be set against its greater risks. If earlier diagnosis is required, transabdominal CVS may be preferable to transcervical CVS.

Table 8 Published data. Information indicating increased risk of vascular disruption when chorionic villus sampling is performed prior to 10 weeks of gestation (70 days)

A. Case studies

Authors	Gestation age (range) at procedure	Limb defects/ procedures	Incidence per 10 000 births
Firth *et al.* (1991)[182]	56–66 days	5/289	173
Brambati *et al.* (1992)[183]	42–49 days	4/249	161
Schloo *et al.* (1992)[184]	≤ 66 days	1/636	16
Hsieh *et al.* (1995)[185]		Total defects: 29	–
	<63 days	20 (68.9%)	
	65–66 days	2	
	70 days	1	
Froster-Iskenius and Baird (1989)[186]	Estimated background risk		5

B. Case–control studies

Authors	Gestation age (range) at procedure	Summary OMLHC*	TLD*	Any TLD*
Mastroiacovo *et al.* (1992)[187]	<70 days	467.2	8.7	19.7
	70–76 days	–	6.5	6.3
	>76 days	–	–	–
Olney *et al.* (1994)[188]	56–84 days	Transverse terminal LD 4.7 (odds ratio) Transverse digital deficiency 6.4 (odds ratio) (trend to earlier gestational age exposed *p* < 0.001)		
Firth *et al.* (1994)[189]	mean: 56 days (49–65)	Absent limb, (humerus/ femur involved)		
	mean: 72 days (51–98)	Terminal phalanx/nail		

OMLHC, oromandibular-limb hypogenesis complex; TLD, transverse limb deficiency; *Incidence per 10 000 births

Clinical trials on early amniocentesis

The non-randomized trials have the majority of procedures reported at 13 and 14 weeks' gestation[42]. Failed or rescheduled procedures ranged from 0–7% in these trials. Laboratory and cytogenetic failures in gestational ages greater than 11 weeks' gestation are usually less than 2%.

To date there has been no large randomized evaluation of early amniocentesis. The two randomized studies have small numbers and have given conflicting results regarding the safety of early amniocentesis when compared with CVS or mid-trimester amniocentesis[193,194] (Table 9). The first study reported a significant increase in spontaneous losses when comparing early amniocentesis and CVS[193]. The excess spontaneous loss after early amniocentesis compared to CVS was 4% with confidence intervals of 1.3–6.7% for the randomized subgroup. The second randomized study found no significant difference in total pregnancy losses between early amniocentesis and mid-trimester amniocentesis[194]. The difference between these studies may be due to several methodological differences including type of procedure being compared, eligibility criteria, size of needle used for early amniocentesis (20 gauge *vs.* 22 gauge) and number of operators (17 *vs.* 3). The incidences of chromosomal abnormalities, congenital anomalies and amniocyte culture failure were similar between the two studies.

Nicolaides and colleagues[193] reported congenital defects in 3.3% and 2.8% of survivors in their total early amniocentesis (EA) and CVS groups, respectively. In the EA group, the incidence of talipes (1.6%) was higher than in the CVS group (0.5%) but this difference was not significant. Talipes equinovarus accounted for 50% of the congenital anomalies in the EA group and 18% in the CVS group. When only randomized patients were included the percentage of talipes was 45% in the EA group and 13% in the CVS group. No other congenital anomaly was reported more than once in the EA group.

Johnson and colleagues[194] found no significant differences in the neonates between early amniocentesis and mid-trimester amniocentesis groups for congenital anomalies, respiratory or musculoskeletal problems. Congenital anomalies were present in 2.4% and 2.6% for the early and mid-trimester amniocenteses respectively. Neonatal respiratory problems were present in 2.2% and 1.6%, respectively. The incidence of musculoskeletal abnormalities was 1% and 2.6%, respectively. Table 10 compares CVS and early amniocentesis techniques.

Comparison of neonatal lung function in fetuses exposed to first-trimester amniocentesis or CVS showed no significant difference between the two groups when functional residual capacity at 2–8 weeks of age was measured. Both groups showed a slightly higher than expected number of functional residual capacities below the 2.5th centile[195]. An increased incidence of other congenital malformations such as talipes and congenital dislocated hips have been recorded following amniocentesis. Crandall and colleagues[41] found no significant difference in congenital malformations detected at birth in patients having amniocentesis at less than 15 weeks' gestation compared with controls at 15–20 weeks' gestation. The incidence of anomalies was 1.8% and 2.2%, respectively. In the early amniocentesis group, seven of the 12 abnormalities involved congenital hip dislocation and subluxation, or genitourinary systems. In the control group, eight of the 30 abnormalities involved genitourinary, congenital hip dislocation and club feet.

There is limited information on the effects of invasive procedures performed at 10–14 weeks of

Table 9 Randomized early amniocentesis studies (see Update section)

	Nicolaides *et al. (1996)*[193]		Johnson *et al. (1996)*[194]	
	EA	*CVS*	*EA*	*MA*
Number	256	262	349	346
Gestational age range (week)	10^{+0}–13^{+0}	10^{+0}–13^{+0}	11^{+0}–12^{+6}	15^{+0}–16^{+6}
Chromosomal anomalies	1.8%	2.2%	2.3%	0.9%
Total pregnancy loss	7.9%*	5.4%*	7.8%‡	7.4%‡
Spontaneous loss	5.8%†	1.8%†	3.7%	5.5%
Congenital anomalies	4.3%	3.1%	2.3%	2.3%
Repeat testing	1.8%	2.5%	0.6%	0
Maternal tissue	–	0.7%	–	
Culture failure	1.8%	0.7%	0.6%	
Mosaic result	–	1.1%	–	

CVS, chorionic villus sampling; EA, early amniocentesis; MA, mid-trimester amniocentesis; *difference % 2.5 (95% CI 1.0 to 6.0); †difference % 4.0 (95% CI 1.3 to 6.7); ‡difference % 0.4 (95% CI 3.6 to 4.4)

Table 10 Comparison of early procedures for prenatal diagnosis

	Chorionic villus sampling (CVS)	Early amniocentesis
Timing	10–11 weeks gestation	11–12 weeks gestation
Risk of miscarriage with no invasive testing (normal ultrasound at 10 weeks, maternal age over 35 years)	Approximately 5%	Approximately 5%
Risk of miscarriage due to procedure alone	Approximately 1%	Approximately 0.5–1%
Chance of obtaining result (from first procedure)	Approximately 96–99%	Between 96–99%
Time for result: culture	Two to four weeks (chromosomes)	Two to four weeks (chromosomes)
rapid direct	24–48 hours	Not available at present
Accuracy of chromosome diagnosis	Highly accurate but higher chance of placental mosaicism being diagnosed	Same accuracy as mid-trimester amniocentesis but greater banding number than CVS
Detection of spina bifida or abdominal wall defects	No*	No* (but the possibility is being researched)
Detection of Down's syndrome and other chromosomal and genetic abnormalities	Yes	Yes
Availability	By choice	Experimental at present
Termination options	Dilatation and evacuation	Dilatation and evacuation

*For patients undergoing chorionic villus sampling and early amniocentesis, at 16–20 weeks gestation maternal serum α-fetoprotein and ultrasound are suggested as a screening test for neural tube defect

gestation on infant morbidity. However, studies are emerging which suggest a higher associated risk for infant morbidity than previously thought[196–199]. Consideration should be given to the effects of such procedures on the infants when balancing relative risks and benefits in early procedures.

The major disadvantages of CVS are related to chorionic mosaicism, possible maternal cell contamination and fetal risks involving pregnancy loss and possibly congenital malformations. The major disadvantages for early amniocentesis are related to fetal risks involving pregnancy loss and possibly congenital malformations. Cytogenetic controversy related to early amniocentesis is less likely but may be dependent on the gestational age at the time of the procedure. Confined mosaicism may be more likely to occur with first-trimester amniocentesis as up to 70% of cells in the amniotic fluid up to 15 weeks' gestation are derived not from the fetus but from the membranes and trophoblasts. Mosaicism has not been reported to cause diagnostic dilemmas for early amniocentesis. The cytogenetic banding quality of early amniocentesis specimens has been reported to be comparable with that of controls at 500–550 bands and even better than long-term cultured chorionic villus sampling at 350–400 bands[200].

Safety and accuracy of prenatal diagnosis in twin gestation

Prenatal diagnosis in twin gestations and higher-order multiple gestations poses particular difficulties in terms of safety and technique of invasive procedures, interpretation of laboratory results, and the dilemmas produced by the finding of discordant abnormality. Prenatal diagnosis by both CVS and amniocentesis can be safely performed in multiple pregnancy with a similar accuracy[201,202]. Although total fetal loss after amniocentesis in a twin pregnancy is at least double that for a singleton, much of this additional risk is probably secondary to the inherent hazards of twins and not procedure-related. In experienced centers, CVS is equally safe and efficacious, and allows an earlier diagnosis that may be beneficial when discordant results are found[203].

A causal relation between the use of methylene blue in second-trimester amniocentesis and the occurrence of jejunal atresia has been suggested[204,205]. Its use is therefore discouraged. Indigo carmine has not been associated with any side-effects or malformations.

Safety and accuracy of fetal blood sampling

No serious maternal complications have been reported. Risks of complications and adverse outcomes depend mainly on the gestational age at the time of the procedure, the operator's experience, and the indication for the procedure. In a low-risk population fetal blood sampling performed by an experienced operator carries about a 1.4% risk of fetal loss before 28 weeks' gestation and a 1.4% risk of perinatal death (after 28 weeks)[206]. In a high-risk population including fetuses with structural anomalies, growth restriction or non-immune hydrops, the overall fetal loss rate can be as high as 25–47% reflecting the natural course of the fetal condition; this risk should be included in patient counseling[207–210]. Bleeding at the puncture site is commonly observed and lasts longer than 1 minute in about 10% of cases. Bradycardia, reported in up to 20% of cases when the umbilical artery is punctured, may necessitate an emergency cesarean section if prolonged[84]. Fetal bradycardia occurred in only 2% of fetuses and feto-maternal hemorrhage was also less likely when blood was sampled from the intrahepatic vein[84]. The cardiac hemodynamic response to fetal blood sampling differs between normally grown and growth-restricted fetuses. This difference may explain the higher rate of complications occurring in the latter group of fetuses after blood sampling[211].

Safety and accuracy of fetal tissue biopsy

Experience with fetal liver biopsy or muscle biopsy is very limited. Prenatal diagnosis by fetal skin biopsy at 15–22 weeks' gestation under guidance of ultrasound is generally a safe procedure. The fetal loss rate following fetal skin biopsy is about 5% to 7%. Premature birth occurs in about 10% of the cases. Moreover, there may be leakage of amniotic fluid and risk of infection. Other reported complications include maternal bleeding, injury to the bladder or bowel of the mother[110]. There have been concerns about scars in the fetus,

but they are small and of no cosmetic consequence when they are visible. Fetal skin biopsy is also reliable, in particular for epidermolysis bulla. However, its accuracy for certain forms of ichthyosis has been questioned[212].

CHOICE OF INVASIVE PROCEDURES

The choice of invasive prenatal diagnostic technique and gestational age timing is very individual. It will vary from patient to patient and is probably influenced by the operator's preference. Many women feel that there is a significant advantage for early prenatal diagnosis resulting in more privacy, safer termination of pregnancy and earlier decrease in anxiety related to pregnancy risks. Others report the emotional cost of CVS in terms of greater number of both spontaneous and selective abortions following CVS, the use of CVS for sex selection, the greater social acceptability of first-trimester abortion, the possibility of increased pressure on women to undergo prenatal diagnosis by health insurance companies, medical professionals and government agencies. All need to be weighed against the advantages of early prenatal diagnosis[213]. Women's prenatal diagnosis preferences for amniocentesis or CVS have been evaluated, indicating the reasoning for choices is variable and is influenced by multiple factors such as ethnicity, number of previous births, and urban or rural habitation[44,45,214,215].

ULTRASOUND GUIDED INVASIVE THERAPY

Most prenatally diagnosed malformations in continuing pregnancies are best managed by medical and surgical therapy in a referral center after planned delivery. However, there are some structural defects with predictable severe developmental consequences that may require intervention *in utero*. Because of the strong association of structural defects and chromosomal abnormalities, it is mandatory to ensure karyotyping is performed before considering surgical interventions. Likewise, other associated anomalies should be excluded with a detailed ultrasound scan before intervention is discussed.

Although much fetal treatment is still experimental, the stage is now set for intrauterine fetal therapy[2,3,216]. Introduction of needles, trocars or fine-gauge endoscopes under ultrasound guidance through the maternal abdomen into the uterine cavity is the current surgical approach for access to the fetus, cord and placenta. A brief outline of these procedures is given below.

Multifetal pregnancy reduction

New technologies and a wider use of ovulation induction agents in the treatment of infertility over the last 10 years have resulted in a worrying increase in the number of multiple gestations. Although twins predominate, higher order pregnancies are also increasing.

Pregnancy complications, neonatal morbidity and mortality are directly related to the order of multiple gestations, primarily because of an increased predisposition to premature delivery. From a social point of view, raising triplets, quadruplets or even quintuplets is very challenging, especially if one or more of the infants is disabled. From a medical and ethical point of view, many would consider fetal reduction in the management of a twin or triplet pregnancy to be a controversial issue[217].

It would be good if the use of assisted reproduction technologies could be further refined to preclude pregnancies of higher order. Until advances in reproductive technology can eliminate this iatrogenic risk, and until progress in perinatology can decrease the threat of early preterm delivery, multifetal pregnancy reduction may be of benefit in an otherwise dismal situation[218].

Multifetal pregnancy reduction was introduced in the mid 1980s[203]. It is a procedure designed to decrease the risk for very premature delivery by reducing the number of live fetuses. It can be performed transcervically, transvaginally, or transabdominally under ultrasound guidance. The latter two approaches have been favored over the past few years. The transabdominal route is generally carried out between 10 and 13 weeks of gestation, whereas the transvaginal technique is used earlier. Injection of a concentrated potassium chloride solution into the thorax of a fetus is the most commonly used method. The pregnancy loss rate after the procedure is about 8–10% in triplets or quadruplets, and is higher for higher order pregnancies[203,219].

Manipulation of amniotic fluid

In the feto-fetal (twin–twin) transfusion syndrome repeated amnioreductions have been advocated to decrease the polyhydramnios-related complications and possibly ameliorate fetal condition[220,221]. With this therapy, an overall survival rate of 49% has been reported[222]. However, the incidence of brain damage in the survivor after late intrauterine death of the monozygous co-twin is about 27% in reported series[220]. More recently, ultrasound guided septostomy or creation of a hole in the intervening membrane as a single therapeutic procedure in gestations with feto-fetal transfusion syndrome has been reported in a limited series with a good perinatal outcome[223]. A multicenter randomized study is ongoing to compare its therapeutic value with serial amniodrainage.

Although ultrasound directed transabdominal amnioinfusion in the second or third trimester has been used mostly to facilitate ultrasound visualization in pregnancies with oligohydramnios, attempts have been made to prevent sequelae of oligohydramnios by serial infusions with promising results[224].

Fetal transfusion therapy

Intraperitoneal transfusion of blood to treat fetal Rh disease removed the conceptual barriers to direct access of the fetus. The development of fetal blood sampling and intravascular fetal blood transfusion for the management of Rh disease has established fetal transfusion therapy[97]. Subsequently, it has expanded to other cytopenias and anemias, including alloimmune thrombocytopenia, maternal autoimmune idiopathic thrombocytopenic purpura (ITP) associated with fetal thrombocytopenia, red blood cell alloimmunization with other factors, and fetal parvovirus B19 infection[225].

Direct injection of drugs to the fetal circulation by cordocentesis has been reported[226].

In utero drainage and shunting procedures

Drainage by ultrasound guided needle aspiration of any large collection of fluid such as fetal ascites, hydrothorax or urine in obstructive uropathy is easily achieved[2]. Serial aspirations will be necessary where fluid is likely to reaccumulate. In this circumstance, introduction of a shunt to continuously drain the fluid into the amniotic cavity may be considered. Shunting of the thorax (thoracoamniotic shunt), abdomen (peritoneal-amniotic shunt) and bladder (vesico-amniotic shunt) are currently the three most rewarding situations for this form of treatment[119,226]. Insertion of a thoraco-amniotic shunt relieves pressure on the developing fetal lungs and reduces the risk of pulmonary hypoplasia[227]. Similarly, drainage of ascites can benefit fetal growth and development. However, all these procedures have certain risks that must be carefully weighed against the expected benefits[228].

Operative fetoscopy

The experience gained in experimental fetal surgery on animals and the technological advances that have made video-endoscopic surgery possible in man have helped the development of ultrasound guided minimally invasive fetoscopic techniques for surgical procedures within the amniotic cavity. This approach has been called operative fetoscopy. Using this modality and ultrasound, percutaneous umbilical cord ligation *in utero* (Figure 7) or Nd : YAG laser coagulation of vascular anastomoses on the chorionic plate (Figure 8) to manage complicated monochorionic multiple gestations have been reported[7,229,230]. In a review on 23 cases of fetoscopic cord ligation, mostly for acardiacs, but also for other abnormal monochorionic twin pregnancies, a neonatal survival rate of 66% was reported. The most significant clinical problem, next to expertise and skills, is the high likelihood of preterm premature rupture of the membranes, complicating about 40% of cases with a majority occurring prior to 32 weeks[231].

Experience with fetoscopic Nd : YAG laser procedures for twin–twin transfusion syndrome (TTS) is accumulating. A 53% fetal survival is achieved with the majority of fetal deaths occurring within 24 hours following over 150 such laser procedures. Neurological morbidity in the children is below 5% at follow-up more than one year after birth[232]. Although this figure is lower than those achieved with any other current therapy, fetal mortality remains high. However, there is much controversy about this procedure because it is thought to be unselective (ablation of all crossing vessels) and yet it has not been proven that it can interrupt the blood flow in the very few deeply located anastomoses in the monochorionic placenta. For these reasons, this may not be the ultimate treatment of choice. None of the proposed therapies for TTS has been, so far, tested in a

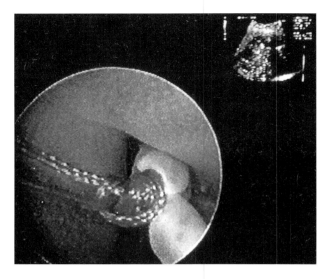

Figure 7 Fetoscopic cord ligation. The umbilical cord of an acardiac twin has been ligated with an extracorporeal knot. The fetoscopic surgeon is continuously backed up by ultrasound images projected by a twin-camera system at the right upper corner of the screen (see also Color plate 23)

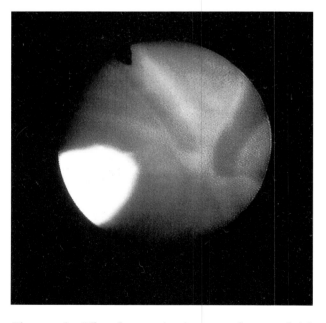

Figure 8 Fiber-fetoscopic image of superficial chorionic plate vessels crossing the intertwin membrane insertion (the white line crossing the image). At 8 o'clock in the image, a 400 μm Nd : YAG laser fiber is inserted to coagulate vessels. The endoscope itself is 1.2 mm in diameter (see also Color plate 24)

randomized study to prove any superiority. Thus, such studies are now urgently needed.

Experience is very limited with a few other reported applications of operative fetoscopy including cystostomy as an alternative to fetal bladder shunting[233], laser ablation of posterior urethral valves[117], devascularization of placental chorioangioma[234] and sacrococcygeal teratoma[235].

As the technique is evolving, future applications of operative fetoscopy are likely to increase.

In utero hematopoietic stem cell transplantation

This is a new experimental therapeutic option for families with increased risk of having a child with certain inherited disorders[6]. Immunological naiveté and the rapidly expanding hematopoietic system in the first-trimester human fetus make therapeutic intervention by intrauterine transplantation a real possibility for those disorders which can be diagnosed early in gestation. Fewer cells are required than in postnatal bone marrow transplantation and therapy can be offered before the pathological sequelae of a disorder become manifest. The hemoglobinopathies, such as α-thalassemia, β-thalassemia, sickle cell anemia, immunological disorders, and many metabolic disorders can potentially benefit by transplantation with hematopoietic stem cells. Transplantation uses guidance of ultrasound to inject fetal stem cells derived from fetal liver and thymus, or T-cell depleted adult bone marrow into the fetal peritoneal cavity. Alternatively, intravascular transplantation can be done by cordocentesis for myeloid disorders when there is no constrain by the narrow window of opportunity which exists with for example the hemoglobinopathies. The results of *in utero* transplantations performed so far are especially encouraging for the immunodeficiency disorders[6,236]. The availability of embryoscopy paves the way for future first-trimester interventions such as gene or cell therapy using the intravascular route[129].

CONCLUSIONS

Amniocentesis performed at 16 to 18 weeks' gestation has been the gold standard approach for prenatal cytogenetic diagnosis. Over the last decade large collaborative studies on chorionic villus sampling have provided information regarding its safety and accuracy. Although first-trimester CVS is now an established alternative to mid-trimester amniocentesis for prenatal diagnosis, there are still some controversies regarding possible associations with limb abnormalities, its usefulness in multiple gestations, and the clinical significance of confined placental mosaicism. These issues have led investigators to study the technical feasibility, safety, and accuracy of amniocentesis performed in the first trimester or early second trimester. Although early amniocentesis appears both safe and efficacious, there are concerns regarding orthopedic abnormalities and the reliability of first-trimester amniotic fluid acetylcholinesterase and AFP levels in the screening of neural tube defects. Other techniques such as coelocentesis and transcervical flushing are being explored and their usefulness, reliability and safety for prenatal diagnosis remain to be established. Thus, future studies have still to address the timing and techniques of prenatal diagnosis.

The inevitable consequence of our increasing knowledge about the fetus and our capability to make early prenatal diagnoses is attempts to treat some of the detected abnormalities. The stage is set for fetal therapy: the final domain and next exciting frontier for perinatologists is *in utero* therapy for the fetus.

UPDATE

Since completion of this chapter, two important randomized studies on early amniocentesis performed at 11 to 13 gestational weeks have been published[237,238]. These studies show that early amniocentesis, even with skilled operators, is associated with an increased risk of fetal loss and talipes equinovarus. Thus, the evidence from these new studies suggests that if an early fetal diagnosis is essential then, unless there are exceptional reasons, it should not be by early amniocentesis.

ACKNOWLEDGEMENTS

T-H.B. and J.A.D. wish to thank the European Commission (Biomed 2 Programme) for its generous financial support of the 'Eurofoetus' research project PL 96 23 83.

References

1. Leschot NJ, Vejerslev LO. Proceedings of the EUCROMIC workshop on prenatal diagnosis. *Eur J Hum Genet* 1997;5(Suppl. 1):1–6
2. Liu DTY, Bui T-H. Fetal therapy: ethical, legal and medical considerations. *Curr Obstet Gynaecol* 1994;4:160–5
3. Luks FI, Deprest JA. Endoscopic fetal surgery: a new alternative? *Eur J Obstet Gynecol Reprod Biol* 1993;52:1–3
4. Quintero RA, Puder KS, Cotton DB. Embryoscopy and fetoscopy. *Obstet Gynecol Clin N Am* 1993;20:563–81
5. Brumfield CG, Atkinson MW. Invasive techniques for fetal evaluation and treatment. *Clin Obstet Gynecol* 1994;37:856–74
6. Jones DRE, Bui T-H, Anderson EM, *et al. In utero* haematopoietic stem cell transplantation: current perspectives and future potential. *Bone Marrow Transpl* 1996;18:831–7
7. Ville Y, Hyett J, Hecher K, *et al.* Preliminary experience with endoscopic laser surgery for severe twin-twin transfusion syndrome. *N Engl J Med* 1995;332:224–7
8. Brock JH, Rodeck CH, Ferguson-Smith MA (eds) *Prenatal Diagnosis and Screening.* London: Churchill Livingstone, 1992
9. Guerina NG. Management strategies for infectious diseases in pregnancy. *Semin Perinatol* 1994;18:305–20
10. Bennett P, Nicolini U. Fetal infections. In Moise KJ, Fisk NM, eds. *Fetal Therapy.* New York: Cambridge University Press, 1997:92–116
11. Hook EB. Rates of chromosome abnormalities at different maternal ages. *Obstet Gynecol* 1981;58:282–5
12. Hook EB, Cross PK, Jackson L, *et al.* Maternal age-specific rates of 47, +21 and other cytogenetic abnormalities diagnosed in the first trimester of pregnancy in chorionic villus biopsy specimens: comparison with rates expected from observations at amniocentesis. *Am J Hum Genet* 1988;42:797–807
13. Hook EB, Cross PK. Maternal age-specific rates of chromosome abnormalities at chorionic villus study: a revision. *Am J Hum Genet* 1989;45:474–7
14. Snijders RJM, Nicolaides KH. *Ultrasound Markers For Fetal Chromosome Defects.* London: Parthenon Publishing, 1995:79
15. Halliday JL, Watson LF, Lumley J, *et al.* New estimates of Down syndrome risks at chorionic villus sampling, amniocentesis, and livebirth in women of advanced maternal age from a uniquely defined population. *Prenat Diagn* 1995;15:455–65
16. MacIntosh MC, Wald NJ, Chard T, *et al.* Selective miscarriage of Down's syndrome fetuses in women aged 35 years and older. *Br J Obstet Gynaecol* 1995;102:798–801
17. D'Alton ME. Prenatal diagnostic procedures. *Semin Perinatol* 1994;18:140–62
18. Anonymous. Chorionic villus sampling and amniocentesis: recommendations for prenatal counseling. Centers for Disease Control and Prevention. *Morbid Mortal Weekly Rep* 1995;44:1–12
19. Dumez Y, Goosens M, Boué J, *et al.* Chorionic villi sampling using rigid forceps under ultrasound control. In Fracarro M, Simoni G, Brambati B, eds. *First Trimester Fetal Diagnosis.* Berlin: Springer-Verlag, 1985:38–45
20. Kennerknecht I, Bauer-Aubele S, Grab D, *et al.* First trimester amniocentesis between the seventh and 13th weeks: evaluation of the earliest possible genetic diagnosis. *Prenat Diagn* 1992;12:595–601
21. Jorgensen FS, Bang J, Lind AM, *et al.* Genetic amniocentesis at 7–14 weeks of gestation. *Prenat Diagn* 1992;12:277–83
22. Bevis DCA. The antenatal prediction of haemolytic disease of the newborn. *Lancet* 1952;1:395–8
23. Steele MW, Breg WR. Chromosome analysis of amniotic-fluid cells. *Lancet* 1966;1:383–5
24. Valenti C, Schutta EJ, Kehaty T. Prenatal diagnosis of Down's syndrome. Lancet 1968;2:220
25. Nadler HL. Antenatal detection of hereditary disorders. *Pediatrics* 1968;42:912–18
26. Bui T-H, Kristoffersson U. Prenatal diagnosis in Sweden: organisation and current issues. *Eur J Hum Genet* 1997;5(Suppl. 1):70–6
27. Bennett PR, Le Van Kim C, Colin Y, *et al.* Prenatal determination of fetal RhD type by DNA amplification. *N Engl J Med* 1993;329:607–10
28. Bennett PR, Warwick R, Vaughan J, *et al.* Prenatal determination of human platelet antigen type using DNA amplification following amniocentesis. *Br J Obstet Gynaecol* 1994;101:246–9
29. Lighten AD, Overton TG, Sepulveda W, *et al.* Accuracy of prenatal determination of RhD type status by polymerase chain reaction with amniotic cells. *Am J Obstet Gynecol* 1995;173:1182–5
30. Khouzami AN, Kickler TS, Bray PF, *et al.* Molecular genotyping of fetal platelet antigens with uncultured amniocytes. *Am J Obstet Gynecol* 1995;173:1202–6
31. Van den Veyver IB, Subramanian SB, Hudson KM, *et al.* Prenatal diagnosis of the RhD fetal blood type on amniotic fluid by polymerase chain reaction. *Obstet Gynecol* 1996;87:419–22

32. Robinson GE, Carr M, Olmstead M, *et al*. Psychological reactions to pregnancy loss after prenatal diagnostic testing. *J Psychosom Obstet Gynecol* 1991; 12:181–92

33. Bombard AT, Powers JF, Carter S, *et al*. Procedure-related fetal losses in transplacental versus non-transplacental genetic amniocentesis. *Am J Obstet Gynecol* 1995;172:868–72

34. Giorlandino C, Mobili L, Bilancioni E, *et al*. Transplacental amniocentesis: is it really a higher-risk procedure? *Prenat Diagn* 1994;14:803–6

35. Nuss S, Brebaum D, Grond-Ginsbach C. Maternal cell contamination in amniotic fluid samples as a consequence of the sampling technique. *Hum Genet* 1994;93:121–4

36. Neilson JP. Prenatal diagnosis in multiple pregnancies. *Curr Opin Obstet Gynecol* 1992;4:280–5

37. Wapner RJ. Genetic diagnosis in multiple pregnancies. *Semin Perinatol* 1995;19:351–62

38. Buscaglia M, Ghisoni L, Bellotti M, *et al*. Genetic amniocentesis in biamniotic twin pregnancies by a single transabdominal insertion of the needle. *Prenat Diagn* 1995;15:17–19

39. van Vugt JM, Nieuwint A, van Geijn HP. Single-needle insertion: an alternative technique for early second-trimester genetic twin amniocentesis. *Fetal Diagn Ther* 1995;10:178–81

40. Bahado-Singh R, Schmitt R, Hobbins JC. New technique for genetic amniocentesis in twins. *Obstet Gynecol* 1992;79:304–7

41. Crandall BF, Kulch P, Tabsh K. Risk assessment of amniocentesis between 11 and 15 weeks: comparison to later amniocentesis controls. *Prenat Diagn* 1994;19:913–19

42. Wilson RD. Early amniocentesis: a clinical review. *Prenat Diagn* 1995;15:1529–73

43. Evans MI, Johnson MP, Holzgreve W. Early amniocentesis. What exactly does it mean? *J Reprod Med* 1994;39:77–8

44. Heckerling PS, Verp MS, Hadro TA. Preferences of pregnant women for amniocentesis or chorionic villus sampling for prenatal testing: comparison of patients' choices and those of a decision-analytic model. *J Clin Epidemiol* 1994;47:1215–28

45. Heckerling PS, Verp MS. A cost-effectiveness analysis of amniocentesis and chorionic villus sampling for prenatal genetic testing. *Med Care* 1994;32: 863–80

46. Wathen NC, Campbell DJ, Kitau MJ, *et al*. Alpha-fetoprotein levels in amniotic fluid from 8 to 18 weeks of pregnancy. *Br J Obstet Gynaecol* 1993;100: 380–2

47. Crandall BF, Chua C. Detecting neural tube defects by amniocentesis between 11 and 15 weeks' gestation. *Prenat Diagn* 1995;15:339–43

48. Sundberg K, Jorgensen FS, Tabor A, *et al*. Experience with early amniocentesis. *J Perinat Med* 1995;23:149–58

49. Jorgensen FS, Sundberg K, Rasmussen-Loft AG, *et al*. Alpha-fetoprotein and acetylcholinesterase activity in first and early second-trimester amniotic fluid. *Prenat Diagn* 1995;15:621–5

50. Dombrowski MP, Isada NB, Johnson MP, *et al*. Modified stylet technique for tenting of amniotic membranes. *Obstet Gynecol* 1996;87:455–6

51. Bravo RR, Shulman LP, Owen PP, *et al*. Transplacental needle passage in early amniocentesis and pregnancy loss. *Obstet Gynecol* 1995;86:437–40

52. Shulman LP, Elias S, Philips OP, *et al*. Early twin amniocentesis prior to 14 weeks gestation. *Prenat Diagn* 1992;12:625–9

53. Kennerknecht I, Kramer S, Grab D, *et al*. Evaluation of amniotic fluid cell filtration: an experimental approach to early amniocentesis. *Prenat Diagn* 1993; 13:247–55

54. Sundberg K, Smidt-Jensen S, Lundsteen C, *et al*. Filtration and recirculation of early amniotic fluid: evaluation of cell cultures from 100 diagnostic cases. *Prenat Diagn* 1993;13:1101–10

55. Byrne DL, Penna L, Marks K, *et al*. First trimester amnifiltration: technical, cytogenetic and pregnancy outcome of 104 consecutive procedures. *Br J Obstet Gynaecol* 1995;102:220–3

56. Frydman R, Pons JC, Borghi E, *et al*. Per-urethral transvesicle first-trimester amniocentesis. *Eur J Obstet Gynecol Reprod Biol* 1993;48:99–101

57. Shalev E, Weiner E, Yanai N, *et al*. Comparison of first-trimester transvaginal amniocentesis with chorionic villus sampling and mid-trimester amniocentesis. *Prenat Diagn* 1994;14:279–83

58. Hahnemann N, Mohr J. Genetic diagnosis in the embryo by means of biopsy from extraembryonic membranes. *Bull Eur Soc Hum Genet* 1968;2:23

59. Kazy Z, Rozovsky IS, Bakharev VA. Chorion biopsy in early pregnancy: a method of early prenatal diagnosis for inherited disorders. *Prenat Diagn* 1972; 2:39–45

60. Kullander S, Sandahl B. Fetal chromosome analysis after transcervical placental biopsies during early pregnancy. *Acta Obstet Gynecol Scand* 1973;52:355–9

61. Hahnemann N. Early prenatal diagnosis: a study of biopsy techniques and cell culturing from extraembryonic membranes. *Clin Genet* 1974;6: 294–306

62. Department of Obstetrics and Gynecology, Tietung Hospital, Anshan Iron and Steel Company. Fetal sex prediction by sex chromatin of chorionic villi cells during early pregnancy. *Chin Med J* 1975;1: 117–26

63. Ward RTH, Modell B, Petrou M, *et al*. A method of chorionic villus sampling in the first trimester of pregnancy under real time ultrasonic guidance. *Br Med J* 1983;286:1542–4

64. Brambati B, Simoni G. Fetal diagnosis of trisomy 21 in the first trimester of pregnancy. *Lancet* 1983; 1:586

65. Old JM, Ward RTH, Karagozlu F, et al. First-trimester fetal diagnosis by chorionic villus sampling for haemoglobinopathies: three cases. Lancet 1983; 2:1414–6

66. Goosens M, Dumez Y, Kaplan L, et al. Prenatal diagnosis of sickle cell anemia in the first trimester. N Engl J Med 1983;309:831–3

67. Pergament E, Ginsburg N, Verlinsky Y, et al. Prenatal Tay-Sachs diagnosis by chorionic villus sampling. Lancet 1983;2:286

68. Grebner EE, Wapner RJ, Barr MA, et al. Prenatal Tay-Sachs diagnosis by chorionic villi sampling. Lancet 1983;2:286–7

69. Holzgreve W, Miny P, Schloo R, et al. International Registry: compilation of data from 24 centres. Prenat Diagn 1990;10:159–67

70. Dalpra L, Nocera G, Tibilett MG, et al. 'Late' chorionic villus sampling: cytogenetic aspects. Prenat Diagn 1993;13:239–46

71. Smidt-Jensen S, Lundsteen C, Lind AM, et al. Transabdominal chorionic villus sampling in the second and third trimesters of pregnancy: chromosome quality, reporting time, and feto-maternal bleeding. Prenat Diagn 1993;13:957–69

72. Cameron AD, Murphy KW, McNay MB, et al. Midtrimester chorionic villus sampling: an alternative approach? Am J Obstet Gynecol 1994;171:1035–7

73. Ko TM, Tseng LH, Hwa HL, et al. Prenatal diagnosis by transabdominal chorionic villus sampling in the second and third trimesters. Arch Gynecol Obstet 1995;256:193–7

74. Shulman LP, Simpson JL, Elias S, et al. Transvaginal chorionic villus sampling using transabdominal ultrasound guidance: a new technique for first-trimester prenatal diagnosis. Fetal Diagn Ther 1993; 8:144–8

75. Lunshof S, Boer K, Leschot NJ, et al. Pregnancy outcome after transcervical CVS with a flexible biopsy forceps: evaluation of risk factors. Prenat Diagn 1995;15:809–16

76. Fortuny A, Borrell A, Soler A, et al. Chorionic villus sampling by biopsy forceps. Results of 1580 procedures from a single centre. Prenat Diagn 1995;15: 541–50

77. Smidt-Jensen S, Hahnemann N. Transabdominal fine needle biopsy from chorionic villi in the first trimester. Prenat Diagn 1984;4:163–9

78. Silverman NS, Sullivan MW, Jungkind DL, et al. Incidence of bacteremia associated with chorionic villus sampling. Obstet Gynecol 1994;84:1021–4

79. Isada NB, Johnson MP, Pryde PG, et al. Technical aspects of transcervical chorionic villus sampling. Fetal Diagn Ther 1994;9:19–28

80. Smidt-Jensen S, Philip J. Comparison of transabdominal and transcervical CVS and amniocentesis: sampling success and risk. Prenat Diagn 1991; 11:529–37

81. Silver RK, MacGregor SN, Muhlbach LH, et al. Congenital malformations subsequent to chorionic villus sampling: outcome analysis of 1048 consecutive procedures. Prenat Diagn 1994;14:421–7

82. Chueh JT, Goldberg JD, Wohlferd MM, et al. Comparison of transcervical and transabdominal chorionic villus sampling loss rates in nine thousand cases from a single center. Am J Obstet Gynecol 1995; 173:1277–82

83. Valenti C. Antenatal detection of hemoglobinopathies. A preliminary report. Am J Obstet Gynecol 1973;115:851–3

84. Nicolini U. Invasive techniques of prenatal diagnosis. Curr Obstet Gynaecol 1992;2:77–84

85. Hobbins JC, Mahoney MJ. In utero diagnosis of hemoglobinopathies. Technique for obtaining fetal blood. N Engl J Med 1974;290:1065–7

86. Rodeck CH, Campbell S. Sampling pure fetal blood by fetoscopy in second trimester of pregnancy. Br Med J 1978;2:728–30

87. Daffos F, Capella-Pavlovsky M, Forestier F. A new procedure for fetal blood sampling in utero: preliminary results of fifty-three cases. Am J Obstet Gynecol 1983;146:985–7

88. Antsaklis AI, Papantoniou NE, Mesogitis SA, et al. Cardiocentesis: an alternative method of fetal blood sampling for the prenatal diagnosis of hemoglobinopathies. Obstet Gynecol 1992;79:630–3

89. Wax JR, Blakemore KJ. Fetal blood sampling. Obstet Gynecol Clin N Am 1993;20:533–62

90. Buscaglia M, Ghisoni L, Bellotti M, et al. Percutaneous umbilical cord sampling: indication changes and procedure loss rate in a nine years' experience. Fetal Diagn Ther 1996;11:106–13

91. Tanemura M, Suzumori K, Yagami Y, et al. Diagnosis of fetal rubella infection with reverse transcription and nested polymerase chain reaction: a study of 34 cases diagnosed in fetuses. Am J Obstet Gynecol 1996;174:578–82

92. Hohlfeld P, Daffos F, Costa JM, et al. Prenatal diagnosis of congenital toxoplasmosis with a polymerase-chain-reaction test on amniotic fluid. N Engl J Med 1994;331:695–9

93. Isada NB, Paar DP, Grossman JH, et al. TORCH infections. Diagnosis in the molecular age. J Reprod Med 1992;37:499–507

94. Shalev E, Zalel Y, Weiner E, et al. The role of cordocentesis in assessment of mosaicism found in amniotic fluid cell culture. Acta Obstet Gynecol Scand 1994;73:119–22

95. Boulot P, Lefort G, Bachelard B, et al. Cordocentesis versus amniocentesis for rapid fetal karyotyping in cases of late referral of women. J Perinat Med 1992; 20:159–61

96. Donner C, Rypens F, Paquet V, et al. Cordocentesis for rapid karyotype: 421 consecutive cases. Fetal Diagn Ther 1995;10:192–9

97. Schumacher B, Moise KJ. Fetal transfusion for red blood cell alloimmunization in pregnancy. *Obstet Gynecol* 1996;88:137–50

98. Nava S, Bocconi L, Zuliani G, *et al*. Aspects of fetal physiology from 18 to 37 weeks' gestation as assessed by blood sampling. *Obstet Gynecol* 1996;87:975–80

99. Shalev E, Blondheim O, Peleg D. Use of cordocentesis in the management of preterm or growth-restricted fetuses with abnormal monitoring. *Obstet Gynecol Surv* 1995;50:839–44

100. Thorpe-Beeston JG, Nicolaides KH. Fetal thyroid function. *Fetal Diagn Ther* 1993;8:60–72

101. Biswas A, Arulkumaran S, Ratnam SS. Disorders of platelets in pregnancy. *Obstet Gynecol Surv* 1994;49:585–94

102. Zosmer N, Vaughan J, Fisk NM. Fetal blood sampling from intrahepatic vein versus cord insertion: effect on pH and blood gases. *Obstet Gynecol* 1993;82:504–8

103. Weiner CP, Okamura K. Diagnostic fetal blood sampling: technique related losses. *Fetal Diagn Ther* 1996;11:169–75

104. Welch CR, Talbert DG, Warwick RM, *et al*. Needle modifications for invasive fetal procedures. *Obstet Gynecol* 1995;85:113–7

105. Okamura K, Murotsuki J, Kosuge S, *et al*. Diagnostic use of cordocentesis in twin pregnancy. *Fetal Diagn Ther* 1994;9:385–90

106. Elias S, Mazur M, Sabbagha R, *et al*. Prenatal diagnosis of harlequin ichthyosis. *Clin Genet* 1980;17:275–80

107. Golbus MS, Sagebiel RW, Filly RA, *et al*. Prenatal diagnosis of congenital bullous ichtyosiform erythroderma (epidermolytic hyperkeratosis) by fetal skin biopsy. *N Engl J Med* 1980;302:93–5

108. Rodeck CH, Eady RAJ, Gosden CM. Prenatal diagnosis of epidermolysis bullosa letalis. *Lancet* 1980;1:949–52

109. Holbrook KA, Smith LT, Elias S. Prenatal diagnosis of genetic skin disease using fetal skin biopsy samples. *Arch Dermatol* 1993;129:1437–54

110. Eady RAJ, Holbrook KA, Blanchet-Bardon C, *et al*. Chair's summary: prenatal diagnosis of skin diseases. In Burgdorf WHC, Katz SI, eds. *Dermatology, Progress and Perspectives*. New York: Parthenon Publishing, 1993:1159–65

111. Murotsuki J, Uehara S, Okamura K, *et al*. Fetal liver biopsy for prenatal diagnosis of carbamoyl phosphate synthetase deficiency. *Am J Perinatol* 1994;11:160–2

112. Evans MI, Hoffman EP, Cadrin C, *et al*. Fetal muscle biopsy: collaborative experience with varied indications. *Obstet Gynecol* 1994;84:913–7

113. Cadrin C, Golbus MS. Fetal tissue sampling: indications, techniques, complications, and experience with sampling of fetal skin, liver, and muscle. *West J Med* 1993;159:269–72

114. Christiano AM, Uitto J. DNA-based prenatal diagnosis of heritable skin diseases. *Arch Dermatol* 1993;129:1455–9

115. Cartolano R, Guerneri S, Fogliani R, *et al*. Prenatal confirmation of trisomy 12 mosaicism by fetal skin biopsy. *Prenat Diagn* 1993;13:1057–9

116. Cendron M, D'Alton ME, Combleholme TM. Prenatal diagnosis and management of the fetus with hydronephrosis. *Semin Perinatol* 1994;18:163–81

117. Quintero RA, Hume R, Smith C, *et al*. Percutaneous fetal cystoscopy and endoscopic fulguration of posterior urethral valves. *Am J Obstet Gynecol* 1995;172:206–9

118. Nicolini U, Tannirandorn Y, Vaughan J, *et al*. Further predictors of renal dysplasia in fetal obstructive uropathy: bladder pressure and biochemistry of 'fresh' urine. *Prenat Diagn* 1991;71:159–66

119. Johnson MP, Bukowski TP, Reitleman C, *et al*. In utero surgical treatment of fetal obstructive uropathy: a new comprehensive approach to identify appropriate candidates for vesicoamniotic shunt therapy. *Am J Obstet Gynecol* 1994;170:1770–9

120. Westin B. Hysteroscopy in early pregnancy. *Lancet* 1954;2:872

121. Mahoney MJ, Hobbins JC. Prenatal diagnosis of chondroectodermal dysplasia (Ellis Van Creveld syndrome) using fetoscopy and ultrasound. *N Engl J Med* 1977;297:258–60

122. Bui T-H, Marsk L, Eklöf O, *et al*. Prenatal diagnosis of chondroectodermal dysplasia with fetoscopy. *Prenat Diagn* 1984;4:155–9

123. Rodeck CH, Kemp JR, Holman CA, *et al*. Direct intravascular fetal blood transfusion by fetoscopy in severe Rhesus isoimmunisation. *Lancet* 1981;1:625–7

124. Quintero RA, Abuhamad A, Hobbins JC, *et al*. Transabdominal thin gauge embryofetoscopy: a technique for early prenatal diagnosis and its use in the diagnosis of a case of Meckel Gruber syndrome. *Am J Obstet Gynecol* 1993;168:1552–7

125. Ginsberg NA, Zbaraz D, Strom C. Transabdominal embryoscopy for the detection of Carpenter syndrome during the first trimester. *J Assist Reprod Genet* 1994;11:373–5

126. Dumez Y, Dommergues M, Gubler MC, *et al*. Meckel Gruber syndrome: prenatal diagnosis at 10 menstrual weeks using embryoscopy. *Prenat Diagn* 1994;14:141–4

127. Hobbins JC, Jones OW, Gottesfeld S, *et al*. Transvaginal ultrasonography and transabdominal embryoscopy in the first trimester diagnosis of Smith-Lemli-Opitz syndrome type II. *Am J Obstet Gynecol* 1994;171:546–9

128. Dommergues M, Lemerrer M, Couly G, *et al*. Prenatal diagnosis of cleft lip at 11 menstrual weeks using embryoscopy in the van der Woude syndrome. *Prenat Diagn* 1995;15:378–81

129. Reece EA, Whetham J, Rotmensch S, *et al*. Gaining access to the embryonic fetal circulation via first-trimester endoscopy: a step into the future. *Obstet Gynecol* 1993;82:876–9

130. Hobbins JC. The future of first-trimester embryoscopy. *Ultrasound Obstet Gynecol* 1996;8:3–4

131. Ville Y, Bernard JP, Doumerc S, *et al*. Transabdominal fetoscopy in fetal anomalies diagnosed by ultrasound in the first trimester of pregnancy. *Ultrasound Obstet Gynecol* 1996;8:11–15

132. Reece EA, Homko C, Goldstein I, *et al*. Toward fetal therapy using needle embryofetoscopy. *Ultrasound Obstet Gynecol* 1995;5:281–5

133. Reece EA. Embryoscopy: new developments in prenatal medicine. *Curr Opin Obstet Gynecol* 1992;4:447–55

134. Reece EA, Homko CJ, Wiznitzer A, *et al*. Needle embryofetoscopy and early prenatal diagnosis. *Fetal Diagn Ther* 1995;10:81–2

135. Jauniaux E, Jurkovic D, Gulbis B, *et al*. Biochemical composition of exocoelomic fluid in early human pregnancy. *Obstet Gynecol* 1991;78:1124–8

136. Wathen NC, Cass PL, Kitau MJ, *et al*. Human chorionic gonadotrophin and alpha-fetoprotein levels in matched samples of amniotic fluid, extraembryonic exocoelomic fluid, and maternal serum in the first trimester of pregnancy. *Prenat Diagn* 1991;11:145–51

137. Wathen NC, Cass PL, Campbell DJ, *et al*. Early amniocentesis: alpha-fetoprotein in amniotic fluid, extraembryonic coelomic fluid and maternal serum between 8 and 13 weeks. *Br J Obstet Gynaecol* 1991;98:866–70

138. Gulbis B, Jauniaux E, Jurkovic D, *et al*. Determination of protein pattern in embryonic cavities of early human pregnancies: a model to understand materno-embryonic exchanges. *Hum Reprod* 1992;7:886–9

139. Jauniaux E, Gulbis B, Jurkovic D, *et al*. Protein and steroid levels in embryonic cavities of early human pregnancy. *Hum Reprod* 1993;8:782–7

140. Jauniaux E, Gulbis B, Jurkovic D, *et al*. Relationship between protein concentrations in embryological fluids and maternal serum and yolk sac size during human early pregnancy. *Hum Reprod* 1994;9:161–6

141. Jauniaux E, Jurkovic D, Lees C, *et al*. In vivo study of diazepam transfer across the first trimester human placenta. *Hum Reprod* 1996;11:889–92

142. Jauniaux E, Lees C, Jurkovic D, *et al*. Transfer of inulin across the first trimester human placenta. *Am J Obstet Gynecol* 1997, in press

143. Jurkovic D, Jauniaux E, Campbell S, *et al*. Coelocentesis: a new technique for early prenatal diagnosis. *Lancet* 1993;341:1623–4

144. Jurkovic D, Jauniaux E, Campbell S, *et al*. Detection of sickle gene by coelocentesis in early

pregnancy: a new approach to prenatal diagnosis of single gene disorders. *Hum Reprod* 1995;10:1287–9

145. Shettles LB. Use of the Y chromosome in prenatal sex determination. *Nature* 1971;230:52

146. Bobrow M, Lewis BV. Unreliability of fetal sexing using cervical material. *Lancet* 1971;2:486

147. Warren R, Sanchez L, Hammond D, *et al*. Prenatal sex determination from exfoliated cells found in cervical mucus. *Am J Hum Genet* 1972;24:22a

148. Griffith-Jones MD, Miller D, Lilford RJ, *et al*. Detection of fetal DNA in transcervical swabs from first trimester pregnancies by gene amplification: a new route to prenatal diagnosis? *Br J Obstet Gynaecol* 1992;99:508–11

149. Morris N, Williamson R. Non-invasive first trimester antenatal diagnosis. *Br J Obstet Gynaecol* 1992;99:446–8

150. Adinolfi M, Davies A, Sharif S, *et al*. Detection of trisomy 18 and Y-derived sequence in fetal nucleated cells obtained by transcervical flushing. *Lancet* 1993;342:403–4

151. Rodeck C, Tutschek B, Serlock J, *et al*. Methods for the transcervical collection of fetal cells during the first trimester of pregnancy. *Prenat Diagn* 1995;15:933–42

152. Bahado-Singh RO, Kliman H, Feng TY, *et al*. First trimester endocervical irrigation: feasibility of obtaining trophoblast cells for prenatal diagnosis. *Obstet Gynecol* 1995;85:461–4

153. Adinolfi M, Sherlock J, Kemp T, *et al*. Prenatal detection of fetal Rh DNA sequences in transcervical samples. *Lancet* 1995;345:318–9

154. National Institute of Child Health and Human Development, National Registry for Amniocentesis Study Group. Mid-trimester amniocentesis for prenatal diagnosis: safety and accuracy. *J Am Med Assoc* 1976;236:1471–6

155. Tabor A, Philip J, Madsen M, *et al*. Randomised controlled trial of genetic amniocentesis in 4606 low-risk women. *Lancet* 1986;1:1287–93

156. Stranc LC, Evans JA, Hamerton JL. Chorionic villus sampling and amniocentesis for prenatal diagnosis. *Lancet* 1997;349:711–4

157. Petrikovsky BM, Kaplan GP. Fetal responses to inadvertent contact with the needle during amniocentesis. *Fetal Diagn Ther* 1995;10:83–5

158. Eller KM, Kuller JA. Porencephaly secondary to fetal trauma during amniocentesis. *Obstet Gynecol* 1995;85:865–7

159. Hershey DW. Ocular injury from amniocentesis. *Ophthalmology* 1993;100:1601–2

160. Anandakumar C, Wong YC, Annapoorna V, *et al*. Amniocentesis and its complications. *Austr NZ J Obstet Gynaecol* 1992;32:97–9

161. Medical Research Council of Canada. Diagnosis of genetic disease by amniocentesis during the

secondtrimester of pregnancy. *Med Res Council Can Report No. 5, Ottawa*

162. Working Party on Amniocentesis. An assessment of the hazards of amniocentesis. *Br J Obstet Gynaecol* 1978;85(Suppl. 2):1–4

163. Hislop A, Fairweather DVI. Amniocentesis and lung growth. An animal experiment with clinical implications. *Lancet* 1982;2:1271–2

164. Milner AD, Hoskyns EW, Hopkin IE. The effects of mid-trimester amniocentesis on lung function in the neonatal period. *Eur J Pediatr* 1992;151:458–60

165. Baird PA, Yee IM, Sadovnick AD. Population-based study of long-term outcomes after amniocentesis. *Lancet* 1994;344:1134–6 [erratum in Lancet 1994;344:1582]

166. Bui T-H, Iselius L, Lindsten J. European collaborative on prenatal diagnosis: mosaicism, pseudomosaicism and single abnormal cells in amniotic fluid cell cultures. *Prenat Diagn* 1984; 4:145–62

167. Canadian Collaborative CVS-Amniocentesis Clinical Trial Group. Multicenter randomized clinical trial of chorion villus sampling and amniocentesis. First report. *Lancet* 1989;1:1–7

168. Lippman A, Tomkins DT, Shine J, *et al.* Canadian multicentre randomised clinical trial of chorion villus sampling and amniocentesis: final report. *Prenat Diagn* 1992;12:385–467

169. Rhoades GG, Jackson LG, Schlesselman SE, *et al.* The safety and efficacy of chorionic villus sampling for early pregnancy diagnosis of cytogenetic abnormalities. *N Engl J Med* 1989;320:609–63

170. Medical Research Council Working Party on the Evaluation of Chorion Villus Sampling. Medical Research Council European trial of chorion villus sampling. *Lancet* 1991;337:1491–9

171. Kuliev A, Jackson L, Froster U, *et al.* Chorionic villus safety. *Am J Obstet Gynecol* 1996;174:807–11

172. Brambati B, Terzian E, Tognoni G. Randomized clinical trial of transabdominal versus transcervical chorionic villus sampling methods. *Prenat Diagn* 1991;11:285–93

173. Jackson LG, Zachary JM, Fowler SE, *et al.* A randomized comparison of transcervical and transabdominal chorionic-villus sampling. *N Engl J Med* 1992;327:594–8

174. Ledbetter DH, Zachary JM, Simpson JL, *et al.* Cytogenetic results from the U.S. Collaborative Study on CVS. *Prenat Diagn* 1992;12:317–45

175. Smidt-Jensen S, Permin M, Philip J, *et al.* Randomized comparison of amniocentesis and transabdominal and transcervical chorionic villus sampling. *Lancet* 1992;340:1237–44

176. Kalousek DK, Howard-Peebles PN, Olsen SB, *et al.* Confirmation of CVS mosaicism in term placentae and high frequency of intrauterine growth retardation associated with confined placental mosaicism. *Prenat Diagn* 1991;11:743–50

177. Kalousek DK, Langlois S, Barrett I, *et al.* Uniparental disomy for chromosome 16 in humans. *Am J Hum Genet* 1993;52:8–16

178. Henderson KG, Shaw TE, Barrett IJ, *et al.* Distribution of mosaicism in human placentae. *Hum Genet* 1996;97:650–4

179. Donnenfeld AE, Librizzi RJ, Dunn LK, *et al.* Chorionic villus sampling followed by amniocentesis in the same pregnancy. *Am J Med Genet* 1993; 45:361–4

180. Ledbetter DH, Engel E. Uniparental disomy in humans: development of an imprinting map and its implications for prenatal diagnosis. *Hum Mol Genet* 1995;4:1757–64

181. Wang BT, Peng W, Cheng KT, *et al.* Chorionic villi sampling: laboratory experience with 4 000 consecutive cases. *Am J Med Genet* 1994;53:307–16

182. Firth HV, Boyd PA, Chamberlain P, *et al.* Severe limb abnormalities after chorion villus sampling at 56–66 days' gestation. *Lancet* 1991;337:762–3

183. Brambati B, Simoni G, Travi M, *et al.* Genetic diagnosis by chorionic villus sampling before 8 gestational weeks: efficiency, reliability, and risks on 317 completed pregnancies. *Prenat Diagn* 1992; 12:789–99

184. Schloo R, Miny O, Holzgreve W, *et al.* Distal limb deficiency following chorionic villus sampling? *Am J Med Genet* 1992;44:404–13

185. Hsieh FH, Shyu MK, Sheu BC, *et al.* Limb defects after chorionic villus sampling. *Obstet Gynecol* 1995; 85:84–88

186. Froster-Iskenius UG, Baird P. Limb reduction defects in over one million consecutive livebirths. *Teratology* 1989;39:127–35

187. Mastroiacovo P, Botto LD, Cavalcanti PD, *et al.* Limb anomalies following chorion villus sampling: a registry based case–control study. *Am J Med Genet* 1992;44:856–64

188. Olney RS, Khoury MJ, Botto LD, *et al.* Limb defects and gestational age at chorionic villus sampling. *Lancet* 1994;344:476

189. Firth HV, Boyd PA, Chamberlain PF, *et al.* Analysis of limb reduction defects in babies exposed to chorionic villus sampling. *Lancet* 1994;343:1069–71

190. Holmes LB. Report of National Institute of Child Health and Human Development Workshop on chorionic villus sampling and limb and other defects, Oct. 20, 1992. *Teratology* 1993;48:7–13

191. Froster UG, Jackson L. Limb defects and chorionic villus sampling: results from an international registry 1992–94. *Lancet* 1996;346:484–5

192. Cutillo DM, Hammond EA, Reeser SL, *et al.* Chorionic villus sampling utilization following reports of a possible association with fetal limb defects. *Prenat Diagn* 1994;14:327–32

193. Nicolaides K, de Lourdes Brizot M, Patel F, *et al.* Comparison of chorionic villus sampling and early

amniocentesis for karyotyping in 1492 singleton pregnancies. *Fetal Diagn Ther* 1996;11:9–15

194. Johnson J, Wilson RD, Winsor E, *et al.* The early amniocentesis study: a randomized clinical trial of early amniocentesis versus midtrimester amniocentesis. *Fetal Diagn Ther* 1996;11:85–93

195. Thompson PJ, Greenough A, Nicolaides KH. Lung function following first trimester amniocentesis or chorion villus sampling. *Fetal Diagn Ther* 1991;6:148–52

196. Greenough A. Congenital abnormalities and antenatal invasive procedures. *Bio Neonate* 1996;70:148–52

197. Yuksel B, Greenough A, Naik S, *et al.* Perinatal lung function and invasive antenatal procedures. *Thorax* 1997;52:181–4

198. Greenough A, Yuksel B, Naik S, *et al.* Lung volume abnormalities in young children and invasive first trimester procedures. *Eur Resp J* 1996;9:466–7

199. Greenough A, Nicolaides KH. Chorionic villus sampling and early amniocentesis for prenatal diagnosis. *Lancet* 1997;349:1395–6

200. Kerber S, Held KR. Early genetic amniocentesis – 4 years' experience. *Prenat Diagn* 1993;13:21–7

201. Ghidini A, Lynch L, Hicks C, *et al.* The risk of second-trimester amniocentesis in twin gestations: a case–control study. *Am J Obstet Gynecol* 1993;169:1013–6.

202. Wapner RJ, Johnson A, Davis G, *et al.* Prenatal diagnosis in twin gestations: a comparison between second-trimester amniocentesis and first-trimester chorionic villus sampling. *Obstet Gynecol* 1993;82:49–56

203. Berkowitz RL, Lynch L, Stone J, *et al.* The current status of multifetal pregnancy reduction. *Am J Obstet Gynecol* 1996;174:1265–72

204. McFadyen I. The dangers of intra-amniotic methylene blue. *Br J Obstet Gynaecol* 1992;99:89–90

205. van der Pol JG, Wolf H, Boer K, *et al.* Jejunal atresia related to the use of methylene blue in genetic amniocentesis in twins. *Br J Obstet Gynaecol* 1992;99:141–3

206. Ghidini A, Sepulveda W, Lockwood CJ, *et al.* Complications of fetal blood sampling. *Am J Obstet Gynecol* 1993;168:1339–44

207. Duchatel F, Oury JF, Mennesson B, *et al.* Complications of diagnostic ultrasound-guided percutaneous umbilical blood sampling: analysis of a series of 341 cases and review of the literature. *Eur J Obstet Gynecol Reprod Biol* 1993;52:95–104

208. Maxwell DJ, Johnson P, Hurley P, *et al.* Fetal blood sampling and pregnancy loss in relation to indications. *Br J Obstet Gynaecol* 1991;98:892–7

209. Westgren M, Stangenberg M, Lingman G. Cordocentesis. *Gynecol Obstet Inv* 1995;40:227–30

210. Wilson RD, Farquharson DF, Wittmann BK, *et al.* Cordocentesis: overall pregnancy loss rate as important as procedure loss rate. *Fetal Diagn Ther* 1994;9:142–8

211. Capponi A, Rizzo G, Rinaldo D, *et al.* Cardiac flow after fetal blood sampling in normally grown and growth-retarded fetuses. *Prenat Diagn* 1995;15:1007–16

212. Arnold ML, Anton-Lambrecht I. Problems in prenatal diagnosis of the ichthyosis congenita group. *Hum Genet* 1985;71:301–11

213. Boss JA. First trimester prenatal diagnosis: earlier is not necessarily better. *J Med Ethics* 1994;20:146–51

214. Burke BM, Kolker A. Clients undergoing chorionic villus sampling versus amniocentesis: contrasting attitudes toward pregnancy. *Health Care Women Int* 1993;14:193–200

215. Halliday J, Lumley J, Watson L. Comparison of women who do and do not have amniocentesis or chorionic villus sampling. *Lancet* 1995;345:704–9

216. Harrison MR. Fetal surgery. *Am J Obstet Gynecol* 1995;174:1255–64

217. Benshushan A, Lewin A, Schenker JG. Multifetal pregnancy reduction: is it always justified? *Fetal Diagn Ther* 1993;8:214–20

218. Rådestad A, Bui T-H, Nygren KG, *et al.* The utilisation rate and pregnancy outcome of multifetal pregnancy reduction in the Nordic countries. *Acta Obstet Gynecol Scand* 1996;75:651–3

219. Evans MI, Dommergues M, Johnson MP, *et al.* Multifetal pregnancy reduction and selective termination. *Curr Opin Obstet Gynecol* 1995;7:126–9

220. Lopriore E, Vandenbussche FPHA, Tiersma ES, *et al.* Twin-to-twin transfusion syndrome: new perspectives. *J Pediatr* 1995;127:675–80

221. Elliott JP, Sawyer AT, Radin TG, *et al.* Large-volume therapeutic amniocentesis in the treatment of hydramnios. *Obstet Gynecol* 1994;84:1025–7

222. Moise KJ. Polyhydramnios: problems and treatment. *Semin Perinatol* 1993;17:197–209

223. Berry DL, Montgomery L, Johnson A, *et al.* Amniotic septostomy for the treatment of the stuck twin sequence. *Am J Obstet Gynecol* 1997;176:519

224. Fisk NM, Ronderos-Dumit D, Soliani A, *et al.* Diagnostic and therapeutic transabdominal amnio-infusion in oligohydramnios. *Obstet Gynecol* 1991;78:270–8

225. Skupski DW, Wolf CFW, Bussel JB. Fetal transfusion therapy. *Obstet Gynecol Surv* 1996;51:181–92

226. Combleholme TM. Invasive fetal therapy: current status and future directions. *Semin Perinatol* 1994;18:385–97

227. Thompson PJ, Greenough A, Nicolaides KH. Respiratory function in infancy following pleuro-amniotic shunting. *Fetal Diagn Ther* 1993;8:79–83

228. Estes JM, Harrison MR. Fetal obstructive uropathy. *Semin Pediatr Surg* 1993;2:129–35

229. Quintero RA, Romero R, Reich H, *et al.* In utero percutaneous umbilical cord ligation in the

management of complicated monochorionic multiple gestations. *Ultrasound Obstet Gynecol* 1996; 8:16–22

230. De Lia JE. Surgery of the placenta and umbilical cord. *Clin Obstet Gynecol* 1996;39:607–25

231. Deprest JA, Evrard VA, Van Ballaer PP, *et al.* Fetoscopic cord ligation. *Eur J Obstet Gynecol Reprod Biol* 1997;in press

232. Ville Y, Hecher K, Gagnon A, *et al.* Endoscopic lazer coagulation in the management of severe twin transfusion system. *Br J Obstet Gynaecol* 1998; in press

233. MacMahon RA, Renou PMM, Shekelton PA, *et al. In utero* cystostomy. *Lancet* 1992;340:234

234. Quintero RA, Reich H, Romero R, *et al. In utero* endoscopic devascularization of a large chorioangioma. *Ultrasound Obstet Gynecol* 1996;8:48–52

235. Hecher K, Hackelöer BJ. Intra-uterine endoscopic lasersurgery for fetal sacrococcygeal teratoma. *Lancet* 1996;347:470

236. Wengler GS, Lanfranchi A, Frusca T, *et al. In utero* transplantation of parental CD34 haematopoietic progenitor cells in a patient with X-linked severe combined immunodeficiency (SCIDXI). *Lancet* 1996;348:1484–7

237. Sundberg K, Bang J, Smidt-Jensen S, *et al.* Randomised study of risk of fetal loss related to early amniocentesis versus chorionic villus sampling. *Lancet* 1997;350:697–703

238. The Canadian Early and Mid-Trimester Amniocentesis Trial (CEMAT) Group. Randomised trial to assess safety and fetal outcome of early and midtrimester amniocentesis. *Lancet* 1998;351: 242–7

Ultrasonographic screening for fetal chromosomal abnormalities in the first and second trimester of pregnancy

18

The-Hung Bui, Roderick F. Hume Jr, Kypros H. Nicolaides and Richard Jaffe

Down's syndrome accounts for about one-third of the cases of severe mental retardation and is the most common pattern of malformations in man[1–3]. It is associated with trisomy of all or part of the long arm of chromosome 21.

There are presently two main approaches to prenatal diagnosis of Down's syndrome. In the first and most commonly practiced approach, women of advanced reproductive age have been offered amniocentesis or chorionic villus sampling (CVS) because the risk for a chromosomally abnormal child, principally Down's syndrome, increases with advanced maternal age[4,5]. These diagnostic investigations for fetal chromosome abnormalities are usually made available to pregnant women 35 years of age or older because at this age the risk for miscarriage associated with the procedures equals or is lower than the risk for aneuploidy[6]. Additionally, a small number of pregnant women also identified as having an increased risk of carrying a fetus with a chromosomal defect due to a previous child with Down's syndrome or other aneuploidy, or a family history of chromosome rearrangement, will be offered the option of amniocentesis or CVS. If all the presumptive mothers over 35 years of age took part in testing by amniocentesis or CVS, at the very most 20–30% of cases with trisomy 21 could be detected[2,3,7–9]. In practice, the number of women of advanced reproductive age who choose to take part in this type of screening program differs considerably in different areas, ranging from 10% to 88%[9–12]. Hence, at best, about 20–25% of cases with Down's syndrome are detected antenatally with this strategy[7–12].

Until recently, there have not been any appropriate means to detect the majority of pregnancies carrying a fetus with trisomy 21. If genetic amniocentesis or CVS were performed on all pregnancies, the risk of miscarriage due to the procedure would be much higher than the probability of an abnormal result, and the costs, both emotional and economical, to detect each affected fetus would therefore be prohibitive. The only possible way to identify the majority of women at risk of having a child with Down's syndrome is by simple, safe mass-screening methods during pregnancy. Thus, in the other and more recently introduced approach to prenatal diagnosis of Down's syndrome, all pregnant women are given the option of a screening test based on the measurement of maternal serum markers or fetal ultrasonographic examination in the first or second trimester of pregnancy. Amniocentesis or CVS, depending on gestational age, is then offered to women with a positive result of the screening test.

Maternal serum screening for Down's syndrome originated with the singular observation of a maternal serum α-fetoprotein level (MSAFP) below the limit of sensitivity in a case of Edward's syndrome (trisomy 18). It was found subsequently that a low MSAFP indicated an increased risk of a chromosome abnormality in the fetus[13]. In about 30% of the pregnancies with trisomy 21, MSAFP was less than 0.5 of the median value. This was not, however, a sufficient increase in detection rate to allow starting maternal serum screening in places where MSAFP screening for neural tube defects was not already performed. However, in 1988 a more effective method was introduced combining three maternal serum markers (AFP, human chorionic gonadotropin (hCG) and unconjugated estriol; 'triple test' or 'triple marker screening') and maternal age to define high-risk pregnancies for further examinations[14]. The calculations showed that about 60% of pregnancies with trisomy 21 could be detected even if the risk pregnancies identified comprised <5% of all pregnant women. This prediction has been subsequently confirmed in prospective studies from numerous centers[15–26].

Routine biochemical screening for Down's syndrome in the second trimester is now widespread. However, because maternal age is a significant risk factor for Down's syndrome, the detection rate by serum screening increases with increasing age. Thus, younger mothers have a higher chance of ending up in the group of low-risk pregnancies even if the fetus has Down's syndrome[15,17]. This has stimulated the search for additional biochemical markers which would bring the detection efficiency to a more practical and useful level[21,24,27-29]. Screening by serum markers and age instead of mere age would lead to a very small increase of births with trisomy 21 to women of advanced reproductive age, if any at all depending on the cut-off levels chosen[26]. However, in many places, these women already have access to a CVS at about 10 weeks of gestation or an early amniocentesis before 15 weeks. They might not accept waiting for the results of the serum screening up to the 17th week and the subsequent late results of the fetal chromosome analysis. Thus, first trimester biochemical or sonographic markers, hopefully also more specific than the present ones, are being searched for[30-44]. If they prove useful, many older mothers may opt for a screening test, and thus often avoid amniocentesis or chorionic villus biopsy, both of which carry a small risk of miscarriage[6].

Several ultrasound markers of Down's syndrome and other chromosomal defects have been reported[45]. The recognition of ultrasonographic signs of fetal aneuploidy provides a potential powerful tool for screening low-risk pregnancies for chromosome disorders because, in many places, the majority of pregnant women undergo ultrasound examination during pregnancy. Moreover, ultrasound has the potential advantage over biochemical markers of providing an immediate result with the possibility to proceed directly to prenatal diagnosis.

The focus of this chapter will be on the current knowledge of sonographic fetometry and specific patterns of malformations or abnormalities associated with the more common chromosomal defects, in particular trisomy 21, as it applies to antenatal ultrasound screening in the low-risk population.

SCREENING FOR CHROMOSOME DEFECTS IN THE SECOND TRIMESTER

A wide range of fetal malformations has been prenatally diagnosed by ultrasound[46]. In many countries ultrasound scanning of the fetus, most often in the mid-trimester, is either an integral part of fetal monitoring during pregnancy[47-50], or is performed for different indications in a majority of pregnancies. This widespread use of ultrasound has increased the awareness of sonographic markers associated with various chromosomal anomalies[45]. However, there is still much controversy over the value of routine ultrasound screening for fetal abnormalities. It has been difficult to assess the accuracy of this screening due to differences in the severity of the malformations, quality of the machines used, characteristics of the investigated population, and expertise of the sonographers in the different studies[47-53]. Other limitations include fetal position, gestational age at which the examination is performed, amount of amniotic fluid, and maternal habitus. Additionally, quality of postnatal ascertainment of abnormalities also accounts for part of the discrepancies in the studies reported[50]. The accuracy of malformation screening tends to be lower in low-risk populations, where sensitivity ranging from 14–85% (average about 51%) and specificity from 98% to more than 99% have been reported, whereas it tends to be higher in high-risk populations where sensitivities ranged from 27–99% (average about 80%) with specificities of 91–100%[46-53]. These results are not surprising because targeted studies are usually performed at referral centers and factors influencing sensitivity and specificity of ultrasonography include the prevalence of an anomaly in the population under investigation. However, it is clear that given good training in ultrasound and scanning performed at 18–20 weeks of gestation, a significant proportion of lethal (Figure 1) or severe abnormalities as well as many less serious defects (Figure 2) can be detected by routine scan in low-risk pregnancies[46-53].

Screening for fetal chromosomal abnormalities by major structural defects

The more frequent chromosomal disorders include trisomy 13 (Patau's syndrome), trisomy 18 (Edwards' syndrome), trisomy 21 (Down's syndrome), monosomy X (Turner's syndrome) and triploidy.

In the first trimester of pregnancy, the best documented ultrasonographic sign of many chromosomal abnormalities is increased nuchal translucency thickness[31] (Figure 3). In the later trimesters, a better definition of fetal anatomy by

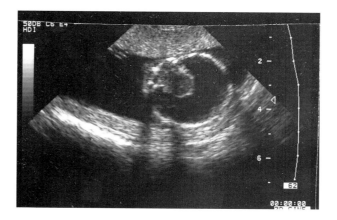

Figure 1　Holoprosencephaly in fetus with trisomy 13

ultrasound allows recognition of patterns of malformations giving important clues to the suspicion of specific chromosomal defects[45]. With few exceptions, consideration should be given to obtaining fetal cells for cytogenetic analysis when structural abnormalities are detected by prenatal

ultrasound, particularly when those anomalies are known to be associated with aneuploidy[45] (Table 1; Figure 1). The likelihood of a chromosome aberration in the fetus will depend not only on the total number of abnormalities identified, but also on the type of structural defects[54,55] (Table 2). The incidence of chromosomal abnormalities increases from 2% in fetuses with only one abnormality or growth retardation to 92% with eight or more abnormalities[55]. In some cases including cystic hygroma (Figure 4), nuchal edema (Figure 5), heart defects, duodenal atresia (Figure 6), and omphalocele (Figure 7) the frequency of chromosomal defects is high even for apparently isolated abnormalities[45] (Table 2). Although ultrasound studies have established that fetuses with multiple structural defects have a high incidence of aneuploidy (see review[45]), sonographic detection of major structural abnormalities in the second trimester appears to be a relatively insensitive tool to screen for fetal chromosome aberrations in the low-risk population. Whereas retrospective studies

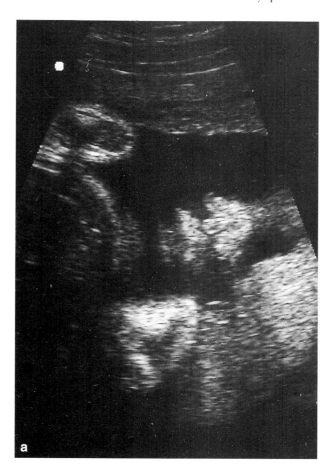

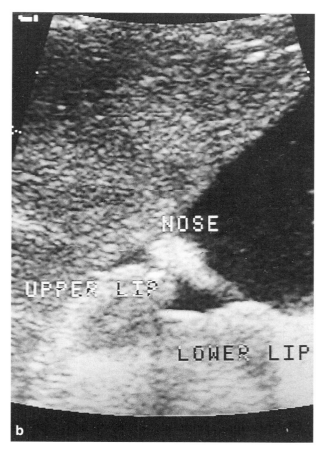

Figure 2　(**a**) Normal face, upper lip and nose in contrast to (**b**) cleft lip, nose, right upper lip and lower lip

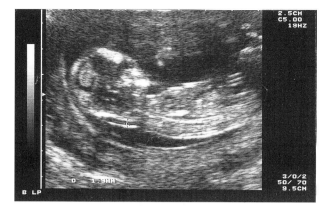

Figure 3 Ultrasonographic picture of a fetus at 12 weeks gestation with nuchal translucency thickness of 1.9 mm

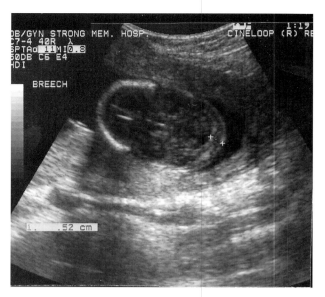

Figure 5 Increased nuchal thickness in fetus with trisomy 21

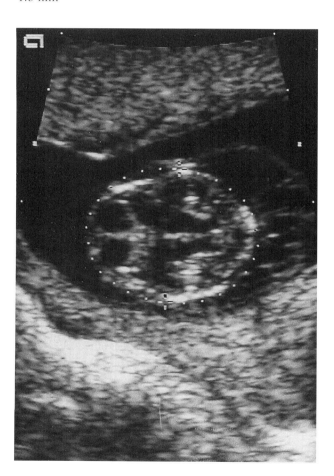

Figure 4 Large cystic hygroma and hypotelorism in fetus with monosomy X

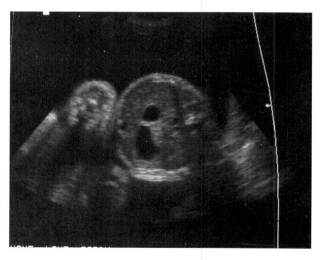

Figure 6 Double bubble indicating small bowel obstruction

from referral centers have shown that most fetuses with trisomy 13 and 18 have major abnormalities detectable by ultrasound, only 33–44% of fetuses with Down's syndrome could be identified through

sonographic detection of structural defects in selected populations[56–59]. In the three studies of routine ultrasound where detection of chromosomal abnormalities was reported, overall about 25% (12 out of 49) fetuses with an abnormal karyotype were detected following the identification of a sonographic abnormality[60–62]. The detection rate was only 16.7% for Down's syndrome in these studies. However, there were indications of improved detection rate with increased screening experience[47,58]. The qualitative nature of structural abnormalities presents a particular problem since

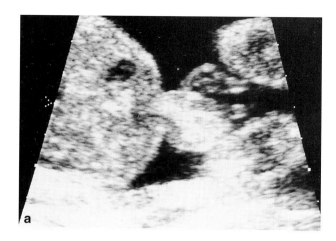 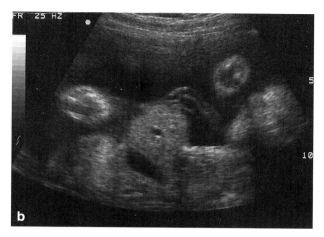

Figure 7 (a) Small omphalocele in fetus with trisomy 13. (b) Large omphalocele in otherwise normal fetus

Table 1 Pattern of abnormalities in common chromosomal defects

Trisomy 21	Brachycephaly, mild ventriculomegaly, flattened face
	Nuchal edema
	Atrioventricular septal defects
	Duodenal atresia with or without hydramnios, echogenic bowel
	Mild hydronephrosis (pyelectasis)
	Limb shortenings, sandal gap
	Clinodactyly or mid-phalanx hypoplasia of fifth finger
Trisomy 18	Brachycephaly (strawberry-shaped head), large choroid plexus cysts
	Corpus callosum agenesis, enlarged cisterna magna
	Facial cleft, micrognathia
	Nuchal edema
	Heart defects
	Diaphragmatic hernia, esophagus atresia, omphalocele
	Renal defects
	Myelomeningocele
	Growth retardation
	Limb shortenings, radial defects, clenched hands
	Talipes, rocker-bottom feet
	Polyhydramnios
Trisomy 13	Holoprosencephaly, associated midline facial defects and cleft
	Microcephaly
	Heart defects
	Omphalocele
	Renal defects, polycystic kidneys
	Postaxial polydactyly, overlapping fingers
	Growth retardation, polyhydramnios
45,X (Turner)	Large nuchal cystic hygroma
lethal type	Generalized edema, pleural effusions, ascites
	Cardiac anomalies
	Mild hydronephrosis (horseshoe kidney?)
Triploidy	Mild ventriculomegaly, micrognathia
	Cardiac defects, myelomeningocele
	Syndactyly, 'hitch-hiker' toe deformity
type 1	Molar placenta, paternally derived extra haploid set of chromosomes
	Fetal death generally before 20 weeks, symmetric growth retardation
type 2	Small placenta, maternally derived extra haploid set of chromosomes
	Early asymmetrical growth retardation, may survive into third trimester

Table 2   Chromosomal defects in fetal abnormalities. Summary of several reports providing data of gestational age at diagnosis and the prevalence of chromosomal defects when the malformation is isolated and when additional abnormalities are present[45]

Malformation	Number	Gestational age (weeks)	Isolated (%)	Multiple (%)
Cerebral ventriculomegaly	690	13–43	2	17
Holoprosencephaly	132	14–38	4	39
Choroid plexus cysts	1806	14–38	1	46
Cranial posterior fossa cyst	101	14–38	0	52
Cleft lip and/or palate	118	15–40	0	51
Micrognathia	65	17–37	–	62
Nuchal cystic hygroma	276	15–38	52	71
Nuchal edema	371	14–38	19	45
Diaphragmatic hernia	173	14–41	2	34
Heart defects	829	?	16	66
Duodenal atresia	44	20–36	38	64
Hyperechogenic bowel	196	13–26	7	42
Omphalocele	475	11–41	13	46
Urinary tract abnormalities	1825	?	3	24
Talipes	127	?	0	33
Small for gestational age	621	?	4	38

the majority of reported studies involved selected populations prior to prenatal diagnosis for mostly advanced maternal age, and the results cannot therefore be transferred to a routine setting.

Minor morphological markers and fetal chromosomal defects

More subtle dysmorphologic and fetometric markers have been used in an attempt to improve the detection rate of Down's syndrome (Table 1). Some of these, such as choroid plexus cysts (Figure 8), pyelectasis (hydronephrosis; Figure 9), nuchal edema (increased nuchal fold thickness; Figure 5) and cerebral ventriculomegaly (Figure 10), have potential for use in screening the low-risk population because they can be relatively easily visualized at the time of the routine scan in the second trimester[45]. Others including echogenic bowel[63] (Figure 11), fronto-thalamic distance[64], hypoplasia and/or clinodactyly of the middle phalanx of the fifth digit[65], presence of simian crease[66], sandal gap[45] (Figure 12) and other skeletal abnormalities (Figure 13) are less readily seen at routine ultrasound and are signs which should be sought in fetuses known to be at increased prior risk or where another sonographic abnormality has been found. One of the main problems with using these markers in the low-risk population is that the majority of studies select high-risk populations, and extrapolation of the associated chromosomal

risks to the low-risk population should be viewed with scepticism. A good example is the controversial significance of choroid plexus cysts which were first identified in 1984 when they were described as a benign transient finding[67]. Subsequently, investigators examined the association of choroid plexus cysts and trisomy 18. Early series seemed to indicate that the risk of trisomy 18 in the presence of choroid plexus cysts was of the order of 10%[68–70]. However, as other large series, including in particular unselected pregnancies, were reported the associated karyotypic abnormality had fallen to less than 1%[45,49,71–73]. A major flaw in most of the early studies was that other risk factors such as raised maternal age, abnormal maternal serum biochemistry or associated malformations were not taken into consideration[72,73].

Further evaluation of the efficacy of minor markers in the detection of chromosomal abnormalities in the low-risk population is needed and care should be taken before applying figures obtained from the high-risk population to the low-risk pregnancy.

Screening for chromosomal defects by increased nuchal skinfold thickness

As many as 80% of infants with Down's syndrome have redundant skin in the posterior neck, possibly due to a previous cystic hygroma[1,74]. Measurements of the nuchal fold are performed in

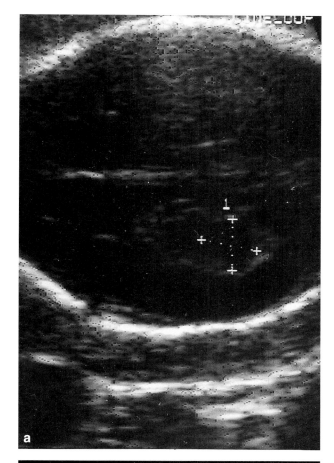

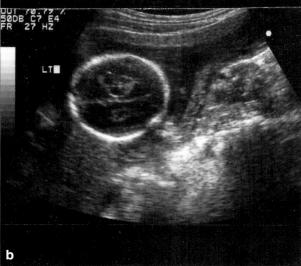

Figure 8 (**a**) and (**b**) Choroid plexus cysts in fetus with trisomy 18

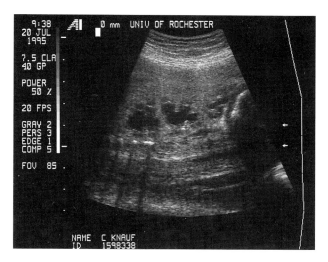

Figure 9 Renal pelvicalyectasis, longitudinal kidney view, in fetus with trisomy 21

the mid-trimester with electronic callipers from the outer skull lining to the outer skin surface using a transverse axial image directed in a suboccipital-

bregmatic plane and including as landmarks the cavum septi pellucidi, cerebral peduncles, cerebellar hemispheres and the cisterna magna (Figure 14). These measurements should be performed carefully, because improper angling can easily produce an incorrect wide value and a false positive result[75]. Abnormal accumulation of fluid behind the fetal neck detected in the second or third trimester can be classified as nuchal cystic hygroma or nuchal edema. In 1985, it was first suggested that nuchal skinfold measurement could be useful in detecting Down's syndrome[76,77]. This sign has been evaluated in a number of studies as a sonographic screening tool in the second trimester (see review[78]). Most series have been retrospectively analyzed with limited value in their conclusions[79]. As can be seen in Table 3, the detection rate varies also considerably in the different prospective series[56,58,80–86]. Although in most series a nuchal fold thickness of 6 mm or more was chosen for a positive test, a more suitable cut-off value may be 5 mm if ultrasound scan is performed in the early second trimester, i.e. between 13 and 18 weeks of gestation[86–88]. Nuchal fold thickness is the best single sonographic marker for the detection of trisomy 21 in the second trimester. However, wide differences in screening efficiency, low reproducibility in many places, costs of ultrasonographic examinations, and the availability of second-trimester biochemical maternal serum markers speak presently against universal screening for Down's syndrome in the second trimester using nuchal skinfold thickness.

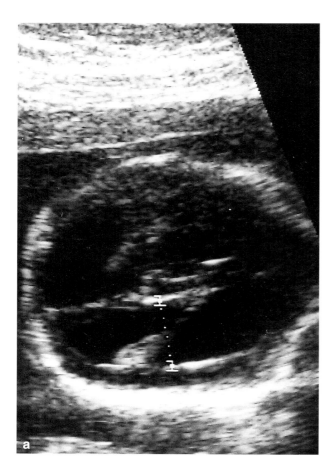
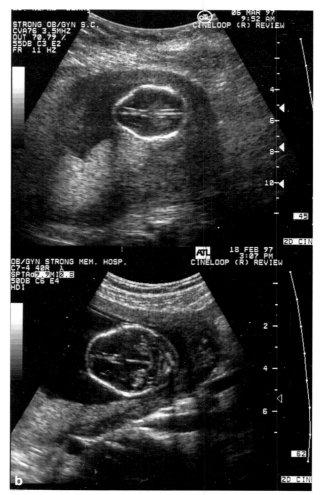

Figure 10 (a) Ventriculomegaly which resolved *in utero* in fetus with trisomy 21. (b) Demonstration of lemon sign (upper panel) and banana sign (lower panel) often seen with hydrocephaly

Fetal long bone measurements and chromosomal defects

Because infants with Down's syndrome have shorter long bones than other infants, the fetal femur length has been used as a sonographic marker for trisomy 21. It is readily obtained and routinely measured when ultrasound is performed after the first trimester. Several parameters have been proposed to identify shorter femur length (FL) including the biparietal diameter (BPD) to FL ratio[89], the ratio of actual to expected FL[56], or the ratio of FL to foot length[90]. A BPD/FL ratio of more than 1.5 SD above the mean, a measured FL/expected FL ratio of 0.91 or less, or a FL/foot length ratio of 0.9 or less have all been associated with Down's syndrome. The inclusion of foot length in a ratio to evaluate long bones does not

seem to improve the detection rate of Down's syndrome[91]. A BPD/FL ratio is gestation-dependent and will vary between studies. However, dividing the actual FL by the value expected for a fetus with the same BPD is independent of gestation. The positive predictive value of a measured FL/expected FL ratio of 0.91 or less has ranged from as high as 1 in 21 to as low as 1 in 644 in different series when applied to the low-risk population with a prevalence of Down's syndrome of 1 in 710. A sensitivity ranging from 12–71% and a false-positive rate from 2–15% have also been reported in different centers[56,90–94]. The explanation for such variations is unclear but may be due, in part, to different maternal age distributions of the populations examined. Thus, the efficiency of these measurements in screening for Down's syndrome is still controversial due to conflicting

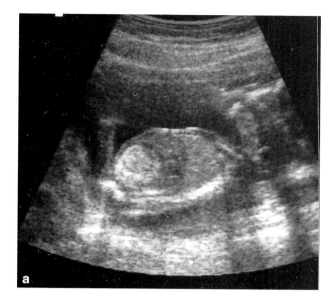

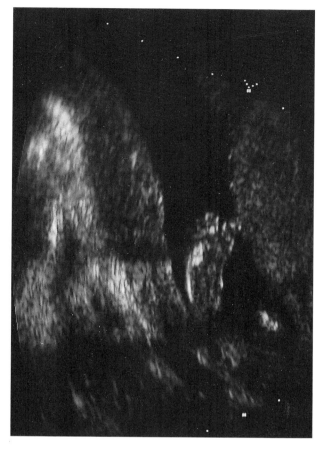

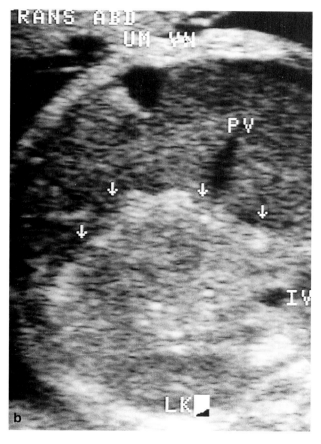

Figure 12 Plantar surface of foot illustrating the persistently widely spaced great toe, sandal foot, in fetus with trisomy 21

Figure 11 (**a**) Hyperechoic bowel, with iliac crest shown, in fetus with trisomy 21. (**b**) Hyperechoic bowel which progressed to meconium peritonitis in fetus found to be homozygous for the delta F 508 mutation cystic fibrosis

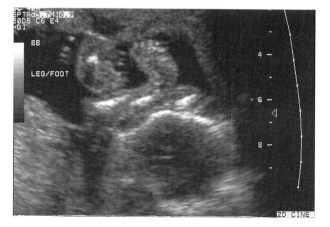

Figure 13 Ultrasonographic demonstration of club foot

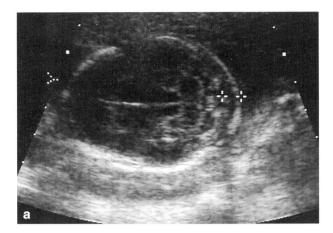

Figure 14 (a) Posterior nuchal thickening in view of cerebellar transverse diameter. (b) Longitudinal view of nuchal edema in fetus with trisomy 21

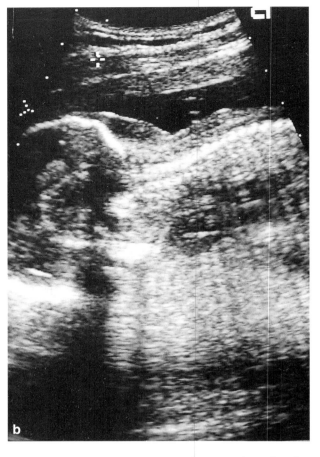

results. For markers whose values approximate a statistical frequency distribution it has been argued that it may be more reliable to use a model to estimate detection and false-positive rates, since most individual prospective evaluation of performance is unlikely to include but a few numbers of trisomy 21 so that the observed detection rate will be an unreliable predictor of the actual rate[95]. On this basis, fetal FL which appears to fit a Gaussian distribution frequency is a weak marker[96].

In a necropsy study it was found that, although short FL would identify about 16% of fetuses with Down's syndrome, the comparable humerus length (HL) measurement would have identified 30% of affected fetuses[97]. Subsequently, a number of studies have reported on the usefulness of this measurement in screening for Down's syndrome.

In most series, the HL shortening was found to be a more sensitive and specific marker than the FL shortening, with an associated 5.4 to 12.8-fold increased risk for Down's syndrome[94,98–100]. Combining the HL and FL resulted in an improved specificity[94,98–100]. However, large prospective studies in low-risk populations using this measurement alone or in combination with other markers are still lacking[78].

Table 3 Detection of Down's syndrome by means of increased fetal nuchal skinfold thickness measured in the second trimester in prospective series

Study	Sensitivity (%)	False positive (%)	PPV (%)
Benacerraf et al., 1987[56]	43 (12/28)	0.1 (4/3816)	75
Nyberg et al., 1990[58]	16 (4/25)	0.3 (1/350)	8*
Ginsberg et al., 1990[80]	41 (5/12)	0 (0/212)	100
Crane and Gray, 1991[81]	75 (12/16)	1.4 (47/3338)	8*
DeVore and Alfi, 1993[82]	20 (7/35)	0.5 (14/2742)	39†
Watson et al., 1994[83]	50 (7/14)	2.0 (27/1382)	21
Donnenfeld et al., 1994[84]	18 (1/13)	1.2 (16/1382)	6
GrandJean et al., 1995[85]	39 (17/44)	8.5 (273/3205)	2*
Borell et al., 1996[86] (≥ 6 mm)	33 (6/18)	0.1 (2/1424)	33*
Borell et al., 1996[86] (≥ 5 mm)	78 (14/18)	2.1 (30/1424)	5*

PPV: positive predictive value; *adjusted to prevalence of Down's syndrome in the general population; †for aneuploidy

Screening for chromosomal defects by combining multiple ultrasound markers

This strategy has been evaluated in a few limited series in high-risk populations[98–104]. It seems clear that the combination of several sonographic markers or biochemical and sonographic markers increases both the sensitivity and specificity of the screening test, thus providing the best approach in screening for Down's syndrome in the second trimester. It allows also the revision of prior risk for Down's syndrome based on maternal age. However, further evaluation of the efficacy of this strategy in the detection of chromosomal abnormalities in the low-risk population is needed and care should be taken before applying figures obtained from the high-risk population to the low-risk pregnancy.

FIRST-TRIMESTER ULTRASOUND SCREENING FOR CHROMOSOMAL DEFECTS

With improved technology, in particular the development of transvaginal probes, it has become possible to examine the fetal anatomy in more detail in the first trimester[105,106], but there are relatively few reports of such programs[107,108]. There are some reports on high-risk populations or specific abnormalities[109,110]. Whether or not it could be considered as an alternative to the second trimester scan is doubtful, in view of the relatively high false-negatives rates reported.

Screening for chromosomal defects by fetal nuchal translucency thickness

During the second and third trimester of pregnancy, abnormal accumulation of fluid behind the fetal neck has been classified as nuchal cystic hygroma or nuchal edema. In the first trimester, the term translucency has been used because it is the ultrasonographic feature observed[30]. Nuchal translucency thickness is obtained with the fetus scanned in a mid-sagittal section as for measurement of fetal crown–rump length; the maximum thickness of the subcutaneous translucency between the skin and the soft tissue over the cervical spine is measured[30]. Repeatability of measurements is of great importance when screening by ultrasound due to possible operator variability. This issue has been addressed in a prospective study including 200 pregnant women in which the variability for intra-observer was found to be 0.54 mm whereas it

was 0.62 mm for inter-observer[111]. Additionally, a large part of the observed variation in measurement could be accounted for by the placement of the callipers rather than the generation of the image. Thus, in practice, the mean of two good measurements rather than one is suggested.

Although the translucency will resolve during the second trimester in most cases, it may evolve into either nuchal edema or cystic hygroma with or without generalized hydrops in a few cases[111]. The underlying mechanisms for the increased nuchal translucency thickness associated with chromosomal defects in the first trimester are not yet well understood, although there is evidence that abnormalities of the heart and great arteries may be implicated[112–114]. Additionally, there is indirect evidence that increased nuchal translucency is an early manifestation of heart failure[115,116].

In the early 1990s, a possible association between increased fetal nuchal translucency thickness and chromosomal defects was reported in 18 small series involving altogether 1698 first-trimester high-risk pregnancies (see review[30]). However, the prevalence of chromosomal defects in these series differed widely, ranging from 19–88%. The variations in results obtained in these different studies may be explained by the definition of the minimal abnormal translucency thickness, ranging from 2 to 10 mm, and by the maternal age distributions of the populations studied which probably differed.

Screening using a combination of maternal age and fetal nuchal translucency thickness in high-risk pregnancies at 10–14 weeks of gestation was first introduced in the early 1990s[30,116–118]. In about 80% of trisomy 21, the nuchal translucency thickness was reported to be above the 95th centile of the normal range. Although similar results were obtained from four different centers[119–122], two studies could identify only 30%[123] and 20%[124], respectively, of the chromosomally aberrant fetuses using >3 mm as the lower cut-off limit for abnormal nuchal translucency thickness. A false-positive rate of 3.2% and 6.5% in the two respective studies were found.

All the early first-trimester screening studies involved a large proportion of high-risk pregnancies and the measurements were not reported in gestation-standardized terms. Thus, the false-positive rates with a nuchal translucency thickness of 3 mm or greater varied from 3.2% to 9.5%, and this may simply reflect gestational differences between centers. In determining whether a given nuchal translucency thickness is increased, it is essential to take gestational age into account since it has been shown in a large study encompassing more than 20 000 pregnancies that the fetal nuchal translucency thickness increases with crown–rump length[125]. The maternal age-adjusted risk for trisomy 21 according to nuchal translucency thickness is shown in Figure 15.

Screening by fetal nuchal translucency thickness in unselected populations

The results of nuchal translucency screening in unselected populations have been reported[125–128]. In one study involving 1704 women with singleton pregnancies[127], only one of three fetuses with trisomy 21 was detected using nuchal translucency thickness $\geq$ 3 mm. However, there were serious flaws in the application of this measurement: in 20% of the cases no measurement was performed, a further 18% of the cases were unsuccessfully measured, and the scans were carried out before 10 weeks of gestation in 28% of the 1127 cases where measurements were made. In the other studies, a majority of fetuses with chromosomal abnormalities could be detected. In the largest study, the screening results of 42 619 completed singleton pregnancies[30] showed that the sensitivity of the test for trisomy 21 was over 80%. Thus, combining maternal age with fetal nuchal translucency thickness at 10–14 weeks of gestation is currently the most sensitive method of screening for chromosomal abnormalities. Additional independent markers may improve the detection rate of trisomy 21 by combining them with maternal age and fetal nuchal translucency thickness. These include fetal heart rate[129], maternal serum free β-hCG, and pregnancy-associated plasma protein A (PAPP-A)[32–42]. It has been estimated that the incorporation of either the fetal heart rate or maternal serum PAPP-A or free β-hCG concentrations into screening using maternal age and fetal nuchal translucency thickness at 10–14

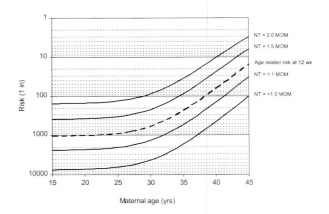

Figure 15 Semilogarithmic graph illustrating estimated risks for fetal trisomies 21 at 12 weeks of gestation on the basis of maternal age alone and maternal age with fetal nuchal translucency thickness expressed as multiples of the appropriate median for crown–rump length (MOM)

weeks of gestation could improve the screening performance for trisomy 21 by about 5%[130,131]. However, more studies are needed to evaluate the cost–benefit of adding more markers to screening by nuchal translucency only.

CONCLUSIONS

Although current common practice is to screen for Down's syndrome in the second trimester, either by maternal age, biochemical maternal serum markers or ultrasonographic examination, a move to earlier screening is anticipated. Presently the combination of maternal age and measurement of fetal nuchal translucency thickness at 10–14 weeks has been shown to have the best test performance in screening for chromosomal abnormalities, with a detection rate for trisomy 21 in excess of 80%. It is possible that better results can be achieved in the future by combined policies with biochemical maternal serum markers.

References

1. Jones KL (ed). Down syndrome. *Smith's Recognizable Patterns of Human Malformation*, 4th edn. Philadelphia: WB Saunders, 1988:10–15

2. Ferguson-Smith MA. Prenatal chromosome analysis and its impact on the birth incidence of chromosome disorders. *Br Med Bull* 1983;39:355–64

3. Cornel MC, Breed ASPM, Beekhuis JR, et al. Down syndrome: effects of demographic factors and prenatal diagnosis on the future of livebirth prevalence. Hum Genet 1993;92:163–8

4. Penrose LS. The relative effects of prenatal and maternal age in mongolism. J Genet 1933;27:219–24

5. Hook EB, Cross PK, Regal RR. The frequency of 47, +21, 47,+18 and 47,+13 at the uppermost extremes of maternal ages: results on 56,094 fetuses studied prenatally and comparisons with data on livebirths. Hum Genet 1984;68:211–20

6. Nicolini U. Invasive techniques of prenatal diagnosis. Curr Obstet Gynaecol 1992;2:77–84

7. Huether CA. Projection of Down syndrome births in the United States 1979–2000 and the potential effects of prenatal diagnosis. Am J Pub Health 1983; 73:1186–9

8. Källén B, Knudsen LB. Effect of maternal age distribution and prenatal diagnosis on the population rates of Down syndrome – a comparative study of 19 populations. Hereditas 1989;110:55–60

9. Olsen CL, Cross PK, Gensburg LJ, et al. The effect of prenatal diagnosis, population ageing, and changing fertility rates on the live birth prevalence of Down syndrome in New York State, 1983–1992. Prenat Diagn 1996;16:991–1002

10. Mikkelsen M. The impact of prenatal diagnosis on the incidence of Down syndrome in Denmark. Birth Defects Orig Art Ser 1992;28:44–51

11. Cornel MC. Variation in prenatal cytogenetic diagnosis: policies in 13 European countries, 1989–1991. EUROCAT Working Group. European Registration of Congenital Anomalies. Prenat Diagn 1994;14:337–44

12. Bui T-H, Kristoffersson U. Prenatal diagnosis in Sweden: organisation and current issues. Eur J Hum Genet 1997;5(Suppl. 1):70–6

13. Merkatz IR, Nitowsky HM, Macri JN, et al. An association between low maternal serum α-fetoprotein and fetal chromosomal abnormalities. Am J Obstet Gynecol 1984;148:886–94

14. Wald NJ, Cuckle HS, Densem JW, et al. Maternal serum screening for Down's syndrome in early pregnancy. Br Med J 1988;297:883–7

15. Haddow JE, Polamaki GE, Knight GJ, et al. Prenatal screening for Down's syndrome with use of maternal serum markers. N Engl J Med 1992;327:588–93

16. Philipps OP, Elias P, Shulman LP, et al. Maternal serum screening for fetal Down's syndrome in women less than 35 years of age using alpha-fetoprotein, hCG and unconjugated estriol: a prospective 2-year study. Obstet Gynecol 1992;80:353–8

17. Wald NJ, Kennard A, Densem JW, et al. Antenatal maternal serum screening for Down's syndrome: results of a demonstration project. Br Med J 1992; 305:391–4

18. Burton BK, Prins GS, Verp MS. A prospective trial of prenatal screening for Down syndrome by means of maternal serum α-fetoprotein, human chorionic gonadotropin, and unconjugated estriol. Am J Obstet Gynecol 1993;169:526–30

19. Cheng EY, Luthy DA, Zebelman AM, et al. A prospective evaluation of a second-trimester screening test for fetal Down syndrome using maternal serum alpha-fetoprotein, hCG, and unconjugated estriol. Obstet Gynecol 1993;81:72–7

20. Dawson AJ, Jones G, Matharu MS, et al. Serum screening for Down's syndrome. Br J Obstet Gynaecol 1993;100:875–7

21. Spencer K, Carpenter P. Prospective study of prenatal screening for Down's syndrome with free β-human chorionic gonadotropin. Br Med J 1993; 307:764–9

22. Wenstrom KD, Williamson RA, Grant SS, et al. Evaluation of multiple marker screening for Down syndrome in a statewide population. Am J Obstet Gynecol 1993;169:793–7

23. Goodburn AF, Yates JRW, Raggart PR. Second-trimester maternal serum screening using alpha-fetoprotein, human chorionic gonadotropin, and unconjugated oestriol: experience of a regional programme. Prenat Diagn 1994;14:391–402

24. Macri JN, Spencer K, Garver K, et al. Maternal serum free beta-hCG screening: results of studies including 480 cases of Down syndrome. Prenat Diagn 1994;14:97–103

25. Piggott M, Wilkinson P, Bennet J. Implementation of an antenatal serum screening programme for Down's syndrome in two districts (Brighton and Eastbourne). J Med Screen 1994;1:45–9

26. Haddow JE, Polamaki GE, Knight GJ, et al. Reducing the need for amniocentesis in women 35 years of age or older with serum markers screening. N Engl J Med 1994;330:1114–8

27. Rotmensch S, Liberti M, Kardana A, et al. Nicked free β-subunit of human chorionic gonadotropin: a potential new marker for Down syndrome screening. Am J Obstet Gynecol 1996;174:609–11

28. Aitken DA, Syvertsen BS, Crossley JA, et al. Heat-stable and immunoreactive placental alkaline phosphatase in maternal serum from Down's syndrome and trisomy 18 pregnancies. Prenat Diagn 1996;16:1051–4

29. Tafas T, Cuckle HS, Nasr S, et al. An automated image analysis method for the measurement of neutrophil alkaline phosphatase in the prenatal screening of Down syndrome. Fetal Diagn Ther 1996;11:254–60

30. Nicolaides KH, Azar G, Byrne D. Fetal nuchal translucency: ultrasound screening for chromosomal defects in first trimester of pregnancy. Br Med J 1992;304:867–9

31. Snijders RJM, Johnson S, Sebire NJ, et al. First-trimester ultrasound screening for chromosomal defects. Ultrasound Obstet Gynecol 1996;7:216–26

32. Wald N, Stone R, Cuckle HS, et al. First trimester concentrations of pregnancy associated plasma

protein A and placental protein 14 in Down's syndrome. *Br Med J* 1992;305:28

33. Brambati B, Macintosh MCM, Teisner B, *et al*. Low maternal serum level of pregnancy associated plasma protein (PAPP-A) in the first trimester in association with abnormal fetal karyotype. *Br J Obstet Gynaecol* 1993;100:324–6

34. Hurley PA, Ward RHT, Teisner B, *et al*. Serum PAPP-A measurements in first-trimester screening for Down's syndrome. *Prenat Diagn* 1993;13:903–8

35. Muller F, Cuckle H, Teisner B, *et al*. Serum PAPP-A levels are depressed in women with fetal Down's syndrome in early pregnancy. *Prenat Diagn* 1993; 13:633–6

36. Bersinger NA, Brizot ML, Johnson A, *et al*. First trimester maternal serum pregnancy-associated plasma protein A and pregnancy-specific β1-glycoprotein in fetal trisomies. *Br J Obstet Gynaecol* 1994;101:970–4

37. Brizot ML, Snijders RJM, Bersinger NA, *et al*. Maternal serum pregnancy associated placental protein A and fetal nuchal translucency thickness for the prediction of fetal trisomies in early pregnancy. *Obstet Gynecol* 1994;84:918–22

38. Ozturk M, Milunsky A, Brambati B, *et al*. Abnormal maternal serum levels of human chorionic gonadotropin free subunits in trisomy 18. *Am J Med Genet* 1990;36:480–3

39. Aitken DA, McCaw G, Crossley JA, *et al*. First-trimester biochemical screening for fetal chromosome abnormalities and neural tube defects. *Prenat Diagn* 1993;13:681–9

40. Macri JN, Kasuuri RV, Krantz DA, *et al*. Maternal serum Down syndrome screening: free beta protein is a more effective marker than human chorionic gonadotropin. *Am J Obstet Gynecol* 1990;163:1248–53

41. Macintosh MC, Iles R, Teisner B, *et al*. Maternal serum human chorionic gonadotropin and pregnancy associated plasma protein A, markers for fetal Down syndrome at 8–14 weeks. *Prenat Diagn* 1994;14:203–8

42. Brizot ML, Snijders RJM, Butler J, *et al*. Maternal serum hCG and fetal nuchal translucency thickness for the prediction of fetal trisomies in the first trimester of pregnancy. *Br J Obstet Gynaecol* 1995; 102:127–32

43. Casals E, Fortuny A, Grudzinskas JG, *et al*. First-trimester biochemical screening for Down syndrome with the use of PAPP-A, AFP, and beta-hCG. *Prenat Diagn* 1996;16:405–10

44. Wald NJ, Kennard A, Hackshaw AK. First trimester serum screening for Down's syndrome. *Prenat Diagn* 1995;15:1227–40

45. Snijders RJM, Nicolaides KH. *Ultrasound Markers for Fetal Chromosome Defects*. London: Parthenon Publishing, 1995

46. Garmel SH, D'Alton ME. Diagnostic ultrasound in pregnancy: an overview. *Semin Perinatol* 1994;18:117–32

47. Levi S, Hyjazi Y, Schaaps JP, *et al*. Sensitivity and specificity of routine antenatal screening for congenital anomalies by ultrasound: the Belgian multicentric study. *Ultrasound Obstet Gynecol* 1991;1: 102–10

48. Tegnander E, Eik-Neis SH, Johansen OJ, *et al*. Prenatal detection of heart defects at the routine fetal examination at 18 weeks in a non-selected population. *Ultrasound Obstet Gynecol* 1995;5:372–80

49. Chitty LS. Ultrasound screening for fetal abnormalities. *Prenat Diagn* 1995;15:1241–57

50. Skupski DW, Newman S, Ederheim T, *et al*. The impact of routine obstetric ultrasonographic screening in low-risk population. *Am J Obstet Gynecol* 1996;175:1142–5

51. Canadian Task Force on the Periodic Health Examination. The periodic health examination, 1992 update: 2. Routine prenatal ultrasound screening. *Can Med Assoc J* 1992;147:627–33

52. Bucher HC, Schmidt JG. Does routine ultrasound screening improve outcome in pregnancy? Meta-analysis of various outcome measures. *Br Med J* 1993;307:13–17

53. Neilson JP. Routine ultrasound in early pregnancy. In Neilson JP, Crowther CA, Hodnett ED, *et al*. eds. *Pregnancy and Childbirth Module of the Cochrane Database of Systematic Reviews*. The Cochrane Library, The Cochrane Collaboration; Issue 1. Oxford: Update Software, 1997

54. Rizzo N, Pittalis MC, Pilu G, *et al*. Prenatal karyotype on malformed fetuses. *Prenat Diagn* 1990;10: 17–23

55. Nicolaides KH, Snijders RJM, Gosden CM, *et al*. Ultrasonically detectable markers of fetal chromosome abnormalities. *Lancet* 1992;340:704–7

56. Benacerraf BR, Gelman R, Frigoletto FD. Sonographic identification of second-trimester fetuses with Down's syndrome. *N Engl J Med* 1987; 317:1371–6

57. Benacerraf BR, Miller WA, Frigoletto FD. Sonographic detection of fetuses with trisomy 13 and 18: accuracy and limitations. *Am J Obstet Gynecol* 1998;158:404–9

58. Nyberg DA, Resta RG, Luthy DA, *et al*. Prenatal sonographic findings of Down syndrome: review of 94 cases. *Obstet Gynecol* 1990;76:370–7

59. Benacerraf BR. Prenatal sonography of autosomal trisomies. *Ultrasound Obstet Gynecol* 1991;1:66–75

60. Chitty LS, Hunt GH, Moore J, *et al*. Effectiveness of routine ultrasonography in detecting fetal structural abnormalities in low risk population. *Br Med J* 1991;303:1165–9

61. Shirley IM, Bottomley F, Robinson VP. Routine radiographer screening for fetal abnormalities by ultrasound in an unselected low risk population. *Br J Radiol* 1992;65:565–9

62. Levi S, Schaaps JP, De Havay P, *et al*. End-result of routine ultrasound screening for congenital

anomalies: the Belgian multicentric study 1984–92. *Ultrasound Obstet Gynecol* 1995;5:366–71

63. Carroll SG, Maxwell DJ. The significance of echogenic areas in the fetal abdomen. *Ultrasound Obstet Gynecol* 1996;7:293–8

64. Bahado-Singh RO, Wyse L, Dorr MA, *et al*. Fetuses with Down syndrome have disproportionately shortened frontal lobe dimension on ultrasonographic examination. *Am J Obstet Gynecol* 1992;167:1009–14

65. Benacerraf BR, Harlow BL, Frigoletto FD. Hypoplasia of the middle phalanx of the fifth digit. A feature of the second trimester fetus with Down syndrome. *J Ultrasound Med* 1990;9:389–94

66. Jeanty P. Prenatal detection of a simian crease. *J Ultrasound Med* 1990;9:131–6

67. Chudleigh P, Pearce JM, Campbell S. The prenatal diagnosis of transient cysts of the fetal choroid plexus. *Prenat Diagn* 1984;4:135–7

68. Nicolaides KH, Rodeck CH, Gosden CM. Rapid karyotyping in non-lethal fetal malformations. *Lancet* 1986;1:283–7

69. Bundy AL, Saltzman DH, Pober B, *et al*. Antenatal sonographic findings in trisomy 18. *J Ultrasound Med* 1986;5:361–4

70. Chitkara U, Cogswell C, Norton K, *et al*. Choroid plexus cysts in the fetus: a benign anatomic variant or pathological entity? Report of 41 cases and review of the literature. *Obstet Gynecol* 1988;72:815–9

71. Gross SJ, Shulman LP, Tolley EA, *et al*. Isolated fetal choroid plexus cysts and trisomy 18: a review and meta-analysis. *Am J Obstet Gynecol* 1995;172:83–7

72. Snijders RJM, Shawa L, Nicolaides KH. Fetal choroid plexus cysts and trisomy 18: assessment of risk based on ultrasound findings and maternal age. *Prenat Diagn* 1994;14:1119–27

73. Gray DL, Winborn RC, Suessen TL, *et al*. Is genetic amniocentesis warranted when isolated choroid plexus cysts are found? *Prenat Diagn* 1996;16:983–90

74. Hall B. Mongolism in newborn infants. *Clin Pediatr* 1966;5:4–12

75. Toi A, Simpson GF, Filly RA. Ultrasonically evident fetal skin thickening: is it specific for Down syndrome? *Am J Obstet Gynecol* 1987;156:150–3

76. Benacerraf BR, Barss VA, Laboda LA. A sonographic sign for the detection in the second trimester of the fetus with Down's syndrome. *Am J Obstet Gynecol* 1985;151:1078–9

77. Benacerraf BR, Frigoletto FD Jr, Laboda LA. Sonographic diagnosis of Down syndrome in the second trimester. *Am J Obstet Gynecol* 1985;153:49–52

78. Benacerraf BR. The second-trimester fetus with Down syndrome: detection using sonographic features. *Ultrasound Obstet Gynecol* 1996;7:147–55

79. Landwehr JB Jr, Johnson MP, Hume RF, *et al*. Abnormal nuchal finding on screening ultrasonography: aneuploidy stratification on the basis of ultrasonographic anomaly and gestational age at detection. *Am J Obstet Gynecol* 1996;175:995–9

80. Ginsberg N, Cadkin A, Pergament E, *et al*. Ultrasonographic detection of second-trimester fetus with trisomy 18 and 21. *Am J Obstet Gynecol* 1990;163:1186–90

81. Crane JP, Gray DL. Sonographically measured nuchal skin-fold thickness as a screening tool for Down syndrome: results of a prospective clinical trial. *Obstet Gynecol* 1991;77:533–6

82. DeVore GR, Alfi O. The association between an abnormal nuchal skin fold, trisomy 21, and ultrasound abnormalities identified during the second trimester of pregnancy. *Ultrasound Obstet Gynecol* 1993;3:387–94

83. Watson WJ, Miller RC, Menard MK, *et al*. Ultrasonographic measurement of fetal nuchal skin to screen for chromosomal abnormalities. *Am J Obstet Gynecol* 1994;170:583–6

84. Donnenfeld AE, Carlson DE, Polamaki GE. Prospective multicenter study of second-trimester nuchal skinfold thickness in unaffected and Down syndrome pregnancies. *Obstet Gynecol* 1994;84:844–7

85. GrandJean H, Sarramon M-F. Association Française pour le Dépistage et la Prévention des Handicaps de l'Enfants Study Group. Sonographic measurement of nuchal skinfold thickness for detection of Down syndrome in the second-trimester fetus: a multicenter prospective study. *Obstet Gynecol* 1995;85:103–6

86. Borrell A, Costa D, Martinez J, *et al*. Early mid-trimester fetal nuchal thickness: effectiveness as a marker of Down syndrome. *Am J Obstet Gynecol* 1996;175:45–9

87. Wilson RD, Venir N, Farquharson DF. Fetal nuchal fluid – physiological or pathological? – in pregnancies less than 17 menstrual weeks. *Prenat Diagn* 1992;12:755–63

88. Gray DL, Crane JP. Optimal nuchal skin-fold thresholds based on gestational age for prenatal detection of Down syndrome. *Am J Obstet Gynecol* 1994;171:1282–6

89. Lockwood C, Benacerraf BR, Krinsky A, *et al*. A sonographic screening method for Down syndrome. *Am J Obstet Gynecol* 1987;157:803–8

90. Johnson MP, Barr M Jr, Treadwell MC, *et al*. Fetal leg and femur/foot length ratio: a marker for trisomy 21. *Am J Obstet Gynecol* 1993;169:557–63

91. GrandJean H, Sarramon M. Femur/foot length ratio for detection of Down syndrome, results of a multicenter prospective study. *Am J Obstet Gynecol* 1995;173:16–9

92. Lockwood CJ, Lynch L, Berkowitz RL. Ultrasonographic screening for the Down syndrome fetus. *Am J Obstet Gynecol* 1991;165:349–52

93. Nyberg DA, Resta RG, Hickok DE, *et al.* Femur length shortening in the detection of Down syndrome: is prenatal screening feasible? *Am J Obstet Gynecol* 1990;162:1247–52

94. Nyberg DA, Resta RG, Luthy DA, *et al.* Humerus and femur length shortening in the detection of Down's syndrome. *Am J Obstet Gynecol* 1993;168:534–8

95. Cuckle H. Biochemical and ultrasound screening for Down's syndrome: rivals or partners. *Ultrasound Obstet Gynecol* 1996;7:236–8

96. Owen J, Wenstrom KD, Hardin JM, *et al.* The utility of fetal biometry as an adjunct to the multiple-marker screening test for Down syndrome. *Am J Obstet Gynecol* 1994;171:1041–6

97. FitzSimmons J, Droste S, Shepard TH, *et al.* Long-bone growth in fetuses with Down syndrome. *Am J Obstet Gynecol* 1989;161:1174–7

98. Rodis JF, Vintzileos AM, Fleming AD, *et al.* Comparison of humerus length with femur length in fetuses with Down syndrome. *Am J Obstet Gynecol* 1991;165:1051–6

99. Benacerraf BR, Neuberg D, Bromley B, *et al.* Sonographic scoring index for prenatal detection of chromosomal abnormalities. *J Ultrasound Med* 1992;11:449–58

100. Biagotti R, Periti E, Cariati E. Humerus and femur length in fetuses with Down syndrome. *Prenat Diagn* 1994;14:429–34

101. Nadal AS, Bromley B, Frigoletto FD, *et al.* Can the presumed risk of autosomal trisomy be decreased in fetuses of older women following a normal sonogram? *J Ultrasound Med* 1995;14:297–302

102. Nyberg DA, Luthy DA, Cheng EY, *et al.* Role of prenatal ultrasonography in women with positive screen for Down syndrome on the basis of maternal serum markers. *Am J Obstet Gynecol* 1995;173:1030–5

103. DeVore GR, Alfi O. The use of color Doppler ultrasound to identify fetuses at increased risk for trisomy 21: an alternative for high-risk patients who decline genetic amniocentesis. *Obstet Gynecol* 1995;85:378–86

104. Vintzileos AM, Campbell WA, Rodis JF, *et al.* The use of second-trimester genetic sonogram in guiding clinical management of patients at increased risk for fetal trisomy 21. *Obstet Gynecol* 1996;87:948–52

105. Cullen MT, Green J, Whetham J, *et al.* Transvaginal ultrasonographic detection of congenital anomalies in the first trimester. *Am J Obstet Gynecol* 1990;163:466–76

106. Timor-Tritsch HE, Monteagudo A, Peisner DB. High-frequency transvaginal sonographic examination for the potential malformation assessment of the 9-week to 14-week fetus. *J Clin Ultrasound* 1992;20:231–8

107. Bronshtein M, Yoffe N, Blumenfeld Z. Detection of fetal abnormalities by ultrasonography: which sonogram, when, by whom, to whom and how many? *Ultrasound Obstet Gynecol* 1991;1(Suppl. 1):125

108. Braithwaite JM, Armstrong MA, Economides DL. Assessment of fetal anatomy at 12–13 weeks of gestation by transabdominal and transvaginal sonography. *Br J Obstet Gynaecol* 1996;103:82–5

109. Rottem S, Bronshtein M. Transvaginal sonographic diagnosis of congenital anomalies between 9 weeks and 16 weeks menstrual age. *J Clin Ultrasound* 1990;18:307–14

110. Achiron R, Tadmor O. Screening for fetal abnormalities during the first trimester of pregnancy: transvaginal versus transabdominal sonography. *Ultrasound Obstet Gynecol* 1991;1:186–91

111. Pandya PP, Altman D, Brizot ML, *et al.* Repeatability of measurement of fetal nuchal translucency thickness. *Ultrasound Obstet Gynecol* 1995;5:334–7

112. Hyett JA, Moscoso G, Nicolaides KH. Cardiac defects in first trimester fetuses with trisomy 18. *Fetal Diagn Ther* 1995;10:381–6

113. Hyett JA, Moscoso G, Nicolaides KH. First trimester nuchal translucency and cardiac septal defects in fetuses with trisomy 21. *Am J Obstet Gynecol* 1995;172:1411–13

114. Hyett JA, Moscoso G, Nicolaides KH. Increased nuchal translucency in trisomy 21 fetuses: relation to narrowing of the aortic isthmus. *Hum Reprod* 1995;10:3049–51

115. Hyett JA, Moscoso G, Papapanagiotou G, *et al.* Abnormalities of the heart and great arteries in chromosomally normal fetuses with increased nuchal translucency thickness at 11–13 weeks of gestation. *Ultrasound Obstet Gynecol* 1996;7:245–50

116. Nicolaides KH, Brizot ML, Snijders RJM. Fetal nuchal translucency thickness: ultrasound screening for fetal trisomy in the first trimester of pregnancy. *Br J Obstet Gynaecol* 1994;101:782–6

117. Pandya PP, Brizot ML, Kuhn P, *et al.* First trimester fetal nuchal translucency thickness and risk for trisomies. *Obstet Gynecol* 1994;84:420–3

118. Pandya PP, Kondylios A, Hilbert L, *et al.* Chromosomal defects and outcome in 1015 fetuses with increased nuchal translucency. *Ultrasound Obstet Gynecol* 1995;5:15–19

119. Comas C, Martinez JM, Ojuel J, *et al.* First-trimester nuchal edema as a marker of aneuploidy. *Ultrasound Obstet Gynecol* 1995;5:26–9

120. Szabo J, Gellen J, Szemere G. First-trimester ultrasound screening for fetal aneuploidy in women over 35 and under 35 years of age. *Ultrasound Obstet Gynecol* 1995;5:161–3

121. Savoldelli G, Binkert G, Achermann J, *et al.* Ultrasound screening for chromosomal anomalies in the first trimester of pregnancy. *Prenatal Diagn* 1993;13:513–18

122. Schulte-Vallentin M, Schindler H. Non-echogenic nuchal oedema as a marker in trisomy 21 screening. *Lancet* 1992;339:1053

123. Brambati B, Cislaghi C, Tului L, *et al*. First-trimester Down's syndrome screening using nuchal translucency: a prospective study. *Ultrasound Obstet Gynecol* 1995;5:9–14

124. Kornman LH, Morssink LP, Beekhuis JR, *et al*. Nuchal translucency cannot be used as a screening test for chromosomal abnormalities in the first trimester of pregnancy in a routine ultrasound practice. *Prenat Diagn* 1996;16:797–805

125. Pandya PP, Goldberg H, Walton B, *et al*. The implementation of first-trimester scanning at 10–13 weeks' gestation and the measurement of fetal nuchal translucency thickness in two maternity units. *Ultrasound Obstet Gynecol* 1995;5:20–5

126. Hafner E, Schuchter K, Philipp K. Screening for chromosomal abnormalities in an unselected population by fetal nuchal translucency. *Ultrasound Obstet Gynecol* 1995;6:330–3

127. Bewley S, Roberts LJ, Mackinson M, *et al*. First trimester fetal nuchal translucency: problems with screening the general population. II. *Br J Obstet Gynaecol* 1995;102:386–8

128. Pandya PP, Snijders RJM, Johnson SJ, *et al*. Screening for fetal trisomies by maternal age and fetal nuchal translucency thickness at 10 to 14 weeks of gestation. *Br J Obstet Gynaecol* 1995;102:957–62

129. Hyett JA, Noble PL, Snijders RJM, *et al*. Fetal heart rate in trisomy 21 and other chromosomal abnormalities at 10–14 weeks of gestation. *Ultrasound Obstet Gynecol* 1996;7:239–44

130. Hyett JA, Noble PL, Snijders RJM, *et al*. Fetal heart rate in trisomy 21 and other chromosomal abnormalities at 10–14 weeks of gestation. *Ultrasound Obstet Gynecol* 1996;7:239–44

131. Noble PL, Abraham HD, Snijders RJM, *et al*. Screening for fetal trisomy 21 in the first trimester of pregnancy: maternal serum free β-hCG and fetal nuchal translucency thickness. *Ultrasound Obstet Gynecol* 1995;6:390–5

Ultrasonography and general screening 19

Kevin J. Gomez, Edilberto Martinez and Joshua A. Copel

With improvements in the neonatal care of extremely premature infants, congenital anomalies have become an increasingly important contributor to perinatal mortality and the cost of neonatal care. Congenital malformations are the leading cause of death in neonates. Because 3% of newborns have major anomalies, which account for 20–30% of perinatal deaths, prenatal detection of congenital anomalies has the potential to alter obstetric management.

The rate of malformations among stillborn fetuses is higher than in the general population, with major malformations occurring in 4–26% of stillborn fetuses. The risk of stillbirth in a subsequent pregnancy is estimated to be about 7%. Of the different organ systems, fetal anomalies of the cardiovascular system constitute the majority of these major malformations[1]. The central nervous system, renal and skeletal system are also frequent sites of anomalies compared to those of other organs[2]. In most instances, fetal death can not be attributed to a malformation, except in those with severe chromosomal defects and congenital cardiac defects. Causes of neonatal deaths from major organ system anomalies are shown in Table 1.

Obstetric ultrasonography is in widespread use for evaluating the fetus and the intrauterine environment. In 1972, Campbell and colleagues[3] reported the first ultrasound prenatal diagnosis of a congenital anomaly with consequent alteration in obstetric management. The American College of Obstetricians and Gynecologists[4] and the American Institute of Ultrasound in Medicine[5] recommend that a fetal anatomy survey to scan for malformations be part of any obstetric ultrasound.

Because of improvements in high-resolution real-time ultrasound, the high level of expertise and training required of ultrasonographers and sonologists, and a high prevalence of anomalies in referral populations, the diagnosis of fetal anomalies has become very reliable. However, the vast majority of malformed fetuses occur in pregnancies not known to have a risk factor.

The detection, treatment, and prevention of congenital anomalies are considered important goals of prenatal care. Antenatal diagnosis of significant fetal anomalies offers a variety of options for the pregnant woman ranging from termination of pregnancy to delivery at a center equipped to perform highly specialized neonatal surgical procedures. Can routine obstetric ultrasound of low-risk obstetric patients be justified?

Considerable controversy surrounds the routine use of ultrasound during pregnancy. The National Institutes of Health Consensus report[6] recommended against routine obstetric ultrasound because of concerns about safety and efficacy in patients

Table 1 Causes of neonatal deaths from major organ system anomalies

Cardiovascular and pulmonary
Hypoplastic left heart syndrome
Transposition of great vessels
Endocardial fibroelastosis
Polysplenia/asplenia syndrome
Diaphragmatic hernia
Cystic adenomatoid malformation
Tracheal agenesis and tracheoesophageal fistula
Pulmonary hypoplasia
Renal
Bilateral agenesis
Bilateral dysplasia
Prune-belly sequence
Infantile polycystic disease
Bilateral hydronephrosis
Central nervous system
Myelocele/spina bifida
Holoprosencephaly
Anencephaly
Hydrocephalus
Hydronencephaly
Musculoskeletal
Caudal regression sequence
Sirenomelia arthrogryposis
Lethal pterygium syndrome
Congenital contractural arachnodactyly
Gastrointestinal
Omphalocele
Gastroschisis
Limb–body wall complex
Intestinal atresias

without specific indications. In contrast, the Royal College of Obstetricians and Gynaecologists recommend routine ultrasound screening in all pregnant patients[7].

DEFINITIONS RELATED TO CONGENITAL ANOMALIES

A birth defect is a non-specific term used to describe any structural abnormality that is present at birth. It is important to group these defects into categories. The distinction between isolated defects and multiple malformations is paramount in causal evaluation as well as counseling about prognosis and recurrence risk.

A congenital anomaly is defined as an abnormality that is present at birth. Congenital anomalies account for 21% of infant mortality[1]. Major anomalies are those with surgical or cosmetic consequences, for example a limb defect. Minor anomalies, despite their diagnostic importance, have little impact on the individual's well-being, for example clinodactyly.

A malformation is a morphologic defect of an organ resulting from an abnormal developmental process. An example of abnormal morphogenesis is seen in incomplete septation of the heart, which results in a ventricular septal defect.

A disruption is a morphologic defect of an organ resulting from an extrinsic breakdown or interference with a normal developmental process. A classic example is the amniotic band that wraps around the developing limb and produces distal amputation. Disruptions are sporadic events.

A deformation is an abnormal form, shape or position of part of the body caused by mechanical forces. Deformations are normal responses to abnormal forces. In the setting of oligohydramnios the fetus may develop a clubfoot due to the mechanical forces of intrauterine constraint.

Dysplasia is an abnormal organization of cells into tissue or tissues and its morphologic result or results. This results from abnormalities of histogenesis. For instance, osteogenesis imperfecta is a dysplasia because the abnormalities are due to a defect in connective tissue. In contrast to malformations and deformities, dysplastic lesions are frequently not confined to a single organ.

A syndrome is a recognizable pattern of structural defects, often with a predictable natural history, that can be identified amongst several patients, and which thus allows diagnosis and classification. An example of a malformation syndrome is Meckel syndrome, characterized by a posterior encephalocele, polycystic kidneys and polydactyly, and inherited in an autosomal recessive fashion.

A sequence is a pattern of multiple anomalies that results from a single identifiable event early in development. We can classify a sequence into different types, depending on the resulting defects. An example is the Potter oligohydramnios sequence. In most cases the single event is the malformation of renal agenesis and the subsequent problems that develop are either a direct or an indirect result of this malformation. Another example is the fetal akinesia sequence, in which the constellation of abnormalities can be related to the lack of fetal movement.

An association refers to certain anomalies which are frequently associated with other anomalies but are not actual syndromes. They typically involve major anomalies with similar timing in organogenesis. An example of this is the VATER association, which is the non-random association of vertebral anomalies, imperforate anus, tracheoesophageal fistula with esophageal atresia, and renal, radial and cardiac defects.

ROUTINE ULTRASOUND IN PREGNANCY

The initial randomized trials comparing routine versus indicated ultrasonography were performed to evaluate several endpoints, such as improved gestational dating and diagnosis of multiple gestations[8-11]. The trial by Eik-Nes and colleagues[8] concluded that screening decreased unnecessary inductions and reduced perinatal morbidity and mortality. These early studies had small numbers of patients, did not include fetal anomaly as a major endpoint, and did not specify the best time in pregnancy to perform the ultrasound. Overall the evidence does not show a significant benefit for the use of screening ultrasound in decreasing the rate of inductions[12-14]. However, in two studies evaluating post-term pregnancies there appeared to be a reduction in the rate of induction[12,14]. In a third study there was no significant change[15].

Although there are numerous evaluations of the ability of ultrasound to detect fetal anomalies in high-risk groups, few studies evaluate the use of routine ultrasound in unselected or low-risk pregnancies. Use of available data is further complicated by varying gestational ages at the time of screening and by the lack of a common definition of a significant anomaly among the various studies. In addition, several of the studies covered in this review are flawed because the total number of fetal anomalies is less than expected based on the sample size. This brings into question the type of follow-up done to verify identification of all neonatal anomalies. The detection rate of fetal anomalies is directly related to postnatal ascertainment of the anomalies. Therefore, in the setting of poor follow-up, the sensitivity of the screening ultrasound would be falsely increased. The overall sensitivity of ultrasound in detecting fetal anomalies ranges from 17–74%[12,13,15–18]. In two studies with high sensitivities of 60.7% and 74%[17,18] the overall rate of detection of anomalies at birth was about half of the usual baseline rate of congenital anomalies of 2–3%. Lower detection rates of 17% and 41% were reported by two studies that appeared to have good postnatal ascertainment, based on 2.4% anomalies detected at birth[16,19].

EFFECTS OF ROUTINE SCREENING

Several randomized trials have been performed comparing routine versus indicated ultrasonography by several endpoints[20] (Table 2).

Studies have shown that with the use of prenatal ultrasound there may be a reduction in perinatal morbidity in neonates with gastrointestinal abnormalities who require early surgical or pediatric interventions[21].

Luck prospectively evaluated the use of ultrasound in 8523 unselected pregnancies at 19 weeks gestation[22]. There were 27 severely crippling or lethal anomalies detected. Of these, 25 resulted in termination of the pregnancy. In addition, early diagnosis influenced the timing and place of delivery in fetuses with cardiac and gastrointestinal anomalies. The authors suggest that detection of an anomaly with offer of termination for those fetuses with severe crippling deformities is cost-effective on the basis of the (British) Department of Health and Social Security's estimate of the cost of maintaining a severely crippled person for 40 years[23].

The evaluation and diagnosis of fetal cardiac anomalies prenatally may result in improved neonatal outcome. Chang and colleagues[24] studied a group of 22 consecutive fetuses who had *in utero* diagnosis of critical left ventricular outflow tract obstruction and had postnatal surgical repair for hypoplastic left heart syndrome. There was only one patient who had metabolic acidosis, and none had cardiac arrest. This was compared with a previous report from the same institution of 89

Table 2 Endpoints used for ultrasound evaluation

Improved gestational age dating
Early recognition of fetal anomalies
Identification of intrauterine growth restriction
Identification of multiple gestations
Reduced perinatal morbidity and mortality
Reduced maternal morbidity

patients with similar lesions, which revealed a prevalence of 45% for metabolic acidosis and 9% for preoperative cardiac arrest. The authors concluded that *in utero* transport of fetuses with suspected ventricular outflow obstruction to a neonatal cardiac surgical center can result in improved neonatal condition and may improve overall survival.

The endpoint of perinatal mortality was recently evaluated in a meta-analysis[25] of four randomized trials of routine versus selective sonography[13–15,26]. This meta-analysis screened 15 935 pregnancies (7992 of which had routine ultrasound compared to 7943 pregnancies which had selective screening). This study revealed a significant decrease in the perinatal mortality in patients of the routine ultrasound group. The authors suggest the decreased perinatal mortality rate may be related to the early detection of fetal anomalies. The most significant contribution to the meta-analysis was made from the Helsinki Ultrasound Trial[13]. In this, 95% of all pregnant women (9310) were prospectively randomized to compare one-stage ultrasound screening with selective examination. The one-stage ultrasound screen was performed at 16–20 weeks gestation and included measurement of biparietal diameter, placental location, gross fetal anomaly, amniotic fluid volume, and fetal number. The ultrasound evaluations were at two institutions. The Helsinki City Hospital performed what appears to have been a basic examination, and the University Hospital performed a targeted examination. Within the screening group, 22.6% had an ultrasound performed even before the screening examination, and 35.6% had one after. In the control group, 70% had ultrasound at some time during pregnancy, with 17.9% obtaining a screening ultrasound in private offices. There were 30 cases of suspected major malformations in the screened group. The rate of diagnosis by ultrasound screen of anomalies observed at delivery or termination revealed sensitivities of 36% at the City Hospital and 76% at the University Hospital. The perinatal mortality was significantly lower in the screened group than in the control group (4.6 of 1000 versus 9.0 of 1000). This 50% decrease in the perinatal mortality rate was mostly due to induced abortions of fetuses in whom malformations had been diagnosed.

The results of the Routine Antenatal Diagnostic Imaging with Ultrasound (RADIUS) trial, the largest randomized clinical trial of routine ultrasound during pregnancy, has rekindled the debate over the use of ultrasound in the low-risk pregnancy[19]. The RADIUS trial was a practice-based study in which 55 744 English speaking women were registered for care at 109 participating practices. Of these, 15 530 (27.9%) ultra-low-risk women were enrolled for the trial. The screened group had ultrasound examinations at 16–22 weeks and again at 31–35 weeks, while the control group only had ultrasound examinations if clinical indications arose during the pregnancy. Any pre-existing reason for ultrasonography such as a family history of ultrasound-detectable congenital anomalies, a planned genetic amniocentesis, or an abnormal α-fetoprotein test was considered an excluding factor from the ultra-low-risk group. The outcome variables of interest were broken down into two groups[19] (Table 3). The primary outcome variable of adverse perinatal outcome, where infants were classified according to the most severe outcome are listed in Table 4[19]. An average of 2.2 scans were performed in the screening group, compared to 0.6 average scans in the control group.

The authors of the RADIUS trial concluded that there was no difference in adverse perinatal outcome between the screened and control group (5.0% versus 4.9%), a conclusion that can not be taken at face value. The adverse outcomes used as outcome variables in the RADIUS trial were heavily weighted towards complications of prematurity, which is, of course, not prevented by ultrasound examinations. The lack of standardized management across the many practices participating in the study may also have obscured some outcome differences. For example, there was a reduction in postdatism and use of tocolytics in the routine sonography group, presumably due to improved gestational dating, although the size of the study did not provide sufficient power to measure related improvements in perinatal and maternal outcomes[27].

The lack of difference in the perinatal mortality differs significantly from the Helsinki Ultrasound

Table 3   Primary and secondary outcome variables

Primary	Secondary
Perinatal mortality	Anomalous infants
Severe neonatal morbidity	SGA infants
Moderate neonatal morbidity	Multiple gestation
Total adverse outcome	Maternal morbidity

SGA, small for gestational age

Table 4   Definitions of adverse perinatal outcomes

Perinatal mortality
   Fetal death up to 28 days of age
Severe morbidity
   Grade IV retinopathy of prematurity
   Bronchopulmonary dysplasia
   Mechanical ventilation required for more than 48 hours
   Intestinal perforation due to necrotizing enterocolitis
   Grade III or IV intraventricular hemorrhage
   Subdural or cerebral hemorrhage
   Spinal cord injury
   Neonatal seizures
   Placement of chest tube
   Documented neonatal sepsis
   Stay of more than 30 days in a special care nursery
Moderate morbidity
   Presumed neonatal sepsis
   Oxygen required for more than 48 hours
   Necrotizing enterocolitis without perforation
   Grade I or II intraventricular hemorrhage
   Fracture of clavicle or other bones
   Facial nerve injury
   Brachial plexus injury
   Stay of more than 5 days in a special care nursery

Trial[13] which found a 50% decrease in the perinatal mortality rate of the screened group compared to the control group (4.6 vs 9.0/1000). This decrease in perinatal mortality was mostly due to induced abortions of the fetuses (61%) in whom malformations had been diagnosed. Use of abortion was much lower among fetuses found to have anomalies in the RADIUS trial (20%)[19] possibly due to the predominance of Midwestern USA practices.

The RADIUS study had a relatively poor detection rate of fetal anomalies, although significantly more anomalies were detected in the routine ultrasound screening group[28] (Table 5). It is unclear why the RADIUS study group had such poor sensitivity to the presence of fetal anomalies prior to 24 weeks gestation (16.6%) compared to combined data from other large studies on routine ultrasound (50.9%)[19]. This discrepancy can partially be explained by the poor detection rate at the non-tertiary care centers[28] (Table 6). The

RADIUS study also included in the definition of what constituted an anomaly some subtle fetal abnormalities which are unlikely to be detectable by ultrasound, and, with mandatory reporting of newborn physical examinations, may have had more complete follow-up than comparable European studies mentioned above.

Evaluation of the secondary outcome variables was disappointing because ultrasound screening did not significantly alter obstetric management in pregnancies complicated by multiple gestations, intrauterine growth restriction and postdatism. This should not be surprising since this trial lacked sufficient power to detect a significant difference in maternal outcomes among the secondary outcome variables. The lack of standard management protocols for these common obstetric complications further ensured that significant findings would be unlikely.

Before the results of the RADIUS trial can be generalized, the highly selective nature of the studied population must be emphasized. Sixty per cent of initially screened patients were excluded from participation largely because of anticipated indicated ultrasounds in that group, and another 45% of the control group required ultrasounds. The authors projected that, based on their results, a policy of two routine prenatal ultrasounds would increase medical costs by over one billion dollars annually. Excluding the scans indicated according to their protocol, however, reduces that number to below $350 million[29]. While this is a significant amount of money, better quality sonograms could be achieved than in the RADIUS trial, with consequent improvements in maternal and neonatal outcomes.

SKILL AND EXPERIENCE

The skill and experience of ultrasonographers and sonologists play a major role in the detection rate of fetal anomalies. The Belgian multicentric study demonstrated an improvement in early detection rates (21–41%) over two time periods (1984–89 compared to 1990–91)[16]. It is also clear that fetal anatomy evaluations performed at tertiary care centers dramatically increases the detection rate of fetal anomalies. The Helsinki trial showed a difference in the detection rates for anomalies (36% versus 77%) when comparing the non-tertiary to tertiary centers[10]. Even in the RADIUS trial, which had lower detection rates, the detection rate of anomalies in the non-tertiary

Table 5 Impact of ultrasound screening on prenatal detection of selected major malformations and gestational ages

Anomaly	Screened (n = 7685)	Control (n = 7596)
Anencephaly	3/3 (100%)	1/2 (50%)
Spina bifida	4/5 (80%)	2/3 (66%)
Other CNS anomaly	2/2 (100%)	2/7 (29%)
Cleft lip, cleft palate	3/10 (30%)	1/7 (14%)
Cystic hygroma	2/2 (100%)	0/1 (0%)
Isolated ventricular septal defect	0/16 (0%)	0/14 (0%)
Isolated atrial septal defect	0/5 (0%)	0/15 (0%)
Complex heart defect	9/21 (43%)	3/14 (21%)
Diaphragmatic hernia	1/1 (100%)	3/5 (60%)
Esophageal atresia/TE fistula	0/3 (0%)	1/3 (33%)
Duodenal atresia	1/1 (100%)	none
Omphalocele	1/1 (100%)	0/1 (0%)
Hydronephrosis	28/29 (97%)	3/7 (43%)
Other renal anomaly	6/6 (100%)	1/3 (33%)
Clubfoot	2/24 (8%)	1/21 (5%)
Miscellaneous major anomaly	3/4 (75%)	1/5 (20%)
< 24 weeks	16.6%	4.9%
< 40 weeks	34.8%	10.4%

CNS, central nervous system; TE, tracheoesophageal

Table 6 Sensitivity of ultrasound detection of fetal anomalies between tertiary and non-tertiary centers

Tertiary (n = 2658)	Non-tertiary (n = 4623)
< 24 weeks 21/57 (37%)	6/65 (12%)

locations was 13%, compared to 35% at the tertiary centers[19].

ACCURACY OF ULTRASOUND IN DETECTION OF ABNORMALITIES IN DIFFERENT SYSTEMS

The accuracy of ultrasound in diagnosing fetal anomalies depends on the anomaly and the organ system involved. Levi and colleagues[2] prospectively evaluated the use of ultrasound in low-risk populations. Levi screened 16 072 pregnancies, among which 381 fetuses had anomalies, and 154 were detected by ultrasound (sensitivity 40.4%, specificity 99.9%). In this study, the ultrasound examination was a stage-2 examination, as recommended by Campbell and Pearce[30], and demonstrated a variation of sensitivities between different organ systems. The highest sensitivities were in neck anomalies (86%), followed by anomalies of the central nervous system (79%) and the urogenital tract (67%). The lowest sensitivities occurred with facial (20%) and cardiac anomalies (24%). This study clearly defined major malformations, which aids in comparisons with other studies. After reviewing their false-negative cases, the authors suggested that additional anomalies, particularly cardiac defects, should have been detected with more specific training and education.

Anomalies of the head and neck have the highest detection rate with prenatal ultrasound. Anomalies such as anencephaly are virtually always diagnosed with ultrasound. The increased sensitivity of ultrasound over the recent past is related particularly to the recognition of abnormalities of fetal cranial anatomy associated with neural tube defects. These findings, as described by Nicolaides and colleagues[31] are related to the Arnold–Chiari malformation, which causes abnormalities in the posterior fossa, concave frontal bones ('lemon sign'), ventriculomegaly, and small head size. When evaluating the posterior fossa, the distorted cerebellum ('banana sign'), inability to visualize the cerebellum, obliteration of the cisterna magna, and an abnormally small cerebellum are further clues to a possible neural tube defect[32] (Tables 7 and 8).

Van Den Hof and colleagues[33] diagnosed open spina bifida in 130 of the 1561 fetuses that were prospectively evaluated because of risk of neural tube defects. They evaluated the diagnostic accuracy of the cranial markers for neural tube defects. There was a correlation between gestational age and these markers. The lemon sign was present in 98% of the fetuses at 24 weeks gestation or less but in only 13% of those greater than 24 weeks gestation. The authors noted cerebellar abnormalities in 95% of cases regardless of gestational age and noted that the alterations in the skull and brain morphology are often more readily attainable than detailed spinal views. Also, they suggest that if the results of the ultrasound examination of the fetal spine, cranium, and cerebellum appear normal, the chance of an undetected lesion must be low; therefore, amniocentesis, with its inherent procedure-related risk, is unnecessary. The results of this study are in agreement with those of several other studies[34,35].

One must realize that the use of cranial and cerebellar signs are subjective and require a high degree of operator skill, which is usually only available at tertiary centers. The sensitivity of ultrasound screening along for neural tube defects in low-risk populations is still uncertain. de Courcy-Wheeler and colleagues[36] evaluated measuring the transverse cerebellar diameter as an objective screen for the detection of spina bifida. The findings of this study showed a sensitivity of 80% in detection of open spina bifida with a 4% false-positive rate.

Other fetal brain anomalies such as hydrocephalus and microcephaly are detectable by ultrasound. However, these conditions may not become diagnosable until the third trimester of pregnancy. In a study by Levi and colleagues[2] only four of 20 cases of fetal hydrocephalus were detected prior to 22 weeks gestation. In addition only two of four cases of microcephaly were diagnosed in the second trimester.

Congenital heart defects are the most common severe congenital anomaly found in live births, with an incidence of 4–5 per 1000 at birth, and account for over 20% of infant mortality due to congenital anomalies[1]. Most children with cardiac disease are born to women who have no historic risk factors. Fifty per cent of prenatally diagnosed cases of congenital heart disease occur in cases referred due to a suspected cardiac defect on a routine ultrasound[37].

It is clear that fetal echocardiography is complex and may be a time-consuming procedure and, as such, may not perform well as a screening test.

Table 7   Lemon sign in spina bifida

Age (weeks)	Incidence, n (%)
16–23	109/110 (99.1)
> 23	2/13 (15.4)

Table 8   Patients with cerebellar signs in open spina bifida (85 cases)

Signs	Nicolaides et al.[33] (n = 21)	Campbell et al.[40] (n = 26)	Pilu et al.[41] (n = 19)	Goldstein et al.[42] (n = 19)
Distorted or small	57%	62%	63%	–
Not visualized	38%	35%	37%	–
Cisternal magna†	95%	–	100%	100%
Normal cerebellum	5%	4%	0%	0%

†Obliterated

However, the four-chamber view is easily obtained and can exclude many malformations. The four-chamber view has been proposed as part of the basic obstetric ultrasound examination by the American Institute of Ultrasound in Medicine because this view may identify fetuses that should be referred for a targeted cardiac examination[5].

Copel and colleagues[37] showed that in experienced hands, the four-chamber view can have a sensitivity of 92% and a specificity of 99.7%. However, this was in a high-risk referral population of which a significant portion of patients were referred for ultrasound evaluation because of an abnormal four-chamber view. They also suggested that including the four-chamber view in the level-I ultrasound examination could improve the screening for cardiac defects.

Vergani and colleagues[38] prospectively screened 5336 unselected pregnancies with the four-chamber view and compared them with 3680 historic controls. The controls had a four-chamber view obtained in 20% of the cases. There were 47 cardiac anomalies identified at 18–20 weeks gestation. Eighty-one per cent of cardiac anomalies were successfully identified in the four-chamber screen group with a specificity of 99.9%, while only 43% were correctly identified in the other group.

A targeted fetal echocardiogram is appropriate for pregnancies at high risk and is usually performed by someone with specialized training in evaluation of the fetal heart. Bromley and colleagues[39] retrospectively evaluated the accuracy of the four-chamber view and fetal echocardiography in patients at high and low risk for cardiac anomalies. There were 39 patients with scans that indicated high risk and 30 with low-risk indications. In the high-risk group, the sensitivity of fetal echocardiography was 82%, and in the low-risk group it was 83%. The four-chamber view had an overall sensitivity of 63% when the high- and low-risk groups were combined. However, the four-chamber view was not evaluated separately in the high- and low-risk populations. The four-chamber view missed cases of tetralogy of Fallot, transposition of the great arteries, ventricular septal defects, and coarctation of the aorta. Because 43% of the fetuses with heart defects were referred for low-risk indications, the authors believe that all obstetric scans performed after 18 weeks gestation should include evaluation of the four-chamber view and the ventricular outflow tracts. Sharland and Allan[40] did a prospective evaluation of the four-chamber view in an unselected population at 10 obstetric units in greater London. During the study period of 32 months, 53 fetuses with congenital heart disease were detected with the four-chamber screen. The overall sensitivity was 77% with a specificity of 99%. The claim of this sensitivity may not be valid since the true denominator is unknown. Of the 53 cases identified, 36 pregnancies were terminated, which significantly lowered the perinatal mortality rate. The authors noted that the percentage of fetuses in whom the four-chamber view was seen at the first attempt increased as the study progressed. The main reasons for not obtaining the four-chamber view were maternal obesity, fetal lie, gestational age less than 18 weeks, and inadequate equipment. The authors suggest that with increasing experience and technology there will be an improvement in screening, so that the number of abnormalities missed is minimal and the majority of referrals to a specialized unit are true positives.

In a study by Tegander and colleagues[41] the low sensitivity of 7% was related to the ascertainment of anomalies well beyond the neonatal period, with a prevalence of 12 per 1000.

Achiron and colleagues[42] prospectively compared the four-chamber view with extended echocardiography. A total of 5347 low-risk pregnancies was included in the study, all seen between 18 and 24 weeks gestation. Eleven defects were diagnosed by the four-chamber view (sensitivity 48%; specificity 99.9%), and a further seven were diagnosed by extended echocardiographic examination (sensitivity 78%; specificity 99.9%). The addition of the extended examination will increase prenatal diagnosis of cardiac anomalies and should be part of standard fetal surveillance.

In a recent study, Stumpflen[43] assessed the prenatal detection of congenital heart disease in an unselected, consecutive group of women with detailed fetal echocardiography. This included the four-chamber view, outflow-tracts, and color-flow mapping with additional Doppler and M-mode investigations done when appropriate. The mean duration of the heart examination for normal cases was about 4 minutes and 3085 consecutive women were evaluated. Of these 2181 (70.7%) were consecutive cases studied without any known risk factors for congenital heart disease. All newborn infants with normal fetal heart scans were examined by a neonatologist. Of the 52 cases of congenital heart disease identified postnatally, 46 were diagnosed prenatally (sensitivity 88.5%, specificity 100%). The group with no risk factors had a detection rate of 15 to 17 cases (sensitivity 88%). Retrospective review of videotape material showed that seven of these 17 cases were detectable in the four-chamber view alone (sensitivity 41%).

Comstock[44] initially reported that the normal fetal cardiac axis was 45 ± 10.4 degrees. Smith[45] prospectively evaluated if a relationship exists between left cardiac axis deviation and fetal anomalies. Those with heart axes greater than 75 degrees to the left were considered to have left axis deviation. Only cases with postnatal follow-up were included. Thirty-four fetuses with left cardiac axis deviation had postnatal follow-up, with 26 found to be abnormal. Twelve of the 34 fetuses were in the low-risk category. Of the 26 abnormal cases, 10 cases (38%) were from the low-risk group. Twenty-one fetuses had cardiac abnormalities and five had extracardiac findings; only three specific cardiac abnormalities predominated among the 21 abnormal hearts: tetralogy of Fallot, transposition of the great vessels, and double outlet right ventricle. The authors suggest that left axis deviation may help identify conotruncal abnormalities, which are not usually detected with the four-chamber view alone.

When evaluating the use of routine ultrasound screening in pregnancy, cardiac anomalies comprise the single largest group of anomalies not detected prenatally. With the use of the four-chamber view, early prenatal diagnosis of congenital heart defects can be made and thus have a great impact on obstetric care. We believe that the four-chamber view, along with eyeballing the cardiac axis, should be a part of every basic ultrasound examination after 18 weeks gestation. Whether or not it is reasonable to include the extended fetal cardiac examination of the outflow tracts as part of the ultrasound screening examination in low-risk pregnancies needs further evaluation because of the specialized training that would be required.

Although the RADIUS study[19] had poor sensitivity for ASDs and VSDs (zero out of 19), the tertiary centers diagnosed 43% of complex cardiac lesions in the ultrasound screening group compared to only 21% in the control group. Of interest, no cardiac lesions, simple or complex, were diagnosed at the non-tertiary centers.

With the use of both ultrasound and maternal serum screening virtually all defects such as omphalocele and gastroschisis should be detectable. In the studies by Ewigman and colleagues[19] and Luck and colleagues[22] 100% of the anterior abdominal wall defects were identified. The diagnosis of other abnormalities such as intestinal obstruction and atresia are less likely in the second trimester, and would, therefore, have a low sensitivity at the usual timing of a routine ultrasound examination.

Renal tract abnormalities are commonly diagnosed prenatally. Twenty-eight of 29 and 99 of 99 cases of obstructive uropathy were detected prenatally in the respective studies by Crane et al. and Luck et al[22]. When looking at ultrasound sensitivity in predicting malformations, inclusion of some minor malformations that border on anatomic variants, such as minor degrees of renal pelvic dilation, can increase the apparent sensitivity. Luck[22] prospectively evaluated the use of ultrasound in 8523 unselected pregnancies at 19 weeks gestation. There were 166 anomalies, of which 140 were detected at 19 weeks gestation (sensitivity 85%; specificity 99.9%). Of the 166 malformations, 105 were of the renal system. This high detection rate was inflated by a high proportion of minor renal anomalies.

GESTATIONAL AGE

The gestational age at which routine screening is performed has an impact on the sensitivity of diagnosed fetal malformations and can alter the management choices available to the patient. The Royal College of Obstetricians and Gynaecologists recommends screening for fetal anomalies at 18–20 weeks gestation[46]. An ultrasound evaluation for fetal anatomy performed at 15–17 weeks may not provide optimal visualization of the fetal anatomy. This may explain in part the lower detection rates (16–41%) in the respective studies by Ewigman and colleagues (RADIUS)[19] and Levi and colleagues[2] which performed ultrasound between 15 and 22 weeks gestation. This can be compared to the better detection rates of 60% and 85% seen in the respective studies from the UK[17,22], which performed ultrasounds at 18–20 weeks.

Hegge and colleagues[47] investigated how often malformations were identified too late in gestation to allow the patient various options including pregnancy termination. There were 23 754 scans, of which 13 849 were in the second or third trimester. About half of the scans were done in the early second trimester for genetic amniocentesis or abnormal maternal serum α-fetoprotein, and the other half were performed later in gestation, often for high-risk indications. Of the 364 fetuses found to have anomalies, 34% were diagnosed at 22 weeks gestation or less, and 66% were diagnosed at 23 weeks gestation or more. Therapeutic options were different if early diagnosis was made. Follow-up of the abnormal fetuses diagnosed at 22 weeks gestation or less showed that 67% were terminated or delivered early for a lethal defect, whereas diagnosis after 22 weeks gestation was associated with 14% termination or early delivery. Of the fetuses that had abnormalities identified after 22 weeks gestation, 56 had no indication for ultrasound prior to 23 weeks gestation, based on the National Institutes of Health Conference criteria[6]. The authors suggest routine ultrasound before 22 weeks gestation because, in their study, patients were much more likely to choose the option of termination when fetal abnormalities were found early enough to permit that option.

SAFETY OF ROUTINE ULTRASOUND

Many clinicians routinely scan their prenatal patients to screen for fetal anomalies, intrauterine growth restriction, multiple gestation, and to confirm gestational dating. This diagnostic use of ultrasound may also lead to an increased frequency of ultrasound examinations in individual pregnancies. With this in mind we must consider whether diagnostic ultrasound improves outcome or increases risk in normal pregnancies.

Frequent ultrasound exposure has been suggested to have adverse effects on fetal growth[48]. Tarantal and Hendrickx[49] observed that when the cynomologus macaque was exposed to frequent prenatal ultrasound there was a reduction in mean birthweight, as well as fetal and neonatal white blood cell count. The macaque and other non-human primates are considered better models for the evaluation of the effects of ultrasound than murine models because of a greater similarity in size and thus distance from transducer to the fetus, although the amount of subcutaneous fat is substantially less in non-human primates than in even the slenderest humans, and the myometrium is also quite thin. In their most recent study Tarantal and colleagues[50] used a MK 600 machine with 7.5 MHz transducer (advanced Technology Laboratories Inc, Bothell, Washington). The ultrasound probe was placed on the abdomen of the macaque with exposure times that were similar to what might occur in clinical practice. Twenty-two animals were involved in the study. Eleven were exposed to diagnostic ultrasound, while the rest had the ultrasound transducer placed on their abdomen with the ultrasound machine set to 'standby', that is, turned on but not emanating sound waves. They then performed both neuro-behavioral and hematologic assessments blinded to study assignment. Their results were a significant decrease in birthweight in the exposed fetuses, which persisted for a month after birth, although no weight differences were apparent thereafter. In addition there was also a significant reduction of the mean white blood cell count, although this was not a consistent finding at all observation points. There was no difference in the postnatal bone marrow aspirates, nor were there influences on the red cell or platelet counts. Similar measurement differences have not been specifically studied in humans, but preliminary data from a randomized clinical trial performed in Winter Haven, Florida, USA, including patients randomized according to presence or absence of ultrasound exposure (including external fetal monitors) fail to support these findings (Hobbins J, personal communication).

Newnham and colleagues[51] screened 2834 women to evaluate the benefits of frequent ultrasound and Doppler velocimetry in a low-risk pregnancy population. An experimental group was assigned to have ultrasound and continuous wave Doppler of the umbilical and arcuate arteries at 18, 24, 28, 34 and 38 weeks, while the control group had a single ultrasound at 18 weeks. They found that the proportion of birthweights below the tenth percentile was significantly higher in the experimental group than in the controls (relative risk 1.35, 95% confidence interval 1.09–1.67). Birthweight below the third percentile was similarly elevated (RR 1.65, 95% CI 1.09–2.49). The mean birthweight of the two groups differed by only 25 grams, however: a difference that is not statistically significant. The authors point out in their discussion that, while the difference is statistically significant, the purpose of the study was to evaluate a different hypothesis, and the effect on birthweight may have been due to chance alone. The authors conclude with a call for a specific prospective evaluation of this possibility, and for caution in the meantime by prudent limitation of ultrasound to those instances when the information gained is likely to be of clinical benefit.

In a recent review of epidemiological studies of human exposure to ultrasound, Salvesen and colleagues[52] did not find any associations between *in utero* ultrasound and childhood maldevelopment. However, in an earlier study the data suggest a possible association between *in utero* ultrasound and subsequent non-right-handedness[53].

EFFECT OF ULTRASOUND ON SURVIVAL RATES OF ANOMALOUS INFANTS

Because of improvements in high resolution ultrasound and higher levels of expertise of individuals performing the examinations, the diagnosis of fetal anomalies has become very reliable, that is, significant false-positive diagnoses are uncommon. The potential benefit of ultrasound in reducing perinatal mortality secondary to early diagnosis of congenital anomalies followed by induced abortions have been discussed. The question arises whether ultrasound screening has an impact on the survival rates of the anomalous infants, particularly those with life-threatening anomalies. Fetuses with severe anomalies are usually offered delivery at tertiary care institutions where specialized pediatric teams can give immediate care with the goal of improving neonatal outcome. Prenatal diagnosis of these anomalies may then help in improving the outcome of these neonates.

There is, at present, only one randomized clinical trial that has looked into this matter. Crane as part of the RADIUS trial[54] did not find a statistically significant difference in the neonatal survival of fetuses with severe anomalies when he compared the routinely screened groups (75%) with the control groups (52%). Unfortunately this study lacks adequate power to detect a difference.

TRANSVAGINAL ULTRASOUND AS A SCREENING TOOL FOR FETAL ANOMALIES

Transvaginal ultrasound (TVS) has become a very useful tool in the evaluation of early gestations. TVS provides a better resolution of the image produced because of the utilization of high frequency probes and the proximity of these probes to the fetus. The higher the frequency of sound, the shallower the depth of penetration but the better the resolution obtained. It has helped in more accurate pregnancy dating and also in the recognition of sonographic markers of chromosomal abnormalities and other malformations[55,56].

A recent publication by D'Ottavio and colleagues[57] reports their experience with the use of TVS as a screening tool for detecting fetal malformations in a selected population of pregnant women. TVS was performed at 14 weeks by several operators with different degrees of experience.

They reported a sensitivity of 53% for TVS in detecting major and minor malformations. A higher detection rate for chromosomal abnormalities was reported (75%). They recommended that early TVS screening be performed in addition to later screening.

Other investigators have reported more encouraging reports when TVS is performed by more experienced operators in highly selected pregnancies[55,58–60]. Yagel and colleagues evaluated whether early TVS can be used alone for the detection of structural abnormalities in the fetus or if it should be followed by a transabdominal ultrasound performed in the late second trimester. The study included 536 pregnant women at risk for birth defects who were evaluated by a TVS at 13 to 16 weeks followed by a TVS at 18 to 20 weeks. Forty-two structural anomalies were identified by TVS. Of these, 24 pregnancies were terminated and one fetus died. The remaining 17 fetuses and the rest of the population had a second ultrasound performed transabdominally at 18 to 20 weeks. This second survey identified eight structural abnormalities that were not noticed by the previous examination. The diagnosed anomaly disappeared in five other cases. Together the scans detected 89% of the abnormal fetuses (41 of 46).

The authors concluded that since 17.4% of anomalies were not detected by early TVS, transabdominal scan should follow the transvaginal evaluation at the most advanced stage of pregnancy at which abortion is still feasible. In a time of fiscal restraint as is currently being experienced in medicine in the USA, such a recommendation becomes difficult to implement. More prospective studies are needed to address the value of TVS as a screening tool for fetal anomalies.

CONCLUSIONS

Fetal malformations are a major factor in perinatal mortality. Therefore detection, treatment, and prevention of congenital anomalies are considered important goals of prenatal care. It is clear from the RADIUS study that only the most experienced sonologist should be screening for fetal anomalies. This is especially true if ultrasound is meant to be cost effective. In addition, ultrasound evaluation should be performed at set times in gestation to gain maximal information and repeated only if the information is likely to be of clinical benefit.

References

1. Centers for Disease Control. Contribution of Birth Defects to Infant Mortality: United States. *Morbid Mortal Wkly Rep* 1989;38:633–5
2. Levi S, Schaaps JP, Defoort P, *et al.* Sensitivity and specificity of routine antenatal screening for congenital anomalies by ultrasound: the Belgian multicentric study. *Ultrasound Obstet Gynecol* 1991;1:102–10
3. Campbell S, Holt EM, Johnstone FD, *et al.* Anencephaly: early ultrasonic diagnosis and active management. *Lancet* 1972;2:1226–7
4. American College of Obstetrics and Gynecology. *Technical Bulletin* 1991:116
5. American Institute of Ultrasound in Medicine. *Guidelines for Obstetrical Scans.* Bethesda: American Institute of Ultrasound in Medicine, 1991
6. Consensus Conference. The use of diagnostic ultrasound imaging during pregnancy. *J Am Med Assoc* 1994;252:669–72
7. Drife JO, Donnai D. *Antenatal Diagnosis of Fetal Abnormalities.* London: Springer-Verlag, 1991:353–7
8. Eik-Nes SH, Okland O, Aure JC, *et al.* Ultrasound screening in pregnancy: a randomized controlled trial. *Lancet* 1984;1:347–54
9. Neilson JP, Munjanja JP, Whitfield CR. Screening for the small-for-dates fetus: a controlled trial. *Br Med J* 1984;289:1179–82
10. Bennett MJ, Little G, Dewhurst J, *et al.* Predictive value of ultrasound measurement in early pregnancy: a randomized controlled trial. *Br J Obstet Gynaecol* 1982;89:338–41
11. Bakketeig LS, Eik-Nes SH, Jacobsen G, *et al.* Randomized controlled trial of ultrasonographic screening in pregnancy. *J Am Med Assoc* 1984;2:207–11
12. LeFevre M, Bain RP, Ewigman BG, *et al.* A randomized trial of prenatal ultrasonographic screening: impact on maternal management and outcome. *Am J Obstet Gynecol* 1993;169:483–90
13. Saari-Kemppainen A, Karjalainen O, Ylostalo P, *et al.* Ultrasound screening and perinatal mortality: controlled trial of systematic one-stage screening in pregnancy. *Lancet* 1990;336:387–91
14. Waldenstrom U, Axelsson O, Nilsson S, *et al.* Effects of routine one-stage ultrasound screening in pregnancy: a randomized controlled trial. *Lancet* 1988;2:585–8
15. Ewigman BG, LeFevre M, Hesser J. A randomized trial of routine prenatal ultrasound. *Obstet Gynecol* 1990;76:189–94
16. Levi S, Schaaps JP, DeHavay P, *et al.* End-result of routine ultrasound screening for congenital anomalies: the Belgium multicentric study 1984–1992. *Ultrasound Obstet Gynecol* 1995;5:366–71
17. Shirley IM, Bottomley F, Robinson VP. Routine radiographer screening for fetal abnormalities by ultrasound in an unselected low risk population. *Br J Radiol* 1992;65:565–9
18. Chitty LS, Hunt GH, Moore J, *et al.* Effectiveness of routine ultrasonography in detecting fetal structural abnormalities in a low risk population. *Br Med J* 1991;303:1165–9
19. Ewigman BG, Crane JP, Frigoletto FD, *et al.* A randomized trial of prenatal ultrasound screening in a low risk population: impact on perinatal outcome. *N Engl J Med* 1993;329:821–7
20. Gomez KJ, Copel JA. Ultrasound screening for fetal structural anomalies. *Curr Opin Obstet Gynecol* 1993;5:204–10
21. Romero R, Ghidini A, Costigan K, *et al.* Prenatal diagnosis of duodenal atresia: does it make any difference? *Obstet Gynecol* 1989;71:739–41
22. Luck CA. Value of routine ultrasound scanning at 19 weeks: a four year study of 8849 deliveries. *Br Med J* 1992;203:1474–8
23. Royal College of Obstetricians and Gynecologists. Working Party Report on Routine Ultrasound Examination in Pregnancy. London: RCOG, 1984:10
24. Chang AC, Huhta JC, Yoon GY, *et al.* Diagnosis, transport and outcome in fetuses with left ventricular outflow tract obstruction. *J Thorac Cardiovasc Surg* 1991;102:841–8
25. Bucher HC, Schmidt JG. Does routine ultrasound scanning improve outcome in pregnancy? Meta-analysis of various outcome measures. *Br Med J* 1993;307:12–17
26. Bakketeig L, Jacobsen G, Brodtkorb C, *et al.* Randomized controlled trial of ultrasonographic screening in pregnancy. *Lancet* 1984;2:207–10
27. Goncalves LF, Romer R. A critical appraisal of the RADIUS study. *Fetus* 1993;3:7–18
28. Crane JP: Routine obstetrical ultrasound screening - is it appropriate? One Day Symposium on Fetal Echo. Stamford Connecticut. November 20, 1993
29. Copel JA, Platt LD, Campbell S. Prenatal ultrasound screening and perinatal outcome (Letter). *N Eng J Med* 1994;330:571
30. Campbell S, Pearce JM. Prenatal diagnosis of fetal structural anomalies by ultrasound. *Clin Obstet Gynecol* 1983;10:75–506

31. Nicolaides KH, Gabbe SC, Campbell S, *et al*. Ultrasound screening for spina bifida: cranial and cerebellar signs. *Lancet* 1984;2:72–4

32. Crane JP. Sonographic detection of neural tube defects. In Sherman E, ed. *Maternal Serum Screening*, New York: Churchill Livingstone, 1992:59–73

33. Van Den Hof MC, Nicolaides KH, Campbell J, *et al*. Evaluation of the lemon and banana sign in one hundred thirty fetuses with open spina bifida. *Am J Obstet Gynecol* 1990;162:322–7

34. Nyberg DA, Nack LA, Hirsch J, *et al*. Abnormalities of fetal cranial contour in sonographic detection of spina bifida: evaluation of the 'lemon' sign. *Radiology* 1988;167:387–93

35. Penso C, Redline RW, Benacerraf BR. A sonographic sign which predicts which fetuses with hydrocephalus have an associated neural tube defect. *J Ultrasound Med* 1987;6:307

36. de Courcy-Wheeler RH, Pomeranz MM, Wald NJ, *et al*. Small fetal cerebellar diameter: a screening test for spina bifida. *Br J Obstet Gynaecol* 1994;101:904–5

37. Copel JA, Pilu G, Green J, *et al*. Fetal echocardiographic screening for congenital heart disease: the importance of the four-chamber view. *Am J Obstet Gynecol* 1987;157:648–55

38. Vergani P, Mariani S, Ghidini A, *et al*. Screening for congenital heart disease with the four-chamber view. *Am J Obstet Gynecol* 1992;167:1000–3

39. Bromley B, Estroff JA, Sanders SP, *et al*. Fetal echocardiography: accuracy and limitations in a population at high and low risk for heart defects. *Am J Obstet Gynecol* 1992;166:1473–81

40. Sharland GK, Allan LDS. Screening for congenital heart disease prenatally: results of a 2 1/2-year study in the South East Thames region. *Br J Obstet Gynaecol* 1992

41. Tegnander E, Eik-Nes SH, Johansen OJ, *et al*. Prenatal detection of heart defects at the routine fetal examination at 18 weeks in a non-selected population. *Ultrasound Obstet Gynecol* 1995;5:372–80

42. Achiron R, Glaser J, Gelernter I, *et al*. Extended fetal echocardiographic examination for detecting cardiac malformations in low risk pregnancies. *Br Med J* 1992;304:671–4

43. Stumpflen I, Stumpflen A, Wimmer M, *et al*. Effect of detailed fetal echocardiography as part of routine prenatal ultrasonographic screening on detection of congenital heart disease source. *Lancet* 1996;348:854–7

44. Comstock CH. Normal fetal heart axis and position. *Obstet Gynecol* 1987;70:255–9

45. Smith RS, Comstock CH, Kirk JS, *et al*. Ultrasonographic left cardiac axis deviation: a marker for fetal anomalies. *Obstet Gynecol* 1995;85:187–91

46. Drife JO, Donnai D. *Antenatal Diagnosis of Fetal Abnormalities*. London: Springer-Verlag, 1991:353–7

47. Hegge FN, Franklin RW, Watson PT, *et al*. An evaluation of the time of discovery of fetal malformations by an indication-based system for ordering obstetrical ultrasound. *Obstet Gynecol* 1989;74:21–4

48. O'Brien WD. Dose dependent effect of ultrasound on fetal weight in mice. *J Ultrasound Med* 1983;2:1–8

49. Tarantal AF, Hendrickx AG. Evaluation of the bioeffects of prenatal ultrasound exposure in the cynomolgus macaque (Macaca Fasicularis): I. Neonatal/infant observations. *Teratology* 1989;39:137–47

50. Tarantal AF, O'Brien WD, Hendrickx AG. Evaluation of the bioeffects of prenatal ultrasound exposure in the cynomolgus macaque (Macaca Fasicularis): III. Developmental and hematologic studies. *Teratology* 1993;47:159–70

51. Newnham JP, Evans SF, Michael CA, *et al*. Effects of frequent ultrasound during pregnancy: a randomized controlled trial. *Lancet* 1993;342:887–91

52. Dslbrdrn KA, Eik-Nes SH. Is ultrasound unsound? A review of epidemiological studies of human exposure to ultrasound. *Ultrasound Obstet Gynecol* 1995;6:293–8

53. Salvesen KA, Vatten LJ, Eik-Nes SH, *et al*. Routine ultrasonography *in utero* and subsequent handedness and neurological development. *Br Med J* 1993;307:159–64

54. Crane *et al*. A randomized trial of prenatal ultrasonographic screening: impact on the detection, management, and outcome of anomalous fetuses. *Am J Obstet Gynecol* 1994;171:392–9

55. Rottem S. IRONFAN – a sonographic window into the natural history of fetal anomalies. *Ultrasound Obstet Gynecol* 1995;5:361

56. Bronshtein M, Blumenfeld Z. Transvaginal sonography detection of findings suggestive of fetal chromosomal anomalies in the first and early second trimester. *Prenat Diagn* 1992;12:587

57. D'Ottavio G *et al*. Pilot screening for fetal malformations: possibilities and limits of transvaginal sonography. *J Ultrasound Med* 1985;14:575–80

58. Cullen MT, Green J, Whethan J, *et al*. Transvaginal ultrasonographic detection of congenital anomalies in the first trimester. *Am J Obstet Gynecol* 1990;163:466

59. Achron R, Tadmor D. Screening for fetal anomalies during the first trimester of pregnancy: transvaginal versus transabdominal sonography. *Ultrasound Obstet Gynecol* 1991;1:186

60. Bonilla-Musales FA, Raga F, Ballester MJ, *et al*. Early detection of embryonic malformations by transvaginal and color Doppler sonography. *J Ultrasound Med* 1994;13:347

Three-dimensional ultrasonography of the embryo and fetus

20

Roger A. Pierson

Imaging technology is a constantly advancing science which provides ever enhanced visualization of the body. As the face of obstetrical practice has been forever changed by the advent of two-dimensional diagnostic ultrasonography, technological sophistication is now being developed into three-dimensional (3-D) ultrasonography which will allow detailed study of the anatomy, physiology and pathophysiology of the embryo and fetus. Advanced 3-D ultrasound imaging will greatly enhance our understanding of the developmental process and the care of pregnant women. Although 3-D ultrasonography is not yet a clinically standard imaging technique, the potential applications are so profound that a basic understanding of the images is essential for maintenance of leading-edge obstetrical care.

Ultrasonography is also extremely important in monitoring the development of the fetus during the second and third trimesters and in the immediately antenatal period. It is hard to imagine obstetrical practice without the ability to acquire detailed knowledge of 'what is going on in there'. However, two-dimensional (2-D) ultrasonography still suffers from several disadvantages which have impeded exploitation of its full potential. Three-dimensional imaging in obstetrics presents an especially difficult problem because of the combined effects of fetal movement, the extreme and ever changing curvature of the pregnant abdomen and the size of the fetus in the middle and later stages of gestation, which is larger than the imaging aperture of the ultrasound transducers.

The recent rapid advances in ultrasound and computer technology have made 3-D ultrasonography approach practicality in clinical settings. There have been nearly constant improvements in image acquisition techniques, reconstruction algorithms, computer power and display technology which have made many previously tedious steps in creating a 3-D image nearly invisible to the clinical ultrasonographer. Volume measurements now may

be made quickly and accurately and surface features are easily evaluated.

In conventional ultrasonography, the operator continuously scans over the fetus, or other structures of interest, in order to build up a mental image of the 3-D structure. One of the tremendous advantages of 3-D imaging is that once the images are acquired and reconstructed, the 3-D image may be rotated to different viewing planes and evaluated without continued scanning of the patient. Therefore, obstetrical examinations may be completed with significantly less scanning time and the physician may repeatedly examine the acquired volumetric data after the patient departs the ultrasound suite.

Three-dimensional ultrasonography is one very important way in which the shortfalls of 2-D imaging may be addressed. The purpose of this chapter is to elucidate the concepts involved in the current generation of 3-D ultrasound techniques and to explore the potential for their use in maternal–fetal medicine.

IMAGING TECHNIQUES

All individuals who work with standard 2-D ultrasonography instinctively know the steps which must occur to perform 3-D ultrasonography. As the ultrasonographer passes the transducer over the pregnant abdomen, he or she interprets the cross-sectional anatomy of the fetus and develops a mental image of 3-D structure in addition to interpreting the specific structures of interest in the 2-D images. To develop 3-D ultrasonography, the same events must occur; however, the ultrasound instrument or a separate computer must acquire, register, assemble, reconstruct and display the 3-D image[1]. There are many techniques for accomplishing this process. In the following discussion, the types of 3-D imaging in most common use in obstetrical ultrasound will be presented, although the list is by no means all-encompassing.

DATA ACQUISITION TECHNIQUES

The first step in any 3-D imaging protocol is to acquire a series of high quality 2-D images. The methods of performing the 3-D data acquisition step are many, but one of the most important components of all techniques is that the acquisition technique must be rapid enough to account for movements of the fetus and the mother. Slow acquisition times induce large artifacts in the final 3-D image. Free-hand techniques which utilize position locators on the transducer are under development for the larger second and third trimester fetuses, while linear and rotational techniques are preferred for first trimester embryos and fetuses.

Free-hand acquisition

The difficulties associated with positioning of second and third trimester fetuses *in utero* make a free-hand approach to 3-D imaging the most attractive in the middle and later stages of gestation. The fetal head and other body parts may be located with conventional 2-D ultrasonography and the plane of scan established. A position locator on the transducer places a simple code at each location where a 2-D image is acquired. This code is used in the registration and reconstruction steps. The images are acquired with arbitrary position under the ultrasonographer's control and may be optimized for view and orientation.

Conceptually, the free-hand method would be optimal for transabdominal scanning of obstetrical patients because of the complexities of fetal position and the curvature of the maternal abdomen. However, free-hand scanning also places the 3-D reconstruction system under the most severe constraints because the exact relative angle and probe position must be determined for each 2-D image that is acquired. Several methods for exact location of the transducer and its position on the abdomen have been developed. They range from acoustic position locators to articulated arms or magnetic field sensors; however, none are in current clinical use[1].

Linear acquisition

Linear frame acquisition is best suited to transabdominal scanning. With the linear technique, a standard clinical transducer is mounted to an apparatus which moves the transducer along a defined axis. The 2-D images are acquired at defined intervals which typically reflect the beam width of the transducer being used. Since the images are acquired in predefined intervals and are parallel to each other, this technique is efficient in both the acquisition and reconstruction steps of 3-D imaging (Figure 1).

Rotational acquisition

Rotational acquisition refers to a method of imaging in which the scan head remains fixed upon a single axis and the images are acquired by rotating the scan head or the entire transducer around the axis. Images are acquired at predetermined degrees of rotation as the acquired images sweep around the axis, typically in a conical fashion. Curvi-linear or linear transducers are typically used with either internal or external apparatuses for rotating the transducer around a central axis. Rotational image acquisition also is well-suited to intravaginal imaging using highly specialized probes to evaluate embryos or fetuses in the first trimester of pregnancy (Figure 2).

Two-dimensional arrays

Two-dimensional arrays utilize a different technique for the acquisition and display of 3-D acoustic data. The multiplanar technique utilizes electronic scanning to create a 2-D array of acoustic energy which moves away from the array in a pyramidal shape[1]. The ultrasound data are then processed in orthogonal planes to yield a thick slab of image data which may be displayed in three dimensions in near real-time. This type of imaging technology is now available clinically and shows great promise in the evaluation of surface features of the embryo and fetus (Figure 3).

THREE-DIMENSIONAL RECONSTRUCTION OF ACQUIRED ULTRASOUND IMAGE DATA

Reconstruction of the 3-D image refers to the registration and display of the 2-D data sets from

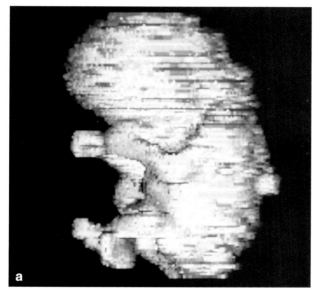

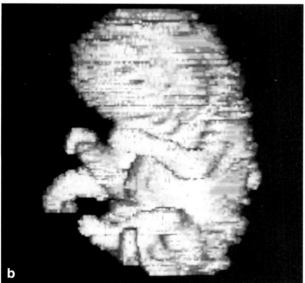

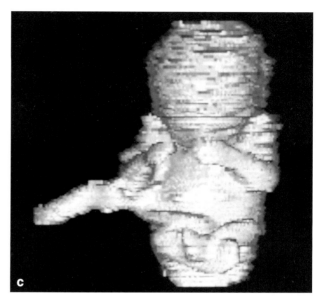

Figure 1 (**a,b,c**) Surface-rendered three-dimensional images of a 12-week gestational age fetus. Individual 2-D images were acquired with a transabdominal transducer in a linear sequence, segmented, reconstructed and surface rendered

the acquired images of the embryo or fetus[2,3]. There are two distinct methods of implementing the data reconstruction. The series of 2-D images, regardless of the method of acquisition, may be segmented to extract the precise information desired before actual 3-D image reconstruction[4–6]. This technique has the advantage of reducing the amount of data that must be manipulated, which allows more efficient rendering of the final image; however, much potentially important data may also be removed from the adjoined structures. The extraction of features or other data for evaluation is also a time-consuming task which must be done manually with most obstetrical applications.

The second technique uses the acquired 2-D images to build a voxel-based volumetric data set by placing each 2-D image in its proper place within the data volume. No assumptions are made regarding the desirability of any of the original data, so no data are lost in the 3-D reconstruction[1,6]. The technique allows for a variety of rendering techniques; however, the data files may be very large and may be difficult to manipulate in near real-time.

RENDERING OF THREE-DIMENSIONAL DATASETS

The reconstructed 3-D data sets must finally be rendered, or translated into a visual form, for viewing of the final image. A variety of techniques are available, but all typically fall into either surface rendering or volume rendering categories[1,4,7]. The choice of rendering technique is highly dependent upon the clinical application of the 3-D image and the method with which the original ultrasonographic data were acquired.

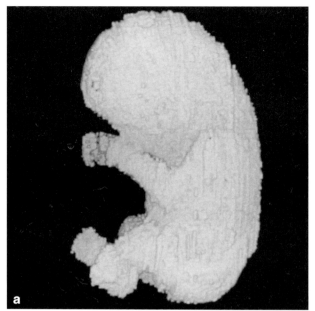

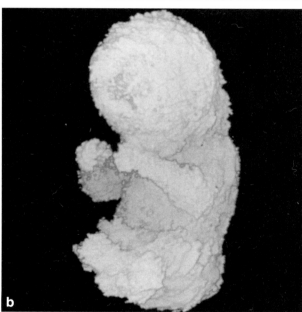

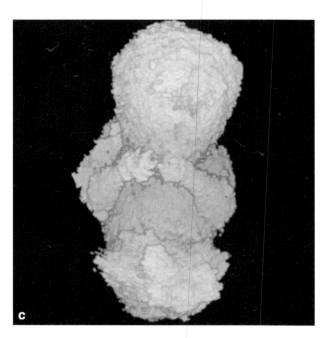

Figure 2 (**a,b,c**) Surface-rendered three-dimensional images of a 12-week gestational age fetus in which the images were acquired with an intravaginal transducer in a rotational sequence, segmented, reconstructed and rendered. Note the improved detail in the surface features compared to the images in Figure 1

image. In surface rendering images, the representations of the surface are shaded and illuminated so that the surface tomography and 3-D relationships of the structures may be appreciated. Directional algorithms are then applied so that the operator may rotate or move the 3-D model to view different aspects of the structures, view the anatomy from differing perspectives or study the inter-relationships among neighbouring structures. This technique is particularly useful for evaluating fetal malformations and congenital anomalies.

Surface rendering techniques

Surface rendering is based upon visualizing the surfaces of the embryos, fetuses or their internal organs. In this approach, the first step is image segmentation or classification of the structures contained within the voxel data[1-6]. A human operator or computerized algorithm analyze each voxel and must determine the structure to which the voxel belongs. Once the boundaries of the structures are classified, either wire-frame models or surface rendering may be used to view the final

Multiplanar image display

Multiplanar viewing is based upon a 3-D voxel-based image which is easily accessible to the display algorithm[1]. Imaging planes are selected from the original volume and may be viewed as reformatted 2-D images. The desired planes are displayed on the viewing screen simultaneously and contain cues to assist in spatial orientation for the examination of the images. This is the system that is currently available for clinical use. Multiplanar visualization may also be accomplished with texture mapping

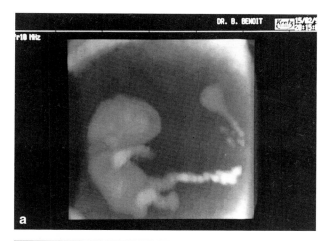

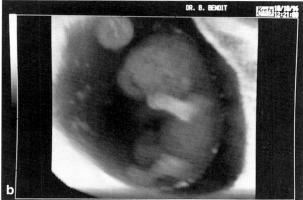

Figure 3 (a,b) Surface-rendered three-dimensional image of a multiplanar scan of a 10-week, 5-day gestational age fetus. Note the echoes representing the amnion and yolk sac in addition to the orientation of the fetus in the uterine cavity. Images courtesy of Dr B. Benoit

techniques[1]. The 3-D image may be displayed as a polyhedron representing the boundaries of the reconstructed volume. As the polyhedron is rotated, its exposed faces may be texture mapped allowing the operator to have immediate image-based spatial location cues.

Volume rendering techniques

Volume rendering presents the operator with all of the 3-D image data after it has been projected onto a 2-D plane, e.g. the computer screen. Volume-based techniques present the fetal anatomy in a semi-translucent manner and conserve all of the original 3-D information. Depth cues may be added to facilitate viewing; however, this may present more problems than the value of the image. One of the most successful applications of the volume rendering technique has been in displaying embryonic and fetal anatomy (Figure 4). This is due to the natural segmentation of the embryo or fetus from the maternal structures by the surrounding amniotic fluid.

APPLICATIONS IN OBSTETRICS

The fluid–tissue interface of the embryo or fetus and the surrounding fluid provides an ideal environment for the application of 3-D ultrasonography. All of the 3-D imaging techniques previously discussed are optimized in obstetrical imaging. Three-dimensional perspectives of the development of the embryo and its transformation to a fetus are striking and will allow detailed study of normal developmental processes and pathophysiologic changes. Enhanced details of the fetal head and face in 3-D provide an imaging perspective that is simply not available with conventional 2-D ultrasonography, even in the most experienced hands.

Three-dimensional ultrasonography of the embryo and early fetus

Ultrasonography is an important part of prenatal care in the first trimester, as well as later stages of gestation. The quality of images produced by the current generation of 2-D ultrasound instruments makes it indispensable for visualizing early obstetrical events. This ability to distinguish extremely fine detail is one of the tenets in the development of 3-D imaging (Figure 5). The underlying quality of the 2-D images is crucial to the success of 3-D imaging. The first trimester of gestation is also the period when 3-D imaging is easiest because the embryo or early fetus is small and typically falls within the imaging aperture of most transabdominal and transvaginal ultrasound transducers.

In the first trimester, 3-D ultrasound volumetric and multiplanar imaging may be used to study the relationships among the embryo, developing placenta and amniotic cavity (Figure 6). In women with leiomyomata, the inter-relationships of placental development and circulation and the fibroid may be assessed and the potential for early embryonic loss evaluated.

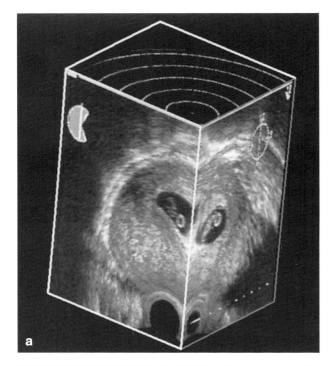

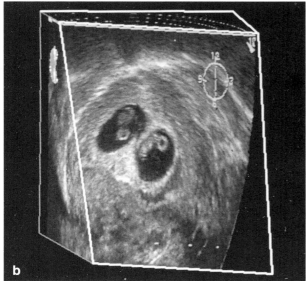

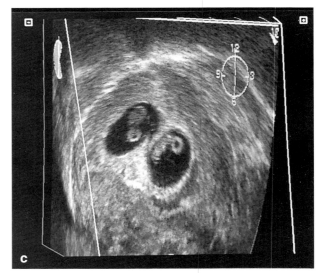

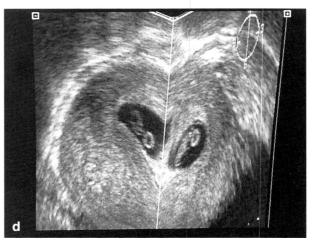

Figure 4 (a,b,c,d) Volume-rendered three-dimensional images of an approximately 7-week gestational age twin pregnancy displayed in different orientations and planes. Notice the relationships among the embryos, developing placentas and uterine environment. Images courtesy of Drs A. Fenster and B. Downey

One particularly exciting application is in the evaluation of embryonic brain cavities as early as 7 to 10 weeks of gestational age[8]. At 7 weeks of gestational age, both hemispheres of the brain and their connections to the third ventricle have been visualized. The study of early embryonic brain development opens a new window on developmental neuroanatomy. Neural tube defects also are perhaps more easily appreciated in three dimensions, with the ability to dissect the volume data to evaluate the extent of the anomaly[9–11]. In

many cases, 3-D ultrasonography would be highly useful in detecting subtle abnormalities, such as cystic hygroma and cleft palate, at very early stages (Figures 7 and 8). These defects would be easily visualized with accurate surface rendering techniques or multiplanar imaging. Abdominal wall defects, such as gastroschisis and skeletal dysplasia, while usually identified with 2-D ultrasonography would be expected to be clearly and unambiguously displayed in 3-D[9,10,12,13]. More severe anomalies, such as segmental agenesis,

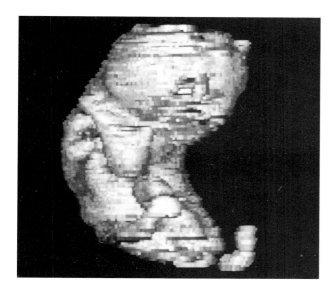

Figure 5 Surface-rendered, linear acquired image of an 8-week gestational age embryo. The cephalic aspect is clearly displayed; the cardiac prominence and limbs are just starting to be recognizable. Craniofacial details remain obscure

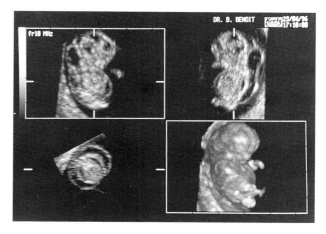

Figure 7 Multiplanar and orthogonal 3-D views of a 9 week gestational age fetus with pathologic changes associated with hydrops. Image planes are indicated by the white line markers. The 3-D image is in the lower right corner. Images courtesy of Dr B. Benoit

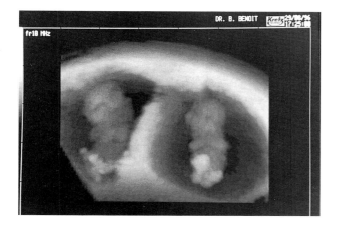

Figure 6 Orthogonal multiplanar view of a 9-week gestational age twin gestation. Embryonic features are discernible and the depth clues provided in this type of image enable excellent three-dimensional visualization. Compare the multiplanar images in this figure with the volumetric images in Figure 4. Images courtesy of Dr B. Benoit

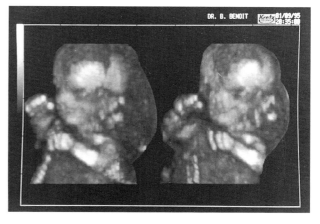

Figure 8 Orthogonal 3-D images of a 12-week gestational age fetus with cystic hygroma associated with trisomy 21. Images courtesy of Dr B. Benoit

Fetal three-dimensional ultrasonography

The fetal head and face of second and third trimester fetuses provide the most dramatic impact in obstetrical scanning. The outlines of the eyes, nose, and lips are easily identified even by inexperienced observers. Three-dimensional scanning may also be used to evaluate the anatomy of the fetal brain, cerebellum and cervical vertebrae[11,14,15] (Figure 9). The structure and location of the ears

would be similarly demonstrated with the improved delineation provided by surface rendering, volume rendering and multiplanar 3-D techniques.

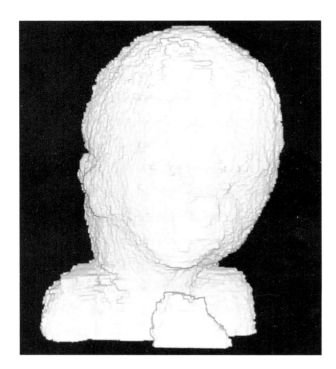

Figure 9 Linear three-dimensional reconstruction of the head of a fetus at 16 weeks of gestational age. Facial details around the eyes, nose and lips are becoming evident, as is the location of the ears

may be more easily evaluated and defects in the ears and lips may be appreciated within their spatial relationships to the surrounding cheeks, nose, mouth, and chin[15]. There is also a significant role for 3-D imaging in counseling patients with fetuses which have craniofacial or other anomalies (Figure 10). The nature and severity of the defect may be clearly communicated visually to the parents and other healthcare providers involved in the patient's care and allow prenatal consultation regarding potential interventions or postnatal corrections.

Multiplanar imaging of the spine appears to be a particularly useful technique. The entire length of the spinal column may be examined for any evidence of spina bifida, as the cervical, thoracic, lumbar and sacral spine may be visualized in all orthogonal planes (Figure 11). Three-dimensional ultrasonography also holds much potential in the evaluation of the developing cardiovascular system. It is anticipated that cardiac lesions such as septal defects and valvular anomalies would be more easily detected and that fetal echocardiography would be a first-line beneficiary of 3-D imaging techniques, especially as small defects may

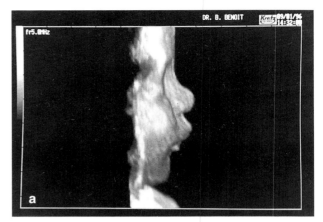

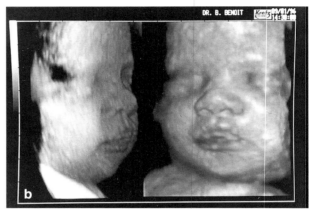

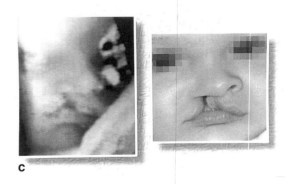

Figure 10 Orthogonal 3-D images of the fetal head and face of a 32-week gestational age fetus. (**a**) Profile. (**b**) Oblique views. Fine details of the facial features may be appreciated in three-dimensional views. (**c**) Near term fetus with a cleft palate demonstrated on an orthogonal surface rendered 3-D ultrasound image (left) and neonate following delivery (right). Images courtesy of Dr B. Benoit

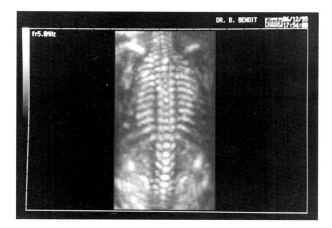

Figure 11 The complete spinal column, ribs, scapulae and some areas of pelvic ossification are clearly demonstrated in this orthogonal 3-D image of a 25-week gestational age fetus. Image courtesy of Dr B. Benoit

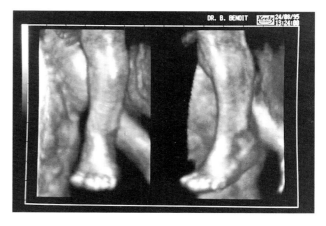

Figure 12 Orthogonal views of the legs and feet of a 25 week gestational age fetus. Detailed examination of the extremities, especially the hands and feet are greatly enhanced with the use of 3-D imaging techniques. Image courtesy of Dr B. Benoit

be evaluated in many different imaging planes without prolonged interactive scanning[11].

The fetal abdomen is expected to be easily evaluated with volumetric imaging; the insertion of the umbilical vein and hepatic circulation holds great potential for early and thorough examination. An early study utilized 3-D ultrasonography to characterize the configuration of the fetal stomach *in utero* in control fetuses; eleven additional fetuses with congenital duodenal obstruction were diagnosed at 29 to 37 weeks of gestation[16,17]. Investigation of the genitourinary system is also possible with 3-D imaging and may be especially useful in detecting renal anomalies and visualization of the external genitalia.

Accurate early prenatal diagnosis of fetal anomalies and malformations may enhance fetal outcomes. Two-dimensional ultrasonography is used routinely in the diagnosis and evaluation of fetal anomalies; however, there are many nooks and crannies in normal and abnormal fetuses that seemingly defy routine investigation. Three-dimensional ultrasonography is expected to solve many of these diagnostic dilemmas by providing the ability to interrogate image planes within the volumetric data that are simply unattainable with conventional 2-D ultrasonography (Figures 11 and 12). In addition, many fetal defects, such as cystic hygroma, the sandal gap between the first and second phalanges of the foot and missing or shortened fifth metacarpals on the hand associated with trisomy 21 may be more easily appreciated

with 3-D ultrasonography and greatly shorten the length of time which must be taken with routine screening ultrasound scans. Volumetric assessment of fetal size is highly desirable in maternal–fetal medicine centers in cases of intrauterine growth restriction. The accurate volumetric assessment of entire third trimester fetuses remains just out of reach of all of the current generation of 3-D techniques, although if the technologic advances continue to occur at the pace of the past decade, 3-D imaging of the whole fetus is within our grasp.

CONCLUSIONS

Although 3-D imaging has been the stuff of dreams since the first ultrasound images were generated, only recently has the technology developed to the point where 3-D imaging in clinical obstetrics has come into the realm of the possible. Three-dimensional ultrasonography remains somewhat shrouded in industrial secrecy and intellectual property protection; however, instruments capable of rendering 3-D images of the embryo and fetus are slowly moving from research laboratories into clinical medicine. It is doubtful that the transition from conventional 2-D ultrasonography into 3-D imaging will take long once physicians become comfortable with computer technology and have confidence in the accuracy of the images that are generated.

Three-dimensional imaging has the potential to make ultrasonography substantially easier to perform and to interpret. However, to be truly useful, 3-D ultrasound imaging must also occur in real-time or near real-time. The imaging steps must take place at the patient's side and be interpreted, at least superficially, in the patient's presence. Ultimately, 3-D ultrasound imaging will make the evaluation of embryos and fetuses easier and more accurate, and progressively earlier and more accurate diagnoses of fetal anomalies will enhance quality of patient care. The volume data available with 3-D ultrasonography will serve the physicians responsible for the care of mothers and their fetuses, and their patients, well as 3-D imaging becomes a routine and efficient tool in obstetrical practice.

ACKNOWLEDGEMENTS

Images used in the chapter were contributed from three different laboratories. Volume rendered images were contributed by Drs Aaron Fenster and Bruce Downey of the Robarts Institute of the University of Western Ontario in London, Ontario, Canada. Multiplanar images were contributed by Dr Bernard Benoit of the Hôpital Archet, Nice, France. Linear and rotational images were provided by the author's laboratory at the University of Saskatchewan, Saskatoon, Canada and reflect the collaboration of John Deptuch, Joel Koehler, Nan Weng and Herb Yang. Original work in the Women's Health Imaging Research Laboratory is funded by the Medical Research Council of Canada.

References

1. Fenster A, Downey DB. 3-D ultrasound imaging: a review. *IEEE Engineer Med Biol* 1996;15: 41–9

2. Prothero JS, Prothero JW. Three-dimensional reconstruction from serial sections. *Computer Biomed Res* 1986;19:361–73

3. Johnson EM, Capowski JJ. Principles of reconstruction and three-dimensional display of serial sections. In Ranney Mize R, ed. *The Microcomputer in Cell and Neurobiology Research.* New York: Elsevier Science, 1985:249–63

4. Muzzolini RE, Yang YH, Pierson RA. Multidimensional texture characterization using robust statistics. *Pattern Recognition* 1993;27:119–34

5. Muzzolini RE, Yang YH, Pierson RA. Multiresolution texture segmentation with application to diagnostic ultrasound images. *Internat Inst Electr Electron Engineers Trans Med Imag (IEEE)* 1993;12: 108–23

6. Muzzolini RE, Yang YH, Pierson RA. Three-dimensional segmentation of volume data. *Internat Inst Electr Electron Engineers Trans Med Imag (IEEE)* 1994;3:488–92

7. Weng N, Yang YH, Pierson RA. 3D surface reconstruction using optical flow for medical imaging. *Proc IEEE Nuclear Sci Symp Med Imaging Conf* 1996; Abstr:158

8. Blaas HG, Eik-Nes SH, Kiserud T, *et al.* Three-dimensional imaging of the brain cavities in human embryos. *Ultrasound Obstet Gynecol* 1995;5:228–32

9. Merz E, Bahlmann F, Weber G. Volume scanning in the evaluation of fetal malformations: a new dimension in prenatal diagnosis. *Ultrasound Obstet Gynecol* 1995;5:222–7

10. Merz E, Bahlmann F, Weber G, *et al.* Three-dimensional ultrasonography in prenatal diagnosis. *J Perinat Med* 1995;23:213–22

11. Mueller GM, Weiner CP, Yankowitz J. Three-dimensional ultrasound in the evaluation of fetal head and spine anomalies. *J Obstet Gynecol* 1996;88: 372–8

12. Steiner H, Spitzer D, Weiss-Wichert PH, *et al.* Three-dimensional ultrasound in prenatal diagnosis of skeletal dysplasia. *Prenat Diagn* 1995;15:373–7

13. Hamper UM, Trapanooto V, Sheth S, *et al.* Three-dimensional US: preliminary clinical experience. *Radiology* 1994;191:397–401

14. Kuo HC, Chang FM, Wu CH, *et al.* The primary application of three-dimensional ultrasonography in obstetrics. *Am J Obstet Gynecol* 1992;166:880–6

15. Devonald KJ, Ellwood DA, Oxon D, *et al.* Volume imaging: three-dimensional appreciation of the fetal head and face. *J Ultrasound Med* 1995;14:919–25

16. Nagata S, Koyanagi T, Fukushima S, *et al.* Change in the three-dimensional shape of the stomach in the developing human fetus. *Early Hum Dev* 1994;37: 27–38

17. Yoshizato T, Koyanagi Y, Nagata S, *et al.* Three-dimensional ultrasound of the fetal stomach: congenital duodenal obstruction *in utero. Early Hum Dev* 1995;14:39–47

Index

abdominal circumference (AC)   50–51, 68
   FL/AC ratio   53, 67, 84
   HC/AC ratio   52, 67, 84
   IUGR diagnosis   67
   macrosomia detection   84
   TC/AC ratio   53, 132
   TCD/AC ratio   53
abdominal cysts   147
abdominal pregnancy   33, 34
abdominal wall defects   143–145
   three-dimensional ultrasonography   322
abortion
   early pregnancy failure   27–28
   incomplete abortion   29
   inevitable abortion   29
   missed abortion   29
   threatened abortion   28–29
abruption, placental   93
absorption   3
acardia-acephalus   235
achondrogenesis type I   183
achondrogenesis type II   183–184
achondroplasia   184
acoustic impedance   3
acrania   108
adnexal mass   32, 33
adnexal ring   32
adrenal function   65
adrenal tumors   150
adrenoblastoma   150
alcohol effects   63
aliasing   6
allantoic cyst   97
alobar holoprosencephaly   112, 118, 120
amino acids, IUGR and   64
amniocentesis   203, 260, 261–263, 277, 287
   early amniocentesis   262–263
     clinical trials   271–273
   mid-trimester amniocentesis   269–270
   multiple gestation and   232
   techniques of   262, 263
amnionicity   94, 228
amniotic band   99
amniotic cavity   25
amniotic fluid   68–69, 99–101
   manipulation of   275
   multiple gestation and   231–232
   volume measurement   99–101, 247–248
   see also oligohydramnios; polyhydramnios
amniotic fluid index (AFI)   100, 220, 248
anembryonic pregnancy   29
anemia   62
   immune fetal hydrops and   222–223
anencephaly   108, 200, 202–203, 204

aneurysm of the vein of Galen   115, 117–118
anterior fontanelle   103, 104
antero-posterior abdominal diameter (APAD)   50
anticardiolipin antibodies   62
antiphospholipid antibodies   62
aorta   37, 156, 162, 166
   coarctation of   162, 164, 169
     surgical repair   169
   overriding aorta   162
aortic atresia   160, 166, 167–168
   surgical repair   168
aortic stenosis   166, 167
   surgical repair   167
aortic valve   155, 160, 162
arachnoid cysts   115, 117
arachnoid granulations, congenital absence of   115
Arnold–Chiari type II malformation   110, 115, 204
array transducers   7–8
   confocal imaging on transmit   7–8
   dynamic focusing on receive   8
   grating lobes   9
   out-of-plane focusing and beam-width artifacts   8–9
   side lobes   9
arthrogryposis multiplex congenita (AMC)   184–185
ascites   147, 217
asphyxiating thoracic dysplasia   185
assisted reproduction techniques (ART), multiple
   gestations and   34, 227, 233
assocation   306
atrial septal defect (ASD)   160, 162, 167
   surgical repair   167
atrioventricular canal defect (AVCD)   168
atrioventricular valves (AV)   158, 160
attenuation see sound propagation in body
axial resolution   4–5

Ballentyne syndrome   224
banana sign   110, 204, 310
band width   2
beam forming   1–2
   frequency and band width   2
beam-width artifacts   8–9
Beckwith–Wiedemann syndrome   119
beta-human chorionic gonadotropin (hCG) assay,
   ectopic pregnancy   30–31
bilateral choroid plexus   39
biometry   47–56
   abdominal circumference (AC)   50–51, 67, 68
   biparietal diameter (BPD)   49, 66–67, 68
   cephalic index (CI)   49
   common errors   55
   estimated fetal weight (EFW)   51–52, 68, 84
   femur length (Fl)   51, 67, 68
   gestational sac   47

head circumference (HC) 49–50, 66–67, 68
  IUGR diagnosis 66–70
  macrosomia detection 84
  morphometric ratios 52–53, 67
  multiple gestation 55
  occipito-frontal diameter (OFD) 49
  ponderal index (PDI) 67
  transverse cerebellar diameter 53, 69
  yolk sac 47
  see also crown-rump length
biophysical profile 72, 248–252
  indications for 252
  interpretation 252
  neuromuscular function 248–249
  non-equivalence of score combinations 250
  performance and scoring of 249–250
biparietal diameter (BPD) 49, 68, 178
  FL/BPD ratio 53, 294
  IUGR diagnosis 66–67
bladder 42, 147
  exstrophy 143, 145, 151
blighted ova 29
blood sampling, fetal 264–266
  safety and accuracy of 274
Bochdalek hernia 133
bones, embryonic development 40–41
  see also skeletal disorders
Brachmann–de Lange syndrome 130, 133
brain 38–40
  anomalies 108–118
    absence of the septi pellucidi 113–114
    agenesis of the corpus callosum 113
    anencephaly 108, 200, 202–203
    aneurysms of the vein of Galen 117–118
    arachnoid cysts 117
    cephalocele 109
    choroid plexus cysts 117
    congenital hydrocephalus 115–117
    Dandy–Walker malformations 114–115
    exencephaly 108
    holoprosencephaly 111–113
    iniencephaly 108–109
    screening for 310
    spinal dysraphism 109–111
  IUGR and 72
  normal anatomy 104–107
    coronal sections 105–106
    sagittal sections 106–107
  three-dimensional ultrasonography 322
bronchial atresia 136–137
bronchogenic cysts 136

calcifications, placenta 90
cardia activity 25, 26–27, 37
  arrhythmia evaluation 158
  fetal heart rate 37
    control of 241–242
    monitoring of 239–240
  prognostic significance 28
  see also heart
cardiomyopathy 163, 164, 168–169
  surgical repair 169

cataracts, fetal 120
caudal regression syndrome 209–210
cavum septi pellucidi 105, 106
  absence of 113–114
central nervous system
  anomalies 107
  embryonic development 27, 38–40
  maturation of 248–249
  see also brain; neural tube; spine
cephalic index (CI) 49
cephalocele 108, 109, 130–131
cerebellum 39, 104, 106
cerebral changes in IUGR 65
cerebro-costo-mandibular syndrome 209
cesarean section
  macrosomia and 81
  multiple gestations 236
chest circumference 131–132
chondrodysplasia punctata 177
chondroectodermal dysplasia 185–186
chorioangioma 93
chorionic mosaicism 270–271, 273
chorionic sac 23
chorionic villus sampling (CVS) 260, 263–264, 269–270, 272–273, 287
  chorionic mosaicism and 270–271, 273
  multiple gestation and 232
  placental mosaicism and 270–271
  techniques of 263–264, 270
chorionicity 94, 228
choroid plexus 39, 104, 106, 115–117
  cysts 117, 292
chromosomal disorders 130
  IUGR and 60
  screening for 288–298
    by major structural defects 288–292
    fetal long bone measurements 294–296
    minor morphological markers 292
    nuchal skinfold thickness 292–293
    nuchal translucency thickness 297–298
  skeletal disorders and 177
  see also individual disorders
cingulate gyrus 106
cisterna magna 106
clavicles 41, 178
  biometry 54
  fractures, macrosomia and 81, 82
cleft lip 120–121
cleft palate 120–121
cloacal exstrophy 143, 145
club feet 178, 204
club hands 178
coarctation of the aorta 162, 164, 169
  surgical repair 169
cocaine 63
coelocentesis 268
color velocity imaging 14–15
compression 11–12
congenital contractures 184–185
congenital cystic adenomatoid malformation (CCAM) 135
congenital diaphragmatic hernia (CDH) 132–134, 143

congenital heart disease   153, 154, 310–312
congestive heart failure   169
conjoined twins   235–236
constructive interference   1
continuous wave Doppler   13
contraction stress testing (CST)   245–247
    interpretation of   246
    performance of   245–246
    predictive value of   246–247
contrast resolution   5
cordocentesis   71–72, 264–265
coronary heart disease, fetal origins hypothesis   72
corpus callosum   105, 106
    agenesis of   107, 109, 111, 113, 115
craniorachischisis   200, 204
crown-rump length (CRL)   199
    at onset of heart activity   37
    early embryo   25–26
    gestational age estimation   26, 48
cystic hygroma   129–130, 289
cystic renal disease   149

D-transposition of the great vessels (DTGA)   166, 169
    surgical repair   169
Dandy–Walker syndrome   109, 114–115
dangling choroid plexus sign   117
de Morsier syndrome   114
decidua   23
deformation   306
destructive interference   1
dextocardia   158–159
diabetes   163
    infant of diabetic mother   163, 170
    macrosomia and   82–83
diamniotic twins   94, 228
diaphragmatic hernia   132–134, 143
diastematomyelia   111, 205
diastrophic dysplasia   186
dichorionic twins   94, 228
diencephalon   38, 39
dilated cardiomyopathy   164, 168
    surgical repair   169
disruption   306
distal femoral epiphysis (DFE)   54
distichiasis-lymphedema syndromes   130
dizygotic twins   94, 227, 228
Doppler ultrasonography   12–20
    continuous wave Doppler   13
    Doppler color flow imaging   14–15
        color velocity imaging   14–15
        power Doppler imaging   15
    Doppler signal processing   15–16
    fetal wellbeing assessment   70–71
    pulsed wave Doppler   13–14
    spectral analysis   16–17
    system controls   20
    umbilical-feto-placental-circulation   18–19,
        252–254
        early detection of placental diseases   19
        placental resistance evaluation   253
    use in multiple gestations   233
    wave form analysis   17–18

see also ultrasound image generation
double decidual sac (DDS)   24, 28, 47
double outlet right ventricle (DORV)   162, 169
    surgical repair   169–170
double stomach bubble   145
Down's syndrome see trisomy 21
drainage procedures   275–276
drug ingestion, maternal
    fetal cardiac anomalies and   154
    IUGR and   63
ductus arteriosus   157, 167
ductus venosus   221
duodenal atresia   145, 289
dye dilution technique   100
dynamic range see ultrasound image generation
dyslipidemia   62
dysostoses   175, 205–206
dysplasia, definition of   175, 306
    see also skeletal disorders
dyssegmental dysplasia   186–187

early pregnancy failure   27–28
Ebstein's anomaly of the tricuspid valve   159, 162, 170
    surgical repair   170
echocardiographic views   153–158, 311
    aortic arch view   156–157
    ductal arch view   157
    four chamber view   54, 155, 311
        abnormalities   158–165
    great vessel view   155–156
        abnormalities   165–167
    inferior vena cava/superior vena cava/right atrium
        (IVC/SVC/RA) view   155
    see also cardiac activity; heart
ectopic pregnancy   23, 28, 30–34
    beta-hCG assay   30–31
    clinical assessment   31
    color Doppler imaging   33
    differential diagnosis   31
    management   33–34
    risk factors   30
    ultrasonographic evaluation   31–33
edema
    nuchal   289, 292
    placenta   219, 220
    skin   217, 219
    triple edema   224
    umbilical cord   97
Edwards' syndrome see trisomy 18
Ellis–van Creveld syndrome   185–186
embryonic development   26–27
    central nervous system   38–40
    early embryonic size   25–26
    gastrointestinal system   42–43
    genitalia   43–44
    heart   37–38
        cardiac activity   26–27, 28, 37
    skeletal system   40–41
    spine   199–201
    three-dimensional ultrasonography   321–323
    urinary tract   41–42
embryonic period   26–27

embryonic pole　25
embryoscopy　267
encephalocele　115, 202, 204
endothelin　63–64
epidermal growth factor　64
epilepsy　63
epiphyses　54
Erb's palsy, macrosomia and　81, 82
estimated fetal weight (EFW)　51–52
　　IUGR diagnosis　68
　　macrosomia detection　84
exencephaly　108
eye anomalies　120

face　118–122
　　anomalies　119–122
　　　　cleft lip and palate　120–121
　　　　eye　120
　　　　mandible　122
　　facial bones　41
　　scanning of　118–119
　　three-dimensional ultrasonography　323–324
falx cerebri　105
Fast Fourier Transform (FFT)　16
feet, skeletal disorders　178
femur length (FL)　51, 68
　　Down's syndrome and　294–296
　　FL/AC ratio　53, 67, 84
　　FL/BPD ratio　53, 294
　　IUGR diagnosis　67
　　macrosomia detection　84
fetal alcohol syndrome　63
fetal growth　68
　　multiple gestation　230–231
　　　　discordant twin growth　231
　　see also biometry; intrauterine growth restriction
　　　　(IUGR)
fetal heart activity see cardiac activity
fetal hydrops see hydrops fetalis
fetal movements　242, 248–249
　　see also non-stress testing
fetal origins hypothesis　72
fetal period　26
fetal sex identification　43–44
fetal transfusion therapy　275
fetal weight estimation see estimated fetal weight
fetal wellbeing assessment　70–72
　　amniotic fluid volume assessment　247–248
　　cordocentesis　71–72
　　Doppler velocimetry　70–71
　　fetal heart rate monitoring　239–240
　　see also biophysical profile; contraction stress
　　　　testing; non-stress testing
feto-placental circulation
　　Doppler waveform analysis　18–19
　　early detection of placental diseases　19
fetoscopy　267, 276–277
fibrin deposits, placenta　90
first arch syndrome　122
fixed lens focusing　7
focal depth of field　1
focusing see ultrasound image generation
Fontan procedure　168, 172

foramen of Morgagni hernia　133
free-hand acquisition　320
frequency　2
Fryns' syndrome　130, 133

gallbladder　42
gastrointestinal system
　　abnormalities　143–147
　　　　abdominal cysts　147
　　　　abdominal wall defects　143–145
　　　　ascites　147
　　　　bowel　146–147
　　embryonic development　42–43
　　herniation into umbilical cord　26, 42
　　see also stomach
gastroschisis　143–144, 312
gastrulation　199
genitalia　43–44
gestational age estimation　23, 47, 54
　　abdominal circumference (AC)　50–51
　　biparietal diameter (BPD)　49
　　cephalic index (CI)　49
　　common errors　55
　　crown-rump length (CRL) 26, 48
　　femur length (FL)　51
　　gestational sac　47
　　head circumference (HC)　49–50
　　multiple gestation　55, 229–230
　　occipito-frontal diameter (OFD)　49
　　orbital diameter　53
　　soft tissue parameters　51
　　TCD/AC ratio　53
　　yolk sac　47
gestational sac　23–24
　　growth of　28, 47
　　role in gestational age estimation　47
glucose, fetal growth and　64, 82–83
Goldenhar syndrome　122, 208, 209
grating lobes　9

Hadlock formula　84
hands, skeletal disorders　178
head circumference (HC)　49–50, 68, 178
　　HC/AC ratio　52, 67, 84
　　IUGR diagnosis　66–67
　　macrosomia detection　84
heart
　　abnormalities　158–172, 289
　　　　clinical significance and surgical repair　167–172
　　　　congenital heart disease　153, 154, 310–312
　　　　non-immune fetal hydrops and　223
　　　　screening for　310–312
　　　　see also individual abnormalities
　　biometry　54
　　embryology　37–38
　　see also cardiac activity; echocardiographic views
heart activity see cardiac activity
hemangioma, umbilical cord　99
hematoma, umbilical cord　97–99
hematopoietic stem cell transplantation　277
hemivertebra　187–188
hepatomegaly　219
hepatosplenomegaly　219

Hirschsprung disease 146
holoprosencephaly 111–113, 114, 118
humerus length, Down's syndrome and 296
hydatiform disease (molar pregnancy) 29–30, 91–93
hydrocephalus 109–111, 114, 115–117
  neural tube defect association 204, 205
hydronephrosis 150–151, 292
hydrops fetalis 135, 136, 137, 217–224
  hemodynamic assessment 220–222
  management
    immune fetal hydrops 222–223
    non-immune fetal hydrops 223–224
  maternal complications 224
  postpartum evaluation 224
  ultrasonographic diagnosis 217–220
hydroureter 150–151
hyperinsulinism, macrosomia and 83
hyperplacentosis 90
hypertension
  fetal origins hypothesis 72
  maternal 62
  see also pre-eclampsia
hypertrophic cardiomyopathy 169
hypoplastic left heart syndrome 160, 162, 166, 168, 170
hypoplastic thorax 178
hypoxia 248–249

idiopathic osteolyses 175
image generation see ultrasound image generation
implantation 23
  abnormalities 88–89
in vitro fertilization, multiple gestation and 227
incomplete abortion 29
inevitable abortion 29
infant of diabetic mother 163, 170
infections
  IUGR and 60
  placental abnormalities 91
inferior vena cava (IVC) 155, 221, 222
iniencephaly 108–109
inionschisis 200, 204
insulin, IUGR and 64
insulin-like growth factor 64
interference 1
interhemispheric fissure 105
interrupted aortic arch 166
interstitial pregnancy 33–34
interventricular foramen (of Monroe) 106
intestine see gastrointestinal system
intrauterine growth restriction (IUGR) 59–70
  decompensated fetus 72
  definition 59–60
  fetal adaptation to 63–65
    metabolic adaptation 64–65
    vascular adaptation 63–64
  fetal cerebral changes 65
  HC/AC ratio and 52
  long term sequelae 72
  management 65–72
    antenatal diagnosis 65–70
    see also fetal wellbeing assessment
  multiple gestation 230–231

pathophysiology 60–63
  cardiovascular disorders 62
  chromosomal disorders 60
  drug effects 63
  hematological disorders 62–63
  immunological disorders 62
  infections 60
  malnutrition 61–62
  placental mosaicism 60
  pregnancy maladaption 60–61

Jarcho–Levin syndrome 208–209
Jeune syndrome 185

kidneys 147
  abnormal position of 149
  biometry 54
  cystic renal disease 149
  embryonic development 41–42
  IUGR and 72
  renal agenesis/hypoplasia 148–149
  renal tumors 150
Klippel–Feil anomaly 206–207, 208
kyphomelic dysplasia 188

Lambda sign 228
Langer–Saldino syndrome 130
laryngel atresia 137
lateral resolution 4–5
lateral ventricles 105, 106
left atrium (LA) 156, 159
left ventricle (LV) 156, 158, 160–161, 164, 166
lemon sign 110, 204, 310
lethal anisospondylic camptomicromelic dwarfism 186
limb–body wall defect 143, 145
limbs 40
linear acquisition 318
liver 42
lobar holoprosencephaly 112–113

macrosomia 81–85
  associated risks 81–82
  definition 81
  detection of 83–84
  management 85
  pathophysiology 82–83
malformations 305, 306
  three-dimensional ultrasonography 325
  see also chromosomal disorders; screening
malnutrition 61–62
mandible 41
  anomalies 122
maternal maladaptation 61
maternal serum α-fetoprotein (MSAFP) 199, 287
maxilla 41
Meckel–Gruber syndrome 109, 114, 119, 306
mesencephalon 38, 39–40
mesoblastic nephroma 150
mesocardia 159
metencephalon 38
microcephaly 109, 111, 112
micrognathia 122
mineralization see ossification

mirror syndrome   224
miscarriage *see* abortion
missed abortion   29
mitral atresia   160, 162, 166, 170
mitral insufficiency   159, 170
mitral stenosis   162, 164
mitral valve   38, 160, 162
molar pregnancies   29–30, 91–93
monoamniotic twins   94, 228
   anomalies   234
monochorionic twins   94, 228
monozygotic twins   227, 228
multifetal pregnancy reduction   233, 275
multiplanar image display   320–321
multiple gestation   23, 34, 227–237
   amniotic fluid volume   231–232
   anomalies   233–236
      acardia-acephalus   235
      conjoined twins   235–236
      monoamniotic twins   234
      polyhydramnios-oligohydramnios sequence
         234–235
      twin transfusion syndrome (TTS)   233–234
      vanishing twins   235
   biometry   55
   chorionicity   228
   diagnosis   227
   fetal growth   230–231
      discordant twin growth   231
   frequency   227–228
   gestational age establishment   55, 229–230
   intrapartum management   236
   membranes   94
   multifetal pregnancy reduction   233, 275
   prenatal diagnosis and   232, 273–274
   presentation   230
   separation anxiety   228
multiple pterygium syndrome   122, 130
multiple vertebral segmentation defects   208–209
MURCS association   207–208
myelocele   109
myeloencephalon   38
myelomeningocele   109, 200, 205
   see also spina bifida
myocarditis   159

neck abnormalities   129–131
   cephalocele   108, 109, 130–131
   cystic hygroma   129–130
   screening for   310
   tumors   130
neoplasms, placenta   93
nephroblastoma   150
neural tube   38, 199–200
   defects   108–111, 200
      associated malformations   204
      screening for   310
      three-dimensional ultrasonography   322
      ultrasonographic findings   204–205
   see also individual defects; spine
non-stress testing   242–245
   indications for   244–245
   interpretation of   242–243

predictive value of   243–244
Noonan syndrome   130
Norwood procedure   168, 170
nuchal edema   289, 292
nuchal skinfold thickness   292–293
nuchal translucency thickness   288, 297–298

occipito-frontal diameter (OFD)   49
oligohydramnios   68–69, 101, 147, 248
   assessment of   247–248
   obstructive uropathy and   150–151
omphalocele   97, 143–144, 289, 312
one centimeter rule (amniotic fluid volume
   measurement)   100
orbital diameter   53, 178
ossification   40–41
   epiphyses   54
   spine   38, 41, 200–201
osteochondrodysplasias   175, 206
osteogenesis   40
osteogenesis imperfecta   188–189
out-of-plane focusing   8–9
overriding aorta   162
oxytocin challenge test (OCT)   245

Patau's syndrome *see* trisomy   13
pelvis, skeletal disorders   181
Pena–Shokeir syndrome   185
penis   44
pericardial effusion   164–165, 219
perinatal mortality   239, 307–308
persistence   12
Pierre Robin syndrome   119, 122
placenta   87–94
   abnormalities   88–93
      abruption   93
      adherence abnormalities   89
      calcifications   90
      fibrin deposits   90
      hydatiform change   91–93
      infarcts   61, 90
      infection   91
      maternal vasculopathy   93
      neoplasms   93
      site of placental attachment   88–89
      thickness   90
      type of implantation   89
   early detection of placental diseases   19
   IUGR and   64, 69
   limitation of placental blood flow   240–241
   placental edema   219, 220
   placental grading   87–88
   placental resistance evaluation   253
   ultrasonographic evaluation of   87–88
      intraplacental villous vessel Doppler ultrasound   71
      see also feto-placental circulation
placenta accreta   89
placenta circummarginata   89
placenta circumvallata   89
placenta extrachorialis   89
placenta increta   89
placenta percreta   89
placenta previa   88–89

placental mosaicism
    chorionic villus sampling and   270–271
    IUGR and   60
pleural effusion   137, 219
polyhydramnios   101, 130, 147, 248
    assessment of   247–248
    brain anomalies and   108–109, 115
    hydrops fetalis and   219–220
    thoracic abnormalities and   133, 134, 135, 136
polyhydramnios-oligohydramnios sequence   234–235
ponderal index (PDI), IUGR diagnosis   67
power Doppler imaging   15
pre-eclampsia   61
pregnancy dating see gestational age estimation
pregnancy maladaption   60–61
prenatal diagnosis   259–269, 307
    choice of invasive procedures   274
    coelocentesis   268
    embryoscopy   267
    fetal blood sampling   264–266, 274
    fetal tissue biopsy   266, 274
    fetal urine sampling   266–267
    fetoscopy   267
    multiple gestation   232, 273–274
    safety and accuracy   269–274
    transcervical flushing   269
    see also amniocentesis; chorionic villus sampling
prosencephalon   38
proximal tibial epiphysis (PTE)   54
prune belly syndrome   135, 151
pseudoascites   217
pseudocampomelia   188
pseudotoxemia   224
pulmonary artery (PA)   155–157, 166, 170, 172
pulmonary atresia   161, 162, 165–167, 170
    surgical repair   170
pulmonary sequestration   136
pulmonary stenosis   166, 170–172
    surgical repair   172
pulmonary valve   155
pulsatility index (PI)   18, 253
    umbilical artery   18–19
pulse repetition frequency (PRF)   13–14, 20
pulsed wave Doppler   13–14
pyelectasis   150, 292

RADIUS trial   308–309, 312
Rastelli procedure   169–170
renal agenesis/hypoplasia   148–149
renal tumors   150
resistance index (RI)   18, 253
resolution see sound propagation in body
reverberations   6
rhombencephalon   38–39
ribs   41
right atrium (RA)   155, 159, 162, 172
right ventricle (RV)   156, 160–164, 166, 170, 172
    double outlet right ventricle   162, 169
        surgical repair   169–170
Robert's syndrome   177
Rossavik growth models   59
rotational acquisition   318

S/D ratio   18, 252–253
sacrococcygeal teratoma   210–211, 224
    differential diagnosis   210
    management and outcome   120–211
scapular biometry   54
scattering   3
schisis association   204
scoliosis   207
screening   305–314
    accuracy of   309–312
    gestational age and   312–313
    routine ultrasound in pregnancy   306–307
        effects of   307–309, 314
        safety of   313
    transvaginal ultrasound as tool   314
    see also chromosomal disorders
semilobar holoprosencephaly   112–113
septi pellucidi see cavum septi pellucidi
sequences   306
sex identification   43–44
shadowing and enhancement   4
Shepard formula   84
short-rib polydactyly syndrome (SRPS)   189–192
shoulder dystocia, macrosomia and   81, 82
shrink wrapped stuck twin   233
shunting procedures   275–276
sickle cell disease   62
side lobes   9
single umbilical artery (SUA)   96–97
situs ambiguous   159
situs inversus   158
skeletal disorders   175–195
    achondrogenesis type I   183
    achondrogenesis type II   183–184
    achondroplasia   184
    arthrogryposis multiplex congenita (AMC)   184–185
    asphyxiating thoracic dysplasia   185
    associated anomalies   182
    chondroectodermal dysplasia   185–186
    classification   175–177
    diagnosis of   177–182
        algorithmic approach   181–182
        hands and feet   178
        long bones   177–178
        pelvis   181
        skull   178
        spine   181
        thorax   178
    diastrophic dysplasia   186
    dyssegmental dysplasia   186–187
    genetics and   177
    hemivertebra   187–188
    kyphomelic dysplasia   188
    osteogenesis imperfecta   188–189
    postnatal evaluation   182–183
    prevalence   175
    short-rib polydactyly syndrome (SRPS)   189–192
    thanatophoric dysplasia   192–195
    see also spine
skeletal system embryology   40–41
skin edema   217,219
Skull   41, 104

biparietal diameter (BPD)   49, 66–67, 68
  cephalic index (CI)   49
  occipito-frontal diameter (OFD)   49
  skeletal disorders   178, 182
small bowel obstruction   146
smoking effects   63
sound propagation in body   1–6
  attenuation   3–4, 10–11
    absorption   3
    acoustic impedance   3
    shadowing and enhancement   4
    specular reflection and scattering   3
  beam forming   1–2
  frequency and band width   2
  interference   1
  resolution   4–5
    contrast resolution   5
    spatial resolution   4–5
  reverberations   6
  speckles   5–6
    under-sampling and aliasing   6
spatial resolution   4–5
speckles   5–6
specular reflection   3
spina bifida   110, 200, 202–205
  associated malformations   204
  screening for   310
  spina bifida occulta   204
  ultrasonographic findings   204–205
spinal dysraphism   109–111, 203–204
  occult spinal dysraphism   204
spine   41, 199–212
  embryonic development   199–201
  ossification   38, 41, 200–201
  skeletal disorders   181, 182
    caudal regression syndrome   209–210
    cerebro-costo-mandibular syndrome   209
    fetal scoliosis   207
    hemivertebra   187–188
    Klippel–Feil anomaly   206–207
    multiple vertebral segmentation defects
      208–209
    MURCS association   207–208
    Sprengel deformity   208
    VATER association   207–208
    Wildervanck syndrome   207
  ultrasonographic examination of   201–202
    three-dimensional ultrasonography   324–325
  see also neural tube
spiral arteries   61, 241
Sprengel deformity   208
stomach   42–43
  abnormalities   145–146
  see also gastrointestinal system
subchorionic hematoma   28–29
subclavian artery supply disruption sequence (SASDS)
  208
superior vena cava (SVC)   155
surface rendering techniques   320
Sylvian fissure   106
symphysis fundal height, IUGR diagnosis   66
syndromes   306
systemic lupus erythematosus   62

telencephalon   38
teratoma, cervical   130
tetralogy of Fallot   162, 164, 172
  surgical repair   172
thanatophoric dysplasia   192–195
thigh circumference   51, 69–70
thoracic abnormalities   131–137
  asphyxiating thoracic dysplasia   185
  bronchial atresia   136–137
  bronchogenic cysts   136
  congenital cystic adenomatoid malformation (CCAM)
    135
  congenital diaphragmatic hernia (CDH)   132–134
  laryngeal atresia   137
  pleural effusion   137
  pulmonary sequestration   136
  skeletal disorders   178
  tracheal atresia   137
thoracic circumference (TC)   131–132
  TC/AC ratio   53, 132
thoracopelvic-phalangeal dystrophy   185
threatened abortion   28–29
three-dimensional ultrasonography   317–326
  applications   321–325
    embryo   321–323
    fetus   323–325
  data acquisition techniques   318
  imaging techniques   317–318
  reconstruction of image data   318–319
  rendering of datasets   319–321
    multiplanar image display   320–321
    surface rendering techniques   320
    volume rendering techniques   321
thrombophilia   63
thrombosis of the umbilical vessels   99
thyroid function   65
time gain compensation   11
tissue biopsy, fetal   266
  safety and accuracy of   274
tobacco effects   63
total anomalous pulmonary venous return (TAPVR)
  159, 172
  surgical repair   172
total intrauterine volume, IUGR and   69
tracheal atresia   137
transabdominal ultrasonography (TAS)   23
transcervical flushing   269
transvaginal ultrasonography (TVS)   23, 103–104
  fetal brain   104
  as screening tool   314
transverse abdominal diameter (TAD)   50
transverse cerebellar diameter (TCD)   53
  IUGR diagnosis   69
  TCD/AC ratio   53
Treacher Collins syndrome   119, 122
tricuspid atresia   161, 172
  surgical repair   172
tricuspid stenosis   161–162, 164
tricuspid valve   38, 155, 161–162
  Ebstein's anomaly   159, 162, 170
    surgical repair   170
triglycerides, IUGR and   64
triple edema   224

triploidy   60, 114, 288
trisomy 4:   130
trisomy 13 (Patau's syndrome)   288
  facial anomalies and   119, 120, 122
  neck anomalies and   130
  screening for   290
  skeletal disorders and   177
trisomy 18 (Edward's syndrome)   60, 133, 287, 288
  brain anomalies and   117
  congenital diaphragmatic hernia and   133, 134
  facial anomalies and   119, 122
  neck anomalies and   130
  screening for   290, 292
  skeletal disorders and   177
trisomy 21 (Down's syndrome)   133, 287–288
  amniocentesis and   261
  brain anomalies and   117
  cardiac anomalies and   162, 168
  facial anomalies and   119
  gastrointestinal disorders and   145, 147
  maternal serum screening test   199
  neck anomalies and   130
  screening for   287–288, 290–297
truncus arteriosus   162, 166–167, 172
  surgical repair   172
tubal pregnancy see ectopic pregnancy
Turner's syndrome   130, 288
twin transfusion syndrome (TTS)   233–234
twin-peak sign   94
twins see mutiple gestation
two-dimensional arrays   320

ultrasound image generation   1, 6–12
 dynamic range   9–12
  compression   11–12
  time gain compensation   11
 focusing   6–9
  with array transducer   7–8
  fixed lens focusing   7
  out-of-plane focusing and beam-width artifacts   8–9
 grating lobes   9
 gray scale system control effects   12
 persistence   12
 side lobes   9
 signal processing chain   6
 see also Doppler ultrasonography; sound propagation
  in body; three-dimensional ultrasonography
umbilical arteries   94–95
 Doppler waveform analysis   18–19, 252–254
  early detection of placental diseases   19
  fetal wellbeing assessment   70–71
  IUGR and   63
  placental resistance evaluation   253

single umbilical artery (SUA)   96–97
umbilical cord   94–99
  amniotic band   99
  fetal intestine herniation into   26, 42
  masses   97–99
  single umbilical artery (SUA)   96–97
  stricture   95
  supernumerary cord vessels   97
  umbilical edema   97
umbilical vein   94–95, 221
under-sampling   6
ureters   147
urinary tract   41–42
  abnormalities   147–151
  obstructive uropathy   150–151
    posterior urethral valve (PUV)   151
    ureteropelvic junction (UPJ)   150
    ureterovesical junction (UVJ)   150–151
  see also bladder, kidneys
urine sampling, fetal   266–267
uterine artery Doppler ultrasound   71

VACTERL syndrome   146, 148
vaginal bleeding   28–29
vaginal delivery, macrosomia and   81
vanishing twins   235
VATER association   207–208
vein of Galen, aneurysm of   115, 117–118
ventricular inversion   160
ventricular septal defect (VSD)   160–164, 166,
  169–170, 172
  surgical repair   172
ventriculomegaly   115–117, 292
vertebrae   41
  hemivertebra   187–188
  multiple vertebral segmentation defects   208–209
  ossification   38, 41, 200, 201
  skeletal disorders   181
  see also spine
volume rendering techniques   321

wavelength   1
Wharton jelly   94–95
Wildervanck syndrome   207
Wilm's tumor   150
Wolf–Hirschhorn syndrome   130

X chromosome deletion   177

yolk sac   24–25, 28, 47

zygosity   94

ROBERT LAMB LIBRARY
INVERCLYDE ROYAL
HOSPITAL